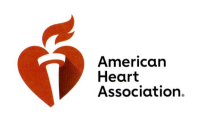

2020

AMERICAN HEART ASSOCIATION
心肺蘇生と救急心血管治療のための
ガイドライン

『Circulation』・第 142 巻・第 16 号・補足資料 2・2020 年 10 月 20 日の補足資料

©2021 American Heart Association
日本語版: Global Speed 2-6-34, Takashima, Nishi-ku, Yokohama-shi, Kanagawa, 220-8515 Japan
登録番号: 0107-03-002847
ISBN: 978-1-61669-943-7. 日本語版 20-2100JP. 発行日：9/21

オリジナルの英語版
2020 American Heart Association Guidelines for CPR and ECC
©2020 American Heart Association

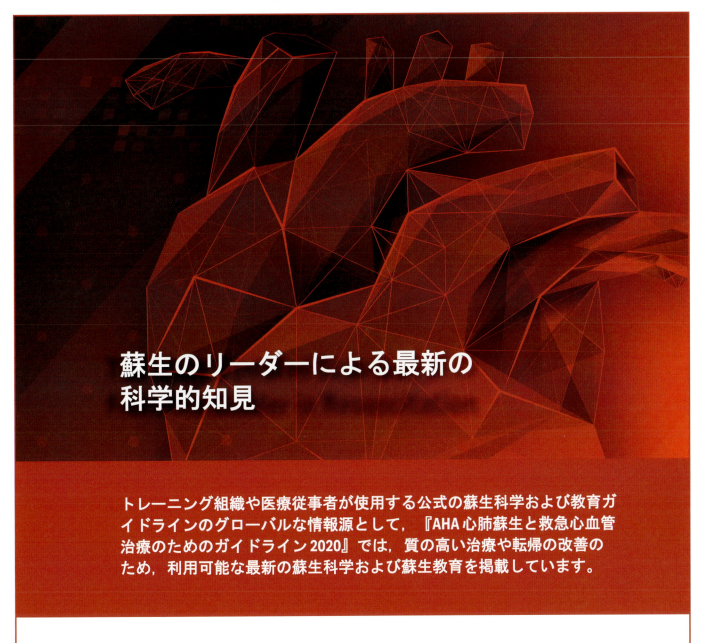

蘇生のリーダーによる最新の科学的知見

トレーニング組織や医療従事者が使用する公式の蘇生科学および教育ガイドラインのグローバルな情報源として，『AHA心肺蘇生と救急心血管治療のためのガイドライン2020』では，質の高い治療や転帰の改善のため，利用可能な最新の蘇生科学および蘇生教育を掲載しています。

以下の公式のガイドラインについて，
今すぐ ECCGuidelines.Heart.org にアクセスしてご確認ください。

- 『AHA心肺蘇生と救急心血管治療のためのガイドライン2020』（印刷版およびデジタル版）
- 『AHA心肺蘇生と救急心血管治療のためのガイドライン2020のハイライト』（17言語版）
- 2020医療従事者向けAHAガイドラインの科学分野に関する現職eラーニングコース
- 『医療従事者向けECCハンドブック2020』（印刷版およびデジタル版）

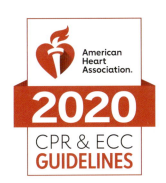

Circulation

補足資料

AHA 心肺蘇生と救急心血管治療のためのガイドライン 2020

第 1 章：要約
「RM Merchant ... 成人一次救命処置と二次救命処置，小児一次救命処置と二次救命処置，新生児救命処置，蘇生教育科学，治療システムの各執筆グループ代表」 S337

第 2 章：エビデンス評価とガイドライン作成
「DJ Magid ... EJ Lavonas」 S358

第 3 章：成人一次救命処置と二次救命処置
「AR Panchal ... 成人一次救命処置と二次救命処置の執筆グループ代表」 S366

第 4 章：小児一次救命処置と二次救命処置
「AA Topjian ... 小児一次救命処置と二次救命処置の共同執筆者代表」 S469

第 5 章：新生児の蘇生
「K Aziz ... J Zaichkin」 S524

第 6 章：蘇生教育科学
「A Cheng ... A Donoghue」 S551

第 7 章：治療システム
「KM Berg ... 成人一次救命処置と二次救命処置，小児一次救命処置と二次救命処置，新生児救命処置，蘇生教育科学の各執筆グループ代表」 S580

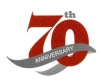
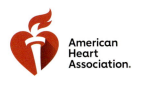

『Circulation』の補足資料

『AHA心肺蘇生と救急心血管治療のためのガイドライン2020』

アメリカ心臓協会救急心血管治療委員会

編集者

Eric J. Lavonas, MD, MS（共同編集者）
David J. Magid, MD, MPH（共同編集者）

副編集者

Eric J. Lavonas, MD, MS
（共同編集者）
David J. Magid, MD, MPH
（共同編集者）
Khalid Aziz, MBBS, MA, MEd（IT）
（新生児執筆グループ長）
Katherine M. Berg, MD
（成人執筆グループ副長）
Adam Cheng, MD（EIT執筆グループ長）
Aaron Donoghue, MD, MSCE
（EIT執筆グループ副長）
Henry C. Lee, MD（新生児執筆グループ副長）
Raina M. Merchant, MD, MSHP
（ECC委員長）
Ashish R. Panchal, MD, PhD
（成人執筆グループ長）
Tia T. Raymond, MD
（小児執筆グループ副長）
Alexis A. Topjian, MD, MSCE
（小児執筆グループ長）

謝辞

AHAはAmber Hoover氏, Melissa Mahgoub氏, Amber Rodriguez氏, およびVeronica Zamora氏, またPaula Blackwell氏, Jenna Joiner氏, Michelle Reneau氏, Kara Robinson氏, Dava Walker氏, Joe Loftin氏, Jody Hundley氏, Julie Scroggins氏, Sarah Johnson氏, Gabrielle Hayes氏からの多大な貢献に心より感謝し, その意をここに表す。

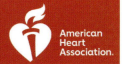

第1章：要約
『AHA 心肺蘇生と救急心血管治療のためのガイドライン 2020』

Raina M. Merchant, MD, MSHP
Alexis A. Topjian, MD, MSCE
Ashish R. Panchal, MD, PhD
Adam Cheng, MD
Khalid Aziz, MBBS, MA, MEd（IT）
Katherine M. Berg, MD
Eric J. Lavonas, MD, MS
David J. Magid, MD, MPH
On behalf of the Adult Basic and Advanced Life Support, Pediatric Basic and Advanced Life Support, Neonatal Life Support, Resuscitation Education Science, and Systems of Care Writing Groups

緒言

『AHA 心肺蘇生 (CPR) と救急心血管治療のためのガイドライン 2020』は，蘇生と救急心血管治療に関するエビデンスベースの推奨事項の包括的なレビューを提供するものである。CPR に関する最初のガイドラインは 1966 年，当時の CPR Committee of the Division of Medical Sciences, National Academy of Sciences—National Research Council により発行された[1]。これは，いくつかの組織や機関からの，トレーニングや対応に関する規格やガイドラインが必要との声を受けたものであった。

それ以来，CPR ガイドラインは AHA により定期的にレビュー，更新，発行されてきた[2-9]。2015 年には，5 年ごとの更新プロセスが，定期的なレビューではなく継続的なエビデンス評価のプロセスを使用するオンライン形式に移管された。これにより，重要な変更点を迅速にレビューし，適切と判断されれば直接ガイドラインに組み込むという大きな変化が起きた。意図したのは，ガイドラインからベッドサイドへの移行をより迅速にする可能性を広げることであった。この 2020 年版ガイドライン文書の作成にあたっては，国際蘇生連絡委員会（ILCOR）やその加盟団体と連携し，臨床的意義が非常に大きいと考えられる科学的問題や新たなエビデンスに特化した，さまざまなエビデンスレベルのレビューを含めた。

最初のガイドラインが発行されてから半世紀を過ぎても，米国や世界の他の国々では，心停止が合併症および死亡の主要な原因となっている。AHA の『Heart Disease and Stroke Statistics—2020 Update』で報告されているように，米国では毎年，院外心停止（OHCA）となった成人 347,000 以上，小児（18 歳未満）7,000 人以上に救急医療サービスが対応している[10]。院内心停止（IHCA）は，成人では心停止 1,000 件中 9.7 件（年間約 292,000 イベント），小児では入院 1,000 件中 2.7 件発生すると推定されている[11]。さらに，米国の新生児の約 1 %には，心肺機能を回復するための集中的な蘇生措置が必要となる[12,13]。

総じて，IHCA の転帰は成人，小児の両方で 2004 年から着実に改善しているものの，OHCA には同様の前進が見られていない[10]。救急医療サービスのケアを受けた OHCA 後に自己心拍再開（ROSC）の見られた成人患者の割合は，2012 年から基本的に変わっていない[10]。

生存率のばらつきの多くは，「救命の連鎖」（図 1）（心停止からの生存の可能性を最大にするために連続して迅速に行う必要のある重要な行動）の強度によるものと考えられる[14]。ガイドラインのこの版では，蘇生転帰に対する回復と生存の重要性を強調するため，6 番目のリンク「リカバリー」がそれぞれの「連鎖」に追加された。また，類似の「救命の連鎖」が，小児の OHCA と，成人と小児の IHCA についても作成された。同様に，新生児の蘇生の成功は，出生前の慎重な評価と準備に始まり，出生時から出生後 28 日までの蘇生および安定化までを含む，一連の統合的な救命手順によって決まる[15]。

キーワード：AHA 科学的提言 ■ 無呼吸 ■ 自動体外式除細動器 ■ 呼気 CO_2 モニター ■ 心肺蘇生 ■ 除細動器 ■ 医療提供（delivery of health care）■ 心エコー法 ■ 同期電気ショック ■ アドレナリン ■ 体外膜型人工肺 ■ 心停止 ■ 輸液，骨髄内 ■ 気管内挿管 ■ 救命処置 ■ 呼吸，人工 ■ ショック，心原性 ■ ショック，敗血症性

© 2020 American Heart Association, Inc.2020

https://www.ahajournals.org/journal/circ

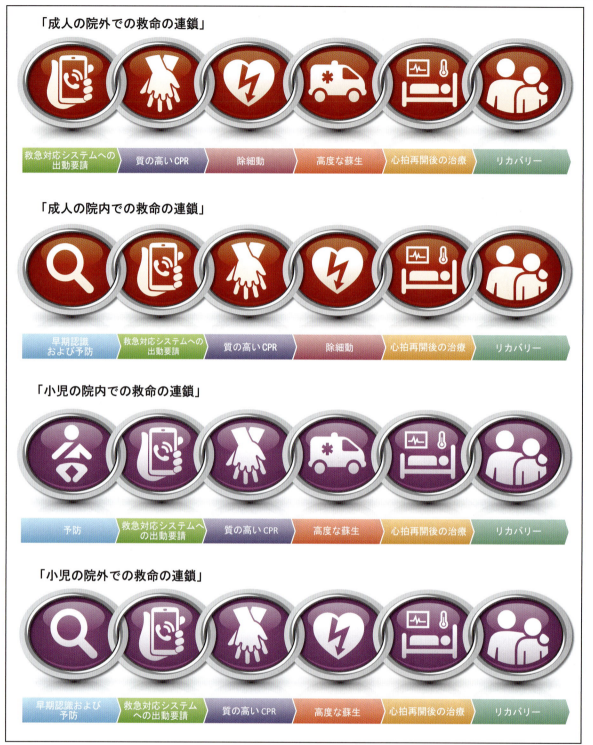

図1. アメリカ心臓協会（American Heart Association, AHA）の「救命の連鎖」
CPR＝心肺蘇生

　この要約ではAHAガイドライン2020の概要と方向性を示すが，このガイドラインはウツタインの生存のための方程式（Utstein Formula for Survival）（図2）を中心にまとめたものである[16]。

　このサマリーの各セクションでは，ガイドラインの各章の適用範囲を記述するとともに，その章での新たな，もしくは更新された推奨事項のうち，最も重要で影響力のあるもののリストを示す。また各セクションには，今後の重要な課題のリストが含まれている。このリストでは，重要な研究課題と，「救命の連鎖」の強化における大きな機会を重点的に取り上げている。本章は詳細な外部の文献引用を含まない。科学的根拠および対応する推奨事項のより詳細なレビューについては，第2～7章を参照されたい[15,17-21]。

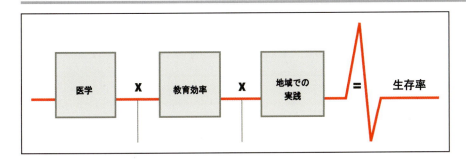

図2. ウツタインの生存のための方程式（Utstein Formula for Survival）。生存率の向上に不可欠な3つの構成要素を強調[16]。

新型コロナウイルス感染症2019（COVID-19）に関するガイダンス

AHAでは他の専門学会とともに，COVID-19感染症が疑われる，あるいは確定した成人，小児，新生児におけるBLS（一次救命処置）とALS（二次救命処置）の暫定的ガイダンスを提供した。エビデンスおよびガイダンスはCOVID-19の状況に応じて変化し続けているため，COVID-19に関する情報はECCガイドラインとは分離したままとする。最新のガイダンスについては，AHAのウェブサイト[22]を参照されたい。

エビデンス評価とガイドライン作成[19]

2020年版ガイドラインは，ILCORおよびILCOR加盟団体と連携して行った詳細なエビデンス評価に基づいている。2020年のプロセスでは，3タイプのエビデンスレビュー（システマティックレビュー，スコーピングレビュー，エビデンスアップデート）を使用した。このそれぞれが文献にまとめられたことにより，ガイドラインの作成が容易になった[23-28]。ILCORのエビデンスレビューでは，「推奨判定，開発，評価の格付」の方法論と用語が使用された[29]。こうしたAHAの治療に関する推奨事項は，標準的なAHAのプロセスと用語体系に沿っているが，これらについては第2章「エビデンス評価とガイドライン作成」[19]で詳細に記述する。

AHAの各執筆グループは，CPRと救急心血管治療に関する最新のすべてのAHAガイドライン[30-41]，関連する『2020 International Consensus on CPR and Emergency Cardiovascular Care Science With Treatment Recommendations』のエビデンス評価と推奨事項[42-48]，および関連するすべてのエビデンス更新ワークシートをレビューして，現在のガイドラインを再確認，更新，廃止すべきか，新たな推奨事項が必要かどうかを決定した。その後，執筆グループは推奨事項を作成，レビュー，承認し，推奨事項のクラス（COR，すなわち強度）とエビデンスレベル（LOE，すなわち質）をそれぞれの推奨事項に割り当てた（本書第2章の表3に概要を示す）[19]。

2020年版ガイドラインには491件の推奨事項（表）が含まれている。蘇生研究の支援における改善が最近行われているにもかかわらず，こうした推奨事項の51％は限定的なデータに基づいており，17％は専門家の見解に基づいている。これは，幅広い研究構想と資金調達機会が必要な今後の課題が依然として蘇生科学に存在することを示す。こうした課題については，患者，家族，蘇生プロセスに関わるチームといった重要なステークホルダーの価値と優先事項に対応する重要性をAHAは認識している。

2020年版ガイドラインはいくつかの集約知識に整理され，具体的なトピックや管理問題に関する情報の個別モジュールに分類されている[49]。それぞれのモジュールの集約知識には，推奨事項の表，簡単な紹介または概要，推奨事項の裏付けとなる解説，ハイパーリンクの参考文献，および必要に応じて，図，アルゴリズムのフローチャート，追加の表が含まれる。

略語

略語	意味／フレーズ
ACLS	二次救命処置（advanced cardiovascular life support）
AED	自動体外式除細動器（automated external defibrillator）
AHA	アメリカ心臓協会（American Heart Association）
ALS	二次救命処置（advanced life support）
BLS	一次救命処置（basic life support）
COR	推奨事項のクラス（Class of Recommendation）
CPR	心肺蘇生（cardiopulmonary resuscitation）
IHCA	院内心停止（in-hospital cardiac arrest）
ILCOR	国際蘇生連絡委員会（International Liaison Committee on Resuscitation）
LOE	エビデンスレベル（Level of Evidence）
OHCA	院外心停止（out-of-hospital cardiac arrest）
PPV	陽圧人工呼吸（positive-pressure ventilation）
ROSC	自己心拍再開（return of spontaneous circulation）

成人一次救命処置と二次救命処置[20]

「第3章：成人一次救命処置と二次救命処置」には，OHCAとIHCAの成人傷病者の治療に関する一連の包括的な推奨事項が含まれる。AHAは「救命の連鎖」の重要なステップを再確認し，「心拍再開後の治療」のセクションに更新されたアルゴリズムを追加して拡大し，回復と生存のために「救命の連鎖」に新たなリンクを導入した。成人の心停止管理における主な重点としては，迅速な認識，CPRの迅速な実施，心室細動および無脈性心室頻拍に対する除細動がある。2010年以降AHAは，まず圧迫を実施してから気道確保，呼吸

表　2020年版ガイドラインの推奨事項

分類	成人一次救命処置と二次救命処置	小児一次救命処置と二次救命処置	新生児の蘇生	蘇生教育科学	治療システム	合計	パーセント
推奨事項のクラス（強さ）							
1（強）	78	53	16	5	9	161	33 %
2a（中）	57	42	14	13	10	135	27 %
2b（弱）	89	30	21	11	6	158	32 %
3：利益なし（中）	15	1	3	0	0	19	4 %
3：有害（強）	11	4	3	0	0	18	4 %
エビデンスレベル（質）							
A	2	1	2	1	0	6	1 %
B-R	37	3	8	7	1	55	11 %
B-NR	57	19	8	5	8	97	20 %
C-LD	123	70	24	15	15	248	51 %
C-EO	31	37	15	1	1	85	17 %
合計	250	130	57	29	25	491	

EO：専門家の見解（expert opinion），LD：限定的なデータ（limited data），NR：非無作為化（nonrandomized），R：無作為化（randomized）

確保を行うことを一般的な対応手順において重視することにより，胸骨圧迫実施までの時間を最短にすることに尽力してきた。2020年版ガイドラインでは引き続き，胸骨圧迫が極めて重要であることを強調し，最新の関連エビデンスを利用した治療の最適化と生存率の向上を図っている。成人の蘇生に関するその他の推奨事項は，「第7章：治療システム」に記載されている[18]。

成人一次救命処置と二次救命処置：重要な新しい推奨事項，更新された推奨事項，および再確認された推奨事項

- 「CPRの再確認」：CPRの実施は長きにわたって心停止管理の特徴となっている。12,500人以上の患者の分析から得られた最新のエビデンス[50]でも，胸骨圧迫の質の重要性とともに，以下の事項が再確認されている。
  - 用手CPR中，救助者は平均的な成人に対して2インチまたは5 cm以上の深さまで胸骨圧迫を行うべきであるが，過度に深く（2.4インチまたは6 cm超）ならないようにする（クラス1，LOE B-NR）[51-54]。
  - 救助者が100〜120回／分のテンポで胸骨圧迫を行うことは妥当である（クラス2a，LOE B-NR）[50,55]。

さらに，新たなシステマティックレビュー[44]から，患者が心停止していない場合は患者への危害のリスクは低いため，心停止が疑われるときに市民救助者がCPRを開始することが推奨される（クラス1，LOE C-LD）[56-59]。

- 「二重連続手動式電気ショック」：突然の心停止が心室細動または無脈性心室頻拍によって生じた場合は，CPRとともに早期の除細動が生存にとって重要となる。しかしながら，除細動に反応しない傷病者に出くわすこともある。二重連続手動式電気ショック（2つの除細動器でほぼ同時に電気ショック実施）が，こうした患者の管理に対する新たな技術的アプローチとして登場している[60-64]。現時点では，治療抵抗性ショック適応リズムに対する二重連続除細動の有用性は確立されていないことが，システマティックレビューによって明らかにされている（クラス2b，LOE C-LD）[48]。

- 「骨髄内（IO）の前に静脈内（IV）」：末梢静脈路は緊急薬物療法を行う際の従来手法であるが，骨髄路の人気が高まり，血管路確保の第一選択として実施件数が増えている。新たなエビデンスでは，静脈路と比較して，骨髄路の有効性にはある程度の不確実性があることが示唆されている[65-69]。したがって，心停止において，薬物投与のためにプロバイダーが最初に静脈路を確保することは妥当である（クラス2a，LOE B-NR）。静脈路の確保が成功しないまたは可能でない場合，骨髄路の確保を検討できる（クラス2b，LOE B-NR）。

- 「早期のアドレナリン投与の再確認」：2つの無作為化試験において[70,71]アドレナリン投与によりROSCと生存率が高まった。これは，心停止患者にはアドレナリンを投与すべきとの推奨事項につながった（クラス1，LOE B-R）[40,72]。アドレナリンが神経学的転帰に及ぼす影響が不確かであること，また投与のタイミングや初期リズムによって転帰にばらつきがあることから，以下の新しい概念が支持された。
  - 投与のタイミングに関しては，ショック不適応リズムを呈する心停止の場合，できるだけ速やかにアドレナリンを投与することが妥当である（クラス2a，C-LD）。

- タイミングに関しては，ショック適応リズムでの心停止の場合，除細動が不成功後にアドレナリンを投与することは妥当としてよい（クラス2b, C-LD）。

成人の心停止アルゴリズムが更新され，非適応リズムの患者に対するアドレナリンの早期投与が強調されている。

- 「個々の蘇生処置に応じた管理」：すべての心停止イベントが同じという訳ではなく，心停止の主因が呼吸器である，妊娠子宮が静脈還流を妨げている，蘇生が生存可能な胎児に関わる場合などは，最適な患者転帰のために特殊な管理が極めて重要になることがある。「特殊な蘇生の状況」のセクションでは，そうした領域の2つ（オピオイド過量投与と妊娠中の心停止）を重点的に取り上げる。
  - オピオイド過量投与：オピオイドの流行により，オピオイド過量投与による呼吸停止や心停止が増加した[73]。この公衆衛生上の危機に対応するため，AHAはオピオイド関連の救急管理のため2つの新しいアルゴリズムを提示している。そこでは，ナロキソンまたはその他の介入に対する患者の反応を待つ間，市民救助者およびトレーニングを受けた救助者が救急対応システムへの出動要請を遅らせてはならないことが強調されている（クラス1, LOE E-O）。また心停止が確認されている，あるいは疑われる患者については，ナロキソンの使用が有益であると証明されていないため，標準的な蘇生処置をナロキソン投与よりも優先し，質の高いCPR（胸骨圧迫および換気）を重視すべきである（クラス1, LOE E-O）[73]。
  - 妊娠中の心停止：AHAが提示する更新された推奨事項および新しいアルゴリズムでは，妊婦と胎児の両方にとっての最良の転帰は，妊婦の蘇生の成功によりもたらされるということが強調されている[74]。妊娠中の心停止に対するチームの計画は，産科，新生児科，救急科，麻酔科，集中治療科，心停止対応チームが協力して作成すべきである（クラス1, LOE C-LD）。心停止の妊婦の処置で優先するのは，質の高いCPRの実施および子宮左方移動による大動静脈圧迫の解除である（クラス1, LOE C-LD）。子宮底がへその高さかへそより上にある妊産婦に通常の蘇生処置＋用手的子宮左方移動を実施し，ROSCが得られなかった場合には，蘇生処置を継続しながら，子宮内容除去の準備に取りかかることが望ましい（クラス1, LOE C-LD）[75-79]。早期に出産させるため（理想的には心停止から5分以内），BLS（一次救命処置）およびACLS（二次救命処置）治療介入を実施しながら，直ちに死戦期帝王切開の準備をすることが妥当である（クラス2a, LOE C-EO）。ただしこのタイミングは，救助者の一連の手技や路用可能な人員数及び（医療）資源によってても論理的に左右される[74]。

- 「ベッドサイドでの超音波検査による予後予測」：携帯型超音波装置のような新しい技術を使用することで，蘇生の中の無駄な要素や蘇生終了の判断におけるガイダンスを提供しようと試みる者は多い。しかしながら，エビデンスをまとめた文献[48]に基づけば，CPR中の予後予測にベッドサイドでの超音波検査を使用することは推奨されない（クラス3：利益なし, LOE C-LD）。この推奨事項は，心停止の治癒可能な原因の識別やROSCの検出に超音波検査を使用することを妨げるものではない。

- 「心拍再開後の治療」：ROSC後の治療は「救命の連鎖」の重要な構成要素であるが，これには包括的，体系的，かつ複数の専門分野にわたるケアのシステムが必要であり，そうしたシステムは心拍再開後患者の治療のために一貫した方法で実施されるべきである（クラス1, LOE B-NR）[40,80]。AHAでは，ROSC後の初期の安定化フェーズとその他の救急処置について説明する新しいアルゴリズムを提示している。主要な考慮事項には，血圧管理，痙攣の監視と治療，目標体温管理が含まれている。

- 「神経学的予後予測の改善」：ROSC後も意識の回復しない心停止生存者では，回復の可能性が高い患者が治療の中止により不良転帰に陥らないようにするため，正確な神経学的予後予測が非常に重要である[81]。神経学的予後予測の多くの面に関する最新のシステマティックレビュー[48]から，心停止後に昏睡状態が続く患者では，神経学的予後予測に集学的アプローチを採用し，単一の所見に基づかないようにすることを推奨する（クラス1, LOE B-NR）[48,81]。このようなプロセスを支援するため，我々は集学的予後予測を可能とするエビデンスベースのガイダンスを作成した。これには以下が含まれる。
  - 心停止後に昏睡状態が続く患者では，薬物投与効果または一時的な所見不良による交絡を防止するために，適度な時間が経過するまで神経学的予後予測を遅らせることを推奨する（クラス1, LOE B-NR）[82]。
  - 心停止後に昏睡状態が続く患者では，個別の予後検査を早期に実施できる場合でも，正常体温に戻ってから72時間以上経過した後に集学的な神経学的予後予測を実施することが妥当である（クラス2a, LOE B-NR）[48]。

また，臨床検査，血清バイオマーカー，電気生理学的検査，および神経画像検査の神経学的予後予測への使用についても，具体的なガイダンスを提供している。

- 回復と生存：最後に，「救命の連鎖」に「心停止からのリカバリー」というリンクを追加した。心停止生存者とその介護者に対して，治療，監視，およびリハビリテーションについて説明した回復生存計者への画を退院時に提供し，心停止の後遺症について説明するとともに，独立した身体的，社会的，精神的，および役割的機能へと治療を転換する必要がある[83]。この概念に対して極めて重要な推奨事項には以下のようなものがある。
  - 心停止からの生存者およびその介護者に対する，不安，うつ状態，心的外傷後ストレス障害，および疲労の体系的な評価を推奨する（クラス 1, LOE B-NR）[83-87]
  - 心停止からの生存者は，退院前に身体的，神経学的，心肺機能的，および認知機能障害に関して，複数のリハビリ評価と治療を受けることが推奨される（クラス 1, LOE C-LD）[83,88-90]。
  - 心停止からの生存者およびその介護者に，医療およびリハビリ治療の推奨事項を採り入れて，求める活動／仕事に復帰するための，包括的かつ集学的な退院計画を提供することが推奨される（クラス 1, LOE C-LD）[83]。

今後の課題

成人の蘇生研究における最も適切な課題には，以下のようなものがある。

- 市民救助者の CPR パフォーマンスを上げるための最適な戦略は？
- 動脈ラインが挿入されている患者では，ある特定の血圧を目標とした CPR により転帰が改善するか？
- 実際の臨床現場において，CPR 中の心電図リズム解析用のアーチファクトフィルタリングアルゴリズムにより，胸骨圧迫の中断が減り，転帰が改善するか？
- ショック適用前の波形解析は転帰の改善につながるか？
- 二重連続除細動や除細動器パッドの代替位置への貼り付けは，ショック適応リズムの心停止における転帰に影響するか？
- 骨髄路による薬物投与は心停止において安全かつ効果的か，また骨髄内挿入部位によって効果は変わるか？
- アドレナリンを心停止後早期に投与した場合，生存率が向上し良好な神経学的転帰が得られるか？
- 心停止中にベッドサイドで心臓超音波検査を行うことで，転帰は改善するか？
- CPR 中に，ある特定の呼気終末二酸化炭素分圧（$ETCO_2$）値を目標とすることは有益か，また $ETCO_2$ がどの程度上昇すれば ROSC が示唆されるか？）
- 体外循環補助を用いた CPR が有益である可能性が最も高いのはどの集団か？
- 心拍再開後患者によく見られるてんかん発作を治療することで患者転帰は改善するか？
- 神経保護薬により，心停止後の良好な神経学的転帰は改善するか？
- 心拍再開後の心原性ショックに対する最も効果的な処置手法は（薬理学的治療，カテーテル治療，植込み型デバイスなど）？
- 目標体温管理は厳格な正常体温と比較して転帰を改善するか？
- 復温前の目標体温管理の最適な継続時間は？
- 目標体温管理での治療後，心拍再開後患者を復温するための最適な手法とは？
- グリア線維性酸性タンパク質，血清タウタンパク質，ニューロフィラメント軽鎖の測定値は，神経学的予後予測に有用か？
- てんかん重積状態，悪性の脳波パターン，および他の脳波パターンをより統一的に定義することで，それらの予後的重要性を研究間でより良好に比較できるか？
- 灰白質／白質比や見かけ上の拡散係数に関する予後予測の一貫した閾値はあるか？
- 心停止からの生存の影響に対する生存者から得られた評価基準とはどのようなものか，また現在の一般的な評価基準や医師から得られた評価基準とどう違うのか？
- 心停止からの生存者に対する病院ベースのプロトコル化された退院計画により，リハビリテーションへのアクセスや照会，患者転帰は向上するか？
- オピオイド関連の心停止で換気ありの CPR を受けている患者において，ナロキソン投与は有益か？
- オピオイド過量投与の大きな原因がフェンタニルおよびフェンタニル類似体である場合，ナロキソンの理想的な初期投与量は？
- 信頼性の高い脈拍チェックができない非医療従事者がオピオイド過量投与疑い例を処置する場合，CPR の開始は有益か？

- 心停止の妊婦に対する死戦期帝王切開の最適なタイミングは？
- 肺塞栓症「疑い」による心停止患者で、蘇生中の緊急血栓溶解療法が効果的な患者とは？

小児一次救命処置と二次救命処置 [21]

2020年版ガイドラインの第4章「小児一次救命処置と二次救命処置」には、小児のOHCAとIHCAの治療（心拍再開後の治療と生存を含む）に関する推奨事項が含まれている。小児の心停止の原因、治療、転帰は、成人の心停止とは異なる。例えば、小児の心停止は呼吸器が原因となることが多い。このガイドラインには新生児期を除く小児のBLSおよびALSに関する推奨事項が含まれており、これらは最も優れた蘇生科学に基づいている。小児のALSに関する推奨事項は、肺高血圧症や先天性心疾患の小児、および心拍再開後の回復状態にある小児の治療を含める形で拡大された。このサマリーでは、心停止後のプロセスや心停止の患者転帰に大きな影響を与えると思われる、小児のBLS、ALSにおける2015年以降の新しい推奨事項と更新された推奨事項を重点的に取り上げる。小児の蘇生に関するその他の推奨事項は、第7章「治療システム」に記載されている。

重要な新しい推奨事項と更新された推奨事項

- 「呼吸数」：小児のCPR中の呼吸数は、小児に関する研究がなかったため、これまでは成人のデータから外挿されていた。現在は、小児におけるCPR中の呼吸数に関する新しいデータを利用できるようになった。限定的なデータではあるが、高度な気道確保器具を挿入している小児では、これまでの推奨よりも高い呼吸数となることが、これらのデータから裏付けられた[91]。高度な気道確保器具を挿入している乳児および小児のCPRを実施する場合は、年齢および臨床状態に応じて、2～3秒ごとに1回（20～30回／分）の呼吸数を目標とすることを妥当としてよい。これらの推奨事項を超える呼吸数は血行動態に悪影響を及ぼす可能性がある（クラス2b、LOE C-LD）[91]。脈拍はあるが呼吸努力がないか不十分な乳児および小児に対して、2～3秒ごとに人工呼吸を1回（20～30回／分）行うことが妥当である（クラス2b、LOE C-LD）[91]。
- 「カフ付き気管チューブ」：カフ付き気管チューブによる挿管により、肺コンプライアンスが低い患者の呼気CO_2モニターおよび換気を改善し、気管チューブ交換の必要性を低下できる。乳児および小児への挿管には、カフなしよりもカフ付きの気管チューブを選択することが妥当である（クラス2a、LOE C-LD）[92-98]。
- 「輪状軟骨圧迫法」：特定の状況下において輪状軟骨圧迫法は有用な場合もあるが、ルーチン使用は咽頭鏡検査での視診やバッグマスク換気による胸の上がりを妨げることがある。臨床研究では、輪状軟骨圧迫法のルーチン使用により最初の挿管成功率が低下することが示されている。小児患者の気管挿管時に、輪状軟骨圧迫法のルーチン使用は推奨されない（クラス3：利益なし、LOE C-LD）[99,100]。輪状軟骨圧迫法を使用する場合、換気の妨げとなったり、挿管の遅れや困難につながるようであれば中止する（クラス3：有害、LOE C-LD）[99,100]。
- 「アドレナリンの早期投与」：CPR中のアドレナリン投与の目標は、冠動脈灌流圧を最適化し、脳灌流圧を維持することである。CPR中のアドレナリンの早期投与は、生存退院率を増加させる可能性がある。小児患者の場合、どのような状況でも、胸骨圧迫の開始から5分以内に初回投与量のアドレナリンを投与することが妥当である（クラス2a、LOE C-LD）[101-104]。
- 「CPRの指針となる拡張期血圧」：心停止時に連続的に観血的動脈圧モニタリングを行っていた患者について、プロバイダーが拡張期血圧を使用してCPRの質を評価することは妥当である（クラス2a、LOE C-LD）[105]。CPR中の理想的な血圧目標値は不明であるが、拡張期血圧は冠動脈血流の主要な原動力であり、動脈ラインが挿入されている場合も介入の指針として使用できる。
- 「心停止後のけいれん発作」：心拍再開後のけいれん発作はよく認められる。多くは非けいれん性発作で、脳波モニタリングでのみ検出可能である。リソースを利用できる場合は、持続的脳症の患者における心停止後のけいれん発作の検出のため継続的な脳波モニタリングが推奨される（クラス1、LOE C-LD）[106-109]。心停止後の臨床的けいれん発作を治療することが推奨される（クラス1、LOE C-LD）[110,111]。専門医と相談のうえ、心停止後の非けいれん性てんかん発作重積状態を治療することは妥当である（クラス2a、LOE C-EO）[110,111]。
- 「回復と生存」：心停止の新たな神経学的後遺症はよく認められるものであり、継続的な評価と介入を行うことで退院後の患者をサポートすべきである。小児の心停止からの生存者はリハビリテーションのため評価することが推奨される（クラス1、LOE C-LD）[112-117]。小児の心停止からの生存者は、少なくとも心停止から1年間は継続的な神経学的評価を受けるよう紹介することが妥当である（クラス2a、LOE C-LD）[81,83,115,117-122]。

- 「敗血症性ショック」：敗血症性ショックの管理に関する前の AHA ガイドラインには，積極的な（20 mL/kg）輸液ボーラス投与が記載され，追加のガイダンスが不足していた。この 2020 年版ガイドラインでは，輸液投与に対してより適したアプローチを推奨し，バソプレシンに関する推奨事項を記載している。
  - 敗血症性ショックの患者において，10 mL/kg または 20 mL/kg で輸液を投与しながら頻回の再評価をすることが妥当である（クラス 2a, LOE C-LD）[123]。プロバイダーは輸液ボーラス投与のたびに患者を再評価し，輸液への反応があるか，体液過剰の徴候があるか確認する必要がある（クラス 1, LOE C-LD）[123-125]。
  - 蘇生に最初に用いる輸液としては，等張晶質液または膠質液のいずれも有効でありうる（クラス 2a, LOE B-R）[126]。蘇生に用いる輸液としては，緩衝液または非緩衝液のいずれも有効でありうる（クラス 2a, LOE B-NR）[127-129]。
  - 輸液抵抗性の敗血症性ショックの乳児および小児において，アドレナリンまたはノルアドレナリンを初回血管作動薬注入として使用することは妥当である（クラス 2a, LOE C-LD）[130-135]。

- 「オピオイド過量投与」：オピオイド過量投与の傷病者のほとんどは成人であるが，年少児は探査行動から，青少年はオピオイド乱用や自傷行為により，オピオイド過量投与となる。オピオイド過量投与により呼吸抑制が起こり，それが呼吸停止，心停止へと進行することがある。小児のオピオイド過量投与管理は，成人の場合と同じである。オピオイド過量投与が疑われ，はっきりとした脈拍を触知できるが普段どおりの呼吸をしていないか，死戦期呼吸のみ（呼吸停止）の患者については，救助者は標準的な小児 BLS または ALS の治療に加え，ナロキソンの筋注または経鼻投与することが妥当である（クラス 2a, LOE B-NR）[136-149]。オピオイドによる致死的な緊急事態にある反応のないすべての患者に対し，標準的な応急処置や医療従事者以外の BLS のプロトコールの補助として，筋肉内または鼻腔内のナロキソンの経験的投与を行うことは妥当としてよい（クラス 2b, LOE C-EO）[137-145,147-150]。市民救助者および医療従事者向けに，新しいオピオイド関連救急アルゴリズムが示されている。

今後の課題

小児の蘇生研究における最も適切な課題には，以下のようなものがある。
- CPR 中の最適な薬剤投与経路は静脈路か，それとも骨髄路か？
- 無脈性心停止においてアドレナリンの初回投与を行う際のタイムフレームは？
- 2 回目以降のアドレナリン投与の投与頻度は？
- CPR 中のリズムチェックの頻度は？
- CPR 中の最適な胸骨圧迫テンポと換気回数は？年齢に依存するか？また高度な気道確保器具を装着している場合は変わるのか？
- OHCA や IHCA において，高度な気道確保器具の装着が有益または有害となる特定の状況はあるか？そうした状況は心停止の原因によって変わるのか？
- 心エコー法により CPR の質や心停止の転帰が改善するか？
- 非心原性の OHCA や IHCA を起こした乳児および小児に対する，体外循環補助を用いた CPR の役割は？
- 心室細動や無脈性心室頻拍に対する除細動の最適なタイミングと投与エネルギーは？
- 小児の IHCA および OHCA の蘇生中止を決断する際に役立つ臨床ツールは？
- 心拍再開後の期間における最適な血圧目標値は？
- 心拍再開後の予後予測のための信頼できる方法とは？
- 心停止後の転帰を改善するためには，どのようなリハビリテーション療法やフォローアップを行うべきか？
- アデノシン抵抗性の上室性頻拍に対して最も効果的で安全な薬剤は？

新生児救命処置 [15]

AHA の 2020 年版ガイドラインの第 5 章「新生児救命処置」[15] では，アルゴリズムに従った進め方についての推奨事項を記載した。それには，予測と準備，分娩時の臍帯管理，最初の行動，心拍数の確認，呼吸補助，胸骨圧迫，血管確保と治療，蘇生の保留または中止，蘇生後のケア，人的因子とパフォーマンスが含まれる。ウツタインの生存のための方程式（Utstein Formula for Survival）との整合性を保ちつつ，2020 年版ガイドラインでは，新生児の蘇生に関する推奨事項の包括的なレビューを提供している。これには，医学文献に発表された研究からの最新のエビデンスや ILCOR によるレビューに基づく，新しい推奨事項と更新された推奨事項が含まれる。

重要な新しい推奨事項と更新された推奨事項

- 「皮膚接触」：蘇生を必要としない健康な新生児を，生後母親と皮膚接触させることは，授乳の向上，体温コントロール，および血糖値の安定に有効な場合がある（クラス 2a, LOE B-R）。コクランのシステマティックレビューから，皮膚接触を受けた健康な乳児は，生後 1～4 カ月に母乳栄養となる可能性が高いことが判明している。さらに，皮膚接触がある方が出生後の血糖が有意に高く，心肺機能の安定性も向上した[151]。

- 「胎便用挿管」：羊水混濁の状態で出生した元気のない新生児（無呼吸または非効果的呼吸を呈する）には，気管吸引の有無を問わず，ルーチンの喉頭鏡検査は推奨されない（クラス 3：利益なし，LOE C-LD）。陽圧人工呼吸（PPV）中に気道閉塞のエビデンスを認めた，羊水混濁の状態で出生した元気のない新生児については，挿管および気管吸引の実施が有益な場合がある（クラス 2a, LOE C-EO）。気管内吸引は，PPV 後に気道閉塞が疑われる場合のみ適応となる[46]。

- 「血管路確保」：出生児に血管路の確保が必要な児では，アクセスルートとして臍静脈が推奨される（クラス 1, LOE C-EO）。静脈路を確保できなければ，骨髄路の使用が妥当な場合がある（クラス 2b, LOE C-EO）。新生児が PPV および胸骨圧迫に反応しない場合は，アドレナリンおよび／または血漿増量剤投与のための血管路確保が必要となる。分娩室では臍静脈カテーテル挿入が推奨される[46,152]。臍静脈が確保できないか，分娩室外で治療が行われている場合は，代わりに骨髄路を選択することができる[46]。

- 「蘇生終了」：蘇生中の新生児の心拍数を検知できず，蘇生の全手順を実施した場合は，蘇生努力の中止について医療チームおよび家族と協議する。このような治療目標の変更を行うのに妥当な時間は，出生後約 20 分である（クラス 1, LOE C-LD）。生後約 20 分まで蘇生努力に反応しなかった新生児における生存の可能性は低い。そのため，治療の方向を変更する前に両親および蘇生チームが協議に参加することを強調しつつ，蘇生努力の中止を決定する時間が示されている[46,153]。

今後の課題

新生児の蘇生研究における最も適切な課題には，以下のようなものがある。

- 分娩時の最適な臍帯管理とは？（特に，呼吸補助が必要と思われる新生児において）
- 蘇生の全段階における最適な酸素管理とは？（PPV 開始時，胸骨圧迫実施時，蘇生後など）
- アドレナリン投与の最適な投与量，タイミング，経路は？
- 循環血液量減少の検出と治療のための最適な管理とは？
- 分娩室以外の部屋では新生児蘇生をどのように変更すべきか？
- プロバイダーおよびチームのパフォーマンスを最適化するための最も効果的な戦略とは？（トレーニング方法，再トレーニングの頻度，およびブリーフィング，デブリーフィング，フィードバックの方法など）

蘇生教育科学 [17]

2020 年版ガイドラインの第 6 章「蘇生教育科学」には，集中的な練習，反復学習，ブースター訓練，チームワークおよびリーダーシップのトレーニング，現場での教育，マネキンの忠実度，CPR フィードバック装置，バーチャルリアリティーやゲーム形式の学習，受講前の準備など，蘇生トレーニングのさまざまな教授システム学（インストラクショナル・デザイン）に関する推奨事項が含まれている[17]。また，市民救助者トレーニングを支援するための教育戦略や，オピオイドの流行に対する取り組みについても取り上げた。第 6 章の第 2 セクションでは，具体的なプロバイダーの考慮事項が教育的介入のインパクトにどのような影響を与えうるかについて説明している。教育格差，CPR を実施する意欲の格差に対処するための推奨事項を提示し，医師の経験と ACLS コースへの参加が心停止の患者転帰にどのように影響するかについて概説した。蘇生教育科学に関するその他の推奨事項は，「第 7 章：治療システム」に記載されている[18]。

重要な新しい推奨事項と更新された推奨事項

- 「ブースター訓練」：蘇生トレーニングに集中学習アプローチを用いる場合は，追加セッションの実施が推奨される（クラス 1, LOE B-R）。現在は蘇生コースのほとんどが集中学習アプローチを取っているが，これは数時間または数日間のトレーニングを 1 回実施した後，1～2 年ごとに再トレーニングを行う方法である[154]。ブースター訓練セッション（既習内容の反復に重点を置いた短時間，頻回のセッション）の蘇生コースへの追加は，12 カ月間の CPR スキル維持の向上に

関連している[155-161]。追加セッションの頻度は，受講者の減少（セッションの頻度が上がるほど減少率も高くなる[155]）や，ブースター訓練の実施を支えるリソースの可用性とのバランスを取るべきである。

- 「反復学習」：蘇生トレーニングには，集中学習アプローチの代わりに反復学習アプローチを用いることが妥当である（クラス 2a, LOE B-R）[162-164]。1～2 日間のコースとなる従来の集中学習アプローチに対し，反復学習アプローチではトレーニングが複数セッションに分かれ，数週間から数カ月おきにセッションが組まれる。各セッションでは新しい学習内容が示され，過去のセッションの内容の反復が含まれることもある[162-164]。反復学習アプローチでは従来の 1～2 日間のコースと比べ，臨床成績と技術的スキル（骨髄針刺入，バッグマスク換気）が向上することが，小児の蘇生トレーニングにおける 2 つの無作為化試験で報告されている[162,164]。新しい内容やスキルが各セッションで提示されるため，コースを完了するにはすべてのセッションへの受講者の参加が必要となる。

- 「集中的な練習および完全習得学習」：スキル習得およびパフォーマンスの向上のため，BLS または ALS コースに，集中的な練習および完全習得学習モデルを組み込むことを考慮してもよい（クラス 2b, LOE B-NR）。集中的な練習は，受講者に（1）個別の達成目標を与え，（2）パフォーマンスに対するフィードバックを即座に提供し，（3）パフォーマンスを改善するための反復の時間を十分に取るトレーニングアプローチである[165]。完全習得学習では，集中的な練習によるトレーニングとテストが使用される。このテストでは一連の基準により，学習するタスクの完全な習得を意味する最低到達基準が設定されている[166]。集中的な練習および完全習得学習モデルをトレーニングに組み込んだ研究では，蘇生スキルにおける受講者のパフォーマンスの向上が示されている[167-174]。反復とそれに対するフィードバックを行い，習熟するための十分な時間を設けることが，転帰の改善に関連する重要な要素となる。

- 「現場でのシミュレーショントレーニング」：従来のトレーニングに加え，現場でのシミュレーションに基づく蘇生トレーニングを実施することが妥当である（クラス 2a, LOE C-LD）。現場でのシミュレーションは，実際の患者治療エリアで行われるシミュレーショントレーニング活動の一形態である[175]。現場トレーニングの 1 つの利点は，受講者にとってより現実的なトレーニング環境が得られるということである。現場トレーニングでは，コミュニケーション，リーダーシップ，役割の割り当て，状況認識など，個々のプロバイダーの技術スキルやチームベースのスキルの開発に重点が置かれることがある[176,177]。他の教育戦略に追加される場合，現場トレーニングは学習および技能結果に良い影響をもたらす[161,164,178-182]。現場トレーニングの利点と，リスクを比較検討するべきである。

- 「市民救助者トレーニング」：自主学習と実践トレーニングを伴うインストラクターが指導するコースとの組み合わせは，市民救助者向けの従来のインストラクターが指導するコースに代わるものとして推奨される。インストラクターが指導するトレーニングが利用できない場合，市民救助者には自主学習トレーニングが推奨される（クラス 1, LOE C-LD）[183-186]。市民救助者（非医療従事者）に対する蘇生トレーニングの主な目標は，OHCA 発生時に，バイスタンダーによる即時の CPR 実施率を上げ，自動体外式除細動器（AED）の使用を増やし，救急対応システムへのタイムリーな通報を促すことである。自主学習やビデオベースの学習をインストラクターが指導するトレーニングと比較した研究では，技能結果における有意差は示されなかった[183-186]。自主学習のトレーニングを増やすことにより，訓練を受けた市民救助者の割合が上昇し，OHCA が発生したときに訓練を受けた市民救助者がいる可能性が高くなる。

- 「学齢期トレーニング」：中高生には，質の高い CPR を実施するトレーニングを行うことが推奨される（クラス 1, LOE C-LD）[187-195]。学齢期に達した子供に対する CPR トレーニングにより，OHCA イベントへの対応に対する自信と前向きな姿勢が養われる[187-195]。この年齢層を CPR トレーニングの対象とすることで，将来的な，地域社会を基本とした，訓練を受けた市民救助者の中核となる人員を育てられる。

- 「CPR トレーニングにおける格差」：CPR トレーニングにおける格差をなくせば，バイスタンダーによる CPR 実施率がこれまで低かった集団でも，バイスタンダーによる CPR 実施率と心停止の転帰を改善できる可能性がある。黒人やヒスパニックが大半を占める地域や，社会経済的ステータスの低い地域では，バイスタンダーによる CPR 実施率や CPR トレーニングの実施率が低くなっている[196-206]。米国では，市民救助者への CPR トレーニングを，特定の人種および民族の集団や地区を対象として，ターゲットに合わせて調整することが推奨される（クラス 1, LOE B-NR）[196-200,207-211]。市民救助者への CPR トレーニングや一般市民の認識を高める努力は，社会経済的地位の低い集団や地区を対象とすることを推奨する（クラス 1, LOE B-NR）[201-206,212-215]。対象を絞ったトレーニングを行う取り組みでは，言語，経済的な問題，情報へのアクセスの悪さなどの障壁を考慮する必要がある。

- 「バイスタンダーによる女性への CPR を妨げる障壁」：女性はバイスタンダーによる CPR を受ける率が低いことが多い。これは，不適切な接触，性的暴行，傷病者にけがを負わせたなど，救助者が非難を受けることを恐れる場合が多いからである。[216,217] 教育的トレーニングおよび一般市民の認識を高める努力を通じて，バイスタンダーによる女性への CPR に対する障壁に対処することは妥当である（クラス 2a, LOE

C-LD）[216-219]。的を絞ったトレーニングにより，こうした障壁が克服され，バイスタンダーによる女性への CPR 実施率が向上する可能性がある。
- 「ACLS（二次救命処置）コースへの参加」：医療従事者が成人の ACLS コースまたは同等のトレーニングを受けることは妥当である（クラス 2a, LOE C-LD）[220-228]。30 年以上にわたり，ACLS コースは最前線の救急処置プロバイダーに対する蘇生トレーニングの重要な要素として認められてきた。ACLS のトレーニングを受けたチームメンバーが 1 人以上いる蘇生チームを編成することで患者転帰が改善することが，最近のシステマティックレビューで判明している[228]。この推奨事項では，救急処置プロバイダーの基礎的なトレーニングとして ACLS コースを使用することが支持されている。

今後の課題

蘇生教育研究における最も適切な課題には，以下のようなものがある。

- 教育的成果やトレーニングにおけるパフォーマンスではなく，実際のパフォーマンスや臨床転帰に最も影響を及ぼす教育的介入とは？
- 最適な転帰を得るためには教授システム学（インストラクショナル・デザイン）をどのように組み合わせ，融合すればよいか？教授システム学（インストラクショナル・デザイン）複合的に使用した場合（現場でのシミュレーショントレーニングを追加セッションとして行うなど）の相乗効果を今後の研究において評価すべきである。
- 蘇生インストラクターを訓練および育成するための最も効果的な方法とは？さまざまなファカルティ・デベロップメント戦略がインストラクターのスキルや受講者の成績に与える影響を，今後の研究において評価すべきである。

治療システム[18]

2020 年版ガイドラインの第 7 章では治療システムに焦点を当て，広範囲の蘇生状況や全年齢の人々に関連する要素を強調している。治療システムのガイドラインは，心停止の予防と早期認識に始まり，蘇生を経て心拍再開後の治療と生存にいたる「救命の連鎖」を中心にまとめられている。OHCA に重点を置く推奨事項には，心停止の認識，CPR，市民による電気ショック，携帯電話技術の使用による第 1 救助者の招集，救急テレコミュニケーターの役割強化を，地域主導により促進することが記載されている。IHCA については，心停止発症リスクのある入院患者の認識および安定化に関する推奨事項がある。その他の推奨事項では，臨床的デブリーフィング，専門の心停止治療センターへの搬送，臓器提供，パフォーマンス測定が取り上げられている。

重要な新しい推奨事項と更新された推奨事項

- 「自主的なバイスタンダーの招集」：救急通報システムは携帯電話のテクノロジーを使用して，CPR または AED の使用を要する事態が発生したことを，付近の自主的なバイスタンダーに通知する必要がある（クラス 1, LOE B-NR）。OHCA 転帰の改善における市民救助者の役割は認識されているものの，大部分の地域でバイスタンダーによる CPR 実施および AED 使用率は低い[229,230]。テキストメッセージや携帯電話アプリなどの携帯電話のテクノロジーは，一般市民でトレーニングを受けた人を近くのイベントに呼び寄せて CPR を手伝ってもらったり，一番近くの AED を持ってくるよう指示したりするのに利用できる[231]。携帯電話アプリによる市民救助者への通知は，バイスタンダーによる応答時間の短縮，バイスタンダーによる CPR 率の向上，除細動までの時間の短縮，および生存から退院にいたる確率の向上をもたらす[47]。この技術のより一層の普及に伴い，さまざまな患者，地域，および地理的背景において，こうした通知が心停止の転帰に与える影響を探る研究が必要となっている。
- 「認知支援ツールおよびチェックリスト」：認知支援ツールを利用して CPR での医療従事者のチームパフォーマンスを改善することが望ましい（クラス 2b, LOE C-LD）。認知支援ツールは，個人やチームが情報を思い出し，タスクを完了し，ガイドラインの推奨事項を遵守するよう支援するために設計されている[232]。例としては，ポケットカード，ポスター，チェックリスト，モバイルアプリ，暗記法などが含まれる。外傷蘇生では認知支援ツールの使用によって蘇生ガイドラインの遵守が向上し，エラーが減少し，生存率が上昇するが[233-236]，心停止での医療チームによるツールの使用について評価した研究はない[47]。
- 「継続的改善のためのデータ」：継続的改善は，蘇生の実施や転帰に関するデータを規律正しく収集，評価することから始まる。組織が心停止患者の治療を行い，治療プロセスデータおよび転帰を収集することは妥当である（クラス 2a, LOE C-LD）。臨床レジストリでは，心停止の実際の管理に関連する治療プロセス（CPR パフォーマンス，除細動の回数）および治療転帰（ROSC，生存）の情報を収集する。レジストリから得られる情報は，治療の質を改善する機会を特定するために使用できる。心停止レジストリを実施した組織や地域では心停止の生存率が向上したことが，最近のシステマティックレビューで判明している[47]。

今後の課題

治療システム研究における最も適切な課題には，以下のようなものがある。

- 特にバイスタンダーによる応答率が低い集団や地域において，CPR の実施および AED の使用に向けた一般市民の意欲を向上させる介入とは？
- ドローンによる AED の配送など，AED をジャストインタイムで配送することにより，タイムリーに除細動を受けられる患者が増え，蘇生転帰が改善するか？
- IHCA リスクの高い患者を正確に識別する臨床基準とは？
- 病院の迅速対応システムや迅速対応チームの理想的な構成要素とは？こうした要素をどのように統合すれば，IHCA 予防に向けた現実的かつ効果的な対応モデルを作成できるか？
- パフォーマンス向上を達成するための，個人，チーム，システムのフィードバックの最適な仕組みとは？
- 地域の CPR および AED プログラムの費用対効果が高くなる状況とは？

ガイドラインの実施

この要約では，ガイドライン策定プロセス，推奨事項，および実践につながる今後の課題について概要を示した。今後の取り組みでは，推奨事項の実施可能性や受容性，費用対効果，および公平性への影響を評価することに重点が置かれる可能性があるが，こうした評価は本書の適用範囲外である。

要約

心停止は依然として，相当数の後遺症および死亡を起こす疾患であり，さまざまな年齢，性別，人種，地理的条件，社会経済的ステータスの個人に広く影響を及ぼす。生存率に多少の改善が見られるものの，この疾患の多大な負荷に対処するためにやるべき作業はまだ多い。このエクゼクティブサマリーでは，2020 年版ガイドラインに含まれる，厳格なエビデンス評価に基づいた新しい推奨事項や更新された推奨事項の概要を示した。

次の 10 年，この疾患への対処に向けて前進を続けるには，「救命の連鎖」をさらに強化し，連携のとれた治療システムを推進する必要がある。2020 年版ガイドラインで特定された今後の課題は，極めて重要な研究課題を指摘するものであるが，これらは対処すべき問題であるとともに，蘇生科学の今後の展開に対して資金提供の機会があることを示すものでもある。ガイドラインの作成は取り組みを進めるための重要な第一歩であり，そうした取り組みが最終的に患者転帰の改善につながるのである。

文献情報

アメリカ心臓協会（AHA）は，本書を以下のとおり引用するよう要請する：Merchant RM, Topjian AA, Panchal AR, Cheng A, Aziz K, Berg KM, Lavonas EJ, Magid DJ; on behalf of the Adult Basic and Advanced Life Support, Pediatric Basic and Advanced Life Support, Neonatal Life Support, Resuscitation Education Science, and Systems of Care Writing Groups. Part 1: executive summary: 2020 American Heart Association Guidelines for Cardiopulmonary Resuscitation and Emergency Cardiovascular Care.. Circulation. 2020;142 (suppl 2): S337-S357. doi: 10.1161/CIR.0000000000000918

謝辞

当執筆グループは，成人一次救命処置と二次救命処置，小児一次救命処置と二次救命処置，新生児救命処置，蘇生教育科学，治療システムの各執筆グループのメンバーに感謝の意を表す。

情報開示

執筆グループの情報開示

執筆グループメンバー	所属	研究助成金	その他の研究支援	講演／謝礼金	鑑定人	株式所有	コンサルタント／顧問	その他
Raina M. Merchant	The University of Pennsylvania	NIH（R01 PI, 心停止に特化したものではない：『Digital Phenotyping and Cardiovascular Health』）*	なし	なし	なし	なし	なし	なし
Khalid Aziz	University of Alberta（Canada）	なし	なし	なし	なし	なし	なし	なし
Katherine M. Berg	Beth Israel Deaconess Medical Center	NHLBI Grant K23 HL128814†	なし	なし	なし	なし	なし	なし
Adam Cheng	Alberta Children's Hospital（Canada）	なし	なし	なし	なし	なし	なし	なし

（続く）

執筆グループの情報開示（続き）

執筆グループメンバー	所属	研究助成金	その他の研究支援	講演／謝礼金	鑑定人	株式所有	コンサルタント／顧問	その他
Eric J. Lavonas	Denver Health Emergency Medicine	BTG Pharmaceuticals（Denver Health（Dr Lavonas の雇用主）は，研究，コールセンター，コンサルティング，教育に関する協定を BTG Pharmaceuticals と締結している。BTG はジゴキシン解毒剤の DigiFab を製造している。Dr Lavonas はボーナスや奨励給を受領しておらず，これらの協定は関連のない製品に関するものである。このガイドラインの作成にあたり，ジゴキシン中毒に関する議論に Dr Lavonas は関与していない。）†	なし	なし	なし	なし	なし	AHA（上級科学編集者）†
David J. Magid	University of Colorado	NIH†；NHLBI†；CMS†；AHA†	なし	なし	なし	なし	なし	AHA（上級科学編集者）†
Ashish R. Panchal	The Ohio State University	なし	なし	なし	なし	なし	なし	なし
Alexis A. Topjian	The Children's Hospital of Philadelphia, University of Pennsylvania	NIH*	なし	なし	なし	なし	なし	なし

この表は，執筆グループの全メンバーに回答および提出が求められる情報開示アンケート（Disclosure Questionnaire）の結果に基づき実在の利益相反または合理的に認定できる利益相反とみなされる可能性のある，執筆グループメンバーの関係を示している。メンバーと該当団体との関係が「顕著」であると考えられるのは，次のいずれかの状況が存在する場合である。（a）当該メンバーが団体から受領する金額が過去いずれの 12 か月間に $10,000 以上であるか，メンバーの総収入の 5 ％以上である。（b）団体の議決権株式の 5 ％以上，またはその団体の公正市場価値の $10,000 以上を保有している。この定義において「重大」に相当するレベルに満たない場合，その関係は「軽度」とみなされる。

*軽度
†重大

レビューアーの情報開示

レビューアー	所属	研究助成金	その他の研究支援	講演／謝礼金	鑑定人	株式所有	コンサルタント／顧問	その他
Aarti Bavare	Baylor College of Medicine	なし	なし	なし	なし	なし	なし	なし
Raúl J. Gazmuri	Rosalind Franklin University of Medicine and Science	Zoll Foundation（受領済み -『Myocardial Effects of Shock Burden During Defibrillation Attempts』。ブタを使用した研究）†。Zoll Foundation（受領済み -『Amplitude Spectral Area to Assess Hemodynamic and Metabolic Interventions during Cardiac Arrest』。ブタを使用した研究）†。Zoll Foundation（『Does Erythropoietin Reduce Adverse Post-Resuscitation Myocardial and Cerebral Effects of Epinephrine Resulting in Improved Survival with Good Neurological Function?』ブタを使用した研究）†	なし	なし	なし	なし	なし	なし
Julia Indik	University of Arizona	なし	なし	なし	なし	なし	なし	なし
Steven L. Kronick	University of Michigan	NIH（Enhancing Pre-Hospital Outcomes for Cardiac Arrest [EPOC]）*	なし	なし	なし	なし	なし	なし

（続く）

レビューアーの情報開示（続き）

レビューアー	所属	研究助成金	その他の研究支援	講演／謝礼金	鑑定人	株式所有	コンサルタント／顧問	その他
Eddy Lang	University of Calgary (Canada)	なし	なし	なし	なし	なし	なし	なし
Alexandra Marquez	Children's Hospital of Philadelphia	Labatt Innovation Fund（「迅速アクセス」ECLSカニューレ展開システムを作成するための機器開発プロジェクトに対する創業資金のグラント（≈25K）†	なし	なし	なし	なし	なし	なし
Mary Ann McNeil	University of Minnesota	なし	なし	なし	なし	なし	なし	なし
Robert D. Nelson	Wake Forest University Health Sciences	なし	なし	なし	なし	なし	なし	なし
Donald H. Shaffner	Johns Hopkins Hospital	なし	なし	なし	なし	なし	なし	なし

この表は，執筆グループの全メンバーに回答および提出が求められる情報開示アンケート（Disclosure Questionnaire）の結果に基づき実在の利益相反または合理的に認定できる利益相反とみなされる可能性のある，執筆グループメンバーの関係を示している。メンバーと該当団体との関係が「顕著」であると考えられるのは，次のいずれかの状況が存在する場合である。（a）当該メンバーが団体から受領する金額が過去いずれの12か月間に$10,000以上であるか，メンバーの総収入の5％以上である，（b）団体の議決権株式の5％以上，またはその団体の公正市場価値の$10,000以上を保有している。この定義において「重大」に相当するレベルに満たない場合，その関係は「軽度」とみなされる。

*軽度
†重大

参考資料

1. National Academy of Sciences. Cardiopulmonary resuscitation. JAMA. 1966;198:372-379.
2. Standards for cardiopulmonary resuscitation (CPR) and emergency cardiac care (ECC), 3: advanced life support. JAMA. 1974;227(suppl):852-860.
3. Standards and guidelines for cardiopulmonary resuscitation (CPR) and emergency cardiac care (ECC). JAMA. 1980;244:453-509.
4. Standards and guidelines for cardiopulmonary resuscitation (CPR) and emergency cardiac care (ECC): National Academy of Sciences—National Research Council. JAMA. 1986;255:2905-2989.
5. Guidelines for cardiopulmonary resuscitation and emergency cardiac care: Emergency Cardiac Care Committee and Subcommittees, American Heart Association, Part I: introduction. JAMA. 1992;268:2171-2183.
6. The American Heart Association in collaboration with the International Liaison Committee on Resuscitation. Guidelines 2000 for Cardiopulmonary Resuscitation and Emergency Cardiovascular Care: Part 6: advanced cardiovascular life support: 7D: the tachycardia algorithms. Circulation. 2000;102(suppl):I158-I165.
7. ECC Committee, Subcommittees, Task Forces of the American Heart Association. 2005 American Heart Association Guidelines for Cardiopulmonary Resuscitation and Emergency Cardiovascular Care. Circulation. 2005;112(suppl):IV1-IV203. doi: 10.1161/CIRCULATIONAHA.105.166550
8. Field JM, Hazinski MF, Sayre MR, Chameides L, Schexnayder SM, Hemphill R, Samson RA, Kattwinkel J, Berg RA, Bhanji F, et al. Part 1: executive summary: 2010 American Heart Association Guidelines for Cardiopulmonary Resuscitation and Emergency Cardiovascular Care. Circulation. 2010;122(suppl 3):S640-S656. doi: 10.1161/CIRCULATIONAHA.110.970889
9. Neumar RW, Shuster M, Callaway CW, Gent LM, Atkins DL, Bhanji F, Brooks SC, de Caen AR, Donnino MW, Ferrer JM, et al. Part 1: executive summary: 2015 American Heart Association Guidelines Update for Cardiopulmonary Resuscitation and Emergency Cardiovascular Care. Circulation. 2015;132(suppl 2):S315-S367. doi: 10.1161/CIR.0000000000000252
10. Virani SS, Alonso A, Benjamin EJ, Bittencourt MS, Callaway CW, Carson AP, Chamberlain AM, Chang AR, Cheng S, Delling FN, et al; on behalf of the American Heart Association Council on Epidemiology and Prevention Statistics Committee and Stroke Statistics Subcommittee. Heart disease and stroke statistics—2020 update: a report from the American Heart Association. Circulation. 2020;141:e139-e596. doi: 10.1161/CIR.0000000000000757
11. Holmberg MJ, Ross CE, Fitzmaurice GM, Chan PS, Duval-Arnould J, Grossestreuer AV, Yankama T, Donnino MW, Andersen LW; American Heart Association's Get With The Guidelines-Resuscitation Investigators. Annual Incidence of Adult and Pediatric In-Hospital Cardiac Arrest in the United States. Circ Cardiovasc Qual Outcomes. 2019;12:e005580. doi: 10.1161/CIRCOUTCOMES.119.005580
12. Perlman JM, Risser R. Cardiopulmonary resuscitation in the delivery room: associated clinical events. Arch Pediatr Adolesc Med. 1995;149:20-25. doi: 10.1001/archpedi.1995.02170130022005
13. Barber CA, Wyckoff MH. Use and efficacy of endotracheal versus intravenous epinephrine during neonatal cardiopulmonary resuscitation in the delivery room. Pediatrics. 2006;118:1028-1034. doi: 10.1542/peds.2006-0416
14. Cummins RO, Ornato JP, Thies WH, Pepe PE. Improving survival from sudden cardiac arrest: the "chain of survival" concept. A statement for health professionals from the Advanced Cardiac Life Support Subcommittee and the Emergency Cardiac Care Committee, American Heart Association. Circulation. 1991;83:1832-1847. doi: 10.1161/01.cir.83.5.1832
15. Aziz K, Lee HC, Escobedo MB, Hoover AV, Kamath-Rayne BD, Kapadia VS, Magid DJ, Niermeyer S, Schmölzer GM, Szyld E, et al. Part 5: neonatal resuscitation: 2020 American Heart Association Guidelines for Cardiopulmonary Resuscitation and Emergency Cardiovascular Care. Circulation. 2020;142(suppl 2):S524-S550. doi: 10.1161/CIR.0000000000000902
16. Søreide E, Morrison L, Hillman K, Monsieurs K, Sunde K, Zideman D, Eisenberg M, Sterz F, Nadkarni VM, Soar J, Nolan JP; Utstein Formula for Survival Collaborators. The formula for survival in resuscitation. Resuscitation. 2013;84:1487-1493. doi: 10.1016/j.resuscitation.2013.07.020
17. Cheng A, Magid DJ, Auerbach M, Bhanji F, Bigham BL, Blewer AL, Dainty KN, Diederich E, Lin Y, Leary M, et al. Part 6: resuscitation education science: 2020 American Heart Association Guidelines for Cardiopulmonary Resuscitation and Emergency Cardiovascular Care. Circulation. 2020;142(suppl 2):S551-S579. doi: 10.1161/CIR.0000000000000903
18. Berg KM, Cheng A, Panchal AR, Topjian AA, Aziz K, Bhanji F, Bigham BL, Hirsch KG, Hoover AV, Kurz MC, et al; on behalf of the Adult Basic and Advanced Life Support, Pediatric Basic and Advanced Life Support, Neonatal Life Support, and Resuscitation Education Science Writing Groups. Part 7: systems of care: 2020 American Heart Association Guidelines for Cardiopulmonary Resuscitation and Emergency Cardiovascular Care. Circulation. 2020;142(suppl 2):S580-S604. doi: 10.1161/CIR.0000000000000899
19. Magid DJ, Aziz K, Cheng A, Hazinski MF, Hoover AV, Mahgoub M, Panchal AR, Sasson C, Topjian AA, Rodriguez AJ, et al. Part 2: evidence evaluation and guidelines development: 2020 American Heart Association Guidelines for Cardiopulmonary Resuscitation and Emergency Cardiovascular Care. Circulation. 2020;142(suppl 2):S358-S365. doi: 10.1161/CIR.0000000000000898
20. Panchal AR, Bartos JA, Cabañas JG, Donnino MW, Drennan IR, Hirsch KG, Kudenchuk PJ, Kurz MC, Lavonas EJ, Morley PT, et al; on behalf of the Adult Basic and Advanced Life Support Writing Group. Part 3: adult basic and advanced life support: 2020 American Heart Association Guidelines for Cardiopulmonary Resuscitation and Emergency

Cardiovascular Care. Circulation. 2020;142(suppl 2):S366-S468. doi: 10.1161/CIR.0000000000000916
21. Topjian AA, Raymond TT, Atkins D, Chan M, Duff JP, Joyner BL Jr, Lasa JJ, Lavonas EJ, Levy A, Mahgoub M, et al; on behalf of the Pediatric Basic and Advanced Life Support Collaborators. Part 4: pediatric basic and advanced life support: 2020 American Heart Association Guidelines for Cardiopulmonary Resuscitation and Emergency Cardiovascular Care. Circulation. 2020;142(suppl 2):S469–S523. doi: 10.1161/CIR.0000000000000901
22. American Heart Association. Coronavirus (COVID-19) resources for CPR training & resuscitation. https://cpr.heart.org/en/resources/coronavirus-covid19-resources-for-cpr-training. Accessed June 24, 2020.
23. International Liaison Committee on Resuscitation. Continuous evidence evaluation guidance and templates. https://www.ilcor.org/documents/continuous-evidence-evaluation-guidance-and-templates. Accessed December 31, 2019.
24. Institute of Medicine (US) Committee of Standards for Systematic Reviews of Comparative Effectiveness Research. Finding What Works in Health Care: Standards for Systematic Reviews. Washington, DC: The National Academies Press; 2011.
25. Tricco AC, Lillie E, Zarin W, O'Brien KK, Colquhoun H, Levac D, Moher D, Peters MDJ, Horsley T, Weeks L, Hempel S, Akl EA, Chang C, McGowan J, Stewart L, Hartling L, Aldcroft A, Wilson MG, Garritty C, Lewin S, Godfrey CM, Macdonald MT, Langlois EV, Soares-Weiser K, Moriarty J, Clifford T, Tunçalp Ö, Straus SE. PRISMA Extension for Scoping Reviews (PRISMA-ScR): Checklist and Explanation. Ann Intern Med. 2018;169:467-473. doi: 10.7326/M18-0850
26. PRISMA. PRISMA for scoping reviews. http://www.prisma-statement.org/Extensions/ScopingReviews. Accessed December 31, 2019.
27. International Liaison Committee on Resuscitation (ILCOR). Continuous evidence evaluation guidance and templates: 2020 evidence update worksheet final. https://www.ilcor.org/documents/continuous-evidence-evaluation-guidance-and-templates#Templates. Accessed December 31, 2019.
28. International Liaison Committee on Resuscitation (ILCOR). Continuous evidence evaluation guidance and templates: 2020 evidence update process final. https://www.ilcor.org/documents/continuous-evidence-evaluation-guidance-and-templates. Accessed December 31, 2019.
29. Guyatt GH, Oxman AD, Vist GE, Kunz R, Falck-Ytter Y, Alonso-Coello P, Schünemann HJ; GRADE Working Group. GRADE: an emerging consensus on rating quality of evidence and strength of recommendations. BMJ. 2008;336:924-926. doi: 10.1136/bmj.39489.470347.AD
30. 2010 American Heart Association Guidelines for Cardiopulmonary Resuscitation and Emergency Cardiovascular Care Science. Circulation. 2010;122(suppl 3):S640-S946.
31. 2015 American Heart Association Guidelines Update for Cardiopulmonary Resuscitation and Emergency Cardiovascular Care. Circulation. 2015;132(suppl 2):S315-S589.
32. Atkins DL, de Caen AR, Berger S, Samson RA, Schexnayder SM, Joyner BL Jr, Bigham BL, Niles DE, Duff JP, Hunt EA, Meaney PA. 2017 American Heart Association Focused Update on Pediatric Basic Life Support and Cardiopulmonary Resuscitation Quality: An Update to the American Heart Association Guidelines for Cardiopulmonary Resuscitation and Emergency Cardiovascular Care. Circulation. 2018;137:e1-e6. doi: 10.1161/CIR.0000000000000540
33. Charlton NP, Pellegrino JL, Kule A, Slater TM, Epstein JL, Flores GE, Goolsby CA, Orkin AM, Singletary EM, Swain JM. 2019 American Heart Association and American Red Cross Focused Update for First Aid: Presyncope: An Update to the American Heart Association and American Red Cross Guidelines for First Aid. Circulation. 2019;140:e931-e938. doi: 10.1161/CIR.0000000000000730
34. Duff JP, Topjian A, Berg MD, Chan M, Haskell SE, Joyner BL Jr, Lasa JJ, Ley SJ, Raymond TT, Sutton RM, Hazinski MF, Atkins DL. 2018 American Heart Association Focused Update on Pediatric Advanced Life Support: An Update to the American Heart Association Guidelines for Cardiopulmonary Resuscitation and Emergency Cardiovascular Care. Circulation. 2018;138:e731-e739. doi: 10.1161/CIR.0000000000000612
35. Duff JP, Topjian AA, Berg MD, Chan M, Haskell SE, Joyner BL Jr, Lasa JJ, Ley SJ, Raymond TT, Sutton RM, Hazinski MF, Atkins DL. 2019 American Heart Association Focused Update on Pediatric Advanced Life Support: An Update to the American Heart Association Guidelines for Cardiopulmonary Resuscitation and Emergency Cardiovascular Care. Circulation. 2019;140:e904-e914. doi: 10.1161/CIR.0000000000000731
36. Duff JP, Topjian AA, Berg MD, Chan M, Haskell SE, Joyner BL Jr, Lasa JJ, Ley SJ, Raymond TT, Sutton RM, et al. 2019 American Heart Association focused update on pediatric basic life support: an update to the American Heart Association guidelines for cardiopulmonary resuscitation and emergency cardiovascular care. Circulation. 2019;140:e915-e921. doi: 10.1161/CIR.0000000000000736
37. Escobedo MB, Aziz K, Kapadia VS, Lee HC, Niermeyer S, Schmölzer GM, Szyld E, Weiner GM, Wyckoff MH, Yamada NK, Zaichkin JG. 2019 American Heart Association Focused Update on Neonatal Resuscitation: An Update to the American Heart Association Guidelines for Cardiopulmonary Resuscitation and Emergency Cardiovascular Care. Circulation. 2019;140:e922-e930. doi: 10.1161/CIR.0000000000000729
38. Kleinman ME, Goldberger ZD, Rea T, Swor RA, Bobrow BJ, Brennan EE, Terry M, Hemphill R, Gazmuri RJ, Hazinski MF, Travers AH. 2017 American Heart Association Focused Update on Adult Basic Life Support and Cardiopulmonary Resuscitation Quality: An Update to the American Heart Association Guidelines for Cardiopulmonary Resuscitation and Emergency Cardiovascular Care. Circulation. 2018;137:e7-e13. doi: 10.1161/CIR.0000000000000539
39. Panchal AR, Berg KM, Cabañas JG, Kurz MC, Link MS, Del Rios M, Hirsch KG, Chan PS, Hazinski MF, Morley PT, Donnino MW, Kudenchuk PJ. 2019 American Heart Association Focused Update on Systems of Care: Dispatcher-Assisted Cardiopulmonary Resuscitation and Cardiac Arrest Centers: An Update to the American Heart Association Guidelines for Cardiopulmonary Resuscitation and Emergency Cardiovascular Care. Circulation. 2019;140:e895-e903. doi: 10.1161/CIR.0000000000000733
40. Panchal AR, Berg KM, Hirsch KG, Kudenchuk PJ, Del Rios M, Cabañas JG, Link MS, Kurz MC, Chan PS, Morley PT, et al. 2019 American Heart Association focused update on advanced cardiovascular life support: use of advanced airways, vasopressors, and extracorporeal cardiopulmonary resuscitation during cardiac arrest: an update to the American Heart Association guidelines for cardiopulmonary resuscitation and emergency cardiovascular care. Circulation. 2019;140:e881-e894. doi: 10.1161/CIR.0000000000000732
41. Panchal AR, Berg KM, Kudenchuk PJ, Del Rios M, Hirsch KG, Link MS, Kurz MC, Chan PS, Cabañas JG, Morley PT, Hazinski MF, Donnino MW. 2018 American Heart Association Focused Update on Advanced Cardiovascular Life Support Use of Antiarrhythmic Drugs During and Immediately After Cardiac Arrest: An Update to the American Heart Association Guidelines for Cardiopulmonary Resuscitation and Emergency Cardiovascular Care. Circulation. 2018;138:e740-e749. doi: 10.1161/CIR.0000000000000613
42. Nolan JP, Maconochie I, Soar J, Olasveengen TM, Greif R, Wyckoff MH, Singletary EM, Aickin R, Berg KM, Mancini ME, et al. Executive summary: 2020 International Consensus on Cardiopulmonary Resuscitation and Emergency Cardiovascular Care Science With Treatment Recommendations. Circulation. 2020;142(suppl 1):S2-S27. doi: 10.1161/CIR.0000000000000890
43. Morley PT, Atkins DL, Finn JC, Maconochie I, Nolan JP, Rabi Y, Singletary EM, Wang TL, Welsford M, Olasveengen TM, et al. Evidence evaluation process and management of potential conflicts of interest: 2020 International Consensus on Cardiopulmonary Resuscitation and Emergency Cardiovascular Care Science With Treatment Recommendations. Circulation. 2020;142(suppl 1):S28-S40. doi: 10.1161/CIR.0000000000000891
44. Olasveengen TM, Mancini ME, Perkins GD, Avis S, Brooks S, Castrén M, Chung SP, Considine J, Couper K, Escalante R, et al; on behalf of the Adult Basic Life Support Collaborators. Adult basic life support: 2020 International Consensus on Cardiopulmonary Resuscitation and Emergency Cardiovascular Care Science With Treatment Recommendations. Circulation. 2020;142(suppl 1):S41-S91. doi: 10.1161/CIR.0000000000000892
45. Maconochie IK, Aickin R, Hazinski MF, Atkins DL, Bingham R, Couto TB, Guerguerian A-M, Nadkarni VM, Ng K-C, Nuthall GA, et al; on behalf of the Pediatric Life Support Collaborators. Pediatric life support: 2020 International Consensus on Cardiopulmonary Resuscitation and Emergency Cardiovascular Care Science With Treatment Recommendations. Circulation. 2020;142(suppl 1):S140-S184. doi: 10.1161/CIR.0000000000000894
46. Wyckoff MH, Wyllie J, Aziz K, de Almeida MF, Fabres J, Fawke J, Guinsburg R, Hosono S, Isayama T, Kapadia VS, et al; on behalf of the Neonatal Life Support Collaborators. Neonatal life support: International Consensus on Cardiopulmonary Resuscitation and Emergency Cardiovascular Care Science With Treatment Recommendations. Circulation. 2020;142(suppl 1):S185-S221. doi: 10.1161/CIR.0000000000000895
47. Greif R, Bhanji F, Bigham BL, Bray J, Breckwoldt J, Cheng A, Duff JP, Gilfoyle E, Hsieh M-J, Iwami T, et al; on behalf of the Education, Implementation, and Teams Collaborators. Education, implementation, and teams: 2020 International Consensus on Cardiopulmonary Resuscitation and Emergency Cardiovascular Care Science With Treatment Recommendations. Circulation. 2020;142(suppl 1):S222-S283. doi: 10.1161/CIR.0000000000000896

48. Berg KM, Soar J, Andersen LW, Böttiger BW, Cacciola S, Callaway CW, Couper K, Cronberg T, D'Arrigo S, Deakin CD, et al; on behalf of the Adult Advanced Life Support Collaborators. Adult advanced life support: 2020 International Consensus on Cardiopulmonary Resuscitation and Emergency Cardiovascular Care Science With Treatment Recommendations. Circulation. 2020;142 (suppl 1):S92-S139. doi: 10.1161/CIR.0000000000000893

49. Levine GN, O'Gara PT, Beckman JA, Al-Khatib SM, Birtcher KK, Cigarroa JE, de Las Fuentes L, Deswal A, Fleisher LA, Gentile F, Goldberger ZD, Hlatky MA, Joglar JA, Piano MR, Wijeysundera DN. Recent Innovations, Modifications, and Evolution of ACC/AHA Clinical Practice Guidelines: An Update for Our Constituencies: A Report of the American College of Cardiology/American Heart Association Task Force on Clinical Practice Guidelines. Circulation. 2019;139:e879-e886. doi: 10.1161/CIR.0000000000000651

50. Considine J, Gazmuri RJ, Perkins GD, Kudenchuk PJ, Olasveengen TM, Vaillancourt C, Nishiyama C, Hatanaka T, Mancini ME, Chung SP, Escalante-Kanashiro R, Morley P. Chest compression components (rate, depth, chest wall recoil and leaning): A scoping review. Resuscitation. 2020;146:188-202. doi: 10.1016/j.resuscitation.2019.08.042

51. Stiell IG, Brown SP, Nichol G, Cheskes S, Vaillancourt C, Callaway CW, Morrison LJ, Christenson J, Aufderheide TP, Davis DP, Free C, Hostler D, Stouffer JA, Idris AH; Resuscitation Outcomes Consortium Investigators. What is the optimal chest compression depth during out-of-hospital cardiac arrest resuscitation of adult patients? Circulation. 2014;130:1962-1970. doi: 10.1161/CIRCULATIONAHA.114.008671

52. Stiell IG, Brown SP, Christenson J, Cheskes S, Nichol G, Powell J, Bigham B, Morrison LJ, Larsen J, Hess E, Vaillancourt C, Davis DP, Callaway CW; Resuscitation Outcomes Consortium (ROC) Investigators. What is the role of chest compression depth during out-of-hospital cardiac arrest resuscitation? Crit Care Med. 2012;40:1192-1198. doi: 10.1097/CCM.0b013e31823bc8bb

53. Edelson DP, Abella BS, Kramer-Johansen J, Wik L, Myklebust H, Barry AM, Merchant RM, Hoek TL, Steen PA, Becker LB. Effects of compression depth and pre-shock pauses predict defibrillation failure during cardiac arrest. Resuscitation. 2006;71:137-145. doi: 10.1016/j.resuscitation.2006.04.008

54. Babbs CF, Kemeny AE, Quan W, Freeman G. A new paradigm for human resuscitation research using intelligent devices. Resuscitation. 2008;77:306-315. doi: 10.1016/j.resuscitation.2007.12.018

55. Hwang SO, Cha KC, Kim K, Jo YH, Chung SP, You JS, Shin J, Lee HJ, Park YS, Kim S, et al. A randomized controlled trial of compression rates during cardiopulmonary resuscitation. J Korean Med Sci. 2016;31:1491-1498. doi: 10.3346/jkms.2016.31.9.1491

56. White L, Rogers J, Bloomingdale M, Fahrenbruch C, Culley L, Subido C, Eisenberg M, Rea T. Dispatcher-assisted cardiopulmonary resuscitation: risks for patients not in cardiac arrest. Circulation. 2010;121:91-97. doi: 10.1161/CIRCULATIONAHA.109.872366

57. Haley KB, Lerner EB, Pirrallo RG, Croft H, Johnson A, Uihlein M. The frequency and consequences of cardiopulmonary resuscitation performed by bystanders on patients who are not in cardiac arrest. Prehosp Emerg Care. 2011;15:282-287. doi: 10.3109/10903127.2010.541981

58. Moriwaki Y, Sugiyama M, Tahara Y, Iwashita M, Kosuge T, Harunari N, Arata S, Suzuki N. Complications of bystander cardiopulmonary resuscitation for unconscious patients without cardiopulmonary arrest. J Emerg Trauma Shock. 2012;5:3-6. doi: 10.4103/0974-2700.93094

59. Tanaka Y, Nishi T, Takase K, Yoshita Y, Wato Y, Taniguchi J, Hamada Y, Inaba H. Survey of a protocol to increase appropriate implementation of dispatcher-assisted cardiopulmonary resuscitation for out-of-hospital cardiac arrest. Circulation. 2014;129:1751-1760. doi: 10.1161/CIRCULATIONAHA.113.004409

60. Beck LR, Ostermayer DG, Ponce JN, Srinivasan S, Wang HE. Effectiveness of Prehospital Dual Sequential Defibrillation for Refractory Ventricular Fibrillation and Ventricular Tachycardia Cardiac Arrest. Prehosp Emerg Care. 2019;23:597-602. doi: 10.1080/10903127.2019.1584256

61. Mapp JG, Hans AJ, Darrington AM, Ross EM, Ho CC, Miramontes DA, Harper SA, Wampler DA; Prehospital Research and Innovation in Military and Expeditionary Environments (PRIME) Research Group. Prehospital Double Sequential Defibrillation: A Matched Case-Control Study. Acad Emerg Med. 2019;26:994-1001. doi: 10.1111/acem.13672

62. Ross EM, Redman TT, Harper SA, Mapp JG, Wampler DA, Miramontes DA. Dual defibrillation in out-of-hospital cardiac arrest: A retrospective cohort analysis. Resuscitation. 2016;106:14-17. doi: 10.1016/j.resuscitation.2016.06.011

63. Emmerson AC, Whitbread M, Fothergill RT. Double sequential defibrillation therapy for out-of-hospital cardiac arrests: The London experience. Resuscitation. 2017;117:97-101. doi: 10.1016/j.resuscitation.2017.06.011

64. Cheskes S, Dorian P, Feldman M, McLeod S, Scales DC, Pinto R, Turner L, Morrison LJ, Drennan IR, Verbeek PR. Double sequential external defibrillation for refractory ventricular fibrillation: the DOSE VF pilot randomized controlled trial. Resuscitation. 2020;150:178-184. doi: 10.1016/j.resuscitation.2020.02.010

65. Granfeldt A, Avis SR, Lind PC, Holmberg MJ, Kleinman M, Maconochie I, Hsu CH, Fernanda de Almeida M, Wang TL, Neumar RW, Andersen LW. Intravenous vs. intraosseous administration of drugs during cardiac arrest: A systematic review. Resuscitation. 2020;149:150-157. doi: 10.1016/j.resuscitation.2020.02.025

66. Feinstein BA, Stubbs BA, Rea T, Kudenchuk PJ. Intraosseous compared to intravenous drug resuscitation in out-of-hospital cardiac arrest. Resuscitation. 2017;117:91-96. doi: 10.1016/j.resuscitation.2017.06.014

67. Kawano T, Grunau B, Scheuermeyer FX, Gibo K, Fordyce CB, Lin S, Stenstrom R, Schlamp R, Jenneson S, Christenson J. Intraosseous Vascular Access Is Associated With Lower Survival and Neurologic Recovery Among Patients With Out-of-Hospital Cardiac Arrest. Ann Emerg Med. 2018;71:588-596. doi: 10.1016/j.annemergmed.2017.11.015

68. Clemency B, Tanaka K, May P, Innes J, Zagroba S, Blaszak J, Hostler D, Cooney D, McGee K, Lindstrom H. Intravenous vs. intraosseous access and return of spontaneous circulation during out of hospital cardiac arrest. Am J Emerg Med. 2017;35:222-226. doi: 10.1016/j.ajem.2016.10.052

69. Nguyen L, Suarez S, Daniels J, Sanchez C, Landry K, Redfield C. Effect of Intravenous Versus Intraosseous Access in Prehospital Cardiac Arrest. Air Med J. 2019;38:147-149. doi: 10.1016/j.amj.2019.02.005

70. Jacobs IG, Finn JC, Jelinek GA, Oxer HF, Thompson PL. Effect of adrenaline on survival in out-of-hospital cardiac arrest: a randomised double-blind placebo-controlled trial. Resuscitation. 2011;82:1138-1143. doi: 10.1016/j.resuscitation.2011.06.029

71. Perkins GD, Ji C, Deakin CD, Quinn T, Nolan JP, Scomparin C, Regan S, Long J, Slowther A, Pocock H, Black JJM, Moore F, Fothergill RT, Rees N, O'Shea L, Docherty M, Gunson I, Han K, Charlton K, Finn J, Petrou S, Stallard N, Gates S, Lall R; PARAMEDIC2 Collaborators. A Randomized Trial of Epinephrine in Out-of-Hospital Cardiac Arrest. N Engl J Med. 2018;379:711-721. doi: 10.1056/NEJMoa1806842

72. Holmberg MJ, Issa MS, Moskowitz A, Morley P, Welsford M, Neumar RW, Paiva EF, Coker A, Hansen CK, Andersen LW, Donnino MW, Berg KM; International Liaison Committee on Resuscitation Advanced Life Support Task Force Collaborators. Vasopressors during adult cardiac arrest: A systematic review and meta-analysis. Resuscitation. 2019;139:106-121. doi: 10.1016/j.resuscitation.2019.04.008

73. Dezfulian C, Orkin AM, Maron BA, Elmer J, Girota S, Gladwin MT, Merchant RM, Panchal AR, Perman SM, Starks M, et al; on behalf of the American Heart Association Council on Cardiopulmonary, Critical Care, Perioperative and Resuscitation; Council on Arteriosclerosis, Thrombosis and Vascular Biology; Council on Cardiovascular and Stroke Nursing; and Council on Clinical Cardiology. Opioid-associated out-of-hospital cardiac arrest: distinctive clinical features and implications for healthcare and public responses: a scientific statement from the American Heart Association. Circulation. In press.

74. Jeejeebhoy FM, Zelop CM, Lipman S, Carvalho B, Joglar J, Mhyre JM, Katz VL, Lapinsky SE, Einav S, Warnes CA, Page RL, Griffin RE, Jain A, Dainty KN, Arafeh J, Windrim R, Koren G, Callaway CW; American Heart Association Emergency Cardiovascular Care Committee, Council on Cardiopulmonary, Critical Care, Perioperative and Resuscitation, Council on Cardiovascular Diseases in the Young, and Council on Clinical Cardiology. Cardiac Arrest in Pregnancy: A Scientific Statement From the American Heart Association. Circulation. 2015;132:1747-1773. doi: 10.1161/CIR.0000000000000300

75. Dijkman A, Huisman CM, Smit M, Schutte JM, Zwart JJ, van Roosmalen JJ, Oepkes D. Cardiac arrest in pregnancy: increasing use of perimortem caesarean section due to emergency skills training? BJOG. 2010;117:282-287. doi: 10.1111/j.1471-0528.2009.02461.x

76. Page-Rodriguez A, Gonzalez-Sanchez JA. Perimortem cesarean section of twin pregnancy: case report and review of the literature. Acad Emerg Med. 1999;6:1072-1074. doi: 10.1111/j.1553-2712.1999.tb01199.x

77. Cardosi RJ, Porter KB. Cesarean delivery of twins during maternal cardiopulmonary arrest. Obstet Gynecol. 1998;92 (4 Pt 2):695-697. doi: 10.1016/s0029-7844 (98)00127-6

78. Rees SG, Thurlow JA, Gardner IC, Scrutton MJ, Kinsella SM. Maternal cardiovascular consequences of positioning after spinal anaesthesia for Caesarean section: left 15 degree table tilt vs. left lateral. Anaesthesia. 2002;57:15-20. doi: 10.1046/j.1365-2044.2002.02325.x
79. Mendonca C, Griffiths J, Ateleanu B, Collis RE. Hypotension following combined spinal-epidural anaesthesia for Caesarean section. Left lateral position vs. tilted supine position. Anaesthesia. 2003;58:428-431. doi: 10.1046/j.1365-2044.2003.03090.x
80. Callaway CW, Donnino MW, Fink EL, Geocadin RG, Golan E, Kern KB, Leary M, Meurer WJ, Peberdy MA, Thompson TM, et al. Part 8: post-cardiac arrest care: 2015 American Heart Association Guidelines Update for Cardiopulmonary Resuscitation and Emergency Cardiovascular Care. Circulation. 2015;132 (suppl 2):S465-482. doi: 10.1161/cir.0000000000000262
81. Geocadin RG, Callaway CW, Fink EL, Golan E, Greer DM, Ko NU, Lang E, Licht DJ, Marino BS, McNair ND, Peberdy MA, Perman SM, Sims DB, Soar J, Sandroni C; American Heart Association Emergency Cardiovascular Care Committee. Standards for Studies of Neurological Prognostication in Comatose Survivors of Cardiac Arrest: A Scientific Statement From the American Heart Association. Circulation. 2019;140:e517-e542. doi: 10.1161/CIR.0000000000000702
82. Samaniego EA, Mlynash M, Caulfield AF, Eyngorn I, Wijman CA. Sedation confounds outcome prediction in cardiac arrest survivors treated with hypothermia. Neurocritical care. 2011;15:113-119. doi: 10.1007/s12028-010-9412-8
83. Sawyer KN, Camp-Rogers TR, Kotini-Shah P, Del Rios M, Gossip MR, Moitra VK, Haywood KL, Dougherty CM, Lubitz SA, Rabinstein AA, Rittenberger JC, Callaway CW, Abella BS, Geocadin RG, Kurz MC; American Heart Association Emergency Cardiovascular Care Committee; Council on Cardiovascular and Stroke Nursing; Council on Genomic and Precision Medicine; Council on Quality of Care and Outcomes Research; and Stroke Council. Sudden Cardiac Arrest Survivorship: A Scientific Statement From the American Heart Association. Circulation. 2020;141:e654-e685. doi: 10.1161/CIR.0000000000000747
84. Wilder Schaaf KP, Artman LK, Peberdy MA, Walker WC, Ornato JP, Gossip MR, Kreutzer JS; Virginia Commonwealth University ARCTIC Investigators. Anxiety, depression, and PTSD following cardiac arrest: a systematic review of the literature. Resuscitation. 2013;84:873-877. doi: 10.1016/j.resuscitation.2012.11.021
85. Presciutti A, Verma J, Pavol M, Anbarasan D, Falo C, Brodie D, Rabbani LE, Roh DJ, Park S, Claassen J, Agarwal S. Posttraumatic stress and depressive symptoms characterize cardiac arrest survivors' perceived recovery at hospital discharge. Gen Hosp Psychiatry. 2018;53:108-113. doi: 10.1016/j.genhosppsych.2018.02.006
86. Presciutti A, Sobczak E, Sumner JA, Roh DJ, Park S, Claassen J, Kronish I, Agarwal S. The impact of psychological distress on long-term recovery perceptions in survivors of cardiac arrest. J Crit Care. 2019;50:227-233. doi: 10.1016/j.jcrc.2018.12.011
87. Lilja G, Nilsson G, Nielsen N, Friberg H, Hassager C, Koopmans M, Kuiper M, Martini A, Mellinghoff J, Pelosi P, Wanscher M, Wise MP, Östman I, Cronberg T. Anxiety and depression among out-of-hospital cardiac arrest survivors. Resuscitation. 2015;97:68-75. doi: 10.1016/j.resuscitation.2015.09.389
88. Nolan JP, Soar J, Cariou A, Cronberg T, Moulaert VR, Deakin CD, Bottiger BW, Friberg H, Sunde K, Sandroni C. European Resuscitation Council and European Society of Intensive Care Medicine 2015 guidelines for post-resuscitation care. Intensive Care Med. 2015;41:2039-2056. doi: 10.1007/s00134-015-4051-3
89. Moulaert VR, Verbunt JA, Bakx WG, Gorgels AP, de Krom MC, Heuts PH, Wade DT, van Heugten CM. 'Stand still., and move on', a new early intervention service for cardiac arrest survivors and their caregivers: rationale and description of the intervention. Clin Rehabil. 2011;25:867-879. doi: 10.1177/0269215511399937
90. Cowan MJ, Pike KC, Budzynski HK. Psychosocial nursing therapy following sudden cardiac arrest: impact on two-year survival. Nurs Res. 2001;50:68-76. doi: 10.1097/00006199-200103000-00002
91. Sutton RM, Reeder RW, Landis WP, Meert KL, Yates AR, Morgan RW, Berger JT, Newth CJ, Carcillo JA, McQuillen PS, Harrison RE, Moler FW, Pollack MM, Carpenter TC, Notterman DA, Holubkov R, Dean JM, Nadkarni VM, Berg RA; Eunice Kennedy Shriver National Institute of Child Health and Human Development Collaborative Pediatric Critical Care Research Network (CPCCRN). Ventilation Rates and Pediatric In-Hospital Cardiac Arrest Survival Outcomes. Crit Care Med. 2019;47:1627-1636. doi: 10.1097/CCM.0000000000003898
92. Chen L, Zhang J, Pan G, Li X, Shi T, He W. Cuffed versus uncuffed endotracheal tubes in pediatrics: a meta-analysis. Open Med (Wars). 2018;13:366-373. doi: 10.1515/med-2018-0055
93. Shi F, Xiao Y, Xiong W, Zhou Q, Huang X. Cuffed versus uncuffed endotracheal tubes in children: a meta-analysis. J Anesth. 2016;30:3-11. doi: 10.1007/s00540-015-2062-4
94. De Orange FA, Andrade RG, Lemos A, Borges PS, Figueiroa JN, Kovatsis PG. Cuffed versus uncuffed endotracheal tubes for general anaesthesia in children aged eight years and under. Cochrane Database Syst Rev. 2017;11:CD011954. doi: 10.1002/14651858.CD011954.pub2
95. Chambers NA, Ramgolam A, Sommerfield D, Zhang G, Ledowski T, Thurm M, Lethbridge M, Hegarty M, von Ungern-Sternberg BS. Cuffed vs. uncuffed tracheal tubes in children: a randomised controlled trial comparing leak, tidal volume and complications. Anaesthesia. 2018;73:160-168. doi: 10.1111/anae.14113
96. de Wit M, Peelen LM, van Wolfswinkel L, de Graaff JC. The incidence of postoperative respiratory complications: A retrospective analysis of cuffed vs uncuffed tracheal tubes in children 0-7 years of age. Paediatr Anaesth. 2018;28:210-217. doi: 10.1111/pan.13340
97. Schweiger C, Marostica PJ, Smith MM, Manica D, Carvalho PR, Kuhl G. Incidence of post-intubation subglottic stenosis in children: prospective study. J Laryngol Otol. 2013;127:399-403. doi: 10.1017/S002221511300025X
98. Dorsey DP, Bowman SM, Klein MB, Archer D, Sharar SR. Perioperative use of cuffed endotracheal tubes is advantageous in young pediatric burn patients. Burns. 2010;36:856-860. doi: 10.1016/j.burns.2009.11.011
99. Kojima T, Laverriere EK, Owen EB, Harwayne-Gidansky I, Shenoi AN, Napolitano N, Rehder KJ, Adu-Darko MA, Nett ST, Spear D, et al; and the National Emergency Airway Registry for Children (NEAR4KIDS) Collaborators and Pediatric Acute Lung Injury and Sepsis Investigators (PALISI). Clinical impact of external laryngeal manipulation during laryngoscopy on tracheal intubation success in critically ill children. Pediatr Crit Care Med. 2018;19:106-114. doi: 10.1097/PCC.0000000000001373
100. Kojima T, Harwayne-Gidansky I, Shenoi AN, Owen EB, Napolitano N, Rehder KJ, Adu-Darko MA, Nett ST, Spear D, Meyer K, Giuliano JS Jr, Tarquinio KM, Sanders RC Jr, Lee JH, Simon DW, Vanderford PA, Lee AY, Brown CA III, Skippen PW, Breuer RK, Toedt-Pingel I, Parsons SJ, Gradidge EA, Glater LB, Culver K, Nadkarni VM, Nishisaki A; National Emergency Airway Registry for Children (NEAR4KIDS) and Pediatric Acute Lung Injury and Sepsis Investigators (PALISI). Cricoid Pressure During Induction for Tracheal Intubation in Critically Ill Children: A Report From National Emergency Airway Registry for Children. Pediatr Crit Care Med. 2018;19:528-537. doi: 10.1097/PCC.0000000000001531
101. Andersen LW, Berg KM, Saindon BZ, Massaro JM, Raymond TT, Berg RA, Nadkarni VM, Donnino MW; American Heart Association Get With the Guidelines-Resuscitation Investigators. Time to Epinephrine and Survival After Pediatric In-Hospital Cardiac Arrest. JAMA. 2015;314:802-810. doi: 10.1001/jama.2015.9678
102. Lin YR, Wu MH, Chen TY, Syue YJ, Yang MC, Lee TH, Lin CM, Chou CC, Chang CF, Li CJ. Time to epinephrine treatment is associated with the risk of mortality in children who achieve sustained ROSC after traumatic out-of-hospital cardiac arrest. Crit Care. 2019;23:101. doi: 10.1186/s13054-019-2391-z
103. Lin YR, Li CJ, Huang CC, Lee TH, Chen TY, Yang MC, Chou CC, Chang CF, Huang HW, Hsu HY, Chen WL. Early Epinephrine Improves the Stabilization of Initial Post-resuscitation Hemodynamics in Children With Non-shockable Out-of-Hospital Cardiac Arrest. Front Pediatr. 2019;7:220. doi: 10.3389/fped.2019.00220
104. Fukuda T, Kondo Y, Hayashida K, Sekiguchi H, Kukita I. Time to epinephrine and survival after paediatric out-of-hospital cardiac arrest. Eur Heart J Cardiovasc Pharmacother. 2018;4:144-151. doi: 10.1093/ehjcvp/pvx023
105. Berg RA, Sutton RM, Reeder RW, Berger JT, Newth CJ, Carcillo JA, McQuillen PS, Meert KL, Yates AR, Harrison RE, Moler FW, Pollack MM, Carpenter TC, Wessel DL, Jenkins TL, Notterman DA, Holubkov R, Tamburro RF, Dean JM, Nadkarni VM; Eunice Kennedy Shriver National Institute of Child Health and Human Development Collaborative Pediatric Critical Care Research Network (CPCCRN) PICqCPR (Pediatric Intensive Care Quality of Cardio-Pulmonary Resuscitation) Investigators. Association Between Diastolic Blood Pressure During Pediatric In-Hospital Cardiopulmonary Resuscitation and Survival. Circulation. 2018;137:1784-1795. doi: 10.1161/CIRCULATIONAHA.117.032270
106. Herman ST, Abend NS, Bleck TP, Chapman KE, Drislane FW, Emerson RG, Gerard EE, Hahn CD, Husain AM, Kaplan PW, LaRoche SM, Nuwer MR, Quigg M, Riviello JJ, Schmitt SE, Simmons LA, Tsuchida TN, Hirsch LJ; Critical Care Continuous EEG Task Force of the American Clinical Neurophysiology Society. Consensus statement on continuous EEG in critically ill adults

and children, part I: indications. J Clin Neurophysiol. 2015;32:87-95. doi: 10.1097/WNP.0000000000000166
107. Abend NS, Topjian A, Ichord R, Herman ST, Helfaer M, Donnelly M, Nadkarni V, Dlugos DJ, Clancy RR. Electroencephalographic monitoring during hypothermia after pediatric cardiac arrest. Neurology. 2009;72:1931-1940. doi: 10.1212/WNL.0b013e3181a82687
108. Topjian AA, Gutierrez-Colina AM, Sanchez SM, Berg RA, Friess SH, Dlugos DJ, Abend NS. Electrographic status epilepticus is associated with mortality and worse short-term outcome in critically ill children. Crit Care Med. 2013;41:215-223. doi: 10.1097/CCM.0b013e3182668035
109. Ostendorf AP, Hartman ME, Friess SH. Early Electroencephalographic Findings Correlate With Neurologic Outcome in Children Following Cardiac Arrest. Pediatr Crit Care Med. 2016;17:667-676. doi: 10.1097/PCC.0000000000000791
110. Brophy GM, Bell R, Claassen J, Alldredge B, Bleck TP, Glauser T, Laroche SM, Riviello JJ Jr, Shutter L, Sperling MR, Treiman DM, Vespa PM; Neurocritical Care Society Status Epilepticus Guideline Writing Committee. Guidelines for the evaluation and management of status epilepticus. Neurocrit Care. 2012;17:3-23. doi: 10.1007/s12028-012-9695-z
111. Topjian AA, Sánchez SM, Shults J, Berg RA, Dlugos DJ, Abend NS. Early Electroencephalographic Background Features Predict Outcomes in Children Resuscitated From Cardiac Arrest. Pediatr Crit Care Med. 2016;17:547-557. doi: 10.1097/PCC.0000000000000740
112. Moler FW, Silverstein FS, Holubkov R, Slomine BS, Christensen JR, Nadkarni VM, Meert KL, Clark AE, Browning B, Pemberton VL, Page K, Shankaran S, Hutchison JS, Newth CJ, Bennett KS, Berger JT, Topjian A, Pineda JA, Koch JD, Schleien CL, Dalton HJ, Ofori-Amanfo G, Goodman DM, Fink EL, McQuillen P, Zimmerman JJ, Thomas NJ, van der Jagt EW, Porter MB, Meyer MT, Harrison R, Pham N, Schwarz AJ, Nowak JE, Alten J, Wheeler DS, Bhalala US, Lidsky K, Lloyd E, Mathur M, Shah S, Wu T, Theodorou AA, Sanders RC Jr, Dean JM; THAPCA Trial Investigators. Therapeutic hypothermia after out-of-hospital cardiac arrest in children. N Engl J Med. 2015;372:1898-1908. doi: 10.1056/NEJMoa1411480
113. Moler FW, Silverstein FS, Holubkov R, Slomine BS, Christensen JR, Nadkarni VM, Meert KL, Browning B, Pemberton VL, Page K, et al; on behalf of the THAPCA Trial Investigators. Therapeutic hypothermia after in-hospital cardiac arrest in children. N Engl J Med. 2017;376:318-329. doi: 10.1056/NEJMoa1610493
114. Slomine BS, Silverstein FS, Page K, Holubkov R, Christensen JR, Dean JM, Moler FW; Therapeutic Hypothermia after Pediatric Cardiac Arrest (THAPCA) Trial Investigators. Relationships between three and twelve month outcomes in children enrolled in the therapeutic hypothermia after pediatric cardiac arrest trials. Resuscitation. 2019;139:329-336. doi: 10.1016/j.resuscitation.2019.03.020
115. Slomine BS, Silverstein FS, Christensen JR, Holubkov R, Telford R, Dean JM, Moler FW; Therapeutic Hypothermia after Paediatric Cardiac Arrest (THAPCA) Trial Investigators. Neurobehavioural outcomes in children after In-Hospital cardiac arrest. Resuscitation. 2018;124:80-89. doi: 10.1016/j.resuscitation.2018.01.002
116. Slomine BS, Silverstein FS, Christensen JR, Page K, Holubkov R, Dean JM, Moler FW. Neuropsychological Outcomes of Children 1 Year After Pediatric Cardiac Arrest: Secondary Analysis of 2 Randomized Clinical Trials. JAMA Neurol. 2018;75:1502-1510. doi: 10.1001/jamaneurol.2018.2628
117. Slomine BS, Silverstein FS, Christensen JR, Holubkov R, Page K, Dean JM, Moler FW; on behalf of the THAPCA Trial Group. Neurobehavioral outcomes in children after out-of-hospital cardiac arrest. Pediatrics. 2016;137:e20153412. doi: 10.1542/peds.2015-3412
118. van Zellem L, Buysse C, Madderom M, Legerstee JS, Aarsen F, Tibboel D, Utens EM. Long-term neuropsychological outcomes in children and adolescents after cardiac arrest. Intensive Care Med. 2015;41:1057-1066. doi: 10.1007/s00134-015-3789-y
119. van Zellem L, Utens EM, Legerstee JS, Cransberg K, Hulst JM, Tibboel D, Buysse C. Cardiac Arrest in Children: Long-Term Health Status and Health-Related Quality of Life. Pediatr Crit Care Med. 2015;16:693-702. doi: 10.1097/PCC.0000000000000452
120. van Zellem L, Utens EM, Madderom M, Legerstee JS, Aarsen F, Tibboel D, Buysse C. Cardiac arrest in infants, children, and adolescents: long-term emotional and behavioral functioning. Eur J Pediatr. 2016;175:977-986. doi: 10.1007/s00431-016-2728-4
121. Topjian AA, Scholefield BR, Pinto NP, Fink EL, Buysse CMP, Haywood K, Maconochie I, Nadkarni VM, de Caen A, Escalante-Kanashiro R, Ng K-C, et al. P-COSCA (Pediatric Core Outcome Set for Cardiac Arrest) in children: an advisory statement from the International Liaison Committee on Resuscitation. Circulation. 2020;142:e000-e000. doi: 10.1161/CIR.0000000000000911
122. Topjian AA, de Caen A, Wainwright MS, Abella BS, Abend NS, Atkins DL, Bembea MM, Fink EL, Guerguerian AM, Haskell SE, Kilgannon JH, Lasa JJ, Hazinski MF. Pediatric Post–Cardiac Arrest Care: A Scientific Statement From the American Heart Association. Circulation. 2019;140:e194-e233. doi: 10.1161/CIR.0000000000000697
123. Inwald DP, Canter R, Woolfall K, Mouncey P, Zenasni Z, O'Hara C, Carter A, Jones N, Lyttle MD, Nadel S, et al; on behalf of PERUKI (Paediatric Emergency Research in the UK and Ireland) and PICS SG (Paediatric Intensive Care Society Study Group). Restricted fluid bolus volume in early septic shock: results of the Fluids in Shock pilot trial. Archives of disease in childhood. 2019;104:426-431. doi: 10.1136/archdischild-2018-314924
124. van Paridon BM, Sheppard C, Garcia Guerra G, Joffe AR; on behalf of the Alberta Sepsis Network. Timing of antibiotics, volume, and vasoactive infusions in children with sepsis admitted to intensive care. Crit Care. 2015;19:293. doi: 10.1186/s13054-015-1010-x
125. Sankar J, Ismail J, Sankar MJ, C P S, Meena RS. Fluid Bolus Over 15-20 Versus 5-10 Minutes Each in the First Hour of Resuscitation in Children With Septic Shock: A Randomized Controlled Trial. Pediatr Crit Care Med. 2017;18:e435-e445. doi: 10.1097/PCC.0000000000001269
126. Medeiros DN, Ferranti JF, Delgado AF, de Carvalho WB. Colloids for the Initial Management of Severe Sepsis and Septic Shock in Pediatric Patients: A Systematic Review. Pediatr Emerg Care. 2015;31:e11-e16. doi: 10.1097/PEC.0000000000000601
127. Balamuth F, Kittick M, McBride P, Woodford AL, Vestal N, Casper TC, Metheney M, Smith K, Atkin NJ, Baren JM, Dean JM, Kuppermann N, Weiss SL. Pragmatic Pediatric Trial of Balanced Versus Normal Saline Fluid in Sepsis: The PRoMPT BOLUS Randomized Controlled Trial Pilot Feasibility Study. Acad Emerg Med. 2019;26:1346-1356. doi: 10.1111/acem.13815
128. Weiss SL, Keele L, Balamuth F, Vendetti N, Ross R, Fitzgerald JC, Gerber JS. Crystalloid Fluid Choice and Clinical Outcomes in Pediatric Sepsis: A Matched Retrospective Cohort Study. J Pediatr. 2017;182:304-310.e10. doi: 10.1016/j.jpeds.2016.11.075
129. Emrath ET, Fortenberry JD, Travers C, McCracken CE, Hebbar KB. Resuscitation With Balanced Fluids Is Associated With Improved Survival in Pediatric Severe Sepsis. Crit Care Med. 2017;45:1177-1183. doi: 10.1097/CCM.0000000000002365
130. Ventura AM, Shieh HH, Bousso A, Góes PF, de Cássia F O Fernandes I, de Souza DC, Paulo RL, Chagas F, Gilio AE. Double-Blind Prospective Randomized Controlled Trial of Dopamine Versus Epinephrine as First-Line Vasoactive Drugs in Pediatric Septic Shock. Crit Care Med. 2015;43:2292-2302. doi: 10.1097/CCM.0000000000001260
131. Ramaswamy KN, Singhi S, Jayashree M, Bansal A, Nallasamy K. Double-Blind Randomized Clinical Trial Comparing Dopamine and Epinephrine in Pediatric Fluid-Refractory Hypotensive Septic Shock. Pediatr Crit Care Med. 2016;17:e502-e512. doi: 10.1097/PCC.0000000000000954
132. Davis AL, Carcillo JA, Aneja RK, Deymann AJ, Lin JC, Nguyen TC, Okhuysen-Cawley RS, Relvas MS, Rozenfeld RA, Skippen PW, Stojadinovic BJ, Williams EA, Yeh TS, Balamuth F, Brierley J, de Caen AR, Cheifetz IM, Choong K, Conway E Jr, Cornell T, Doctor A, Dugas MA, Feldman JD, Fitzgerald JC, Flori HR, Fortenberry JD, Graciano AL, Greenwald BM, Hall MW, Han YY, Hernan LJ, Irazuzta JE, Iselin E, van der Jagt EW, Jeffries HE, Kache S, Katyal C, Kissoon N, Kon AA, Kutko MC, MacLaren G, Maul T, Mehta R, Odetola F, Parbuoni K, Paul R, Peters MJ, Ranjit S, Reuter-Rice KE, Schnitzler EJ, Scott HF, Torres A Jr, Weingarten-Arams J, Weiss SL, Zimmerman JJ, Zuckerberg AL. American College of Critical Care Medicine Clinical Practice Parameters for Hemodynamic Support of Pediatric and Neonatal Septic Shock. Crit Care Med. 2017;45:1061-1093. doi: 10.1097/CCM.0000000000002425
133. Lampin ME, Rousseaux J, Botte A, Sadik A, Cremer R, Leclerc F. Noradrenaline use for septic shock in children: doses, routes of administration and complications. Acta Paediatr. 2012;101:e426-e430. doi: 10.1111/j.1651-2227.2012.02725.x
134. Deep A, Goonasekera CD, Wang Y, Brierley J. Evolution of haemodynamics and outcome of fluid-refractory septic shock in children. Intensive Care Med. 2013;39:1602-1609. doi: 10.1007/s00134-013-3003-z
135. Weiss SL, Peters MJ, Alhazzani W, Agus MSD, Flori HR, Inwald DP, Nadel S, Schlapbach LJ, Tasker RC, Argent AC, Brierley J, Carcillo J, Carrol ED, Carroll CL, Cheifetz IM, Choong K, Cies JJ, Cruz AT, De Luca D, Deep A, Faust SN, De Oliveira CF, Hall MW, Ishimine P, Javouhey E, Joosten KFM, Joshi P, Karam O, Kneyber MCJ, Lemson J, MacLaren G, Mehta NM, Møller MH, Newth CJL, Nguyen TC, Nishisaki A, Nunnally ME, Parker MM, Paul RM, Randolph AG, Ranjit S, Romer LH, Scott HF, Tume LN, Verger JT,

Williams EA, Wolf J, Wong HR, Zimmerman JJ, Kissoon N, Tissieres P. Surviving Sepsis Campaign International Guidelines for the Management of Septic Shock and Sepsis-Associated Organ Dysfunction in Children. Pediatr Crit Care Med. 2020;21:e52-e106. doi: 10.1097/PCC.0000000000002198
136. Kelly LK, Porta NF, Goodman DM, Carroll CL, Steinhorn RH. Inhaled prostacyclin for term infants with persistent pulmonary hypertension refractory to inhaled nitric oxide. J Pediatr. 2002;141:830-832. doi: 10.1067/mpd.2002.129849
137. Kerr D, Kelly AM, Dietze P, Jolley D, Barger B. Randomized controlled trial comparing the effectiveness and safety of intranasal and intramuscular naloxone for the treatment of suspected heroin overdose. Addiction. 2009;104:2067-2074. doi: 10.1111/j.1360-0443.2009.02724.x
138. Wanger K, Brough L, Macmillan I, Goulding J, MacPhail I, Christenson JM. Intravenous vs subcutaneous naloxone for out-of-hospital management of presumed opioid overdose. Acad Emerg Med. 1998;5:293-299. doi: 10.1111/j.1553-2712.1998.tb02707.x
139. Barton ED, Colwell CB, Wolfe T, Fosnocht D, Gravitz C, Bryan T, Dunn W, Benson J, Bailey J. Efficacy of intranasal naloxone as a needleless alternative for treatment of opioid overdose in the prehospital setting. J Emerg Med. 2005;29:265-271. doi: 10.1016/j.jemermed.2005.03.007
140. Robertson TM, Hendey GW, Stroh G, Shalit M. Intranasal naloxone is a viable alternative to intravenous naloxone for prehospital narcotic overdose. Prehosp Emerg Care. 2009;13:512-515. doi: 10.1080/10903120903144866
141. Cetrullo C, Di Nino GF, Melloni C, Pieri C, Zanoni A. [Naloxone antagonism toward opiate analgesic drugs. Clinical experimental study]. Minerva Anestesiol. 1983;49:199-204.
142. Osterwalder JJ. Naloxone-for intoxications with intravenous heroin and heroin mixtures-harmless or hazardous? A prospective clinical study. J Toxicol Clin Toxicol. 1996;34:409-416. doi: 10.3109/15563659609013811
143. Sporer KA, Firestone J, Isaacs SM. Out-of-hospital treatment of opioid overdoses in an urban setting. Acad Emerg Med. 1996;3:660-667. doi: 10.1111/j.1553-2712.1996.tb03487.x
144. Stokland O, Hansen TB, Nilsen JE. [Prehospital treatment of heroin intoxication in Oslo in 1996]. Tidsskr Nor Laegeforen. 1998;118:3144-3146.
145. Buajordet I, Naess AC, Jacobsen D, Brørs O. Adverse events after naloxone treatment of episodes of suspected acute opioid overdose. Eur J Emerg Med. 2004;11:19-23. doi: 10.1097/00063110-200402000-00004
146. Cantwell K, Dietze P, Flander L. The relationship between naloxone dose and key patient variables in the treatment of non-fatal heroin overdose in the prehospital setting. Resuscitation. 2005;65:315-319. doi: 10.1016/j.resuscitation.2004.12.012
147. Boyd JJ, Kuisma MJ, Alaspää AO, Vuori E, Repo JV, Randell TT. Recurrent opioid toxicity after pre-hospital care of presumed heroin overdose patients. Acta Anaesthesiol Scand. 2006;50:1266-1270. doi: 10.1111/j.1399-6576.2006.01172.x
148. Nielsen K, Nielsen SL, Siersma V, Rasmussen LS. Treatment of opioid overdose in a physician-based prehospital EMS: frequency and long-term prognosis. Resuscitation. 2011;82:1410-1413. doi: 10.1016/j.resuscitation.2011.05.027
149. Wampler DA, Molina DK, McManus J, Laws P, Manifold CA. No deaths associated with patient refusal of transport after naloxone-reversed opioid overdose. Prehosp Emerg Care. 2011;15:320-324. doi: 10.3109/10903127.2011.569854
150. Kelly AM, Kerr D, Dietze P, Patrick I, Walker T, Koutsogiannis Z. Randomised trial of intranasal versus intramuscular naloxone in prehospital treatment for suspected opioid overdose. Med J Aust. 2005;182:24-27.
151. Moore ER, Bergman N, Anderson GC, Medley N. Early skin-to-skin contact for mothers and their healthy newborn infants. Cochrane Database Syst Rev. 2016;11:CD003519. doi: 10.1002/14651858.CD003519.pub4
152. de Almeida MF, Guinsburg R, Velaphi S, Aziz K, Perlman JM, Szyld E, Kim HS, Hosono S, Liley HG, Mildenhall L, et al. Intravenous vs. intraosseous administration of drugs during cardiac arrest: International Liaison Committee on Resuscitation (ILCOR) Neonatal Life Support Task Force. 2019. https://costr.ilcor.org/document/intravenous-vs-intraosseous-administration-of-drugs-during-cardiac-arrest-nls-task-force-systematic-review-costr. Updated February 20, 2020. Accessed March 2, 2020.
153. Foglia EE, Weiner G, de Almeida MF, Liley HG, Aziz K, Fabres J, Fawke J, Hosono S, Isayama T, Kapadia VS, et al. Impact of duration of intensive resuscitation (NLS #895): systematic review: International Liaison Committee on Resuscitation (ILCOR) Neonatal Life Support Task Force. 2020. https://costr.ilcor.org/document/impact-of-duration-of-intensive-resuscitation-nls-896-systematic-review. Updated February 19, 2020. Accessed March 1, 2020.
154. Cheng A, Nadkarni VM, Mancini MB, Hunt EA, Sinz EH, Merchant RM, Donoghue A, Duff JP, Eppich W, Auerbach M, Bigham BL, Blewer AL, Chan PS, Bhanji F; American Heart Association Education Science Investigators; and on behalf of the American Heart Association Education Science and Programs Committee, Council on Cardiopulmonary, Critical Care, Perioperative and Resuscitation; Council on Cardiovascular and Stroke Nursing; and Council on Quality of Care and Outcomes Research. Resuscitation Education Science: Educational Strategies to Improve Outcomes From Cardiac Arrest: A Scientific Statement From the American Heart Association. Circulation. 2018;138:e82-e122. doi: 10.1161/CIR.0000000000000583
155. Anderson R, Sebaldt A, Lin Y, Cheng A. Optimal training frequency for acquisition and retention of high-quality CPR skills: A randomized trial. Resuscitation. 2019;135:153-161. doi: 10.1016/j.resuscitation.2018.10.033
156. Lin Y, Cheng A, Grant VJ, Currie GR, Hecker KG. Improving CPR quality with distributed practice and real-time feedback in pediatric healthcare providers – A randomized controlled trial. Resuscitation. 2018;130:6-12. doi: 10.1016/j.resuscitation.2018.06.025
157. O'Donnell CM, Skinner AC. An evaluation of a short course in resuscitation training in a district general hospital. Resuscitation. 1993;26:193-201. doi: 10.1016/0300-9572(93)90179-t
158. Oermann MH, Kardong-Edgren SE, Odom-Maryon T. Effects of monthly practice on nursing students' CPR psychomotor skill performance. Resuscitation. 2011;82:447-453. doi: 10.1016/j.resuscitation.2010.11.022
159. Kardong-Edgren S, Oermann MH, Odom-Maryon T. Findings from a nursing student CPR study: implications for staff development educators. J Nurses Staff Dev. 2012;28:9-15. doi: 10.1097/NND.0b013e318240a6ad
160. Nishiyama C, Iwami T, Murakami Y, Kitamura T, Okamoto Y, Marukawa S, Sakamoto T, Kawamura T. Effectiveness of simplified 15-min refresher BLS training program: a randomized controlled trial. Resuscitation. 2015;90:56-60. doi: 10.1016/j.resuscitation.2015.02.015
161. Sullivan NJ, Duval-Arnould J, Twilley M, Smith SP, Aksamit D, Boone-Guercio P, Jeffries PR, Hunt EA. Simulation exercise to improve retention of cardiopulmonary resuscitation priorities for in-hospital cardiac arrests: A randomized controlled trial. Resuscitation. 2015;86:6-13. doi: 10.1016/j.resuscitation.2014.10.021
162. Patocka C, Cheng A, Sibbald M, Duff JP, Lai A, Lee-Nobbee P, Levin H, Varshney T, Weber B, Bhanji F. A randomized education trial of spaced versus massed instruction to improve acquisition and retention of paediatric resuscitation skills in emergency medical service (EMS) providers. Resuscitation. 2019;141:73-80. doi: 10.1016/j.resuscitation.2019.06.010
163. Patocka C, Khan F, Dubrovsky AS, Brody D, Bank I, Bhanji F. Pediatric resuscitation training-instruction all at once or spaced over time? Resuscitation. 2015;88:6-11. doi: 10.1016/j.resuscitation.2014.12.003
164. Kurosawa H, Ikeyama T, Achuff P, Perkel M, Watson C, Monachino A, Remy D, Deutsch E, Buchanan N, Anderson J, Berg RA, Nadkarni VM, Nishisaki A. A randomized, controlled trial of in situ pediatric advanced life support recertification ("pediatric advanced life support reconstructed") compared with standard pediatric advanced life support recertification for ICU frontline providers*. Crit Care Med. 2014;42:610-618. doi: 10.1097/CCM.0000000000000024
165. Ericsson KA. Deliberate practice and the acquisition and maintenance of expert performance in medicine and related domains. Acad Med. 2004;79 (suppl):S70-81. doi: 10.1097/00001888-200410001-00022
166. McGaghie WC. When I say … mastery learning. Med Educ. 2015;49:558-559. doi: 10.1111/medu.12679
167. Magee MJ, Farkouh-Karoleski C, Rosen TS. Improvement of Immediate Performance in Neonatal Resuscitation Through Rapid Cycle Deliberate Practice Training. J Grad Med Educ. 2018;10:192-197. doi: 10.4300/JGME-D-17-00467.1
168. Diederich E, Lineberry M, Blomquist M, Schott V, Reilly C, Murray M, Nazaran P, Rourk M, Werner R, Broski J. Balancing Deliberate Practice and Reflection: A Randomized Comparison Trial of Instructional Designs for Simulation-Based Training in Cardiopulmonary Resuscitation Skills. Simul Healthc. 2019;14:175-181. doi: 10.1097/SIH.0000000000000375
169. Braun L, Sawyer T, Smith K, Hsu A, Behrens M, Chan D, Hutchinson J, Lu D, Singh R, Reyes J, Lopreiato J. Retention of pediatric resuscitation performance after a simulation-based mastery learning session: a

multicenter randomized trial. Pediatr Crit Care Med. 2015;16:131-138. doi: 10.1097/PCC.0000000000000315
170. Cordero L, Hart BJ, Hardin R, Mahan JD, Nankervis CA. Deliberate practice improves pediatric residents' skills and team behaviors during simulated neonatal resuscitation. Clin Pediatr (Phila). 2013;52:747-752. doi: 10.1177/0009922813488646
171. Hunt EA, Duval-Arnould JM, Chime NO, Jones K, Rosen M, Hollingsworth M, Aksamit D, Twilley M, Camacho C, Nogee DP, Jung J, Nelson-McMillan K, Shilkofski N, Perretta JS. Integration of in-hospital cardiac arrest contextual curriculum into a basic life support course: a randomized, controlled simulation study. Resuscitation. 2017;114:127-132. doi: 10.1016/j.resuscitation.2017.03.014
172. Hunt EA, Duval-Arnould JM, Nelson-McMillan KL, Bradshaw JH, Diener-West M, Perretta JS, Shilkofski NA. Pediatric resident resuscitation skills improve after "rapid cycle deliberate practice" training. Resuscitation. 2014;85:945-951. doi: 10.1016/j.resuscitation.2014.02.025
173. Jeffers J, Eppich W, Trainor J, Mobley B, Adler M. Development and Evaluation of a Learning Intervention Targeting First-Year Resident Defibrillation Skills. Pediatr Emerg Care. 2016;32:210-216. doi: 10.1097/PEC.0000000000000765
174. Reed T, Pirotte M, McHugh M, Oh L, Lovett S, Hoyt AE, Quinones D, Adams W, Gruener G, McGaghie WC. Simulation-Based Mastery Learning Improves Medical Student Performance and Retention of Core Clinical Skills. Simul Healthc. 2016;11:173-180. doi: 10.1097/SIH.0000000000000154
175. Kurup V, Matei V, Ray J. Role of in-situ simulation for training in healthcare: opportunities and challenges. Curr Opin Anaesthesiol. 2017;30:755-760. doi: 10.1097/ACO.0000000000000514
176. Goldshtein D, Krensky C, Doshi S, Perelman VS. In situ simulation and its effects on patient outcomes: a systematic review. BMJ Simulation and Technology Enhanced Learning. 2020;6:3-9. doi: 10.1136/bmjstel-2018-000387
177. Rosen MA, Hunt EA, Pronovost PJ, Federowicz MA, Weaver SJ. In situ simulation in continuing education for the health care professions: a systematic review. J Contin Educ Health Prof. 2012;32:243-254. doi: 10.1002/chp.21152
178. Steinemann S, Berg B, Skinner A, DiTulio A, Anzelon K, Terada K, Oliver C, Ho HC, Speck C. In situ, multidisciplinary, simulation-based teamwork training improves early trauma care. J Surg Educ. 2011;68:472-477. doi: 10.1016/j.jsurg.2011.05.009
179. Clarke SO, Julie IM, Yao AP, Bang H, Barton JD, Alsomali SM, Kiefer MV, Al Khulaif AH, Aljahany M, Venugopal S, Bair AE. Longitudinal exploration of in situ mock code events and the performance of cardiac arrest skills. BMJ Simul Technol Enhanc Learn. 2019;5:29-33. doi: 10.1136/bmjstel-2017-000255
180. Rubio-Gurung S, Putet G, Touzet S, Gauthier-Moulinier H, Jordan I, Beissel A, Labaune JM, Blanc S, Amamra N, Balandras C, Rudigoz RC, Colin C, Picaud JC. In situ simulation training for neonatal resuscitation: an RCT. Pediatrics. 2014;134:e790-e797. doi: 10.1542/peds.2013-3988
181. Saqe-Rockoff A, Ciardiello AV, Schubert FD. Low-Fidelity, In-Situ Pediatric Resuscitation Simulation Improves RN Competence and Self-Efficacy. J Emerg Nurs. 2019;45:538-544.e1. doi: 10.1016/j.jen.2019.02.003
182. Katznelson JH, Wang J, Stevens MW, Mills WA. Improving Pediatric Preparedness in Critical Access Hospital Emergency Departments: Impact of a Longitudinal In Situ Simulation Program. Pediatr Emerg Care. 2018;34:17-20. doi: 10.1097/PEC.0000000000001366
183. Reder S, Cummings P, Quan L. Comparison of three instructional methods for teaching cardiopulmonary resuscitation and use of an automatic external defibrillator to high school students. Resuscitation. 2006;69:443-453. doi: 10.1016/j.resuscitation.2005.08.020
184. Roppolo LP, Pepe PE, Campbell L, Ohman K, Kulkarni H, Miller R, Idris A, Bean L, Bettes TN, Idris AH. Prospective, randomized trial of the effectiveness and retention of 30-min layperson training for cardiopulmonary resuscitation and automated external defibrillators: The American Airlines Study. Resuscitation. 2007;74:276-285. doi: 10.1016/j.resuscitation.2006.12.017
185. de Vries W, Turner NM, Monsieurs KG, Bierens JJ, Koster RW. Comparison of instructor-led automated external defibrillation training and three alternative DVD-based training methods. Resuscitation. 2010;81:1004-1009. doi: 10.1016/j.resuscitation.2010.04.006
186. Saraç L, Ok A. The effects of different instructional methods on students' acquisition and retention of cardiopulmonary resuscitation skills. Resuscitation. 2010;81:555-561. doi: 10.1016/j.resuscitation.2009.08.030
187. Zeleke BG, Biswas ES, Biswas M. Teaching Cardiopulmonary Resuscitation to Young Children (<12 Years Old). Am J Cardiol. 2019;123:1626-1627. doi: 10.1016/j.amjcard.2019.02.011
188. Schmid KM, García RQ, Fernandez MM, Mould-Millman NK, Lowenstein SR. Teaching Hands-Only CPR in Schools: A Program Evaluation in San José, Costa Rica. Ann Glob Health. 2018;84:612-617. doi: 10.9204/aogh.2367
189. Li H, Shen X, Xu X, Wang Y, Chu L, Zhao J, Wang Y, Wang H, Xie G, Cheng B, et al. Bystander cardiopulmonary resuscitation training in primary and secondary school children in China and the impact of neighborhood socioeconomic status: A prospective controlled trial. Medicine (Baltimore). 2018;97:e12673. doi: 10.1097/MD.0000000000012673
190. Paglino M, Contri E, Baggiani M, Tonani M, Costantini G, Bonomo MC, Baldi E. A video-based training to effectively teach CPR with long-term retention: the ScuolaSalvaVita.it ("SchoolSavesLives.it") project. Intern Emerg Med. 2019;14:275-279. doi: 10.1007/s11739-018-1946-3
191. Magid KH, Heard D, Sasson C. Addressing Gaps in Cardiopulmonary Resuscitation Education: Training Middle School Students in Hands-Only Cardiopulmonary Resuscitation. J Sch Health. 2018;88:524-530. doi: 10.1111/josh.12634
192. Andrews T, Price L, Mills B, Holmes L. Young adults' perception of mandatory CPR training in Australian high schools: a qualitative investigation. Austr J Paramedicine. 2018;15. doi: 10.33151/ajp.15.2.577
193. Aloush S, Tubaishat A, ALBashtawy M, Suliman M, Alrimawi I, Al Sabah A, Banikhaled Y. Effectiveness of Basic Life Support Training for Middle School Students. J Sch Nurs. 2019;35:262-267. doi: 10.1177/1059840517753879
194. Gabriel IO, Aluko JO. Theoretical knowledge and psychomotor skill acquisition of basic life support training programme among secondary school students. World J Emerg Med. 2019;10:81-87. doi: 10.5847/wjem.j.1920-8642.2019.02.003
195. Brown LE, Carroll T, Lynes C, Tripathi A, Halperin H, Dillon WC. CPR skill retention in 795 high school students following a 45-minute course with psychomotor practice. Am J Emerg Med. 2018;36:1110-1112. doi: 10.1016/j.ajem.2017.10.026
196. Brookoff D, Kellermann AL, Hackman BB, Somes G, Dobyns P. Do blacks get bystander cardiopulmonary resuscitation as often as whites? Ann Emerg Med. 1994;24:1147-1150. doi: 10.1016/s0196-0644(94)70246-2
197. Vadeboncoeur TF, Richman PB, Darkoh M, Chikani V, Clark L, Bobrow BJ. Bystander cardiopulmonary resuscitation for out-of-hospital cardiac arrest in the Hispanic vs the non-Hispanic populations. Am J Emerg Med. 2008;26:655-660. doi: 10.1016/j.ajem.2007.10.002
198. Anderson ML, Cox M, Al-Khatib SM, Nichol G, Thomas KL, Chan PS, Saha-Chaudhuri P, Fosbol EL, Eigel B, Clendenen B, Peterson ED. Rates of cardiopulmonary resuscitation training in the United States. JAMA Intern Med. 2014;174:194-201. doi: 10.1001/jamainternmed.2013.11320
199. Fosbøl EL, Dupre ME, Strauss B, Swanson DR, Myers B, McNally BF, Anderson ML, Bagai A, Monk L, Garvey JL, Bitner M, Jollis JG, Granger CB. Association of neighborhood characteristics with incidence of out-of-hospital cardiac arrest and rates of bystander-initiated CPR: implications for community-based education intervention. Resuscitation. 2014;85:1512-1517. doi: 10.1016/j.resuscitation.2014.08.013
200. Blewer AL, Schmicker RH, Morrison LJ, Aufderheide TP, Daya M, Starks MA, May S, Idris AH, Callaway CW, Kudenchuk PJ, Vilke GM, Abella BS; Resuscitation Outcomes Consortium Investigators. Variation in Bystander Cardiopulmonary Resuscitation Delivery and Subsequent Survival From Out-of-Hospital Cardiac Arrest Based on Neighborhood-Level Ethnic Characteristics. Circulation. 2020;141:34-41. doi: 10.1161/CIRCULATIONAHA.119.041541
201. Mitchell MJ, Stubbs BA, Eisenberg MS. Socioeconomic status is associated with provision of bystander cardiopulmonary resuscitation. Prehosp Emerg Care. 2009;13:478-486. doi: 10.1080/10903120903144833
202. Vaillancourt C, Lui A, De Maio VJ, Wells GA, Stiell IG. Socioeconomic status influences bystander CPR and survival rates for out-of-hospital cardiac arrest victims. Resuscitation. 2008;79:417-423. doi: 10.1016/j.resuscitation.2008.07.012
203. Chiang WC, Ko PC, Chang AM, Chen WT, Liu SS, Huang YS, Chen SY, Lin CH, Cheng MT, Chong KM, Wang HC, Yang CW, Liao MW, Wang CH, Chien YC, Lin CH, Liu YP, Lee BC, Chien KL, Lai MS, Ma MH. Bystander-initiated CPR in an Asian metropolitan: does the socioeconomic status matter? Resuscitation. 2014;85:53-58. doi: 10.1016/j.resuscitation.2013.07.033
204. Moncur L, Ainsborough N, Ghose R, Kendal SP, Salvatori M, Wright J. Does the level of socioeconomic deprivation at the location of cardiac arrest in an English region influence the likelihood of receiving bystander-initiated

cardiopulmonary resuscitation? Emerg Med J. 2016;33:105-108. doi: 10.1136/emermed-2015-204643
205. Dahan B, Jabre P, Karam N, Misslin R, Tafflet M, Bougouin W, Jost D, Beganton F, Marijon E, Jouven X. Impact of neighbourhood socio-economic status on bystander cardiopulmonary resuscitation in Paris. Resuscitation. 2017;110:107-113. doi: 10.1016/j.resuscitation.2016.10.028
206. Brown TP, Booth S, Hawkes CA, Soar J, Mark J, Mapstone J, Fothergill RT, Black S, Pocock H, Bichmann A, Gunson I, Perkins GD. Characteristics of neighbourhoods with high incidence of out-of-hospital cardiac arrest and low bystander cardiopulmonary resuscitation rates in England. Eur Heart J Qual Care Clin Outcomes. 2019;5:51-62. doi: 10.1093/ehjqcco/qcy026
207. Liu KY, Haukoos JS, Sasson C. Availability and quality of cardiopulmonary resuscitation information for Spanish-speaking population on the Internet. Resuscitation. 2014;85:131-137. doi: 10.1016/j.resuscitation.2013.08.274
208. Yip MP, Ong B, Tu SP, Chavez D, Ike B, Painter I, Lam I, Bradley SM, Coronado GD, Meischke HW. Diffusion of cardiopulmonary resuscitation training to chinese immigrants with limited english proficiency. Emerg Med Int. 2011;2011:685249. doi: 10.1155/2011/685249
209. Meischke H, Taylor V, Calhoun R, Liu Q, Sos C, Tu SP, Yip MP, Eisenberg D. Preparedness for cardiac emergencies among Cambodians with limited English proficiency. J Community Health. 2012;37:176-180. doi: 10.1007/s10900-011-9433-z
210. Sasson C, Haukoos JS, Bond C, Rabe M, Colbert SH, King R, Sayre M, Heisler M. Barriers and facilitators to learning and performing cardiopulmonary resuscitation in neighborhoods with low bystander cardiopulmonary resuscitation prevalence and high rates of cardiac arrest in Columbus, OH. Circ Cardiovasc Qual Outcomes. 2013;6:550-558. doi: 10.1161/CIRCOUTCOMES.111.000097
211. Sasson C, Haukoos JS, Ben-Youssef L, Ramirez L, Bull S, Eigel B, Magid DJ, Padilla R. Barriers to calling 911 and learning and performing cardiopulmonary resuscitation for residents of primarily Latino, high-risk neighborhoods in Denver, Colorado. Ann Emerg Med. 2015;65:545-552. e2. doi: 10.1016/j.annemergmed.2014.10.028
212. Blewer AL, Ibrahim SA, Leary M, Dutwin D, McNally B, Anderson ML, Morrison LJ, Aufderheide TP, Daya M, Idris AH, et al. Cardiopulmonary resuscitation training disparities in the United States J Am Heart Assoc. 2017;6:e006124. doi: 10.1161/JAHA.117.006124
213. Abdulhay NM, Totolos K, McGovern S, Hewitt N, Bhardwaj A, Buckler DG, Leary M, Abella BS. Socioeconomic disparities in layperson CPR training within a large U.S. city. Resuscitation. 2019;141:13-18. doi: 10.1016/j.resuscitation.2019.05.038
214. Sasson C, Keirns CC, Smith DM, Sayre MR, Macy ML, Meurer WJ, McNally BF, Kellermann AL, Iwashyna TJ. Examining the contextual effects of neighborhood on out-of-hospital cardiac arrest and the provision of bystander cardiopulmonary resuscitation. Resuscitation. 2011;82:674-679. doi: 10.1016/j.resuscitation.2011.02.002
215. Root ED, Gonzales L, Persse DE, Hinchey PR, McNally B, Sasson C. A tale of two cities: the role of neighborhood socioeconomic status in spatial clustering of bystander CPR in Austin and Houston. Resuscitation. 2013;84:752-759. doi: 10.1016/j.resuscitation.2013.01.007
216. Becker TK, Gul SS, Cohen SA, Maciel CB, Baron-Lee J, Murphy TW, Youn TS, Tyndall JA, Gibbons C, Hart L, Alviar CL; Florida Cardiac Arrest Resource Team. Public perception towards bystander cardiopulmonary resuscitation. Emerg Med J. 2019;36:660-665. doi: 10.1136/emermed-2018-208234
217. Perman SM, Shelton SK, Knoepke C, Rappaport K, Matlock DD, Adelgais K, Havranek EP, Daugherty SL. Public Perceptions on Why Women Receive Less Bystander Cardiopulmonary Resuscitation Than Men in Out-of-Hospital Cardiac Arrest. Circulation. 2019;139:1060-1068. doi: 10.1161/CIRCULATIONAHA.118.037692
218. Blewer AL, McGovern SK, Schmicker RH, May S, Morrison LJ, Aufderheide TP, Daya M, Idris AH, Callaway CW, Kudenchuk PJ, Vilke GM, Abella BS; Resuscitation Outcomes Consortium (ROC) Investigators. Gender Disparities Among Adult Recipients of Bystander Cardiopulmonary Resuscitation in the Public. Circ Cardiovasc Qual Outcomes. 2018;11:e004710. doi: 10.1161/CIRCOUTCOMES.118.004710
219. Kramer CE, Wilkins MS, Davies JM, Caird JK, Hallihan GM. Does the sex of a simulated patient affect CPR? Resuscitation. 2015;86:82-87. doi: 10.1016/j.resuscitation.2014.10.016
220. Camp BN, Parish DC, Andrews RH. Effect of advanced cardiac life support training on resuscitation efforts and survival in a rural hospital. Ann Emerg Med. 1997;29:529-533. doi: 10.1016/s0196-0644(97)70228-2
221. Dane FC, Russell-Lindgren KS, Parish DC, Durham MD, Brown TD. In-hospital resuscitation: association between ACLS training and survival to discharge. Resuscitation. 2000;47:83-87. doi: 10.1016/s0300-9572(00)00210-0
222. Lowenstein SR, Sabyan EM, Lassen CF, Kern DC. Benefits of training physicians in advanced cardiac life support. Chest. 1986;89:512-516. doi: 10.1378/chest.89.4.512
223. Makker R, Gray-Siracusa K, Evers M. Evaluation of advanced cardiac life support in a community teaching hospital by use of actual cardiac arrests. Heart Lung. 1995;24:116-120. doi: 10.1016/s0147-9563(05)80005-6
224. Moretti MA, Cesar LA, Nusbacher A, Kern KB, Timerman S, Ramires JA. Advanced cardiac life support training improves long-term survival from in-hospital cardiac arrest. Resuscitation. 2007;72:458-465. doi: 10.1016/j.resuscitation.2006.06.039
225. Pottle A, Brant S. Does resuscitation training affect outcome from cardiac arrest? Accid Emerg Nurs. 2000;8:46-51. doi: 10.1054/aaen.1999.0089
226. Sanders AB, Berg RA, Burress M, Genova RT, Kern KB, Ewy GA. The efficacy of an ACLS training program for resuscitation from cardiac arrest in a rural community. Ann Emerg Med. 1994;23:56-59. doi: 10.1016/s0196-0644(94)70009-5
227. Sodhi K, Singla MK, Shrivastava A. Impact of advanced cardiac life support training program on the outcome of cardiopulmonary resuscitation in a tertiary care hospital. Indian J Crit Care Med. 2011;15:209-212. doi: 10.4103/0972-5229.92070
228. Lockey A, Lin Y, Cheng A. Impact of adult advanced cardiac life support course participation on patient outcomes-A systematic review and meta-analysis. Resuscitation. 2018;129:48-54. doi: 10.1016/j.resuscitation.2018.05.034
229. Girotra S, van Diepen S, Nallamothu BK, Carrel M, Vellano K, Anderson ML, McNally B, Abella BS, Sasson C, Chan PS; CARES Surveillance Group and the HeartRescue Project. Regional Variation in Out-of-Hospital Cardiac Arrest Survival in the United States. Circulation. 2016;133:2159-2168. doi: 10.1161/CIRCULATIONAHA.115.018175
230. Zijlstra JA, Stieglis R, Riedijk F, Smeekes M, van der Worp WE, Koster RW. Local lay rescuers with AEDs, alerted by text messages, contribute to early defibrillation in a Dutch out-of-hospital cardiac arrest dispatch system. Resuscitation. 2014;85:1444-1449. doi: 10.1016/j.resuscitation.2014.07.020
231. Berglund E, Claesson A, Nordberg P, Djärv T, Lundgren P, Folke F, Forsberg S, Riva G, Ringh M. A smartphone application for dispatch of lay responders to out-of-hospital cardiac arrests. Resuscitation. 2018;126:160-165. doi: 10.1016/j.resuscitation.2018.01.039
232. Fletcher KA, Bedwell WL. Cognitive aids: design suggestions for the medical field. Proc Int Symp Human Factors Ergonomics Health Care. 2014;3:148-152. doi: 10.1177/2327857914031024
233. Fitzgerald M, Cameron P, Mackenzie C, Farrow N, Scicluna P, Gocentas R, Bystrzycki A, Lee G, O'Reilly G, Andrianopoulos N, Dziukas L, Cooper DJ, Silvers A, Mori A, Murray A, Smith S, Xiao Y, Stub D, McDermott FT, Rosenfeld JV. Trauma resuscitation errors and computer-assisted decision support. Arch Surg. 2011;146:218-225. doi: 10.1001/archsurg.2010.333
234. Bernhard M, Becker TK, Nowe T, Mohorovicic M, Sikinger M, Brenner T, Richter GM, Radeleff B, Meeder PJ, Büchler MW, Böttiger BW, Martin E, Gries A. Introduction of a treatment algorithm can improve the early management of emergency patients in the resuscitation room. Resuscitation. 2007;73:362-373. doi: 10.1016/j.resuscitation.2006.09.014
235. Kelleher DC, Carter EA, Waterhouse LJ, Parsons SE, Fritzeen JL, Burd RS. Effect of a checklist on advanced trauma life support task performance during pediatric trauma resuscitation. Acad Emerg Med. 2014;21:1129-1134. doi: 10.1111/acem.12487
236. Lashoher A, Schneider EB, Juillard C, Stevens K, Colantuoni E, Berry WR, Bloem C, Chadbunchachai W, Dharap S, Dy SM, Dziekan G, Gruen RL, Henry JA, Huwer C, Joshipura M, Kelley E, Krug E, Kumar V, Kyamanywa P, Mefire AC, Musafir M, Nathens AB, Ngendahayo E, Nguyen TS, Roy N, Pronovost PJ, Khan IQ, Razzak JA, Rubiano AM, Turner JA, Varghese M, Zakirova R, Mock C. Implementation of the World Health Organization Trauma Care Checklist Program in 11 Centers Across Multiple Economic Strata: Effect on Care Process Measures. World J Surg. 2017;41:954-962. doi: 10.1007/s00268-016-3759-8

Circulation

第 2 章：エビデンス評価とガイドライン作成
『AHA 心肺蘇生と救急心血管治療のためのガイドライン2020』

要旨：『AHA 心肺蘇生と救急心血管治療のためのガイドライン2020』は，国際蘇生連絡委員会と連携して行った詳細なエビデンス評価に基づいている。成人一次救命処置と二次救命処置，小児一次救命処置と二次救命処置，新生児救命処置，蘇生教育科学，および治療システムの各執筆グループは，推奨事項を作成，レビュー，承認し，推奨事項のクラス（強度）とエビデンスレベル（質）をそれぞれの推奨事項に割り当てた。2020年版ガイドラインはいくつかの集約知識に整理され，具体的なトピックや管理問題に関する情報の個別モジュールに分類されている。2020年版ガイドラインは，そのトピックの専門家によるブラインドピアレビューを受けており，AHA Science Advisory and Coordinating Committee と AHA Executive Committee によるレビューと発行承認も得ている。AHA は利益相反に関する厳格な方針と手順により，ガイドラインの作成におけるバイアスのリスクや不適切な影響を最小限に抑えている。ガイドライン作成プロセスのいずれかの部分に関与した者は全員，商業的な関係およびそれ以外の潜在的利益相反について，すべて開示している。

David J. Magid, MD, MPH
Khalid Aziz, MBBS, MA, MEd（IT）
Adam Cheng, MD
Mary Fran Hazinski, RN, MSN
Amber V. Hoover, RN, MSN
Melissa Mahgoub, PhD
Ashish R. Panchal, MD, PhD
Comilla Sasson, MD, PhD
Alexis A. Topjian, MD, MSCE
Amber J. Rodriguez, PhD
Aaron Donoghue, MD, MSCE
Katherine M. Berg, MD
Henry C. Lee, MD
Tia T. Raymond, MD
Eric J. Lavonas, MD, MS

緒言

この章では，『AHA 心肺蘇生（CPR）と救急心血管治療（ECC）のためのガイドライン 2020』の作成プロセスについて説明する。エビデンス評価のプロセス，ガイドライン文書の形式，AHA 執筆グループの編成，ガイドラインの作成，レビュー，承認プロセス，および潜在的利益相反の管理について記載する。

方法論とエビデンスレビュー

2020年版ガイドラインは，CPR と ECC に関する指針を包括的かつ簡潔にまとめたものを提示する目的で作成された。成人一次救命処置と二次救命処置，小児一次救命処置と二次救命処置，新生児救命処置，蘇生教育科学，および治療システムに関するガイドラインは，国際蘇生連絡委員会（ILCOR）と連携して行った詳細なエビデンス評価に基づいているが，これについては『2020 International Consensus on CPR and ECC Science With Treatment Recommendations (CoSTR)』に詳述されている[1-7]。

AHA はエビデンスレビュープロセスにおいて，ILCOR タスクフォースおよび ILCOR 加盟団体と提携した。方法論の専門家で構成される ILCOR Scientific Advisory Committee により，エビデンス評価に対する方法論的ガバナンスのプロセスが作成された。『AHA 心肺蘇生と救急心血管治療のためのガイドラインアップデート 2015』は主にシステマティックレビューに頼っていたが，2020年版ガイドラインでは 3 タイプのエビデンスレビュー（システマティックレビュー，スコーピングレビュー，エビデンスアップデート）が使用された。このそれぞれがエビデンスとして記述

キーワード：AHA 科学的提言 ■ 心停止 ■ エビデンス評価 ■ 蘇生

© 2020 American Heart Association, Inc.

https://www.ahajournals.org/journal/circ

表1. 推奨事項の強度とエビデンス確実性評価の基準に関するGRADEの用語[34]

推奨事項の強度			
強い推奨 = AHAによる推奨		弱い推奨 = AHAによる提案	
効果の確実性に関する評価基準			
研究デザイン	効果の確実性（当初のレベル）	レベルを下げる要因	レベルを上げる要因
無作為化試験	高または中	バイアスのリスク	大きな効果
観察研究	低またはごく低い	非一貫性	用量反応性
		非直接性	すべての交絡因子が提示された効果を減少させる，あるいは，効果がないという結果が出た場合にスプリアス効果を示唆する
		不精確さ	
		出版バイアス	

GRADE：推奨判定，開発，評価の格付

され公表されたことにより，ガイドラインの作成が容易になった[4,8]。

システマティックレビュー

エビデンスレビューの第1タイプはシステマティックレビューである。これは，National Academy of Medicine の推奨事項に従い[9]，推奨判定，開発，評価の格付（Grading of Recommendations Assessment, Development and Evaluation, GRADE）ワーキンググループによって提案された方法論的アプローチを用いて行われた[10]。各 ILCOR タスクフォースは，対処すべき問題の特定と優先順位付けを，PICOST（population, intervention, comparator, outcome, study design, time frame，集団，介入，比較，転帰，研究デザイン，期間）フォーマットを用いて行い[11]，報告すべき重要な成果を決定した。関連文献の詳細な検索は，MEDLINE, Embase, Cochrane Library の各データベースで行い，特定された文献をふるい分けて詳細評価を行った。

システマティックレビューのレビューアー 2 人が，それぞれの関連研究についてバイアスリスクの評価を行った。その際，無作為化比較試験（RCT）にはコクランおよび GRADE の基準[12]，診断精度の研究には Quality Assessment of Diagnostic Accuracy Studies（QUADAS）-2 の基準[13]，治療や予後における問題を報告する観察研究や介入研究には GRADE の基準を用いた[10]。科学的バイアスの評価に加え，コクランのバイアスリスクツールでは，資金源と研究著者の潜在的利益相反についても考慮される。レビューアーは，すべての研究成果に関する情報を盛り込んだエビデンスプロファイルテーブルを作成した[14]。エビデンスの質（効果の推定に対する信頼度）は，研究の方法論と GRADE ドメイン（バイアス，非一貫性，非直接性，不精確さ，出版バイアス）[10]（表 1 および 2）に基づいて，高，中，低，非常に低い，に分類された[15]。レビューアーの評価の差を解消できなかったときは，Scientific Advisory Committee を代表するタスクフォースとの議論や合意形成により解消し，それでも意見が一致しない点は，より大きな ILCOR タスクフォースにより解消した。

ILCOR タスクフォースは研究およびシステマティックレビューによる分析をレビュー，議論，討議し，科学的提言に関する合意事項，および，それぞれの成果について特定されたエビデンスとエビデンスの質をまとめた文書について，草稿を作成した。合意が形成された場合は，合意による治療推奨事項をタスクフォースが作成した。推奨事項には「強」または「弱」の表示を行った。また推奨事項は，ある治療や予後予測ツール，診断的検査を推奨するか，それに反対するものとなるが，エビデンスの確実性にも言及した。さらに，各トピックの要約にはPICOST での問題点と，正当化およびエビデンスから決断を導き出すための枠組みを示すセクションが含まれており，タスクフォースが考慮した価値観や意向事項を記録するとともに，今後の課題のリストを示した。PICOST の作成やCoSTR 提言の草稿作成など，複数の段階で一般市民の意見を求めた[4]。CoSTR 提言を仕上げる際には，タスクフォースによりすべてのパブリックコメントが検討された。2020 年の CoSTR 提言はすべて，各トピックの専門家 5 人以上によるピアレビューを受け，ILCOR 理事会の承認を受けてから発行された。

スコーピングレビュー

エビデンスレビューの第 2 タイプはスコーピングレビューである。スコーピングレビューの目的は，具体的なトピックに関連する入手可能な研究エビデンスの概要を示し，システマティックレビューの成果を推奨できるだけの十分なエビデンスが特定されているかどうかを判断することである。スコーピングレビューとシステマティックレビューの違いの 1 つは，スコーピングレビューがより広範な選択基準を取るのに対し，従来のシステマティックレビューでは狭い，明確に定義された問題に対処するということである。システマティックレビューから治療推奨事項が作成されることがあるのに対し，スコーピングレビューから新たな ILCOR 治療推奨事項や，既存の ILCOR 治療推奨事項の変更が生じることはない。

スコーピングレビューの方法論は『Preferred Reporting Items for Systematic Reviews and Meta-analyses

表2. GRADE の用語 [34]

バイアスのリスク	無作為化試験における限界には，対象者割り付けが隠蔽されない，盲検化されていない，患者および転帰イベントの説明が不十分，選択的な転帰報告バイアス，および良い結果を得るための早期の試験停止などがある。観察研究における限界には，適切な適応条件が適用されない，曝露および転帰の測定における不備，交絡を十分制御できていない，不完全なフォローアップなどがある。
非一貫性	結果の非一貫性に関する基準には次のようなものがある：点推定が研究間で大きく異なる，CI のオーバーラップがほとんどまったく見られない，異質性の検定における P 値が低い，I^2 が大きい（研究間の差に起因する点推定のばらつきの尺度）。value; and the I^2 is large (a measure of variation in point estimates resulting from among-study differences).
非直接性	非直接性の原因には，対照集団が異なる研究からのデータ（IHCA でなく OHCA，小児でなく成人など），介入が異なる（圧迫・換気比が異なる等），転帰が異なる，間接的な比較などがある。
不精確さ	イベント発生率が低い場合やサンプルサイズが小さい場合は，一般的に CI が広がって不精確となる。
出版バイアス	出版バイアスの原因には，否定的な研究を発表したくないという傾向や，企業からの資金提供を受けた研究の影響などがある。ファンネルプロットが非対称の場合は，出版バイアスの疑いが強まる。
優れた取り組みに関する提言	ガイドラインパネルでは，研究エビデンスの正式なレビューに適さない特定のトピックに関するガイダンスの発行が必要と考えることがよくある。その理由は，トピックに関する研究が見つかりそうになかったり，そうした研究が非倫理的または実行不可能と考えられるためである。グレードを付与しない，優れた取り組みに関する提言の発行基準には，次のようなものがある：推奨されるガイダンスの利益が有害性を上回るという圧倒的な確実性があり，具体的な根拠が得られている，提言は特定の対象集団に対して明確で実用的なものでなければならない，ガイダンスが必要とみなされても，具体的に伝わるものでなければ一部のプロバイダーに見落とされる可能性がある，推奨事項はガイダンスの対象となる特定の対象者がすぐに実施できるものでなければならない。

GRADE：推奨判定，開発，評価の格付，IHCA：院内心停止，OHCA：院外心停止

『(PRISMA) Extension for Scoping Reviews』に基づくものとした [8,16,17]。各タスクフォースはレビューが必要な問題を特定し，PICOST フォーマットで示した。その後，MEDLINE，Embase，およびコクランのデータベースを検索し，関連文献を特定した。スコーピングレビューの実施者はデータを抽出し，サマリーテーブルを作成した。タスクフォースは次に，研究とエビデンステーブルをレビューし，合意によるエビデンスの要約と，タスクフォースの見識の概要を作成した。各トピックの要約とタスクフォースの見識の概要は，スコーピングレビュー一式とともに，一般市民によるレビューや意見を募るため ILCOR ウェブサイトに掲載された [4]。最終版は当該タスクフォースの CoSTR 発表論文の付録に収録され，その要約が本文に記載された。

エビデンスアップデート

エビデンスアップデートは，2020 年 CoSTR および 2020 年版ガイドラインを支える第 3 タイプのレビューである。このレビューは，システマティックレビューもスコーピングレビューも行われていない問題に使用される。エビデンスアップデートは，AHA 執筆グループのメンバー，AHA のボランティア，および ILCOR 加盟団体のボランティアによって実施された。エビデンスアップデートのレビューアーは PubMed を使用して，MEDLINE データベースにインデックスされている英語文献の検索を行った。過去のレビューにおける検索式が利用できる場合はそれを使用した。MEDLINE データベース以外の検索は任意とし，レビューアーの裁量に任せた。レビューアーは関連する新しい研究，ガイドライン，システマティックレビューを特定し，エビデンスアップデートワークシートへの記入を行った（研究課題，検索式，新しいエビデンスの要約表など）[8]。ILCOR Science Advisory Committee の委員長によるレビュー後，エビデンスアップデートワークシートは関連する 2020 年 CoSTR タスクフォース発行論文の付録に収録され，本文中でも引用された。

ガイドラインの形式

過去の ECC ガイドラインとは異なり，2020 年版ガイドラインはいくつかの集約知識に整理され，具体的なトピックや管理問題に関する情報の個別モジュールに分類されている [18]。それぞれのモジュールの集約知識には，推奨事項の表，簡単な紹介または概要，推奨事項の裏付けとなる解説，および必要に応じて，図，アルゴリズムのフローチャート，追加の表が含まれる。ハイパーリンクの付いた参考文献が示されており，迅速なアクセスとレビューがしやすくなっている。

AHA ガイドライン執筆グループの編成

ガイドラインの各執筆グループには必要な専門知識と多様性を持ったメンバーが含まれるよう AHA は尽力している。より広い範囲の医学会を代表するものとなるよう，さまざまな経歴，北米の地理的地域，性別，人種，民族，考え方，診療範囲から専門家を選んでいる。蘇生への関心および一般に認められた専門知識を持つボランティアを執筆グループの委員長が指名し，それを AHA ECC Committee が選定，AHA Manuscript Oversight Committee が承認する。「成人一次救命処置と二次救命処置」執筆グループには，救急医学，集中治療，心臓学，中毒学，神経学，救急医療サービス，教育，研究，公衆衛生の専門家が含まれる。「小児一次

表3. 患者ケアにおける臨床上の戦略，介入，治療，または診断検査への推奨事項のクラスとエビデンスレベルの適用（2019年5月更新）*

患者ケアにおける臨床上の戦略，介入，治療，または診断検査への推奨事項のクラスとエビデンスレベルの適用（2019年5月更新）*

推奨事項のクラス（強さ）

クラス1（強い） 利益＞＞＞リスク

推奨事項文に適した表現例：
- 推奨される
- 適応／有用／有効／有益である
- 実施／投与（など）すべきである
- 比較に基づく有効性の表現例†：
  – 治療Bよりも治療／治療戦略Aが推奨される／適応である
  – 治療Bよりも治療Aを選択すべきである

クラス2a（中等度） 利益＞＞リスク

推奨事項文に適した表現例：
- 妥当である
- 有用／有効／有益でありうる
- 比較に基づく有効性の表現例†：
  – 治療Bよりも治療／治療戦略Aがおそらく推奨される／適応である
  – 治療Bよりも治療Aを選択することが妥当である

クラス2b（弱い） 利益≧リスク

推奨事項文に適した表現例：
- 妥当としてよい／よいだろう
- 考慮してもよい／よいだろう
- 有用性／有効性が不明／不明確／不確実である、あるいは十分に確立されていない

クラス3：利益なし（中等度） 利益＝リスク
（一般にLOE AまたはBの使用に限る）

推奨事項文に適した表現例：
- 推奨しない
- 適応／有用／有効／有益ではない
- 実施／投与（など）すべきでない

クラス3：有害（強い） リスク＞利益

推奨事項文に適した表現例：
- 有害な可能性がある
- 有害となる
- 合併症発生率／死亡率の上昇を伴う
- 実施／投与（など）すべきでない

エビデンスレベル（質）‡

レベルA
- 複数のRCTから得られた質の高いエビデンス‡
- 質の高いRCTのメタアナリシス
- 質の高い症例登録試験によって裏付けられた1件以上のRCT

レベルB-R （無作為化）
- 1件以上のRCTから得られた質が中等度のエビデンス‡
- 質が中等度のRCTのメタアナリシス

レベルB-NR （非無作為化）
- 1件以上の綿密にデザインされ、適切に実施された非無作為化試験、観察研究、または症例登録試験から得られた質が中等度のエビデンス‡
- そのような試験のメタアナリシス

レベルC-LD （限定的なデータ）
- デザインまたは実施に限界がある無作為化または非無作為化観察研究または症例登録試験
- そのような試験のメタアナリシス
- ヒトを対象にした生理学的試験または反応機構研究

レベルC-EO （専門家の見解）
- 臨床経験に基づく専門家の見解のコンセンサス

CORおよびLOEは個別に決定する（CORとLOEのあらゆる組み合わせが可能）。

LOE Cの推奨事項は、その推奨事項が弱いことを意味するわけではない。ガイドラインが扱っている重要な医療上の問題の多くは、臨床試験の対象となっていない。RCTが行われていなくても、特定の検査あるいは治療法の有用性／有効性について、臨床上非常に明確なコンセンサスが得られている場合がある。

* 介入の成果または結果を記述すべきである（臨床転帰の改善、または診断精度の向上、または予後情報の増加）。

† 比較に基づく有効性の推奨事項（COR 1および2a、LOE AおよびBのみ）に関してその推奨事項の裏付けとなる試験は、評価する治療または治療戦略を直接比較しているものでなければならない。

‡ 標準化され、広く用いられていて、望ましくは検証されている複数のエビデンス評価ツールを活用する、システマティックレビューについてはエビデンスレビュー委員会を設けるなど、質を評価する方法は進化している。

COR：推奨事項のクラス（Class of Recommendation），EO：専門家の見解（expert opinion），LD：限定的なデータ（limited data），LOE：エビデンスレベル（Level of Evidence），NR：非無作為化（nonrandomized），R：無作為化（randomized），RCT：無作為化比較試験（randomized controlled trial）。

このツールは『ガイドラインアップデート2015』で最初に公表されてから、すべてのAHA ECCガイドラインと重点的アップデートで使用されている[35]。

救命処置と二次救命処置」執筆グループは、集中治療専門医、心臓集中治療専門医、心臓専門医、救急医および救急看護師を含む小児科医で構成される。「新生児救命処置」執筆グループには、臨床医学、教育、研究、公衆衛生で経験を積んだ新生児専門医と看護師が含まれる。「蘇生教育科学」執筆グループは、蘇生教育、臨床医学（小児、集中治療、救急医学）、看護学、プレホスピタルケア、医療サービスおよび教育研究の専門家で構成される。「治療システム」執筆グループには、臨床医学、教育、研究、公衆衛生の専門家が含まれる。任命される前に、執筆グループのメンバーは関連する産業との関係性の開示を完了した。また執筆グループのメンバーは、潜在的利益相反の管理に関するAHAの要求事項をすべて遵守した。

ガイドラインの作成、レビュー、承認

AHAの各執筆グループは、CPRとECCに関する最新のすべてのAHAガイドライン[19-30]、関連する2020年CoSTRのエビデンスと推奨事項[1-3,6,7]、および関連するすべてのエビデンスアップデートワークシートをレビューして、現在のガイドラインを再確認、修正、廃止すべきか、新たな推奨事項が必要かどうかを決定した。その後、

執筆グループは推奨事項を作成，レビュー，承認し，推奨事項のクラス（COR）（すなわち強度）とエビデンスレベル（LOE）（すなわち質）をそれぞれの推奨事項に割り当てた（表3）．2020年版ガイドラインの各記事は，AHAが指名したそのトピックの専門家5人によるブラインドピアレビューを受けた。任命される前に，ピアレビューのレビューアーは全員，産業との関係性およびそれ以外の潜在的な利益相反の開示を求められ，すべての開示内容をAHAスタッフがレビューした。ピアレビューのレビューアーによるフィードバックは草稿形式のガイドラインに対して行い，最終形式のガイドラインに対しても再度行った。ガイドラインはすべて，AHA Science Advisory and Coordinating Committee と AHA Executive Committee により，レビューおよび発行承認された。

潜在的利益相反の管理

AHAとILCORは利益相反に関する厳格な方針と手順により，CoSTRおよびAHAガイドラインの作成におけるバイアスのリスクや不適切な影響を最小限に抑えている。両組織とも，2020年のエビデンス評価および文書作成プロセス全体を通じてこれらの方針[31-33]に従い，このプロセスのいずれかの部分に関与した者は全員，商業的な関係およびそれ以外の（知的利益相反を含む）潜在的利益相反について，執筆グループ参加前と執筆グループ活動中の両時点において，すべて開示している。こうした開示のレビューは，タスクフォースの委員長とメンバー，執筆グループの委員長とメンバー，コンサルタント，ピアレビューのレビューアーを任命する前に行った。AHAの利益相反方針に沿う形で，ILCORおよびAHAの各執筆グループの委員長と大半のメンバーには，関連する利益相反がないことが求められた。執筆グループのメンバーは，関連する利益相反のある推奨事項に対しては原稿作成や投票を行っていない。付録1に，執筆グループメンバーの開示情報を記載する。ピアレビューのレビューアーも，産業との関係性およびそれ以外の潜在的な利益相反の開示を求められた。これらの開示については付録2に記載する。

文献情報

アメリカ心臓協会（AHA）は，本書を以下のとおり引用するよう要請する：Magid DJ, Aziz K, Cheng A, Hazinski MF, Hoover AV, Mahgoub M, Panchal AR, Sasson C, Topjian AA, Rodriguez AJ, Donoghue A, Berg KM, Lee HC, Raymond T, Lavonas EJ. Part 2: evidence evaluation and guidelines development: 2020 American Heart Association Guidelines for Cardiopulmonary Resuscitation and Emergency Cardiovascular Care. Circulation. 2020;142(suppl 2):S358–S365. doi: 10.1161/CIR.0000000000000898

情報開示

付録1. 執筆グループの情報開示

執筆グループメンバー	所属	研究助成金	その他の研究支援	講演／謝礼金	鑑定人	株式所有	コンサルタント／顧問	その他
David J. Magid	University of Colorado	NIH†；NHLBI†；CMS†；AHA†	なし	なし	なし	なし	なし	アメリカ心臓協会（American Heart Association, AHA）（上級科学編集者）†
Khalid Aziz	University of Alberta Pediatrics	なし	なし	なし	なし	なし	なし	給与：University of Alberta†
Katherine M. Berg	Beth Israel Deaconess Medical Center Pulmonary and Critical Care	NHLBI Grant K23 HL128814†	なし	なし	なし	なし	なし	なし
Adam Cheng	Alberta Children's Hospital（Canada）	なし	なし	なし	なし	なし	なし	なし
Aaron Donoghue	The Children's Hospital of Philadelphia, University of Pennsylvania School of Medicine	なし	なし	なし	Atkinson, Haskins, Nellis, Brittingham, Gladd & Fiasco*	なし	なし	なし
Mary Fran Hazinski	Vanderbilt University School of Nursing	なし	なし	なし	なし	なし	アメリカ心臓協会（American Heart Association†, AHA）	なし
Amber V. Hoover	American Heart Association	なし	なし	なし	なし	なし	なし	なし

（続く）

付録 1. （続き）

執筆グループメンバー	所属	研究助成金	その他の研究支援	講演／謝礼金	鑑定人	株式所有	コンサルタント／顧問	その他
Eric J. Lavonas	Denver Health Emergency Medicine	BTG Pharmaceuticals（Denver Health（Dr Lavonas の雇用主）は，研究，コールセンター，コンサルティング，教育に関する協定を BTG Pharmaceuticals と締結している。BTG はジゴキシン解毒剤の DigiFab を製造している。Dr Lavonas はボーナスや奨励給を受領しておらず，これらの協定は関連のない製品も含まれる。このガイドラインの作成にあたり，ジゴキシン中毒に関する議論に Dr Lavonas は関与していない。）†	なし	なし	なし	なし	なし	アメリカ心臓協会（American Heart Association, AHA）（上級科学編集者）†
Henry C. Lee	Stanford University	NICHD（R01 グラント（妊娠期間のごく早期に生まれた乳児に対する集中治療の調査）の研究主宰者）*	なし	なし	なし	なし	なし	なし
Melissa Mahgoub	American Heart Association	なし	なし	なし	なし	なし	なし	なし
Ashish R. Panchal	The Ohio State University Wexner Medical Center Emergency Medicine	なし	なし	なし	なし	なし	なし	なし
Tia T. Raymond	Medical City Children's Hospital Congenital Heart Surgery Unit	なし	なし	なし	なし	なし	なし	なし
Amber J. Rodriguez	American Heart Association National Center Emergency Cardiovascular Care	なし	なし	なし	なし	なし	なし	なし
Comilla Sasson	American Heart Association	なし	なし	なし	なし	なし	なし	なし
Alexis A. Topjian	The Children's Hospital of Philadelphia, University of Pennsylvania School of Medicine Anesthesia and Critical Care	なし	なし	なし	なし	なし	なし	なし

　この表は，執筆グループの全メンバーに回答および提出が求められる情報開示アンケート（Disclosure Questionnaire）の結果に基づき実在の利益相反または合理的に認定できる利益相反とみなされる可能性のある，執筆グループメンバーの関係を示している。メンバーと該当団体との関係が「重大」であると考えられるのは，次のいずれかの状況が存在する場合である。（a）当該メンバーが団体から受領する金額が過去いずれの 12 か月間に $10,000 以上であるか，メンバーの総収入の 5 ％以上である。（b）団体の議決権株式の 5 ％以上，またはその団体の公正市場価値の $10,000 以上を保有している。この定義において「重大」に相当するレベルに満たない場合，その関係は「軽度」とみなされる。
　*軽度
　†重大

付録 2. レビューアーの情報開示

レビューアー	所属	研究助成金	その他の研究支援	講演／謝礼金	鑑定人	株式所有	コンサルタント／顧問	その他
Fredrik Folke	Gentofte University Hospital (Denmark)	なし	なし	なし	なし	なし	なし	なし
Joel Lexchin	University Health Network, Toronto (Canada)	なし	なし	なし	なし	なし	なし	なし
Robert T. Mallet	University North Texas Health Science Center	なし	なし	なし	なし	なし	アメリカ心臓協会（American Heart Association, AHA）（蘇生研究を支援する助成金への応募を審査する研究セクションでの業務）*	なし
Mary Ann McNeil	University of Minnesota	なし	なし	なし	なし	なし	なし	なし
Taylor Sawyer	Seattle Children's Hospital/University of Washington	なし	なし	なし	なし	なし	なし	なし
Will Smith	Wilderness and Emergency Medicine Consulting (WEMC)	なし	なし	なし	なし	なし	なし	なし
Lorrel E. B. Toft	University of Nevada Reno	なし	なし	なし	なし	なし	なし	なし

この表は、執筆グループの全メンバーに回答および提出が求められる情報開示アンケート（Disclosure Questionnaire）の結果に基づき実在の利益相反または合理的に認定できる利益相反とみなされる可能性のある、執筆グループメンバーの関係を示している。メンバーと該当団体との関係が「顕著」であると考えられるのは、次のいずれかの状況が存在する場合である。（a）当該メンバーが団体から受領する金額が過去いずれの 12 か月間に $10,000 以上であるか、メンバーの総収入の 5％以上である、（b）団体の議決権株式の 5％以上、またはその団体の公正市場価値の $10,000 以上を保有している。この定義において「重大」に相当するレベルに満たない場合、その関係は「軽度」とみなされる。

*軽度
†重大

参考資料

1. Berg KM, Soar J, Andersen LW, Böttiger BW, Cacciola S, Callaway CW, Couper K, Cronberg T, D'Arrigo S, Deakin CD, et al; on behalf of the Adult Advanced Life Support Collaborators. Adult advanced life support: 2020 International Consensus on Cardiopulmonary Resuscitation and Emergency Cardiovascular Care Science With Treatment Recommendations. Circulation. 2020;142 (suppl 1):S92-S139. doi: 10.1161/CIR.0000000000000893
2. Greif R, Bhanji F, Bigham BL, Bray J, Breckwoldt J, Cheng A, Duff JP, Gilfoyle E, Hsieh M-J, Iwami T, et al; on behalf of the Education, Implementation, and Teams Collaborators. Education, implementation, and teams: 2020 International Consensus on Cardiopulmonary Resuscitation and Emergency Cardiovascular Care Science With Treatment Recommendations. Circulation. 2020;142 (suppl 1):S222-S283. doi: 10.1161/CIR.0000000000000896
3. Maconochie IK, Aickin R, Hazinski MF, Atkins DL, Bingham R, Couto TB, Guerguerian A-M, Nadkarni VM, Ng K-C, Nuthall GA, et al; on behalf of the Pediatric Life Support Collaborators. Pediatric life support: 2020 International Consensus on Cardiopulmonary Resuscitation and Emergency Cardiovascular Care Science With Treatment Recommendations Circulation. 2020;142 (suppl 1):S140-S184. doi: 10.1161/CIR.0000000000000894
4. Morley PT, Atkins DL, Finn JC, Maconochie I, Nolan JP, Rabi Y, Singletary EM, Wang TL, Welsford M, Olasveengen TM, et al. Evidence evaluation process and management of potential conflicts of interest: 2020 International Consensus on Cardiopulmonary Resuscitation and Emergency Cardiovascular Care Science With Treatment Recommendations. Circulation. 2020;142 (suppl 1):S28-S40. doi: 10.1161/CIR.0000000000000891
5. Nolan JP, Maconochie I, Soar J, Olasveengen TM, Greif R, Wyckoff MH, Singletary EM, Aickin R, Berg KM, Mancini ME, et al. Executive summary: 2020 International Consensus on Cardiopulmonary Resuscitation and Emergency Cardiovascular Care Science With Treatment Recommendations. Circulation. 2020;142 (suppl 1):S2-S27. doi: 10.1161/CIR.0000000000000890
6. Olasveengen TM, Mancini ME, Perkins GD, Avis S, Brooks S, Castrén M, Chung SP, Considine J, Couper K, Escalante R, et al; on behalf of the Adult Basic Life Support Collaborators. Adult basic life support: 2020 International Consensus on Cardiopulmonary Resuscitation and Emergency Cardiovascular Care Science With Treatment Recommendations. Circulation. 2020;142 (suppl 1):S41-S91. doi: 10.1161/CIR.0000000000000892
7. Wyckoff MH, Wyllie J, Aziz K, de Almeida MF, Fabres J, Fawke J, Guinsburg R, Hosono S, Isayama T, Kapadia VS, et al; on behalf of the Neonatal Life Support Collaborators. Neonatal life support: 2020 International Consensus on Cardiopulmonary Resuscitation and Emergency Cardiovascular Care Science With Treatment Recommendations. Circulation. 2020;142 (suppl 1):S185-S221. doi: 10.1161/CIR.0000000000000895
8. International Liaison Committee on Resuscitation. Continuous evidence evaluation guidance and templates. https://www.ilcor.org/documents/continuous-evidence-evaluation-guidance-and-templates. Accessed December 31, 2019.
9. Institute of Medicine (US) Committee of Standards for Systematic Reviews of Comparative Effectiveness Research. Finding What Works in Health Care: Standards for Systematic Reviews. Washington, DC: The National Academies Press; 2011.
10. GRADE Working Group. 5.2.1. Study limitations (risk of bias). In: Schünemann HJ, Brożek J, Guyatt G, Oxman A., eds. GRADE Handbook. 2013. https://gdt.gradepro.org/app/handbook/handbook.html. Accessed December 31, 2019.
11. Cochrane Training. Chapter 5: defining the review questions and developing criteria for including studies. In: O'Connor D, Higgins J, Green S, eds. Cochrane Handbook for Systematic Reviews of Interventions. Version 5.1.0. 2011. https://handbook-5-1.cochrane.org/chapter_5/5_defining_the_review_question_and_developing_criteria_for.htm. Accessed December 31, 2019.
12. Cochrane Training. Chapter 8: assessing risk of bias in included studies. In: Higgins JPT, Altman DG, Sterne J, eds. Cochrane Handbook for Systematic Reviews of Interventions. Version 5.1.0. 2011. https://handbook-5-1.cochrane.org/chapter_8/8_assessing_risk_of_bias_in_included_studies.htm. Accessed December 31, 2019.
13. Whiting PF, Rutjes AW, Westwood ME, Mallett S, Deeks JJ, Reitsma JB, Leeflang MM, Sterne JA, Bossuyt PM; QUADAS-2 Group. QUADAS-2: a revised tool for the quality assessment of diagnostic accuracy studies. Ann Intern Med. 2011;155:529-536. doi: 10.7326/0003-4819-155-8-201110180-00009
14. Evidence Prime. GRADEpro GDT—an introduction to the system. https://gdt.gradepro.org/app/help/user_guide/index.html. Accessed December 31, 2019.
15. Schünemann HJ, Oxman AD, Brozek J, Glasziou P, Jaeschke R, Vist GE, Williams JW Jr, Kunz R, Craig J, Montori VM, Bossuyt P, Guyatt GH; GRADE Working Group. Grading quality of evidence and

15. strength of recommendations for diagnostic tests and strategies. BMJ. 2008;336:1106-1110. doi: 10.1136/bmj.39500.677199.AE
16. Tricco AC, Lillie E, Zarin W, O'Brien KK, Colquhoun H, Levac D, Moher D, Peters MDJ, Horsley T, Weeks L, Hempel S, Akl EA, Chang C, McGowan J, Stewart L, Hartling L, Aldcroft A, Wilson MG, Garritty C, Lewin S, Godfrey CM, Macdonald MT, Langlois EV, Soares-Weiser K, Moriarty J, Clifford T, Tunçalp Ö, Straus SE. PRISMA extension for scoping reviews (PRISMA-ScR): checklist and explanation. Ann Intern Med. 2018;169:467-473. doi: 10.7326/M18-0850
17. PRISMA. PRISMA for scoping reviews. http://www.prisma-statement.org/Extensions/ScopingReviews. Accessed December 31, 2019.
18. Levine GN, O'Gara PT, Beckman JA, Al-Khatib SM, Birtcher KK, Cigarroa JE, de Las Fuentes L, Deswal A, Fleisher LA, Gentile F, Goldberger ZD, Hlatky MA, Joglar JA, Piano MR, Wijeysundera DN. Recent innovations, modifications, and evolution of ACC/AHA clinical practice guidelines: an update for our constituencies: a report of the American College of Cardiology/American Heart Association Task Force on Clinical Practice Guidelines. Circulation. 2019;139:e879-e886. doi: 10.1161/CIR.0000000000000651
19. Field JM, Hazinski MF, Sayre MR, Chameides L, Schexnayder SM, Hemphill R, Samson RA, Kattwinkel J, Berg RA, Bhanji F, et al. Part 1: executive summary: 2010 American Heart Association Guidelines for Cardiopulmonary Resuscitation and Emergency Cardiovascular Care. Circulation. 2010;122 (suppl 3):S640-S656. doi: 10.1161/CIRCULATIONAHA.110.970889
20. Neumar RW, Shuster M, Callaway CW, Gent LM, Atkins DL, Bhanji F, Brooks SC, de Caen AR, Donnino MW, Ferrer JM, et al. Part 1: executive summary: 2015 American Heart Association Guidelines Update for Cardiopulmonary Resuscitation and Emergency Cardiovascular Care. Circulation. 2015;132 (suppl 2):S315-S367. doi: 10.1161/CIR.0000000000000252
21. Kleinman ME, Goldberger ZD, Rea T, Swor RA, Bobrow BJ, Brennan EE, Terry M, Hemphill R, Gazmuri RJ, Hazinski MF, Travers AH. 2017 American Heart Association focused update on adult basic life support and cardiopulmonary resuscitation quality: an update to the American Heart Association Guidelines for Cardiopulmonary Resuscitation and Emergency Cardiovascular Care. Circulation. 2018;137:e7-e13. doi: 10.1161/CIR.0000000000000539
22. Escobedo MB, Aziz K, Kapadia VS, Lee HC, Niermeyer S, Schmölzer GM, Szyld E, Weiner GM, Wyckoff MH, Yamada NK, Zaichkin JG. 2019 American Heart Association focused update on neonatal resuscitation: an update to the American Heart Association Guidelines for Cardiopulmonary Resuscitation and Emergency Cardiovascular Care. Circulation. 2019;140:e922-e930. doi: 10.1161/CIR.0000000000000729
23. Panchal AR, Berg KM, Cabañas JG, Kurz MC, Link MS, Del Rios M, Hirsch KG, Chan PS, Hazinski MF, Morley PT, Donnino MW, Kudenchuk PJ. 2019 American Heart Association focused update on systems of care: dispatcher-assisted cardiopulmonary resuscitation and cardiac arrest centers: an update to the American Heart Association Guidelines for Cardiopulmonary Resuscitation and Emergency Cardiovascular Care. Circulation. 2019;140:e895-e903. doi: 10.1161/CIR.0000000000000733
24. Panchal AR, Berg KM, Hirsch KG, Kudenchuk PJ, Del Rios M, Cabañas JG, Link MS, Kurz MC, Chan PS, Morley PT, et al. 2019 American Heart Association focused update on advanced cardiovascular life support: use of advanced airways, vasopressors, and extracorporeal cardiopulmonary resuscitation during cardiac arrest: an update to the American Heart Association guidelines for cardiopulmonary resuscitation and emergency cardiovascular care. Circulation. 2019;140:e881-e894. doi: 10.1161/CIR.0000000000000732
25. Panchal AR, Berg KM, Kudenchuk PJ, Del Rios M, Hirsch KG, Link MS, Kurz MC, Chan PS, Cabañas JG, Morley PT, Hazinski MF, Donnino MW. 2018 American Heart Association focused update on advanced cardiovascular life support use of antiarrhythmic drugs during and immediately after cardiac arrest: an update to the American Heart Association Guidelines for Cardiopulmonary Resuscitation and Emergency Cardiovascular Care. Circulation. 2018;138:e740-e749. doi: 10.1161/CIR.0000000000000613
26. Atkins DL, de Caen AR, Berger S, Samson RA, Schexnayder SM, Joyner BL Jr, Bigham BL, Niles DE, Duff JP, Hunt EA, Meaney PA. 2017 American Heart Association focused update on pediatric basic life support and cardiopulmonary resuscitation quality: an update to the American Heart Association Guidelines for Cardiopulmonary Resuscitation and Emergency Cardiovascular Care. Circulation. 2018;137:e1-e6. doi: 10.1161/CIR.0000000000000540
27. Charlton NP, Pellegrino JL, Kule A, Slater TM, Epstein JL, Flores GE, Goolsby CA, Orkin AM, Singletary EM, Swain JM. 2019 American Heart Association and American Red Cross focused update for first aid: presyncope: an update to the American Heart Association and American Red Cross Guidelines for First Aid. Circulation. 2019;140:e931-e938. doi: 10.1161/CIR.0000000000000730
28. Duff JP, Topjian A, Berg MD, Chan M, Haskell SE, Joyner BL Jr, Lasa JJ, Ley SJ, Raymond TT, Sutton RM, Hazinski MF, Atkins DL. 2018 American Heart Association focused update on pediatric advanced life support: an update to the American Heart Association Guidelines for Cardiopulmonary Resuscitation and Emergency Cardiovascular Care. Circulation. 2018;138:e731-e739. doi: 10.1161/CIR.0000000000000612
29. Duff JP, Topjian AA, Berg MD, Chan M, Haskell SE, Joyner BL Jr, Lasa JJ, Ley SJ, Raymond TT, Sutton RM, Hazinski MF, Atkins DL. 2019 American Heart Association focused update on pediatric advanced life support: an update to the American Heart Association Guidelines for Cardiopulmonary Resuscitation and Emergency Cardiovascular Care. Circulation. 2019;140:e904-e914. doi: 10.1161/CIR.0000000000000731
30. Duff JP, Topjian AA, Berg MD, Chan M, Haskell SE, Joyner BL Jr, Lasa JJ, Ley SJ, Raymond TT, Sutton RM, et al. 2019 American Heart Association focused update on pediatric basic life support: an update to the American Heart Association guidelines for cardiopulmonary resuscitation and emergency cardiovascular care. Circulation. 2019;140:e915-e921. doi: 10.1161/CIR.0000000000000736
31. American Heart Association. Conflict of interest policy. https://www.heart.org/en/about-us/statements-and-policies/conflict-of-interest-policy. Accessed December 31, 2019.
32. American Heart Association. MOC policies and procedures regarding relationships with industry for writing group members. https://professional.heart.org/idc/groups/ahamah-public/@wcm/@sop/@spub/documents/downloadable/ucm_495614.pdf. Accessed April 30, 2020.
33. American College of Cardiology Foundation, American Heart Association. Methodology manual and policies from the ACCF/AHA task force on practice guidelines. 2010. https://professional.heart.org/idc/groups/ahamah-public/@wcm/@sop/documents/downloadable/ucm_319826.pdf. Accessed April 30, 2020.
34. Soar J, Maconochie I, Wyckoff MH, Olasveengen TM, Singletary EM, Greif R, Aickin R, Bhanji F, Donnino MW, Mancini ME, Wyllie JP, Zideman D, Andersen LW, Atkins DL, Aziz K, Bendall J, Berg KM, Berry DC, Bigham BL, Bingham R, Couto TB, Böttiger BW, Borra V, Bray JE, Breckwoldt J, Brooks SC, Buick J, Callaway CW, Carlson JN, Cassan P, Castrén M, Chang WT, Charlton NP, Cheng A, Chung SP, Considine J, Couper K, Dainty KN, Dawson JA, de Almeida MF, de Caen AR, Deakin CD, Drennan IR, Duff JP, Epstein JL, Escalante R, Gazmuri RJ, Gilfoyle E, Granfeldt A, Guerguerian AM, Guinsburg R, Hatanaka T, Holmberg MJ, Hood N, Hosono S, Hsieh MJ, Isayama T, Iwami T, Jensen JL, Kapadia V, Kim HS, Kleinman ME, Kudenchuk PJ, Lang E, Lavonas E, Liley H, Lim SH, Lockey A, Lofgren B, Ma MH, Markenson D, Meaney PA, Meyran D, Mildenhall L, Monsieurs KG, Montgomery W, Morley PT, Morrison LJ, Nadkarni VM, Nation K, Neumar RW, Ng KC, Nicholson T, Nikolaou N, Nishiyama C, Nuthall G, Ohshimo S, Okamoto D, O'Neil B, Yong-Kwang Ong G, Paiva EF, Parr M, Pellegrino JL, Perkins GD, Perlman J, Rabi Y, Reis A, Reynolds JC, Ristagno G, Roehr CC, Sakamoto T, Sandroni C, Schexnayder SM, Scholefield BR, Shimizu N, Skrifvars MB, Smyth MA, Stanton D, Swain J, Szyld E, Tijssen J, Travers A, Trevisanuto D, Vaillancourt C, Van de Voorde P, Velaphi S, Wang TL, Weiner G, Welsford M, Woodin JA, Yeung J, Nolan JP, Hazinski MF. 2019 International Consensus on Cardiopulmonary Resuscitation and Emergency Cardiovascular Care Science With Treatment Recommendations: summary from the Basic Life Support; Advanced Life Support; Pediatric Life Support; Neonatal Life Support; Education, Implementation, and Teams; and First Aid Task Forces. Circulation. 2019;140:e826-e880. doi: 10.1161/CIR.0000000000000734
35. Morrison LJ, Gent LM, Lang E, Nunnally ME, Parker MJ, Callaway CW, Nadkarni VM, Fernandez AR, Billi JE, Egan JR, et al. Part 2: evidence evaluation and management of conflicts of interest: 2015 American Heart Association Guidelines Update for Cardiopulmonary Resuscitation and Emergency Cardiovascular Care. Circulation. 2015;132(suppl 2):S368-S382. doi: 10.1161/CIR.0000000000000253

Circulation

第3章：成人一次救命処置と二次救命処置
AHA 心肺蘇生と救急心血管治療のためのガイドライン 2020

Ashish R. Panchal, MD, PhD, Chair
Jason A. Bartos, MD, PhD
José G. Cabañas, MD, MPH
Michael W. Donnino, MD
Ian R. Drennan, ACP, PhD (C)
Karen G. Hirsch, MD
Peter J. Kudenchuk, MD
Michael C. Kurz, MD, MS
Eric J. Lavonas, MD, MS
Peter T. Morley, MBBS
Brian J. O'Neil, MD
Mary Ann Peberdy, MD
Jon C. Rittenberger, MD, MS
Amber J. Rodriguez, PhD
Kelly N. Sawyer, MD, MS
Katherine M. Berg, MD, Vice Chair
On behalf of the Adult Basic and Advanced Life Support Writing Group

成人の救命処置について覚えておくべき 10 のポイント

1. 市民救助者は，心停止イベントを認識すると同時に迅速に救急対応システムに通報し，心肺蘇生（CPR）を開始する必要がある。
2. 質の高い CPR の実施には，適切な深さとテンポの胸骨圧迫を行いながら，圧迫の中断を最小限にすることが含まれる。
3. 突然の心停止が心室細動または無脈性心室頻拍によって引き起こされる場合，早期除細動と同時に質の高い CPR を行うことが生存に不可欠である。
4. アドレナリン投与と同時に質の高い CPR を行うと，特にショック非適応リズム患者の生存率が向上する。
5. すべての心停止イベントが同一ではないことを認識することは，最適な患者転帰にとって重要であり，多くの状態（電解質異常，妊娠，心臓手術後など）には専門的治療が必要とされる。
6. オピオイドの流行で，オピオイド関連の院外心停止が増加しているが，ケアの中心は救急対応システムへの通報と質の高い CPR の実施であることに変わりはない。
7. 心拍再開後の治療は救命の連鎖の重要な要素であり，最適な患者転帰のためには，包括的，体系的，かつ複数の専門分野にわたるシステムが一貫した方法で実施される必要がある。
8. 最適な機能的および神経学的転帰を確実にするため，自己心拍再開後に指示に従わないすべての患者には，目標体温管理を迅速に開始する必要がある。
9. 脳損傷のある心停止生存者では，回復の可能性が高い患者が治療の中止により不良転帰に陥らないようにするため，正確な神経学的予後予測が非常に重要である。
10. 心停止生存者とその介護者に対して，治療，監視，およびリハビリテーションについて説明した回復生存者への計画を退院時に提供し，自宅および外来への治療の転換を最適化する必要がある。

前文

2015 年，米国で救急医療サービス（EMS）要員により対応された，非外傷性の院外心停止（OHCA）を経験した成人は，約 350,000 人にのぼった[1]。OHCA 患者のうち，初回入院で生存した割合は約 10.4 %，良好な機能状態で生存した割合は 8.2 %であった。OHCA からの蘇生を成功させる主な要因は，市民救助者による心肺蘇生（CPR）と，自動体外式除細動器（AED）の公共利用である。最近は増加しているが，市民救助者による CPR を受けた成人は 39.2 %のみで，一般市民が AED を使用した事例はわずか 11.9 %である[1]。OHCA からの生存率は，米国の各地

キーワード： AHA 科学的ステートメント ■ 無呼吸 ■ 心肺蘇生 ■ 除細動器 ■ 医療の提供 ■ 電気ショック ■ 心停止 ■ 救命処置

© 2020 American Heart Association, Inc.

https://www.ahajournals.org/journal/circ

域と EMS 機関では大きく異なる[2,3]。有意な改善後は，2012 年以降 OHCA からの生存率は横ばい状態である。

米国の病院に収容された成人の約 1.2 %は，院内心停止（IHCA）を起こしている[1]。これらの患者のうち，生存して退院した割合は 25.8 %，退院時に良好な機能状態を呈した割合は生存者の 82 %であった。IHCA からの生存率は着実に向上しているが，改善の余地はまだ多く残っている。

国際蘇生連絡委員会（ILCOR）の生存のための方程式では，良好な蘇生転帰のための 3 つの重要な要素（健全な蘇生科学に基づくガイドライン，市民救助者と蘇生プロバイダーの効果的な教育，適切に機能する救命の連鎖の実施）を重視している[4]。

これらのガイドラインは，利用可能な最良の蘇生科学に基づいており，成人患者のための一次救命処置（BLS）と二次救命処置（ALS）の推奨事項が記載されている。「主要な概念」で紹介した救命の連鎖が，ここでは心停止からの回復中の生存の重要な要素を強調するために拡張されており，さまざまな分野の医療専門家による連携した取り組み，OHCA の場合は市民救助者，救急指令者，および第 1 救助者による連携した取り組みが必要となる。また，蘇生プロバイダーのトレーニングに関する具体的な推奨事項は「第 6 章：蘇生教育科学」，治療システムに関する推奨事項は「第 7 章：治療システム」に記載されている。

緒言
ガイドラインの範囲

これらのガイドラインは主に，成人の BLS と ALS の最新の概要を探している北米の医療従事者，および蘇生科学と現在の知識不足に関するより詳細な情報を求めている人々を対象としている。青少年の BLS は成人のガイドラインに従う。『アメリカ心臓協会（AHA）心肺蘇生と救急心血管治療のためのガイドライン 2020』のこの章には，心停止中の成人（心停止が迫っている生命を脅かす状態にある成人を含む）と，心停止からの蘇生が成功した後の成人の臨床ケアに関する推奨事項が記載されている。

推奨事項の中には，CPR トレーニングを受けている市民救助者や，受けていない市民救助者，さらに蘇生装置をほとんどまたはまったく利用できない市民救助者に直接関連したものもあれば，より高度な蘇生トレーニングを受けていて，蘇生薬や蘇生装置へのアクセスの有無にかかわらず実施でき，病院内または病院外で働く人に関連したものもある。一部の治療の推奨事項には，自己心拍再開（ROSC）後，または蘇生が失敗した場合の医療と意思決定が含まれている。重要なことは，将来の蘇生の成功率を高めるために，チームのデブリーフィングと体系的なフィードバックに関連する推奨事項が提供されていることである。

執筆グループの組織

成人の救命処置執筆グループには，救急医療，救命医療，心臓病学，毒物学，神経学，EMS，教育，研究，公衆衛生の経歴を持つ多様な専門家グループと，コンテンツ専門家，AHA スタッフ，AHA 上級科学編集者が含まれていた。各推奨事項は，執筆グループによって作成され，正式に承認された。

AHA には，ガイドライン作成における偏見や不適切な影響のリスクを最小限に抑えるための厳格な利益相反方針と手順がある。執筆グループのメンバーは，任命の前にすべての利害関係とその他の考えうる（知的を含む）利益相反を明らかにした。これらの手順の詳細については「第 2 章：エビデンス評価とガイドライン作成」に記載されている。執筆グループのメンバーの公開情報は，付録 1 に記載する。

方法論とエビデンスレビュー

これらのガイドラインは，ILCOR および関連する ILCOR メンバー評議会と連携して実施された広範なエビデンス評価に基づいている。2020 年のプロセスでは，3 種類のエビデンスレビュー（システマティックレビュー，スコーピングレビュー，エビデンスアップデート）が使用された。これらが個々に文献の説明となり，ガイドライン作成に役立った。これらの方法に関するより包括的な説明は，「第 2 章：エビデンス評価とガイドライン作成」に記載されている。

推奨事項のクラスとエビデンスレベル

すべての AHA ガイドラインと同様に，2020 年の各推奨事項には，エビデンスの強さと一貫性，代替治療オプション，および患者と社会への影響に基づいて，推奨事項のクラス（COR）が割り当てられている（表 1）。エビデンスレベル（LOE）は，利用可能なエビデンスの質，量，関連性，一貫性に基づいている。執筆グループは推奨事項ごとに，特定の推奨事項の文言と COR および LOE の割り当てについて協議し，承認した。COR を決定する際に，執筆グループは LOE と，システムの問題，経済的要因，および公平性，受容性，実現可能性などの倫理的要因を含むその他の要因を考慮した。COR と LOE の決定に使用される特定の基準を含む，これらのエビデンスレビュー方法の詳細については，「第 2 章：エビデンス評価とガイドライン作成」に記載されている。成人一次救命処置と二次救命処置執筆グループのメンバーは，これらの推奨事項に対する最終的な権限を持ち，正式に承認した。

表1. 患者ケアにおける臨床上の戦略，介入，治療，または診断検査への推奨事項のクラスとエビデンスレベルの適用（2019年5月更新）

推奨事項のクラス（強さ）	エビデンスレベル（質）‡
クラス1（強い） 利益＞＞＞リスク 推奨事項文に適した表現例： • 推奨される • 適応／有用／有効／有益である • 実施／投与（など）すべきである • 比較に基づく有効性の表現例†： 　－ 治療Bよりも治療／治療戦略Aが推奨される／適応である 　－ 治療Bよりも治療Aを選択すべきである	**レベルA** • 複数のRCTから得られた質の高いエビデンス‡ • 質の高いRCTのメタアナリシス • 質の高い症例登録試験によって裏付けられた1件以上のRCT
クラス2a（中等度） 利益＞＞リスク 推奨事項文に適した表現例： • 妥当である • 有用／有効／有益でありうる • 比較に基づく有効性の表現例†： 　－ 治療Bよりも治療／治療戦略Aがおそらく推奨される／適応である 　－ 治療Bよりも治療Aを選択することが妥当である	**レベルB-R** （無作為化） • 1件以上のRCTから得られた質が中等度のエビデンス‡ • 質が中等度のRCTのメタアナリシス
クラス2b（弱い） 利益≧リスク 推奨事項文に適した表現例： • 妥当としてよい／よいだろう • 考慮してもよい／よいだろう • 有用性／有効性は不明／不明確／不確実である，あるいは十分に確立されていない	**レベルB-NR** （非無作為化） • 1件以上の綿密にデザインされ，適切に実施された非無作為化試験，観察研究，または症例登録試験から得られた質が中等度のエビデンス‡ • そのような試験のメタアナリシス
クラス3：利益なし（中等度） 利益＝リスク （一般にLOE AまたはBの使用に限る） 推奨事項文に適した表現例： • 推奨しない • 適応／有用／有効／有益ではない • 実施／投与（など）すべきでない	**レベルC-LD** （限定的なデータ） • デザインまたは実施に限界がある無作為化または非無作為化観察研究または症例登録試験 • そのような試験のメタアナリシス • ヒトを対象にした生理学的試験または反応機構研究
クラス3：有害（強い） リスク＞利益 推奨事項文に適した表現例： • 有害な可能性がある • 有害となる • 合併症発生率／死亡率の上昇を伴う • 実施／投与（など）すべきでない	**レベルC-EO** （専門家の見解） • 臨床経験に基づく専門家の見解のコンセンサス

CORおよびLOEは個別に決定する（CORとLOEのあらゆる組み合わせが可能）。

LOE Cの推奨事項は，その推奨事項が弱いことを意味するわけではない。ガイドラインが扱っている重要な医療上の問題の多くは，臨床試験の対象となっていない。RCTが行われていなくても，特定の検査あるいは治療法の有用性／有効性について，臨床上非常に明確なコンセンサスが得られている場合がある。

* 介入の成果または結果を記述すべきである（臨床転帰の改善，または診断精度の向上，または予後情報の増加）。

† 比較に基づく有効性の推奨事項（COR 1および2a，LOE AおよびBのみ）に関してその推奨事項の裏付けとなる試験は，評価する治療または治療戦略を直接比較しているものでなければならない。

‡ 標準化され，広く用いられていて，望ましくは検証されている複数のエビデンス評価ツールを活用する，システマティックレビューについてはエビデンスレビュー委員会を設けるなど，質を評価する方法は進化している。

COR：推奨事項のクラス（Class of Recommendation），EO：専門家の見解（expert opinion），LD：限定的なデータ（limited data），LOE：エビデンスレベル（Level of Evidence），NR：非無作為化（nonrandomized），R：無作為化（randomized），RCT：無作為化比較試験（randomized controlled trial）。

残念ながら，蘇生研究のデザインと資金援助が改善しているにもかかわらず，蘇生科学のエビデンスベースの全体的な確実性は低い。これらのガイドラインに記載されている250の推奨事項のうち，レベルAのエビデンス（複数の無作為化比較試験［RCT］から得られた質の高いエビデンス，または質の高い症例登録試験によって裏付けられた1件以上のRCT）によって裏付けられる推奨事項は2つのみである。レベルBの無作為化エビデンス（1件以上のRCTから得られた中等度のエビデンス）によって裏付けられる推奨事項は37，レベルBの非無作為化エビデンスによって裏付けられる推奨事項は57である。推奨事項の大部分はレベルCのエビデンスに基づいており，限られたデータに基づいているものが123，専門家の意見に基づいているものが31である。その結果，推奨事項の強さは最適よりも弱い。これらのガイドラインには，78のクラス1（強い）推奨事項，57のクラス2a（中等度）推奨事項，89のクラス2b（弱い）推奨事項が含まれている。さらに，15の推奨事項がクラス3：利益なし，11の推奨事項がクラス3：有害に指定されている。蘇生の臨床試験が切に必要とされている。

ガイドラインの構成

2020年版の各ガイドラインは知識チャンク（大きな塊）に分けられ，特定のトピックまたは管理の問題に関する個別の情報モジュールにグループ化されている。[5] 各モジュール型知識チャンク（大きな塊）には，CORとLOEについてAHAの標準的な用語を使用した推奨事項の表が含まれている。簡単な緒言または短い概要は，推奨事項を重要な背景情報や包括的な管理または治療の概念と関連付けて説明するために記載している。推奨事項の解説では，推奨事項を裏付ける理論的根拠と主要な研究データを明確にしている。必要に応じて，フローチャートまたは追加の表を含めた。簡単に参照して確認できるように，ハイパーリンクされた参照資料も記載している。

文書のレビューと承認

各『ガイドライン2020』文書は，匿名の査読のために，AHAが指名した5名の対象分野の専門家に提出した。すべての査読者は，任命の前に業界との関係と利益相反を明らかにし，その内容をAHAのスタッフがレビューした。査読者からのフィードバックは，草稿形式のガイドラインと最終形式のガイドラインで提供された。すべてのガイドラインは，AHA Science Advisory and Coordinating Committee および AHA Executive Committee がレビューし，公開を承認した。査読者の公開情報は，付録2に記載する。

参考資料

1. Virani SS, Alonso A, Benjamin EJ, Bittencourt MS, Callaway CW, Carson AP, Chamberlain AM, Chang AR, Cheng S, Delling FN, et al: on behalf of the American Heart Association Council on Epidemiology and Prevention Statistics Committee and Stroke Statistics Subcommittee.Heart disease and stroke statistics—2020 update: a report from the American Heart Association.Circulation.2020;141:e139-e596. doi: 10.1161/CIR.0000000000000757
2. Okubo M, Schmicker RH, Wallace DJ, Idris AH, Nichol G, Austin MA, Grunau B, Wittwer LK, Richmond N, Morrison LJ, Kurz MC, Cheskes S, Kudenchuk PJ, Zive DM, Aufderheide TP, Wang HE, Herren H, Vaillancourt C, Davis DP, Vilke GM, Scheuermeyer FX, Weisfeldt ML, Elmer J, Colella R, Callaway CW; Resuscitation Outcomes Consortium Investigators. Variation in Survival After Out-of-Hospital Cardiac Arrest Between Emergency Medical Services Agencies.JAMA Cardiol.2018;3:989-999. doi: 10.1001/jamacardio.2018.3037
3. Zive DM, Schmicker R, Daya M, Kudenchuk P, Nichol G, Rittenberger JC, Aufderheide T, Vilke GM, Christenson J, Buick JE, Kaila K, May S, Rea T, Morrison LJ; ROC Investigators.Survival and variability over time from out of hospital cardiac arrest across large geographically diverse communities participating in the Resuscitation Outcomes Consortium.Resuscitation.2018;131:74-82. doi: 10.1016/j.resuscitation.2018.07.023
4. Søreide E, Morrison L, Hillman K, Monsieurs K, Sunde K, Zideman D, Eisenberg M, Sterz F, Nadkarni VM, Soar J, Nolan JP; Utstein Formula for Survival Collaborators.The formula for survival in resuscitation.Resuscitation.2013;84:1487-1493. doi: 10.1016/j.resuscitation.2013.07.020
5. Levine GN, O'Gara PT, Beckman JA, Al-Khatib SM, Birtcher KK, Cigarroa JE, de Las Fuentes L, Deswal A, Fleisher LA, Gentile F, Goldberger ZD, Hlatky MA, Joglar JA, Piano MR, Wijeysundera DN. Recent Innovations, Modifications, and Evolution of ACC/AHA Clinical Practice Guidelines: An Update for Our Constituencies: A Report of the American College of Cardiology/American Heart Association Task Force on Clinical Practice Guidelines.Circulation.2019;139:e879-e886. doi: 10.1161/CIR.0000000000000651

略語

ACD	能動圧迫-減圧（active compression-decompression）
ACLS	二次救命処置（advanced cardiovascular life support）
ADC	見かけ上の拡散係数（apparent diffusion coefficient）
AED	自動体外式除細動器（automated external defibrillator）
AHA	アメリカ心臓協会（American Heart Association）
ALS	二次救命処置（advanced life support）
aOR	調節後のオッズ比（adjusted odds ratio）
AV	房室（atrioventricular）
BLS	一次救命処置（basic life support）
COR	推奨事項のクラス（Class of Recommendation）
CoSTR	International Consensus on Cardiopulmonary Resuscitation and Emergency Cardiovascular Care Science With Treatment Recommendations
CPR	心肺蘇生（cardiopulmonary resuscitation）
CT	コンピュータ断層撮影（computed tomography）
DWI	拡散強調画像（diffusion-weighted imaging）
ECG	心電図（electrocardiogram）
ECPR	体外循環補助を用いた心肺蘇生（extracorporeal cardiopulmonary resuscitation）
EEG	脳波図（electroencephalogram）
EMS	救急医療サービス（emergency medical services）
$ETCO_2$	呼気終末二酸化炭素（分圧）（end-tidal carbon dioxide）
ETI	気管挿管（endotracheal intubation）
GWR	灰白質／白質比（gray-white ratio）
ICU	集中治療室（intensive care unit）
IHCA	院内心停止（in-hospital cardiac arrest）
ILCOR	国際蘇生連絡委員会（International Liaison Committee on Resuscitation）
IO	骨内（intraosseous）
ITD	インピーダンス閾値器具（impedance threshold device）
IV	静脈内（intravenous）
LAST	局所麻酔薬全身毒性（local anesthetic systemic toxicity）
LOE	エビデンスレベル（Level of Evidence）
MAP	平均動脈圧（mean arterial pressure）
MRI	磁気共鳴画像法（magnetic resonance imaging）
NSE	ニューロン特異的エノラーゼ（neuron-specific enolase）
OHCA	院外心停止（out-of-hospital cardiac arrest）
$Paco_2$	動脈血二酸化炭素分圧（arterial partial pressure of carbon dioxide）
PCI	経皮的冠動脈インターベンション（percutaneous coronary intervention）
PE	肺塞栓症（pulmonary embolism）
PMCD	死戦期帝王切開（perimortem cesarean delivery）
無脈性VT	無脈性心室頻拍（pulseless ventricular tachycardia）
RCT	無作為化比較試験（randomized controlled trial）
ROSC	自己心拍再開（return of spontaneous circulation）
S100B	S100カルシウム結合タンパク質（S100 calcium binding protein）
SGA	声門上気道（supraglottic airway）

（続く）

SSEP	体性感覚誘発電位	(somatosensory evoked potential)
STEMI	ST上昇型心筋梗塞	(ST-segment elevation myocardial infarction)
SVT	上室性頻拍	(supraventricular tachycardia)
TCA	三環系抗うつ薬	(tricyclic antidepressant)
TOR	蘇生終了	(termination of resuscitation)
TTM	目標体温管理	(targeted temperature management)
VF	心室細動	(ventricular fibrillation)
VT	心室頻拍	(ventricular tachycardia)

主要な概念

成人の心停止の概念の概要

成人の心停止からの生存と回復は，複雑なシステムが連携して機能し，傷病者にとって最良の転帰を確保できるかどうかで決まる。成人の心停止イベントの主な焦点には，迅速な認識，CPRの迅速な実施，ショック適応の悪性リズムの除細動，およびROSC後の支持療法と基礎原因の治療が含まれる。このアプローチでは，成人のほとんどの突然の心停止が心臓を原因としており，特に心筋梗塞と電気障害によるものであることを認識している。だが主要な原因が心臓でない心停止（例えば，呼吸不全，中毒物質の摂取，肺塞栓症［PE］，溺死）も多く認められ，そのような場合，救助者が可逆的な基礎原因の治療を検討することが重要である[1]。非心原性病因の中には，特に院内でよく見られるものがある。オピオイド過量投与などの他の非心原性病因は，院外で急増している[2]。心停止の場合，救助者は通報し，CPRを実施して冠状動脈と脳の血流を回復し，心室細動（VF）または心室頻拍（VT）が存在する場合はAEDを使用して直接治療するように指示される。蘇生の成功の大部分は，質の高いCPRと除細動の実施によって達成されるが，考えうる基礎原因に対する特定の治療が役立つ場合もある。

成人の救命の連鎖

プロバイダーの心停止管理の主な焦点は，転帰を改善するために必要なすべての重要手順を最適化することである。これには，救急対応システムへの通報，質の高いCPRと早期除細動の実施，ALS介入，慎重な予後予測を含むROSC後の効果的な処置，回復中および生存中の補助が含まれる。これらの活動はすべて，それぞれの生存を可能にする教育，トレーニング，機器，消耗品，およびコミュニケーションをサポートする組織的インフラストラクチャを必要とする。したがって，こうしたケアの多様な側面それぞれが，心停止傷病者の最終的な機能的生存に寄与することを認識している。

蘇生の原因，プロセス，および転帰は，OHCAとIHCAで大きく異なり，それぞれの救命の連鎖に反映されている（図1）。OHCAでは，傷病者のケアは地域の関与と対応に依存している。地域住民は，心停止を認識して119番（または緊急対応番号）に通報し，CPR（トレーニングを受けていない市民救助者が実施する胸骨圧迫

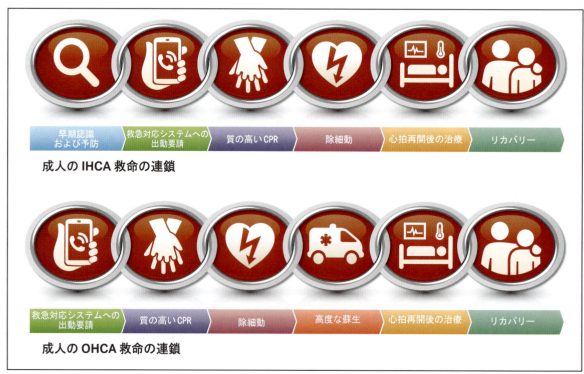

図1. 2020年アメリカ心臓協会IHCAおよびOHCAに対する救命の連鎖。
CPR：心肺蘇生（cardiopulmonary resuscitation），IHCA：院内心停止（in-hospital cardiac arrest），OHCA：院外心停止（out-of-hospital cardiac arrest）。

のみのCPRを含む）を実施して，AEDを使用することが重要である[3,4]。その後，救急医療要員が現場に呼ばれ，蘇生を継続し，安定化と根本的治療のために患者を搬送する。一方，IHCAの重要な側面は監視と予防である。病院で心停止が発生した場合には，複数の専門分野にわたる強力なアプローチが存在し，これには医療専門家チームによる対応，CPRの実施，迅速な除細動，ALS処置の開始，ROSC後のケアの継続が含まれる。IHCAの転帰は，OHCAの転帰より全体的に優れている[5]。その理由は，効果的な蘇生開始の遅れが短いためだと考えられる。

　成人のOHCAとIHCAの救命の連鎖は，治療システムの進化と回復および生存の重要な役割を強調するように更新され，新しい鎖が追加されている。この「リカバリー」の鎖は，心停止後の生存者と家族の両方にとっての，重症疾患の急性期治療の終了から複数のリハビリテーション（短期および長期の両方）にいたる長期に及ぶ回復と生存の道のりを強調している。この新しい鎖は，心停止の生存者とその介護者がケアを病院から自宅に移行して，役割と社会的機能に戻る際に，回復をサポートし，期待について話し合い，治療，監視，およびリハビリテーションに対処する計画を提供するための治療システムが必要であることを認めている。

参考資料

1. Lavonas EJ, Drennan IR, Gabrielli A, Heffner AC, Hoyte CO, Orkin AM, Sawyer KN, Donnino MW. Part 10: special circumstances of resuscitation: 2015 American Heart Association Guidelines Update for Cardiopulmonary Resuscitation and Emergency Cardiovascular Care. Circulation. 2015;132(suppl 2):S501–S518. doi: 10.1161/CIR.0000000000000264
2. Dezfulian C, Orkin AM, Maron BA, Elmer J, Girota S, Gladwin MT, Merchant RM, Panchal AR, Perman SM, Starks M, van Diepen S, Lavonas EJ; on behalf of the American Heart Association Council on Cardiopulmonary, Critical Care, Perioperative and Resuscitation; Council on Arteriosclerosis, Thrombosis and Vascular Biology; Council on Cardiovascular and Stroke Nursing; and Council on Clinical Cardiology. Opioid-associated out-of-hospital cardiac arrest: distinctive clinical features and implications for healthcare and public responses: a scientific statement from the American Heart Association. Circulation. In press.
3. Sayre MR, Berg RA, Cave DM, Page RL, Potts J, White RD; American Heart Association Emergency Cardiovascular Care Committee. Hands-only (compression-only) cardiopulmonary resuscitation: a call to action for bystander response to adults who experience out-of-hospital sudden cardiac arrest: a science advisory for the public from the American Heart Association Emergency Cardiovascular Care Committee. Circulation. 2008;117:2162–2167. doi: 10.1161/CIRCULATIONAHA.107.189380
4. Kleinman ME, Brennan EE, Goldberger ZD, Swor RA, Terry M, Bobrow BJ, Gazmuri RJ, Travers AH, Rea T. Part 5: adult basic life support and cardiopulmonary resuscitation quality: 2015 American Heart Association Guidelines Update for Cardiopulmonary Resuscitation and Emergency Cardiovascular Care. Circulation. 2015;132(suppl 2):S414–S435. doi: 10.1161/CIR.0000000000000259
5. Virani SS, Alonso A, Benjamin EJ, Bittencourt MS, Callaway CW, Carson AP, Chamberlain AM, Chang AR, Cheng S, Delling FN, et al; on behalf of the American Heart Association Council on Epidemiology and Prevention Statistics Committee and Stroke Statistics Subcommittee. Heart disease and stroke statistics—2020 update: a report from the American Heart Association. Circulation. 2020;141:e139–e596. doi: 10.1161/CIR.0000000000000757

蘇生の手順
心停止の認識

心停止の認識に関する推奨事項		
COR	LOE	推奨事項
1	C-LD	1. 傷病者が意識消失／無反応で，無呼吸または異常な呼吸（死戦期呼吸のみ）の場合，市民救助者はその傷病者が心停止状態とみなすべきである。
1	C-LD	2. 傷病者が意識消失／無反応で，無呼吸または異常な呼吸（死戦期呼吸のみ）の場合，医療従事者は10秒以内に脈拍を確認する必要がある。はっきりした脈拍を触知できない場合，その傷病者が心停止状態とみなすべきである。

「概要」

市民救助者によるCPRで，心停止からの生存率が2～3倍向上する[1]。心停止した患者にCPRを実施することの利点は，意識はないが心停止を起こしていない人に胸骨圧迫を実施する潜在的なリスクを上回る。こうした患者ではCPRによる負傷のリスクは低いことが示されている[2]。

　脈拍の検出はすべての救助者にとって難しいものであり，そのためCPRが遅延したり，場合によっては心停止した患者に対してCPRがまったく実行されない可能性があることがこれまでに示されている[3]。したがって，市民救助者による心停止の認識は，傷病者の意識レベルと呼吸努力に基づいて行われる。医療従事者による心停止の認識には脈拍チェックが含まれるが，脈拍の検出努力を長引かせないことの重要性が強調されている。

「推奨事項の裏付けとなる解説」

1. 死戦期呼吸は，ゆっくりかつ不規則で，換気を行っても効果がないあえぎ呼吸を特徴とする。市民救助者が死戦期呼吸を説明する用語はさまざまで，「異常な呼吸」，「いびき呼吸」，「あえぎ呼吸」などが使用される[4]。死戦期呼吸は頻繁に見られ，OHCAの傷病者の最大40％から60％で認められると報告されている[5]。市民救助者が患者を心停止していないと誤診する一般的な理由として，死戦期呼吸の存在が挙げられている[6]。患者の反応がなく，呼吸をしていない，あるいは呼吸が異常な場合，市民救助者は患者が心停止を起こしていると想定し，通報して直ちにCPRを開始する必要がある。これらの2つの基準（患者の反応と呼吸の評価）により，心停止を起こした患者のかなりの割合を迅速に特定でき，市民救助者はCPRを即座に開始できることが示されている。さらに，意識はないが心停止していない患者で胸骨圧迫を開始した場合に重大な有害事象が発生する割合は低い[2]。有害事象としては，胸骨圧迫の領

域の痛み（8.7％），骨折（肋骨および鎖骨）（1.7％），横紋筋融解（0.3％）などが認められたが，内臓損傷は報告されていない[2]。
2. 蘇生努力の開始時や，連続で行うCPRサイクルの合間に脈拍をチェックする際，CPRの遅延が長引く可能性がある。医療従事者は脈拍チェックに手間取ったり[7,8]脈拍があるかどうかの判断に苦労したりすることがある[7-9]。ただし，循環の検知方法として呼吸や咳，または体動のチェックのほうが脈拍チェックより優れているとするエビデンスはない[10]。したがって，医療従事者は脈拍をすばやくチェックし，はっきりとした脈拍が触知できない場合は胸骨圧迫を開始するように指示されている[9,11]。

このトピックは，直近で2010年に正式なエビデンスレビューを受けている[3]。

参考資料

1. Sasson C, Rogers MA, Dahl J, Kellermann AL.Predictors of survival from out-of-hospital cardiac arrest: a systematic review and meta-analysis. Circ Cardiovasc Qual Outcomes.2010;3:63-81. doi: 10.1161/CIRCOUTCOMES.109.889576
2. Olasveengen TM, Mancini ME, Perkins GD, Avis S, Brooks S, Castrén M, Chung SP, Considine J, Couper K, Escalante R, et al; on behalf of the Adult Basic Life Support Collaborators.Adult basic life support: 2020 International Consensus on Cardiopulmonary Resuscitation and Emergency Cardiovascular Care Science With Treatment Recommendations.Circulation.2020;142 (suppl 1):S41-S91. doi: 10.1161/CIR.0000000000000892
3. Berg RA, Hemphill R, Abella BS, Aufderheide TP, Cave DM, Hazinski MF, Lerner EB, Rea TD, Sayre MR, Swor RA.Part 5: adult basic life support: 2010 American Heart Association Guidelines for Cardiopulmonary Resuscitation and Emergency Cardiovascular Care.Circulation.2010;122 (suppl 3):S685-S705. doi: 10.1161/CIRCULATIONAHA.110.970939
4. Riou M, Ball S, Williams TA, Whiteside A, Cameron P, Fatovich DM, Perkins GD, Smith K, Bray J, Inoue M, O'Halloran KL, Bailey P, Brink D, Finn J. 'She's sort of breathing': What linguistic factors determine call-taker recognition of agonal breathing in emergency calls for cardiac arrest? Resuscitation.2018;122:92-98. doi: 10.1016/j.resuscitation.2017.11.058
5. Fukushima H, Imanishi M, Iwami T, Seki T, Kawai Y, Norimoto K, Urisono Y, Hata M, Nishio K, Saeki K, Kurumatani N, Okuchi K. Abnormal breathing of sudden cardiac arrest victims described by laypersons and its association with emergency medical service dispatcher-assisted cardiopulmonary resuscitation instruction.Emerg Med J. 2015;32:314-317. doi: 10.1136/emermed-2013-203112
6. Brinkrolf P, Metelmann B, Scharte C, Zarbock A, Hahnenkamp K, Bohn A. Bystander-witnessed cardiac arrest is associated with reported agonal breathing and leads to less frequent bystander CPR.Resuscitation.2018;127:114-118. doi: 10.1016/j.resuscitation.2018.04.017
7. Eberle B, Dick WF, Schneider T, Wisser G, Doetsch S, Tzanova I. Checking the carotid pulse check: diagnostic accuracy of first responders in patients with and without a pulse.Resuscitation.1996;33:107-116. doi: 10.1016/s0300-9572(96)01016-7
8. Moule P. Checking the carotid pulse: diagnostic accuracy in students of the healthcare professions.Resuscitation.2000;44:195-201. doi: 10.1016/s0300-9572(00)00139-8
9. Ochoa FJ, Ramalle-Gómara E, Carpintero JM, García A, Saralegui I. Competence of health professionals to check the carotid pulse.Resuscitation.1998;37:173-175. doi: 10.1016/s0300-9572(98)00055-0
10. Perkins GD, Stephenson B, Hulme J, Monsieurs KG.Birmingham assessment of breathing study (BABS).Resuscitation.2005;64:109-113. doi: 10.1016/j.resuscitation.2004.09.007
11. Mather C, O'Kelly S. The palpation of pulses.Anaesthesia. 1996;51:189-191. doi: 10.1111/j.1365-2044.1996.tb07713.x

蘇生の開始

蘇生の開始に関する 推奨事項：市民救助者（訓練を受けていない，または訓練を受けている）		
COR	LOE	推奨事項
1	B-NR	1. 訓練を受けた市民救助者は，最低限の処置として，心停止傷病者に対して胸骨圧迫を行う必要がある。
1	C-LD	2. 救助者が1人の場合は，心停止を特定したら最初に救急対応システムに出動を要請し，ただちにCPRを開始する必要がある。
1	C-LD	3. 患者が心停止していない場合でも患者に危害が及ぶリスクは低いため，心停止が疑われるときは市民救助者がCPRを開始することが推奨される。
2a	C-LD	4. 胸骨圧迫と換気（人工呼吸）によるCPRの訓練を受けた市民救助者の場合，成人のOHCAに対して胸骨圧迫に加えて換気（人工呼吸）を行うことは妥当である。

「概要」

心停止が認識された後，救命の連鎖は救急対応システムへの出動要請とCPRの開始を継続する。CPRの迅速な開始は，おそらく生存と神経学的転帰を改善するための最も重要な介入である。救急対応システムへの出動要請とCPRの開始を同時に実行することが理想である。モバイルデバイスの使用が普及し，アクセスのしやすさが向上している現代では，救助者が1人でも，通報して電話をスピーカーモードにしたまま通話を継続し，ただちにCPRを開始することで，救急対応システムへの出動要請とCPRの開始を同時に実行できる。1人のみの救助者がEMSに通報するために傷病者から離れなければならないというまれな状況では，優先されるのは迅速なEMSへの出動要請で，その後すぐに傷病者の元に戻ってCPRを開始する必要がある。

既存のエビデンスでは，心停止を起こしていると誤って特定された患者へのCPRが有害となる可能性は低いことを示唆している[1]。全体的に見て，心停止に対してCPRを開始する有益性は，心停止していない患者が負傷する比較的低いリスクを上回る。心停止が認識された後の蘇生の最初の処置は，市民救助者と医療従事者で類似しており，早期のCPRが優先される。市民救助者は，プロセスを簡素化してCPRの開始を促進するために，胸骨圧迫のみのCPRを実施する場合がある一方で，医療従事者は胸骨圧迫と換気を実施する場合がある（図2-4）。

「推奨事項の裏付けとなる解説」

1. CPRは心停止の患者にとって最も重要な介入であり，胸骨圧迫は迅速に実施すべきである。胸骨圧迫はCPRの最も重要な要素であるため，市民救助者が人工呼吸を実施する訓練を受けていない，または実施を躊躇する場合は，胸骨圧迫のみのアプローチが

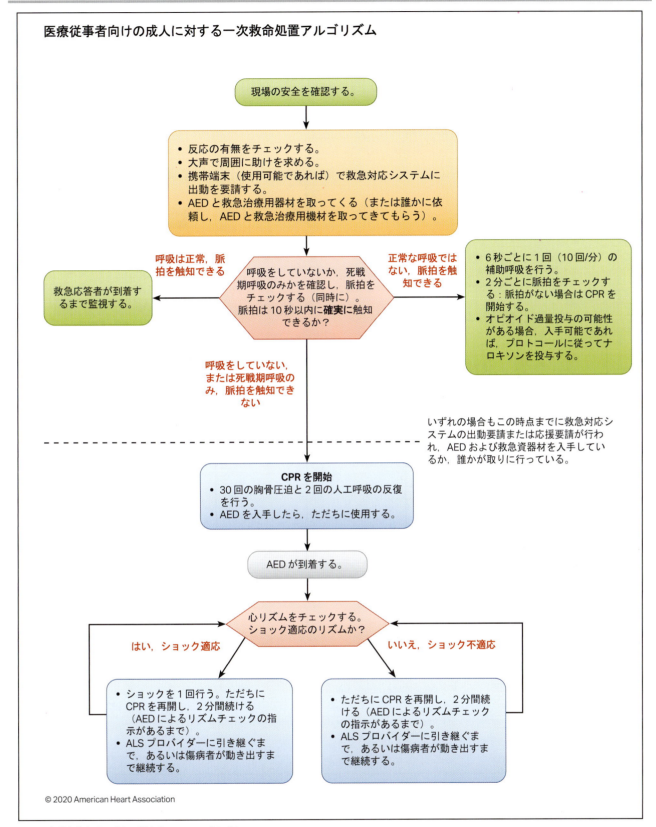

図 2. 医療従事者向けの成人に対する BLS アルゴリズム。
AED：自動体外式除細動器（automated external defibrillator），ALS：二次救命処置（advanced life support），BLS：一次救命処置（basic life support），CPR：心肺蘇生（cardiopulmonary resuscitation）。

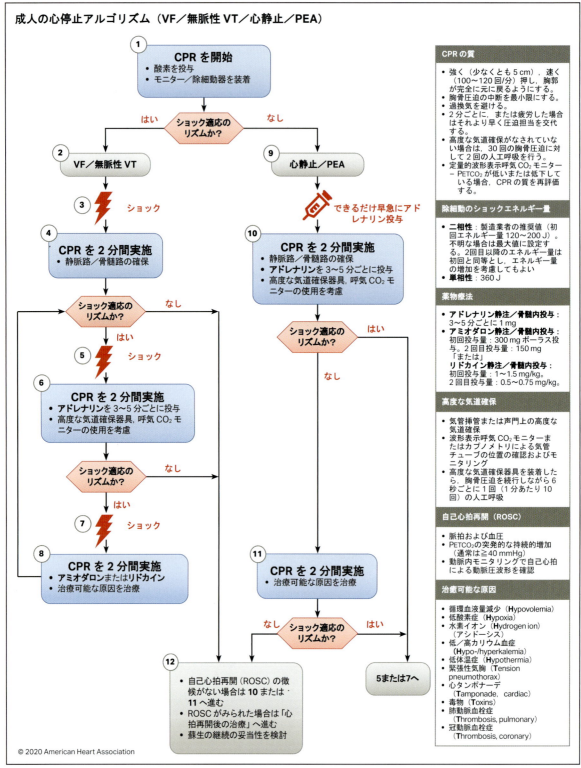

図3. 成人の心停止アルゴリズム。
CPR：心肺蘇生（cardiopulmonary resuscitation），PEA：無脈性電気活動（pulseless electrical activity），無脈性VT：無脈性心室頻拍（pulseless ventricular tachycardia），VF：心室細動（ventricular fibrillation）。

成人の心停止循環アルゴリズム

CPRを開始
- 酸素を投与
- モニター／除細動器を装着

心リズムのチェック — VF／pVTの場合ショック — **自己心拍再開（ROSC）** → 心拍再開後の治療

2分ごとに：
- CPRを続行する
- CPRの質をモニタリングする

薬物療法
静脈路／骨髄路の確保
アドレナリンを3〜5分ごとに反復投与
治療抵抗性VF／pVTの場合はアミオダロンまたはリドカインを投与

高度な気道確保器具を考慮
定量的波形表示呼気CO₂モニター

治療可能な原因を治療

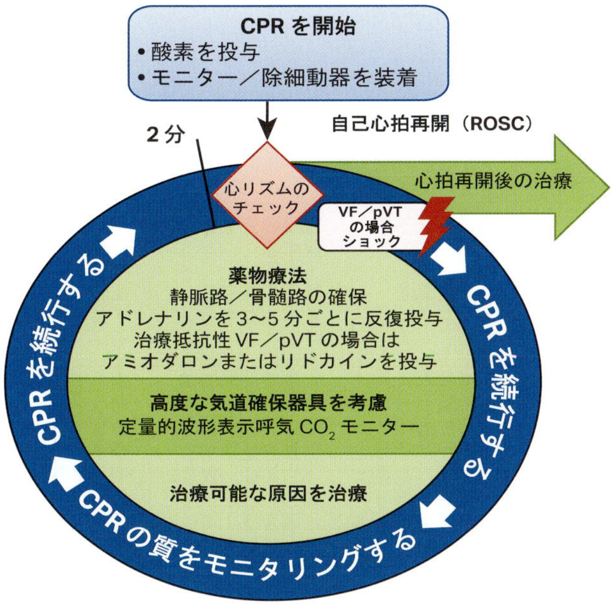

CPRの質
- 強く（≧5 cm）、速く（100〜120回/分）押し、胸郭が完全に元に戻るようにする。
- 胸骨圧迫の中断を最小限にする。
- 過換気を避ける。
- 2分ごとに、または疲労した場合はそれより早く胸骨圧迫担当者を交代する。
- 高度な気道確保器具が装着されていない場合は、30回の胸骨圧迫に対して2回の人工呼吸を行う。
- 定量的波形表示呼気 CO_2 モニター
  – $PETCO_2$ が低いまたは低下している場合、CPRの質を再評価する。

除細動のショックエネルギー量
- **二相性：** 製造業者の推奨値（初回エネルギー量120〜200 J）。不明な場合は最大値に設定する。2回目以降のエネルギー量は初回と同等とし、より大きなエネルギー量を考慮してもよい。
- **単相性：** 360 J

薬物療法
- **アドレナリン静注／骨髄内投与：** 3〜5分ごとに1 mg
- **アミオダロン静注／骨髄内投与：** 初回投与量：300 mgボーラス投与。2回目投与量：150 mg。
  「または」
- **リドカイン静注／骨髄内投与：** 初回投与量：1〜1.5 mg/kg。2回目投与量：0.5〜0.75 mg/kg。

高度な気道確保器具
- 気管挿管または声門上気道確保
- 波形表示呼気 CO_2 モニターまたはカプノメトリによる気管チューブの位置の確認およびモニタリング
- 高度な気道確保器具を装着したら、胸骨圧迫を続行しながら6秒ごとに1回（10回/分）の人工呼吸

自己心拍再開（ROSC）
- 脈拍および血圧
- $PETCO_2$ の突発的な持続的増加（通常は≧40 mm Hg）
- 動脈内モニタリングで自己心拍による動脈圧波形を確認

治療可能な原因
- 循環血液量減少（**H**ypovolemia）
- 低酸素症（**H**ypoxia）
- 水素イオン（アシドーシス）（**H**ydrogen ion (acidosis)）
- 低／高カリウム血症（**H**ypo-/hyperkalemia）
- 低体温症（**H**ypothermia）
- 緊張性気胸（**T**ension pneumothorax）
- 心タンポナーデ（**T**amponade, cardiac）
- 毒物（**T**oxins）
- 肺動脈血栓症（**T**hrombosis, pulmonary）
- 冠動脈血栓症（**T**hrombosis, coronary）

© 2020 American Heart Association

図4．成人の心停止循環アルゴリズム。
CPR：心肺蘇生（cardiopulmonary resuscitation），無脈性VT：無脈性心室頻拍（pulseless ventricular tachycardia），VF：心室細動（ventricular fibrillation）。

適切である。CPR手順を胸骨圧迫から開始することで、最初の胸骨圧迫までの時間が最小限になった[2-4]。市民救助者における胸骨圧迫のみのCPRが全国的に普及したことにより、日本ではOHCA後の良好な神経学的転帰を伴う生存率が増加した。CPRを実施する市民救助者が増加したためだと考えられる[5]。胸骨圧迫の際に最初に衣服を脱がせる必要はなく、できる限り迅速に圧迫を開始すべきである。

2. CPRの開始と救急対応システムへの出動要請の最適なタイミングは、2020年のILCORシステマティックレビューで評価された[1]。17,000を超えるOHCAイベントを対象とした観察研究では、「先に通報」戦略と「先にCPR」戦略のいずれでも同様の結果が報告された[6]。モバイルデバイスが普及している現代では、EMSへの出動要請とCPRの開始を同時に実行することが理想的である。

3. 4件の観察研究[7-10]で、心停止していない患者が市民救助者によるCPRを受けた場合の転帰が報告されている。後に心停止していなかったと判断された患者でも、CPRによる深刻な有害性は認められなかった[1]。これは、心停止している患者にCPRを行わないリスクが有意であることと対照的であり、

心停止が疑われる場合にCPRを実施することを強く支持するリスク対利益比となる。

4. 一部の観察研究では，胸部圧迫のみを受けた心停止傷病者と比較して，従来のCPR（圧迫と換気）を受けた心停止傷病者で転帰が改善されたことが認められている[5,11,12]。他の観察研究では，従来のCPRを受けた患者と，圧迫のみのCPRを受けた患者の転帰に違いはないと報告している[11,13-21]。従来のCPRの潜在的な有益性を考慮すると，市民救助者が適切に訓練されている場合は，圧迫と同時に換気を実施することが奨励されるべきである。従来のCPRを実施する際の胸骨圧迫と人工呼吸の比率に関するデータの詳細なレビューについては，「換気および胸骨圧迫と人工呼吸の比率」で説明している。

これらの推奨事項は，「2020 ILCOR Consensus on CPR and Emergency Cardiovascular Care Science With Treatment Recommendations」（CoSTR）で支持されている。[1]

蘇生の開始に関する推奨事項：医療従事者

COR	LOE	推奨事項
1	C-LD	1. 医療従事者が1人の場合は，換気ではなく胸骨圧迫から開始する必要がある。
2a	C-LD	2. 心原性か非心原性かを問わず，心停止を起こしたすべての成人患者に対して医療従事者が胸骨圧迫と換気を実施することは妥当である。

「推奨事項の裏付けとなる解説」

1. 『心肺蘇生と救急心血管治療のためのガイドライン2010』では，トレーニングを受けた救助者は人工呼吸ではなく胸骨圧迫からCPR手順を開始して（気道確保，人工呼吸，循環補助の順序ではなく，循環補助，気道確保，人工呼吸の順序），胸骨圧迫開始までの時間を最小限にするという大きな変更があった。このアプローチは新しい文献によって再度支持されており，2020年のILCORシステマティックレビューに要約されている（表2）[1-4]。推奨手順に従って，トレーニングを受けた救助者はまず胸骨圧迫を開始してから，酸素化および換気のための口対マスク人工呼吸またはバッグマスクを用いた人工呼吸を実施する。マネキンを用いた研究で，換気ではなく胸骨圧迫から開始することで，胸骨圧迫[3,23]，補助呼吸[4]，および最初のCPRサイクル完了までの時間が短縮されることが明らかになっている[4]。

2. 医療従事者は胸骨圧迫および換気の両方を実施するためのトレーニングを受ける。動脈血酸素含量はCPRの時間が延長するにつれて減少すると考えられるため，換気補助を伴わない長時間の胸骨圧迫の実施は，従来のCPR（胸骨圧迫＋人工呼吸）ほど有効でない。この懸念は，特に呼吸原性心停止の場合に当てはまる[11]。トレーニングを受け理解している医療従事者が最も可能性の高い心停止の原因に応じて次の救命手順を調整することは現実的である。

これらの推奨事項は，BLSに関する2020年のCoSTRで支持されている[1]。

表2. 成人のBLS手順[22]

手順	訓練を受けていない市民救助者	訓練を受けた市民救助者	医療従事者
1	現場の安全を確保する	現場の安全を確保する	現場の安全を確保する
2	反応の有無をチェックする。	反応の有無をチェックする。	反応の有無をチェックする。
3	大声で周囲に助けを求める自分で119番に通報するか，誰かに通報を依頼する（電話または電話を持った通報者は傷病者の脇に留まり，電話をスピーカーモードにする）。	大声で周囲に助けを求め，救急対応システムの出動を要請する（119番，救急対応）。誰かが応じた場合は，可能な限り電話を傷病者の脇に置くようにする。	大声で周囲に助けを求め，蘇生チームを要請する。医療従事者はこの時点，または呼吸と脈拍を確認した後に蘇生チームを要請できる。
4	救急指令者*の指示に従う。	呼吸をしていないか，死戦期呼吸のみかを確認する。呼吸をしていない場合は，CPRと圧迫を開始する。	呼吸をしていないか，死戦期呼吸のみかを確認し，脈拍を確認する（理想的には同時に）。通常呼吸および脈拍がないことを確認し，心停止と判断するとすぐに，医療従事者1人または救助者より派遣された別の人物が，AED／救急治療用器材を作動し，持ってくる必要がある。
5	救急指令者の指示に従って，呼吸をしていないか，死戦期呼吸のみかを確認する。	救急指令者の質問に答え，その指示に従う。	ただちにCPRを開始し，使用可能な場合はAED／除細動器を使用する。
6	救急指令者の指示に従う。	別の人物がいる場合は，AEDを取ってこさせる。	その人物が戻ると，2人法のCPRを行い，AED／除細動器を使用する。

AED：自動体外式除細動器（automated external defibrillator），BLS：一次救命処置（basic life support），CPR：心肺蘇生（cardiopulmonary resuscitation）。

*「救急指令者」と「通信司令員」の用語は，多くの場合に同義として使用される。

参考資料

1. Olasveengen TM, Mancini ME, Perkins GD, Avis S, Brooks S, Castrén M, Chung SP, Considine J, Couper K, Escalante R, et al; on behalf of the Adult Basic Life Support Collaborators.Adult basic life support: 2020 International Consensus on Cardiopulmonary Resuscitation and Emergency Cardiovascular Care Science With Treatment Recommendations.Circulation.2020;142 (suppl 1):S41-S91. doi: 10.1161/CIR.0000000000000892
2. Lubrano R, Cecchetti C, Bellelli E, Gentile I, Loayza Levano H, Orsini F, Bertazzoni G, Messi G, Rugolotto S, Pirozzi N, Elli M. Comparison of times of intervention during pediatric CPR maneuvers using ABC and CAB sequences: a randomized trial.Resuscitation.2012;83:1473-1477. doi: 10.1016/j.resuscitation.2012.04.011
3. Sekiguchi H, Kondo Y, Kukita I. Verification of changes in the time taken to initiate chest compressions according to modified basic life support guidelines.Am J Emerg Med.2013;31:1248-1250. doi: 10.1016/j.ajem.2013.02.047
4. Marsch S, Tschan F, Semmer NK, Zobrist R, Hunziker PR, Hunziker S. ABC versus CAB for cardiopulmonary resuscitation: a prospective, randomized simulator-based trial.Swiss Med Wkly.2013;143:w13856. doi: 10.4414/smw.2013.13856
5. Iwami T, Kitamura T, Kiyohara K, Kawamura T. Dissemination of Chest Compression-Only Cardiopulmonary Resuscitation and Survival After Out-of-Hospital Cardiac Arrest.Circulation.2015;132:415-422. doi: 10.1161/CIRCULATIONAHA.114.014905
6. Kamikura T, Iwasaki H, Myojo Y, Sakagami S, Takei Y, Inaba H. Advantage of CPR-first over call-first actions for out-of-hospital cardiac arrests in nonelderly patients and of noncardiac aetiology.Resuscitation.2015;96:37-45. doi: 10.1016/j.resuscitation.2015.06.027
7. White L, Rogers J, Bloomingdale M, Fahrenbruch C, Culley L, Subido C, Eisenberg M, Rea T. Dispatcher-assisted cardiopulmonary resuscitation: risks for patients not in cardiac arrest.Circulation.2010;121:91-97. doi: 10.1161/CIRCULATIONAHA.109.872366
8. Haley KB, Lerner EB, Pirrallo RG, Croft H, Johnson A, Uihlein M. The frequency and consequences of cardiopulmonary resuscitation performed by bystanders on patients who are not in cardiac arrest.Prehosp Emerg Care.2011;15:282-287. doi: 10.3109/10903127.2010.541981
9. Moriwaki Y, Sugiyama M, Tahara Y, Iwashita M, Kosuge T, Harunari N, Arata S, Suzuki N. Complications of bystander cardiopulmonary resuscitation for unconscious patients without cardiopulmonary arrest.J Emerg Trauma Shock.2012;5:3-6. doi: 10.4103/0974-2700.93094
10. Tanaka Y, Nishi T, Takase K, Yoshita Y, Wato Y, Taniguchi J, Hamada Y, Inaba H. Survey of a protocol to increase appropriate implementation of dispatcher-assisted cardiopulmonary resuscitation for out-of-hospital cardiac arrest.Circulation.2014;129:1751-1760. doi: 10.1161/CIRCULATIONAHA.113.004409
11. Kitamura T, Iwami T, Kawamura T, Nagao K, Tanaka H, Hiraide A; Implementation Working Group for All-Japan Utstein Registry of the Fire and Disaster Management Agency.Bystander-initiated rescue breathing for out-of-hospital cardiac arrests of noncardiac origin.Circulation.2010;122:293-299. doi: 10.1161/CIRCULATIONAHA.109.926816
12. Ogawa T, Akahane M, Koike S, Tanabe S, Mizoguchi T, Imamura T. Outcomes of chest compression only CPR versus conventional CPR conducted by lay people in patients with out of hospital cardiopulmonary arrest witnessed by bystanders: nationwide population based observational study.BMJ.2011;342:c7106. doi: 10.1136/bmj.c7106
13. Svensson L, Bohm K, Castrèn M, Pettersson H, Engerström L, Herlitz J, Rosenqvist M. Compression-only CPR or standard CPR in out-of-hospital cardiac arrest.N Engl J Med.2010;363:434-442. doi: 10.1056/NEJMoa0908991
14. Rea TD, Fahrenbruch C, Culley L, Donohoe RT, Hambly C, Innes J, Bloomingdale M, Subido C, Romines S, Eisenberg MS.CPR with chest compression alone or with rescue breathing.N Engl J Med.2010;363:423-433. doi: 10.1056/NEJMoa0908993
15. Iwami T, Kawamura T, Hiraide A, Berg RA, Hayashi Y, Nishiuchi T, Kajino K, Yonemoto N, Yukioka H, Sugimoto H, Kakuchi H, Sase K, Yokoyama H, Nonogi H. Effectiveness of bystander-initiated cardiac-only resuscitation for patients with out-of-hospital cardiac arrest.Circulation.2007;116:2900-2907. doi: 10.1161/CIRCULATIONAHA.107.723411
16. Kitamura T, Iwami T, Kawamura T, Nagao K, Tanaka H, Berg RA, Hiraide A; Implementation Working Group for All-Japan Utstein Registry of the Fire and Disaster Management Agency.Time-dependent effectiveness of chest compression-only and conventional cardiopulmonary resuscitation for out-of-hospital cardiac arrest of cardiac origin.Resuscitation.2011;82:3-9. doi: 10.1016/j.resuscitation.2010.09.468
17. Ong ME, Ng FS, Anushia P, Tham LP, Leong BS, Ong VY, Tiah L, Lim SH, Anantharaman V. Comparison of chest compression only and standard cardiopulmonary resuscitation for out-of-hospital cardiac arrest in Singapore. Resuscitation.2008;78:119-126. doi: 10.1016/j.resuscitation.2008.03.012
18. SOS-KANTO Study Group.Cardiopulmonary resuscitation by bystanders with chest compression only (SOS-KANTO): an observational study.Lancet.2007;369:920-926. doi: 10.1016/S0140-6736 (07)60451-6
19. Bobrow BJ, Spaite DW, Berg RA, Stolz U, Sanders AB, Kern KB, Vadeboncoeur TF, Clark LL, Gallagher JV, Stapczynski JS, LoVecchio F, Mullins TJ, Humble WO, Ewy GA.Chest compression-only CPR by lay rescuers and survival from out-of-hospital cardiac arrest.JAMA.2010;304:1447-1454. doi: 10.1001/jama.2010.1392
20. Olasveengen TM, Wik L, Steen PA.Standard basic life support vs. continuous chest compressions only in out-of-hospital cardiac arrest.Acta Anaesthesiol Scand.2008;52:914-919. doi: 10.1111/j.1399-6576.2008.01723.x
21. Panchal AR, Bobrow BJ, Spaite DW, Berg RA, Stolz U, Vadeboncoeur TF, Sanders AB, Kern KB, Ewy GA.Chest compression-only cardiopulmonary resuscitation performed by lay rescuers for adult out-of-hospital cardiac arrest due to non-cardiac aetiologies.Resuscitation.2013;84:435-439. doi: 10.1016/j.resuscitation.2012.07.038
22. Kleinman ME, Brennan EE, Goldberger ZD, Swor RA, Terry M, Bobrow BJ, Gazmuri RJ, Travers AH, Rea T. Part 5: adult basic life support and cardiopulmonary resuscitation quality: 2015 American Heart Association Guidelines Update for Cardiopulmonary Resuscitation and Emergency Cardiovascular Care.Circulation.2015;132 (suppl 2):S414-S435. doi: 10.1161/CIR.0000000000000259
23. Kobayashi M, Fujiwara A, Morita H, Nishimoto Y, Mishima T, Nitta M, Hayashi T, Hotta T, Hayashi Y, Hachisuka E, Sato K. A manikin-based observational study on cardiopulmonary resuscitation skills at the Osaka Senri medical rally.Resuscitation.2008;78:333-339. doi: 10.1016/j.resuscitation.2008.03.230

気道確保

「緒言」

適切な換気と酸素化を促進するには，気道開通が不可欠である。患者の気道の確保と維持に関して，ある手技を他の手技よりも支持する質の高いエビデンスはないが，救助者は各手技の長所と短所を認識し，それぞれに必要なスキルの習熟度を維持する必要がある。救助者は，適切な気道確保には複数のアプローチが必要になる可能性があることを認識すべきである。気道の開通性と適切な換気および酸素化を確認するために，患者を常に監視する必要がある。心停止患者の気道確保についてさまざまな戦略を比較した研究はない。気道戦略の有効性を調べるエビデンスの多くは，X線検査と死体を用いた研究に由来する。

気道確保に関する 推奨事項

COR	LOE	推奨事項
1	C-EO	1. 医療従事者は，頭頸部に外傷を認めない傷病者に対しては頭部後屈―あご先挙上法を用いて気道を確保する。
1	C-EO	2. トレーニングを受けていて，胸骨圧迫と換気の両方を行う自信がある市民救助者は，頭頸部に外傷を認めない傷病者に対しては頭部後屈―あご先挙上法を用いて気道を確保する。
2b	C-EO	3. 気道補助用具（口咽頭エアウェイや鼻咽頭エアウェイなど）の使用は，咳嗽反射・咽頭反射のない無意識の（無反応の）患者ではバッグマスクによる換気が容易になるため合理的な場合がある。
2a	C-EO	4. 頭蓋底骨折または重度の凝固障害が判明しているか，または疑われる場合には，鼻咽頭エアウェイより口咽頭エアウエイが望ましい。
3：利益なし	C-LD	5. 成人の心停止に対する輪状軟骨圧迫法のルーチン使用は推奨されない。

「推奨事項の裏付けとなる解説」

1 および 2. 非心停止研究および放射線学的研究で，頭部後屈―あご先挙上法が気道確保に効果的であることが示されている[2-5]。心停止中の気道確保について，頭部後屈―あご先挙上法を他の気道確保手技と比較した研究はない。

3. 心停止中のその使用の有効性を調査したエビデンスはないが，口咽頭エアウエイと鼻咽頭エアウエイを使用することで，舌による気道閉鎖を防止でき，気道開通を維持して適切な換気を促進できる。ただし挿入が不適切な場合，舌が中咽頭の後ろに移動して気道閉塞を引き起こす可能性がある[6,7]。

4. 頭蓋底骨折または重度の凝固障害が判明しているか，または疑われる場合での鼻咽頭エアウェイと比較した口咽頭エアウエイの有益性は，臨床試験では評価されていない。ただし，鼻咽頭エアウェイには外傷のリスクがあるため，口咽頭エアウエイが望ましい。頭蓋底骨折患者において鼻咽頭エアウエイの頭蓋内挿入が複数例報告されている[8,9]。

5. 輪状軟骨圧迫法が心停止患者の換気を促進する，または誤嚥のリスクを低減するというエビデンスはない。非心停止患者に輪状軟骨圧迫法を使用すると，バッグマスク換気の実施中，誤嚥および胃への送気を防止できる可能性があるという複数のエビデンスがある[10-13]。しかし，輪状軟骨圧迫法によって換気や，声門上気道デバイス（SGA）の留置または挿管が阻害されたり[14-20]，挿管中の気道損傷リスクが増大する可能性もある[21]。

このトピックは，直近で2010年に正式なエビデンスレビューを受けている[22]。

頭頸部外傷後における気道確保に関する 推奨事項

COR	LOE	推奨事項
1	C-EO	1. 頸椎損傷が疑われる場合，医療従事者は頭部を後屈させない下顎挙上法で気道を確保する。
1	C-EO	2. 頭頸部に外傷が認められる状況で，下顎挙上法と気道補助器具の挿入で気道を確保できない場合は，頭部後屈―あご先挙上法を実施する。
3：有害	C-LD	3. 頭頸部に外傷が認められる状況では，トレーニングを受けていない救助者による固定具の使用は有害になる可能性があるため，市民救助者は固定具を使用してはならない。

「推奨事項の裏付けとなる解説」

1. 医療従事者は，気道を確保する前に脊髄損傷の可能性を考慮するべきである。脊髄損傷が疑われる場合，またはその可能性を除外できない場合は，頭部後屈―あご先挙上法ではなく下顎挙上法を使用して気道を確保する[2]。

2. 気道開通の維持と適切な換気と酸素化の実施は，CPR中の優先事項である。下顎挙上法や気道補助器具の挿入を行っても気道を確保できず，換気が起こらない場合は，頭部後屈―あご先挙上法が唯一の気道確保法になると考えられる。このような場合，気道確保の必要性は心停止患者のさらなる脊髄損傷のリスクを上回るため，脊髄損傷の可能性がある場合でもこの手技を使用する必要がある。

3. 脊髄損傷が疑われる場合，またはその可能性を除外できない場合，救助者は用手的に脊椎運動制限を維持すべきであり，固定具

を使用してはならない。用手で安定させると，適切な換気と気道確保を行いながら，患者ケア中の頸椎の動きを減少させることができる[23,24]。脊椎固定具を使用すると，気道開通の維持[25,26]および適切な換気の実施が困難になる場合がある。

このトピックは，直近で2010年に正式なエビデンスレビューを受けている[22]。

参考資料

1. Deleted in proof.
2. Elam JO, Greene DG, Schneider MA, Ruben HM, Gordon AS, Hustead RF, Benson DW, Clements JA, Ruben A. Head-tilt method of oral resuscitation. JAMA. 1960;172:812–815. doi: 10.1001/jama.1960.03020080042011
3. Guildner CW. Resuscitation—opening the airway: a comparative study of techniques for opening an airway obstructed by the tongue. JACEP. 1976;5:588–590. doi: 10.1016/s0361-1124(76)80217-1
4. Greene DG, Elam JO, Dobkin AB, Studley CL. Cinefluorographic study of hyperextension of the neck and upper airway patency. JAMA. 1961;176:570–573. doi: 10.1001/jama.1961.03040200006002
5. Ruben HM, Elam JO, Ruben AM, Greene DG. Investigation of upper airway problems in resuscitation.1. Studies of pharyngeal x-rays and performance by laymen. Anesthesiology. 1961;22:271–279. doi: 10.1097/00000542-196103000-00017
6. Kim HJ, Kim SH, Min JY, Park WK. Determination of the appropriate oropharyngeal airway size in adults: Assessment using ventilation and an endoscopic view. Am J Emerg Med. 2017;35:1430–1434. doi: 10.1016/j.ajem.2017.04.029
7. Kim HJ, Kim SH, Min NH, Park WK. Determination of the appropriate sizes of oropharyngeal airways in adults: correlation with external facial measurements: A randomised crossover study. Eur J Anaesthesiol. 2016;33:936–942. doi: 10.1097/EJA.0000000000000439
8. Schade K, Borzotta A, Michaels A. Intracranial malposition of nasopharyngeal airway. J Trauma. 2000;49:967–968. doi: 10.1097/00005373-200011000-00032
9. Muzzi DA, Losasso TJ, Cucchiara RF. Complication from a nasopharyngeal airway in a patient with a basilar skull fracture. Anesthesiology. 1991;74:366–368. doi: 10.1097/00000542-199102000-00026
10. Salem MR, Wong AY, Mani M, Sellick BA. Efficacy of cricoid pressure in preventing gastric inflation during bag-mask ventilation in pediatric patients. Anesthesiology. 1974;40:96–98. doi: 10.1097/00000542-197401000-00026
11. Lawes EG, Campbell I, Mercer D. Inflation pressure, gastric insufflation and rapid sequence induction. Br J Anaesth. 1987;59:315–318. doi: 10.1093/bja/59.3.315
12. Petito SP, Russell WJ. The prevention of gastric inflation-a neglected benefit of cricoid pressure. Anaesth Intensive Care. 1988;16:139–143. doi: 10.1177/0310057X8801600202
13. Moynihan RJ, Brock-Utne JG, Archer JH, Feld LH, Kreitzman TR. The effect of cricoid pressure on preventing gastric insufflation in infants and children. Anesthesiology. 1993;78:652–656. doi: 10.1097/00000542-199304000-00007
14. Brimacombe J, White A, Berry A. Effect of cricoid pressure on ease of insertion of the laryngeal mask airway. Br J Anaesth. 1993;71:800–802. doi: 10.1093/bja/71.6.800
15. Allman KG. The effect of cricoid pressure application on airway patency. J Clin Anesth. 1995;7:197–199. doi: 10.1016/0952-8180(94)00048-9
16. Hartsilver EL, Vanner RG. Airway obstruction with cricoid pressure. Anaesthesia. 2000;55:208–211. doi: 10.1046/j.1365-2044.2000.01205.x
17. Hocking G, Roberts FL, Thew ME. Airway obstruction with cricoid pressure and lateral tilt. Anaesthesia. 2001;56:825–828. doi: 10.1046/j.1365-2044.2001.02133.x
18. Turgeon AF, Nicole PC, Trépanier CA, Marcoux S, Lessard MR. Cricoid pressure does not increase the rate of failed intubation by direct laryngoscopy in adults. Anesthesiology. 2005;102:315–319. doi: 10.1097/00000542-200502000-00012
19. Asai T, Goy RW, Liu EH. Cricoid pressure prevents placement of the laryngeal tube and laryngeal tube-suction II. Br J Anaesth. 2007;99:282–285. doi: 10.1093/bja/aem159
20. McNelis U, Syndercombe A, Harper I, Duggan J. The effect of cricoid pressure on intubation facilitated by the gum elastic bougie. Anaesthesia. 2007;62:456–459. doi: 10.1111/j.1365-2044.2007.05019.x
21. Carauna E, Chevret S, Pirracchio R. Effect of cricoid pressure on laryngeal view during prehospital tracheal intubation: a propensity-based analysis. Emerg Med J. 2017;132–137. doi: doi: 10.1136/emermed-2016-205715
22. Berg RA, Hemphill R, Abella BS, Aufderheide TP, Cave DM, Hazinski MF, Lerner EB, Rea TD, Sayre MR, Swor RA. Part 5: adult basic life support: 2010 American Heart Association Guidelines for Cardiopulmonary Resuscitation and Emergency Cardiovascular Care. Circulation. 2010;122(suppl 3):S685–S705. doi: 10.1161/CIRCULATIONAHA.110.970939
23. Majernick TG, Bieniek R, Houston JB, Hughes HG. Cervical spine movement during orotracheal intubation. Ann Emerg Med. 1986;15:417–420. doi: 10.1016/s0196-0644(86)80178-0
24. Lennarson PJ, Smith DW, Sawin PD, Todd MM, Sato Y, Traynelis VC. Cervical spinal motion during intubation: efficacy of stabilization maneuvers in the setting of complete segmental instability. J Neurosurg. 2001;94(suppl):265–270. doi: 10.3171/spi.2001.94.2.0265
25. Hastings RH, Wood PR. Head extension and laryngeal view during laryngoscopy with cervical spine stabilization maneuvers. Anesthesiology. 1994;80:825–831. doi: 10.1097/00000542-199404000-00015
26. Gerling MC, Davis DP, Hamilton RS, Morris GF, Vilke GM, Garfin SR, Hayden SR. Effects of cervical spine immobilization technique and laryngoscope blade selection on an unstable cervical spine in a cadaver model of intubation. Ann Emerg Med. 2000;36:293–300. doi: 10.1067/mem.2000.109442

質の高いCPRの指標

「緒言」

質の高いCPRは，ショック適応のリズムへの除細動と並んで，心停止している患者にとって最も重要な救命処置である。研究が進むにつれて，最適なCPRを構成する要素に関するエビデンスは進化し続けている。質の高いCPRについては，胸骨圧迫の中断を最小限に抑える，適切なテンポと深さの圧迫を行う，圧迫と圧迫の間に胸部にもたれかからない，過度の換気を避けるなど，多くの重要な要素が定義されている[1]。ただし，対照試験が比較的不足しており，観察研究によるエビデンスが相反することもある。非常に多くのことが同時に発生し，それらの効果において相互作用する可能性があるため，個々のCPRの質の指標または介入の効果を評価するのは難しい。例えば，圧迫のテンポと圧迫の深さはどちらも良好な転帰に関連付けられているが，これらの変数は互いに逆相関しているため，一方を改善すると他方が悪化する可能性がある[1-3]。CPRの質の高い介入は「バンドル（包括的治療）」で適用されることが多いため，特定の指標の有益性を確認するのが困難である。フィードバック器具を使用し，圧迫の深さや胸骨圧迫の割合などのCPR指標に関するデータを収集するセンターやEMSシステムがますます増えているため，これらの推奨事項はこうしたデータにより継続的に更新されると思われる。

CPRの位置と場所に関する 推奨事項		
COR	LOE	推奨事項
1	C-LD	1. 胸骨圧迫を実施する場合は，傷病者の胸部中央（胸骨の下半分）の真上に片方の手のひらの付け根を置き，もう一方の手をその上に置いて，両手が重なるようにする。
1	C-EO	2. 質の高いCPRをその場所で安全かつ効果的に実施できる限り，蘇生法は通常，患者を発見した場所でそのまま実施する。
2a	C-LD	3. 可能であれば，硬い表面で，傷病者を仰臥位にしてCPRを実施することが望ましい。
2b	C-LD	4. 傷病者を仰臥位にできない場合，特に入院中で高度な気道確保器具を挿入している場合は，伏臥位のままCPRを行うことを検討してもかまわない。

「推奨事項の裏付けとなる解説」

1. 2020年のILCORシステマティックレビューで，合計57例の患者を対象に，蘇生プロセスと転帰に対する手の位置の影響を調査した研究が3件見つかった[4]。蘇生の転帰に違いは認められなかったが，2件の研究では，胸骨の下から3分の1の位置で行った圧迫を胸骨の中央で行った圧迫と比較したところ，生理学的パラメーター（ピーク動脈圧，平均動脈圧［MAP］，呼気終末二酸化炭素［$ETCO_2$］）の改善が認められた[5,6]。3件目の研究では違いは認められなかった[7]。X線検査により，左心室は通常，乳頭間線（胸骨の下半分に対応）に位置することがわかっている[8]。ただし，乳頭間線より下に手を置くと，剣状突起が圧迫される可能性がある[9]。マネキンを用いた研究で得られたデータは相反するが，利き手または非利き手が胸骨と接触しているかどうかは問題ではないと思われる[10,11]。

2. 蘇生を開始する前に傷病者を移動する必要があるかどうかを判断する際の主な考慮事項は，傷病者が発見された場所と位置で質の高いCPRを実施できるかどうか，およびその安全性である。これは，蘇生を継続しながら患者を病院に移送するかどうか，またはそのタイミングを判断することとは別の問題である。

3. CPRの効果は，傷病者が仰臥位で，救助者が傷病者の胸の横にひざまずく（院外の場合）か，ベッドの横に立つ（院内の場合）ことで最大になると思われる[12]。胸骨圧迫は，傷病者を硬い表面に寝かせた状態で行うのが最も効果的だと考えらる[13,14]。マネキンを用いた研究では，病院のマットレスで実施したCPRで，一般的に許容可能な胸部圧迫が得られることが認められている。

4. 以前のシステマティックレビューでは，腹臥位で実施されたCPRの症例報告22件（手術室で21件，集中治療室［ICU］で1件）で，22例中10例の患者の生存が確認されている[15]。難治性IHCA患者6例による小規模な症例集積研究では，腹臥位で土嚢付きのボードを使用して胸骨圧迫を行ったところ，CPR中の血行動態は改善したが，ROSCには至らなかった[16]。腹臥位でのCPRの有効性は立証されていないが，非常に限定的なエビデンスにより，患者を仰臥位にできない場合，またはこれが安全に行われるまで，腹臥位でCPRを実施するほうがCPRを実施しないよりも効果的な場合があることが示唆されている。

推奨事項1，2および3は，BLSに関する2020年のCoSTRで支持されている[4]。推奨事項4は，直近で2010年に正式なエビデンスレビューを受けている[17]。

圧迫の割合と中断に関する 推奨事項		
COR	LOE	推奨事項
1	C-LD	1. 成人の心停止では，ショック前後の胸骨圧迫中断をできるだけ短くすべきである。
1	C-LD	2. 医療従事者は，リズムチェック中の脈拍チェックにかかる時間を最小限に抑える必要がある（10秒以内）。救助者は明確な脈拍を触知できない場合は，胸骨圧迫を再開すべきである。
2a	B-R	3. 救助者が2人以上いる場合は，胸骨圧迫の質が低下しないよう，およそ2分ごと（あるいは30：2の割合で行う胸骨圧迫と換気の約5サイクル後）に胸骨圧迫を交代することが妥当である。
2a	B-R	4. いかなる状況においても，成人の心停止に対するショック施行直後の胸骨圧迫再開は妥当である。
2a	C-LD	5. 心停止を起こし，高度な気道確保器具を使用せずにCPRを受けている成人に対し，胸骨圧迫中断で2回の人工呼吸を1回につき1秒以上かけて行うことは妥当である。
2b	C-LD	6. 成人の心停止では，胸骨圧迫の割合を60％以上としたCPRの実施を妥当としてよい。

「推奨事項の裏付けとなる解説」

1. 観察研究によるエビデンスでは，ショック適応のリズムを伴う患者に対する胸骨圧迫の割合を高めることで，転帰が改善することが示されている[18,19]。特に，圧迫中断を短くすることでROSCが増加すると報告されている[20-22]。

2. この推奨事項は，CPRの中断を最小限に抑え，胸骨圧迫の割合を60％以上に維持するという全体的な原則に基づいたものであり，この原則は転帰の改善に関連する[18,19,23]。

3. 胸骨圧迫の深さは，CPRの開始から90～120秒後に低下し始めるが，その時間枠の中で圧迫のテンポが大幅に低下することはない[24]。マネキンを使用した無作為化試験では，1分ごとに交代した場合と2分ごとに交代した場合での質の高い圧迫の割合に差は見られなかった[25]。このアプローチにより胸骨圧迫の質が維持されること，および通常はリズム解析のためにCPRが中断されることから，指名された胸骨圧迫担当者を2分ごとに交代する方法は妥当といえる。
4. 1000例を超える患者が登録された2件のRCTでは，除細動後のリズム解析のためにCPRを中断した場合の生存率改善は認められていない[26,27]。観察研究では，ショック後ただちに胸骨圧迫を再開しなかった場合は，ROSCが低下することが示されている[28,29]。
5. 胸骨圧迫の割合を60％以上とすることは蘇生転帰の改善に関連するため，換気目的の圧迫の中断はできる限り短くする必要がある[18,19,23]。
6. 2015年のシステマティックレビューでは，研究間の有意な均一性が示されており，一部の研究（すべてではない）では，生存から退院にいたる確率の向上が胸骨圧迫の割合を高めることに関連すると報告されている[18,19,23]。2件の研究では，胸骨圧迫の割合を高めることが，生存率の低下に関連付けられている[2,30]。圧迫のテンポおよび深さと，除細動や気道確保，投薬などの共介入も重要であり，胸骨圧迫の割合と相互に作用する可能性がある。パフォーマンスの高いEMSシステムでは，60％以上を目標としており，80％以上が目標となる頻度も高い。

推奨事項1および4は，BLSに関する2020年のCoSTRで支持されている[4]。推奨事項2，3，5，6は，直近で2015年に正式なエビデンスレビューを受けている[31]。

圧迫の深さとテンポに関する 推奨事項

COR	LOE	推奨事項
1	B-NR	1. 用手CPR中，救助者は平均的な成人に対して2インチまたは5cm以上の深さまで胸骨圧迫を行うべきであるが，過度に深く（2.4インチまたは6cm超）ならないようにする。
2a	B-NR	2. 心停止を起こした成人傷病者において，救助者が100～120回/分のテンポで胸骨圧迫を行うことは妥当である。
2a	C-LD	3. 心停止を起こした成人では，胸郭が完全に元に戻るようにするため，圧迫と圧迫の間は救助者が胸部にもたれないようにすると有益な場合がある。
2b	C-EO	4. 胸骨圧迫と戻り／弛緩の時間がほぼ等しくなる胸骨圧迫は，妥当としてよい。

「推奨事項の裏付けとなる解説」

1. 2020年のILCORによるスコーピングレビュー[32]では，12件の研究（患者数12,500人超）で，胸骨圧迫の要素に目を向けていることが確認されている。その複数の研究において，圧迫の深さを5cm以上とした場合は，4cm未満とした場合と比較して，生存から退院にいたる確率や除細動の成功など，転帰の改善がみられる[3,20,33,34]。
2. このレビュー[32]では，13件の研究（患者数15,000人超）が圧迫のテンポに注目したことが確認された。結果には多少のばらつきが見られ，高い圧迫のテンポと転帰との関連性を示したのは，成人を対象とした3件の観察研究のみである[1,35,36]。100回のテンポと120回のテンポを比較したのは，292人の患者を対象としたRCTのみであるが[37]，成人において圧迫のテンポを100回/分から120回/分に変更するよう推奨するに足るエビデンスは示されていない。3件の研究では，テンポが速くなると深さが低下することが報告されており，CPRの質を単独の指標のみで評価する際の注意点が強調されている[1-3]。
3. このILCORのレビュー[32]では，胸骨圧迫の解放速度と生存率の関連性について，2件の観察研究の結果に一貫性が見られないことが確認されており，一方の研究では関連性がないとされているのに対し，他方の研究では，解放速度が速い方が生存率は向上するとされている[38,39]。胸郭の不十分な戻りは，胸腔内圧の上昇と冠動脈灌流圧の低下に関連付けられている[40,41]。
4. CPRのデューティサイクルとは，圧迫と減圧のサイクルにかかる合計時間に占める圧迫時間の割合を指す。2010年のガイドラインでは，主に実践での実現が容易と受け止められるという観点から，50％のデューティサイクル，つまり圧迫と減圧にかける時間が等しくなるようにすることが推奨されていた。とりわけ，院外VFによる心停止を発症した成人患者（生存退院率43％）を対象とした臨床研究では，蘇生中に認められたデューティサイクルの平均は39％であった[42]。小児を対象とした研究でも平均デューティサイクルは40％であり，臨床現場ではデューティサイクルが短くなるのが一般的であることが示されている[43]。多数の動物実験では，デューティサイクルが50％未満のときに血流量の増加と転帰の改善が認められているが，最適なデューティサイクルは不明である。現在のところ既存の推奨事項を変更するに足るエビデンスは不十分であり，さらなる調査を必要とする課題が残されている。

推奨事項1，2および3は，BLSに関する2020年のCoSTRで支持されている[4]。推奨事項4は，直近で2010年に正式なエビデンスレビューを受けている[44]。

CPR フィードバックおよびモニタリングに関する推奨事項		
COR	LOE	推奨事項
2b	B-R	1. リアルタイムで CPR 能力を最適化するために，CPR 中の視聴覚的なフィードバック器具の使用を妥当としてよい。
2b	C-LD	2. CPR の質のモニタリングおよび最適化が可能であれば，動脈血圧または呼気終末 CO_2 などの生理学的パラメータの使用を妥当としてよい。when feasible to monitor and optimize CPR quality.

「推奨事項の裏付けとなる解説」

1. 2020 年の ILCOR によるシステマティックレビューでは，ほとんどの研究では，リアルタイムフィードバックと患者転帰の改善の間に有意な関連性は見られないことが認められている[4]。ただし，有意な有害性が見られた研究も認められず，一部では生存率における臨床的に重要な改善が示されている。最近のある RCT では，圧迫の深さおよび戻りに関する聴覚的なフィードバックにより，IHCA からの生存退院が 25.6 ％上昇したと報告されている（54 ％対 28.4 ％，P<0.001）[45]。

2. AHA の Get With The Guidelines-Resuscitation 登録から取得したデータの解析では，$ETCO_2$ または拡張期血圧を使用して CPR の質をモニタリングした場合，ROSC の確率（オッズ比：1.22, 95 ％信頼区間：1.04〜1.34, P=0.017）が向上することが示されている[46]。成人患者を対象とした観察研究（IHCA および OHCA）では，圧迫の深さが 10 mm 増加するごとに $ETCO_2$ が 1.4 mm Hg 増加すると報告されている[47]。2018 年の $ETCO$ のシステマティックレビュー（$ETCO_2$ を ROSC の予後指標として使用[48]）では，カットオフ値にばらつきが見られるが，一般的に転帰不良に関連付けられるのは 10 mm Hg 未満であり，20 mm Hg を超える場合は，10 mm Hg 未満の場合よりも ROSC との強い関連性が認められた。高い $ETCO_2$ と ROSC の関連性，および圧迫が深いほど $ETCO_2$ が高くなるという事実を組み合わせると，少なくとも値が 10 mm Hg 以上，理想的には 20 mm Hg 以上となる目標圧迫を設定することが有用であることが示唆される。挿管されていない患者においては，$ETCO_2$ の妥当性と信頼性は十分に確立されていない。可能な場合は，観血的動脈内血圧モニタリングを実施することで，CPR の取り組みを評価およびガイドするのに役立つ場合がある。心停止中に拡張期血圧モニタリングを行うことで，ROSC が向上する[46]とされているが，具体的な圧力を示唆するヒトのデータは不十分である。

これらの推奨事項は，BLS および ALS に関する 2020 年の CoSTR で支持されている[4,49]。

参考資料

1. Idris AH, Guffey D, Pepe PE, Brown SP, Brooks SC, Callaway CW, Christenson J, Davis DP, Daya MR, Gray R, Kudenchuk PJ, Larsen J, Lin S, Menegazzi JJ, Sheehan K, Sopko G, Stiell I, Nichol G, Aufderheide TP; Resuscitation Outcomes Consortium Investigators.Chest compression rates and survival following out-of-hospital cardiac arrest.Crit Care Med.2015;43:840–848. doi: 10.1097/CCM.0000000000000824
2. Vadeboncoeur T, Stolz U, Panchal A, Silver A, Venuti M, Tobin J, Smith G, Nunez M, Karamooz M, Spaite D, Bobrow B. Chest compression depth and survival in out-of-hospital cardiac arrest.Resuscitation.2014;85:182–188. doi: 10.1016/j.resuscitation.2013.10.002
3. Stiell IG, Brown SP, Christenson J, Cheskes S, Nichol G, Powell J, Bigham B, Morrison LJ, Larsen J, Hess E, Vaillancourt C, Davis DP, Callaway CW; Resuscitation Outcomes Consortium (ROC) Investigators.What is the role of chest compression depth during out-of-hospital cardiac arrest resuscitation? Crit Care Med.2012;40:1192–1198. doi: 10.1097/CCM.0b013e31823bc8bb
4. Olasveengen TM, Mancini ME, Perkins GD, Avis S, Brooks S, Castrén M, Chung SP, Considine J, Couper K, Escalante R, et al; on behalf of the Adult Basic Life Support Collaborators.Adult basic life support: 2020 International Consensus on Cardiopulmonary Resuscitation and Emergency Cardiovascular Care Science With Treatment Recommendations.Circulation.2020;142(suppl 1):S41-S91. doi: 10.1161/CIR.0000000000000892
5. Cha KC, Kim HJ, Shin HJ, Kim H, Lee KH, Hwang SO.Hemodynamic effect of external chest compressions at the lower end of the sternum in cardiac arrest patients.J Emerg Med.2013;44:691–697. doi: 10.1016/j.jemermed.2012.09.026
6. Orlowski JP.Optimum position for external cardiac compression in infants and young children.Ann Emerg Med.1986;15:667–673. doi: 10.1016/s0196-0644(86)80423-1
7. Qvigstad E, Kramer-Johansen J, Tømte Ø, Skålhegg T, Sørensen Ø, Sunde K, Olasveengen TM.Clinical pilot study of different hand positions during manual chest compressions monitored with capnography.Resuscitation.2013;84:1203–1207. doi: 10.1016/j.resuscitation.2013.03.010
8. Shin J, Rhee JE, Kim K. Is the inter-nipple line the correct hand position for effective chest compression in adult cardiopulmonary resuscitation? Resuscitation.2007;75:305–310. doi: 10.1016/j.resuscitation.2007.05.003
9. Kusunoki S, Tanigawa K, Kondo T, Kawamoto M, Yuge O. Safety of the inter-nipple line hand position landmark for chest compression.Resuscitation.2009;80:1175–1180. doi: 10.1016/j.resuscitation.2009.06.030
10. Nikandish R, Shahbazi S, Golabi S, Beygi N. Role of dominant versus non-dominant hand position during uninterrupted chest compression CPR by novice rescuers: a randomized double-blind crossover study.Resuscitation.2008;76:256–260. doi: 10.1016/j.resuscitation.2007.07.032
11. Kundra P, Dey S, Ravishankar M. Role of dominant hand position during external cardiac compression.Br J Anaesth.2000;84:491–493. doi: 10.1093/oxfordjournals.bja.a013475
12. Handley AJ, Handley JA.Performing chest compressions in a confined space.Resuscitation.2004;61:55–61. doi: 10.1016/j.resuscitation.2003.11.012
13. Nishisaki A, Nysaether J, Sutton R, Maltese M, Niles D, Donoghue A, Bishnoi R, Helfaer M, Perkins GD, Berg R, Arbogast K, Nadkarni V. Effect of mattress deflection on CPR quality assessment for older children and adolescents.Resuscitation.2009;80:540–545. doi: 10.1016/j.resuscitation.2009.02.006
14. Noordergraaf GJ, Paulussen IW, Venema A, van Berkom PF, Woerlee PH, Scheffer GJ, Noordergraaf A. The impact of compliant surfaces on in-hospital chest compressions: effects of common mattresses and a backboard.Resuscitation.2009;80:546–552. doi: 10.1016/j.resuscitation.2009.03.023
15. Brown J, Rogers J, Soar J. Cardiac arrest during surgery and ventilation in the prone position: a case report and systematic review.Resuscitation.2001;50:233–238. doi: 10.1016/s0300-9572 (01)00362-8
16. Mazer SP, Weisfeldt M, Bai D, Cardinale C, Arora R, Ma C, Sciacca RR, Chong D, Rabbani LE.Reverse CPR: a pilot study of CPR in the prone position.Resuscitation.2003;57:279–285. doi: 10.1016/s0300-9572 (03)00037-6
17. Cave DM, Gazmuri RJ, Otto CW, Nadkarni VM, Cheng A, Brooks SC, Daya M, Sutton RM, Branson R, Hazinski MF. Part 7: CPR techniques and devices: 2010 American Heart Association Guidelines for Cardiopulmonary Resuscitation and Emergency Cardiovascular Care.Circulation.2010;122:S720–728. doi: 10.1161/CIRCULATIONAHA.110.970970
18. Talikowska M, Tohira H, Finn J. Cardiopulmonary resuscitation quality and patient survival outcome in cardiac arrest: A systematic review and meta-analysis.Resuscitation.2015;96:66–77. doi: 10.1016/j. resuscitation.2015.07.036
19. Christenson J, Andrusiek D, Everson-Stewart S, Kudenchuk P, Hostler D, Powell J, Callaway CW, Bishop D, Vaillancourt C, Davis D, Aufderheide TP, Idris A, Stouffer JA, Stiell I, Berg R; Resuscitation Outcomes Consortium Investigators.Chest compression fraction determines survival in patients with out-of-hospital ventricular fibrillation.Circulation.2009;120:1241–1247. doi: 10.1161/CIRCULATIONAHA.109.852202
20. Edelson DP, Abella BS, Kramer-Johansen J, Wik L, Myklebust H, Barry AM, Merchant RM, Hoek TL, Steen PA, Becker LB.Effects of compression depth and pre-shock pauses predict defibrillation failure during cardiac arrest. Resuscitation.2006;71:137–145. doi: 10.1016/j.resuscitation.2006.04.008

21. Eftestøl T, Sunde K, Steen PA. Effects of interrupting precordial compressions on the calculated probability of defibrillation success during out-of-hospital cardiac arrest. Circulation. 2002;105:2270–2273. doi: 10.1161/01.cir.0000016362.42586.fe
22. Cheskes S, Schmicker RH, Christenson J, Salcido DD, Rea T, Powell J, Edelson DP, Sell R, May S, Menegazzi JJ, Van Ottingham L, Olsufka M, Pennington S, Simonini J, Berg RA, Stiell I, Idris A, Bigham B, Morrison L; Resuscitation Outcomes Consortium (ROC) Investigators. Perishock pause: an independent predictor of survival from out-of-hospital shockable cardiac arrest. Circulation. 2011;124:58–66. doi: 10.1161/CIRCULATIONAHA.110.010736
23. Vaillancourt C, Everson-Stewart S, Christenson J, Andrusiek D, Powell J, Nichol G, Cheskes S, Aufderheide TP, Berg R, Stiell IG; Resuscitation Outcomes Consortium Investigators. The impact of increased chest compression fraction on return of spontaneous circulation for out-of-hospital cardiac arrest patients not in ventricular fibrillation. Resuscitation. 2011;82:1501–1507. doi: 10.1016/j.resuscitation.2011.07.011
24. Sugerman NT, Edelson DP, Leary M, Weidman EK, Herzberg DL, Vanden Hoek TL, Becker LB, Abella BS. Rescuer fatigue during actual in-hospital cardiopulmonary resuscitation with audiovisual feedback: a prospective multicenter study. Resuscitation. 2009;80:981–984. doi: 10.1016/j.resuscitation.2009.06.002
25. Manders S, Geijsel FE. Alternating providers during continuous chest compressions for cardiac arrest: every minute or every two minutes? Resuscitation. 2009;80:1015–1018. doi: 10.1016/j.resuscitation.2009.05.014
26. Jost D, Degrange H, Verret C, Hersan O, Banville IL, Chapman FW, Lank P, Petit JL, Fuilla C, Migliani R, et al; and the DEFI 2005 Work Group. DEFI 2005: a randomized controlled trial of the effect of automated external defibrillator cardiopulmonary resuscitation protocol on outcome from out-of-hospital cardiac arrest. Circulation. 2010;121:1614–1622. doi: 10.1161/CIRCULATIONAHA.109.878389
27. Beesems SG, Berdowski J, Hulleman M, Blom MT, Tijssen JG, Koster RW. Minimizing pre- and post-shock pauses during the use of an automatic external defibrillator by two different voice prompt protocols. A randomized controlled trial of a bundle of measures. Resuscitation. 2016;106:1–6. doi: 10.1016/j.resuscitation.2016.06.009
28. Rea TD, Helbock M, Perry S, Garcia M, Cloyd D, Becker L, Eisenberg M. Increasing use of cardiopulmonary resuscitation during out-of-hospital ventricular fibrillation arrest: survival implications of guideline changes. Circulation. 2006;114:2760–2765. doi: 10.1161/CIRCULATIONAHA.106.654715
29. Bobrow BJ, Clark LL, Ewy GA, Chikani V, Sanders AB, Berg RA, Richman PB, Kern KB. Minimally interrupted cardiac resuscitation by emergency medical services for out-of-hospital cardiac arrest. JAMA. 2008;299:1158–1165. doi: 10.1001/jama.299.10.1158
30. Cheskes S, Schmicker RH, Rea T, Powell J, Drennan IR, Kudenchuk P, Vaillancourt C, Conway W, Stiell I, Stub D, Davis D, Alexander N, Christenson J; Resuscitation Outcomes Consortium investigators. Chest compression fraction: A time dependent variable of survival in shockable out-of-hospital cardiac arrest. Resuscitation. 2015;97:129–135. doi: 10.1016/j.resuscitation.2015.07.003
31. Kleinman ME, Brennan EE, Goldberger ZD, Swor RA, Terry M, Bobrow BJ, Gazmuri RJ, Travers AH, Rea T. Part 5: adult basic life support and cardiopulmonary resuscitation quality: 2015 American Heart Association Guidelines Update for Cardiopulmonary Resuscitation and Emergency Cardiovascular Care. Circulation. 2015;132 (suppl 2):S414–S435. doi: 10.1161/CIR.0000000000000259
32. Considine J, Gazmuri RJ, Perkins GD, Kudenchuk PJ, Olasveengen TM, Vaillancourt C, Nishiyama C, Hatanaka T, Mancini ME, Chung SP, Escalante-Kanashiro R, Morley P. Chest compression components (rate, depth, chest wall recoil and leaning): A scoping review. Resuscitation. 2020;146:188–202. doi: 10.1016/j.resuscitation.2019.08.042
33. Stiell IG, Brown SP, Nichol G, Cheskes S, Vaillancourt C, Callaway CW, Morrison LJ, Christenson J, Aufderheide TP, Davis DP, Free C, Hostler D, Stouffer JA, Idris AH; Resuscitation Outcomes Consortium Investigators. What is the optimal chest compression depth during out-of-hospital cardiac arrest resuscitation of adult patients? Circulation. 2014;130:1962–1970. doi: 10.1161/CIRCULATIONAHA.114.008671
34. Babbs CF, Kemeny AE, Quan W, Freeman G. A new paradigm for human resuscitation research using intelligent devices. Resuscitation. 2008;77:306–315. doi: 10.1016/j.resuscitation.2007.12.018
35. Kilgannon JH, Kirchhoff M, Pierce L, Aunchman N, Trzeciak S, Roberts BW. Association between chest compression rates and clinical outcomes following in-hospital cardiac arrest at an academic tertiary hospital. Resuscitation. 2017;110:154–161. doi: 10.1016/j.resuscitation.2016.09.015
36. Abella BS, Sandbo N, Vassilatos P, Alvarado JP, O'Hearn N, Wigder HN, Hoffman P, Tynus K, Vanden Hoek TL, Becker LB. Chest compression rates during cardiopulmonary resuscitation are suboptimal: a prospective study during in-hospital cardiac arrest. Circulation. 2005;111:428–434. doi: 10.1161/01.CIR.0000153811.84257.59
37. Hwang SO, Cha KC, Kim K, Jo YH, Chung SP, You JS, Shin J, Lee HJ, Park YS, Kim S, et al. A randomized controlled trial of compression rates during cardiopulmonary resuscitation. J Korean Med Sci. 2016;31:1491–1498. doi: 10.3346/jkms.2016.31.9.1491
38. Cheskes S, Common MR, Byers AP, Zhan C, Silver A, Morrison LJ. The association between chest compression release velocity and outcomes from out-of-hospital cardiac arrest. Resuscitation. 2015;86:38–43. doi: 10.1016/j.resuscitation.2014.10.020
39. Kovacs A, Vadeboncoeur TF, Stolz U, Spaite DW, Irisawa T, Silver A, Bobrow BJ. Chest compression release velocity: Association with survival and favorable neurologic outcome after out-of-hospital cardiac arrest. Resuscitation. 2015;92:107–114. doi: 10.1016/j.resuscitation.2015.04.026
40. Yannopoulos D, McKnite S, Aufderheide TP, Sigurdsson G, Pirrallo RG, Benditt D, Lurie KG. Effects of incomplete chest wall decompression during cardiopulmonary resuscitation on coronary and cerebral perfusion pressures in a porcine model of cardiac arrest. Resuscitation. 2005;64:363–372. doi: 10.1016/j.resuscitation.2004.10.009
41. Zuercher M, Hilwig RW, Ranger-Moore J, Nysaether J, Nadkarni VM, Berg MD, Kern KB, Sutton R, Berg RA. Leaning during chest compressions impairs cardiac output and left ventricular myocardial blood flow in piglet cardiac arrest. Crit Care Med. 2010;38:1141–1146. doi: 10.1097/CCM.0b013e3181ce1fe2
42. Johnson BV, Johnson B, Coult J, Fahrenbruch C, Blackwood J, Sherman L, Kudenchuk P, Sayre M, Rea T. Cardiopulmonary resuscitation duty cycle in out-of-hospital cardiac arrest. Resuscitation. 2015;87:86–90. doi: 10.1016/j.resuscitation.2014.11.008
43. Wolfe H, Morgan RW, Donoghue A, Niles DE, Kudenchuk P, Berg RA, Nadkarni VM, Sutton RM. Quantitative analysis of duty cycle in pediatric and adolescent in-hospital cardiac arrest. Resuscitation. 2016;106:65–69. doi: 10.1016/j.resuscitation.2016.06.003
44. Berg RA, Hemphill R, Abella BS, Aufderheide TP, Cave DM, Hazinski MF, Lerner EB, Rea TD, Sayre MR, Swor RA. Part 5: adult basic life support: 2010 American Heart Association Guidelines for Cardiopulmonary Resuscitation and Emergency Cardiovascular Care. Circulation. 2010;122 (suppl 3):S685–S705. doi: 10.1161/CIRCULATIONAHA.110.970939
45. Goharani R, Vahedian-Azimi A, Farzanegan B, Bashar FR, Hajiesmaeili M, Shojaei S, Madani SJ, Gohari-Moghaddam K, Hatamian S, Mosavinasab SMM, Khoshfetrat M, Khabiri Khatir MA, Miller AC; MORZAK Collaborative. Real-time compression feedback for patients with in-hospital cardiac arrest: a multi-center randomized controlled clinical trial. J Intensive Care. 2019;7:5. doi: 10.1186/s40560-019-0357-5
46. Sutton RM, French B, Meaney PA, Topjian AA, Parshuram CS, Edelson DP, Schexnayder S, Abella BS, Merchant RM, Bembea M, Berg RA, Nadkarni VM; American Heart Association's Get With The Guidelines–Resuscitation Investigators. Physiologic monitoring of CPR quality during adult cardiac arrest: A propensity-matched cohort study. Resuscitation. 2016;106:76–82. doi: 10.1016/j.resuscitation.2016.06.018
47. Sheak KR, Wiebe DJ, Leary M, Babaeizadeh S, Yuen TC, Zive D, Owens PC, Edelson DP, Daya MR, Idris AH, Abella BS. Quantitative relationship between end-tidal carbon dioxide and CPR quality during both in-hospital and out-of-hospital cardiac arrest. Resuscitation. 2015;89:149–154. doi: 10.1016/j.resuscitation.2015.01.026
48. Paiva EF, Paxton JH, O'Neil BJ. The use of end-tidal carbon dioxide ($ETCO_2$) measurement to guide management of cardiac arrest: A systematic review. Resuscitation. 2018;123:1–7. doi: 10.1016/j.resuscitation.2017.12.003
49. Berg KM, Soar J, Andersen LW, Böttiger BW, Cacciola S, Callaway CW, Couper K, Cronberg T, D'Arrigo S, Deakin CD, et al; on behalf of the Adult Advanced Life Support Collaborators. Adult advanced life support: 2020 International Consensus on Cardiopulmonary Resuscitation and Emergency Cardiovascular Care Science With Treatment Recommendations. Circulation. 2020;142 (suppl 1):S92–S139. doi: 10.1161/CIR.0000000000000893

換気および胸骨圧迫と人工呼吸の比率

「緒言」

脈拍のある無呼吸患者に対しては，補助呼吸を実施することが重要である。心停止の患者に対する補助換気の相対的な寄与については，議論が分かれている。

動脈血酸素含量は CPR の時間が延長するにつれて減少すると考えられるため，換気補助を伴わない長時間の胸骨圧迫の実施は，従来のCPR（胸骨圧迫＋人工呼吸）ほど有効でないと懸念される。この懸念は，特に呼吸原性心停止の場合に当てはまる。これらの研究のほとんどは，EMS が短時間で対応した心原性と推定される心停止患者を対象にしていた。それ以上換気を行わないことで有害になると思われる時間閾値が存在すると予想されるため，その知見があらゆる場面に一般化できるかを慎重に検討しなければならない[1]。

高度な気道確保器具の留置後は，胸骨圧迫を継続することで胸骨圧迫の割合が高くなるが，適切な換気の実施が困難になる。圧迫と換気を同時に行うことは避ける必要があるが[2]，換気のための中断を入れずに胸骨圧迫を実施することは妥当な選択肢と考えられる[3]。最近発表されたRCT による裏付けはないが，声門上気道確保器具（SGA）を使用すると，気管チューブを使用した場合よりも心停止中の換気効率が低下するため，複雑さが増す要因となる[4,5]。

心停止時の換気の基本に関する 推奨事項

COR	LOE	推奨事項
2a	C-LD	1. 心停止中の成人に対して，1 回換気量が約 500〜600 mL，または胸の上りを目視で確認できる程度の換気を実施することは妥当である。
2a	C-EO	2. 高度な気道確保器具を留置していない患者には，口対口またはバッグマスク換気による人工呼吸を行うことが妥当である。
2b	C-EO	3. 補助呼吸を行う場合は，1 秒かけて 1 回息を吹き込み，「通常の」（深くない）息をつき，1 秒かけて次の補助呼吸を行うことを妥当としてよい。
3：有害	C-LD	4. 救助者は，CPR 中の過剰な換気（呼吸回数が多すぎる，または換気量が大きすぎる）を避ける必要がある。

「推奨事項の裏付けとなる解説」

1. 胸の上がりを目視で確認できる 1 回換気量（約 500〜600 mL）は，過度の膨張または胃膨満のリスクを最小限に抑えながら適切な換気を実施できることが，複数の研究で報告されている[6-9]。
2. 口対口の人工呼吸とバッグマスク換気のどちらでも，傷病者に対して酸素と換気が提供される[10]。口対口人工呼吸を行うには，傷病者の気道を確保し，鼻をつまみ，覆うように口と口を密着させ，人工呼吸を実施する。
3. 深くではなくいつもどおりの息を吸い込むことで，救助者はめまいや頭のふらつきを防ぐと同時に，傷病者の肺の過膨張を防止できる。人工呼吸を難しくする主な原因は，気道を十分に確保できないことにある[11]。このため，1 回目の人工呼吸を行ったときに傷病者の胸の上がりがみられない場合は，頭部後屈—あご先挙上法を行ってから，2 回目の人工呼吸を行う。1 秒という推奨事項は，CPR の中断をできる限り短時間にとどめるためである。
4. 過度の換気は不必要であり，胃膨満や逆流，誤嚥をもたらすおそれがある[12,14]。過剰な換気は，胸腔内圧の上昇，心臓への静脈還流の低下，および心拍出量の低下を招くため有害となる可能性がある[14]。

このトピックは，直近で 2010 年に正式なエビデンスレビューを受けている[15]。

心停止時の換気の基本に関する推奨事項：特殊な状況

COR	LOE	推奨事項
2a	C-LD	1. 傷病者の口を通じた換気が不可能な場合，または現実的でない場合は，口対鼻人工呼吸の実施が妥当である。
2b	C-EO	2. 気管瘻を有する傷病者が補助呼吸を必要とする場合，口対気管切開孔またはフェイスマスク（小児に推奨）対気管切開孔の人工呼吸法を妥当としてよい。

「推奨事項の裏付けとなる解説」

1. 外傷や体位，密閉状態の確保の困難により，傷病者の口を通じた換気が不可能な場合は，口対鼻人工呼吸が必要になる場合がある。症例集積研究では，成人への口対鼻人工呼吸は実施可能，安全かつ有効であることが示されている[16]。
2. 気管瘻を有する患者に対して効果的な換気を実施するには，口対気管切開孔による補助呼吸，または丸い小児用フェイスマスクにより気管切開孔との完全な密着状態を作るバッグマスク法のいずれかを使用して，気管切開孔を通じた換気が必要になる場合がある。口対気管切開孔人工呼吸法が安全，有効，あるいは実施可能であるとのエビデンスは発表されていない。ある研究によると，喉頭摘出術患者が小児用フェイスマスクを使用したところ，開口部付近の密閉度は標準的な換気マスクよりも良好であった[17]。

このトピックは，直近で 2010 年に正式なエビデンスレビューを受けている[15]。

自己心拍がある場合の換気に関する推奨事項

COR	LOE	推奨事項
2b	C-LD	1. 自己心拍再開を示す（強い脈拍を容易に触知できる）成人の傷病者に換気補助が必要な場合，医療従事者は 6 秒ごとに約 1 回，または 1 分あたり約 10 回の人工呼吸を妥当としてよい。

「推奨事項の裏付けとなる解説」

1. 成人患者に対する補助呼吸のレビューが最後に行われた 2010 年以降、従来の推奨事項の変更を支持するエビデンスは示されていない。換気補助を必要とする重篤患者の研究では、10 回/分のバッグマスク換気により、挿管前の低酸素イベントの減少が認められた[18]。

このトピックは、直近で 2010 年に正式なエビデンスレビューを受けている[15]。

胸骨圧迫と人工呼吸の比率に関する推奨事項：ALS

COR	LOE	推奨事項
2a	B-R	1. 高度な気道確保器具（声門上器具または気管チューブ）の留置前に、医療従事者が胸骨圧迫 30 回と人工呼吸 2 回の反復を伴う CPR を実施することは妥当である。
2b	B-R	2. 高度な気道確保器具の留置前に、EMS プロバイダーが継続的な胸骨圧迫を行いながら、10 回/分（6 秒ごとに 1 回）の非同期的人工呼吸を行うことは妥当としてよい。
2b	C-LD	3. 高度な気道確保器具が留置されている場合、胸骨圧迫を継続しながら 6 秒ごとに 1 回（10 回/分）の人工呼吸を行うことは妥当としてよい。
2b	C-LD	4. 目撃されたショック適応の OHCA に対して、一連の治療の一環として、最初は中断を最小限に抑えた胸骨圧迫（換気を遅らせる）を実施することは妥当としてよい。

「推奨事項の裏付けとなる解説」

1. 2017 年の ILCOR システマティックレビューでは、30 回の圧迫に対して 2 回の人工呼吸という比率が、他の比率よりも優れた生存率につながることが認められている。これは、2018 年に AHA によって再確認された推奨事項である[19,20]。このような研究のほとんどは、「一連の」心停止治療として調査を行っているため、改善が胸骨圧迫と人工呼吸の比率に起因するのか判断することは不可能である。この比率は、大規模な OHCA の RCT によって裏付けられており、30：2（圧迫の中断は 5 秒未満）という比率を使用した場合、少なくとも継続的な胸骨圧迫と同等の成果が得られている[21]。

2. ある大規模な試験では、圧迫を中断せずに 10 回/分の換気速度で治療を行った OHCA 患者の集団と、挿管前に 30：2 の比率で換気を行った集団を比較した場合、生存率および良好な神経学的転帰を伴う生存率は同様であった[21]。

3. 2017 年のシステマティックレビューでは、ヒトを対象とした 1 件の観察研究と 10 件の動物実験において、高度な気道確保器具留置後に複数の換気速度を比較していることが認められている[22]。10 回/分の換気速度による明確な有益性は認められていないが、他の速度の優位性も確認されていない。2017 年の ILCOR システマティックレビューでは、この推奨事項を変更すべき新たなエビデンスは認められておらず、『2017 AHA Focused Update on Adult BLS and CPR Quality: An Update to the AHA Guidelines for CPR and Emergency Cardiovascular Care』で繰り返されている[19,20]。

4. 2017 年の ILCOR システマティックレビューでは、中断を最小限に抑えた胸骨圧迫を含む一連の治療を支持する観察研究から得られたエビデンスは確実性が非常に低い（主に結果が未調整）ものの、そのようなアプローチをすでに実施しているシステムでは、そのまま継続してもよいと結論付けている[19]。

このような推奨事項は、成人の BLS および CPR の質に関するガイドラインに対して行われた 2017 年の重点的アップデートで支持されている[20]。

参考資料

1. Kleinman ME, Brennan EE, Goldberger ZD, Swor RA, Terry M, Bobrow BJ, Gazmuri RJ, Travers AH, Rea T. Part 5: adult basic life support and cardiopulmonary resuscitation quality: 2015 American Heart Association Guidelines Update for Cardiopulmonary Resuscitation and Emergency Cardiovascular Care.Circulation.2015;132(suppl 2):S414–S435. doi: 10.1161/CIR.0000000000000259
2. Krischer JP, Fine EG, Weisfeldt ML, Guerci AD, Nagel E, Chandra N. Comparison of prehospital conventional and simultaneous compression–ventilation cardiopulmonary resuscitation.Crit Care Med.1989;17:1263–1269. doi: 10.1097/00003246-198912000-00005
3. Jabre P, Penaloza A, Pinero D, Duchateau FX, Borron SW, Javaudin F, Richard O, de Longueville D, Bouilleau G, Devaud ML, Heidet M, Lejeune C, Fauroux S, Greingor JL, Manara A, Hubert JC, Guihard B, Vermylen O, Lievens P, Auffret Y, Maisondieu C, Huet S, Claessens B, Lapostolle F, Javaud N, Reuter PG, Baker E, Vicaut E, Adnet F. Effect of Bag-Mask Ventilation vs Endotracheal Intubation During Cardiopulmonary Resuscitation on Neurological Outcome After Out-of-Hospital Cardiorespiratory Arrest: A Randomized Clinical Trial.JAMA.2018;319:779–787. doi: 10.1001/jama.2018.0156
4. Benger JR, Kirby K, Black S, Brett SJ, Clout M, Lazaroo MJ, Nolan JP, Reeves BC, Robinson M, Scott LJ, Smartt H, South A, Stokes EA, Taylor J, Thomas M, Voss S, Wordsworth S, Rogers CA.Effect of a Strategy of a Supraglottic Airway Device vs Tracheal Intubation During Out-of-Hospital Cardiac Arrest on Functional Outcome: The AIRWAYS-2 Randomized Clinical Trial.JAMA.2018;320:779–791. doi: 10.1001/jama.2018.11597
5. Wang HE, Schmicker RH, Daya MR, Stephens SW, Idris AH, Carlson JN, Colella MR, Herren H, Hansen M, Richmond NJ, Puyana JCJ, Aufderheide TP, Gray RE, Gray PC, Verkest M, Owens PC, Brienza AM, Sternig KJ, May SJ, Sopko GR, Weisfeldt ML, Nichol G. Effect of a Strategy of Initial Laryngeal Tube Insertion vs Endotracheal Intubation on 72-Hour Survival in Adults With Out-of-Hospital Cardiac Arrest: A Randomized Clinical Trial. JAMA.2018;320:769–778. doi: 10.1001/jama.2018.7044
6. Wenzel V, Keller C, Idris AH, Dörges V, Lindner KH, Brimacombe JR.Effects of smaller tidal volumes during basic life support ventilation in patients with respiratory arrest: good ventilation, less risk? Resuscitation.1999;43:25–29. doi: 10.1016/s0300-9572(99)00118-5
7. Baskett P, Nolan J, Parr M. Tidal volumes which are perceived to be adequate for resuscitation.Resuscitation.1996;31:231–234. doi: 10.1016/0300-9572(96)00994-x
8. Dörges V, Ocker H, Hagelberg S, Wenzel V, Idris AH, Schmucker P. Smaller tidal volumes with room-air are not sufficient to ensure adequate oxygenation during bag-valve-mask ventilation.Resuscitation.2000;44:37–41. doi: 10.1016/s0300-9572(99)00161-6
9. Dörges V, Ocker H, Hagelberg S, Wenzel V, Schmucker P. Optimisation of tidal volumes given with self-inflatable bags without additional oxygen. Resuscitation.2000;43:195–199. doi: 10.1016/s0300-9572(99)00148-3
10. Wenzel V, Idris AH, Banner MJ, Fuerst RS, Tucker KJ.The composition of gas given by mouth-to-mouth ventilation during CPR. Chest.1994;106:1806–1810. doi: 10.1378/chest.106.6.1806
11. Safar P, Escarraga LA, Chang F. Upper airway obstruction in the unconscious patient.J Appl Physiol.1959;14:760–764. doi: 10.1152/jappl.1959.14.5.760

12. Berg MD, Idris AH, Berg RA.Severe ventilatory compromise due to gastric distention during pediatric cardiopulmonary resuscitation. Resuscitation.1998;36:71-73. doi: 10.1016/s0300-9572 (97)00077-4
13. Deleted in proof.
14. AufderheideTP,SigurdssonG,PirralloRG,YannopoulosD,McKniteS,vonBriesenC, SparksCW,ConradCJ,ProvoTA,LurieKG.Hyperventilation-inducedhypotension during cardiopulmonary resuscitation.Circulation.2004;109:1960-1965. doi: 10.1161/01.CIR.0000126594.79136.61
15. Berg RA, Hemphill R, Abella BS, Aufderheide TP, Cave DM, Hazinski MF, Lerner EB, Rea TD, Sayre MR, Swor RA.Part 5: adult basic life support: 2010 American Heart Association Guidelines for Cardiopulmonary Resuscitation and Emergency Cardiovascular Care.Circulation.2010;122 (suppl 3):S685-S705. doi: 10.1161/CIRCULATIONAHA.110.970939
16. Ruben H. The immediate treatment of respiratory failure.Br J Anaesth.1964;36:542-549. doi: 10.1093/bja/36.9.542
17. Bhalla RK, Corrigan A, Roland NJ.Comparison of two face masks used to deliver early ventilation to laryngectomized patients.Ear Nose Throat J. 2004;83:414, 416.
18. Casey JD, Janz DR, Russell DW, Vonderhaar DJ, Joffe AM, Dischert KM, Brown RM, Zouk AN, Gulati S, Heideman BE, et al; and the PreVent Investigators and the Pragmatic Critical Care Research Group.Bag-mask ventilation during tracheal intubation of critically ill adults.N Engl J Med.2019;380:811-821. doi: 10.1056/NEJMoa1812405
19. Ashoor HM, Lillie E, Zarin W, Pham B, Khan PA, Nincic V, Yazdi F, Ghassemi M, Ivory J, Cardoso R, Perkins GD, de Caen AR, Tricco AC; ILCOR Basic Life Support Task Force.Effectiveness of different compression-to-ventilation methods for cardiopulmonary resuscitation: A systematic review. Resuscitation.2017;118:112-125. doi: 10.1016/j.resuscitation.2017.05.032
20. Kleinman ME, Goldberger ZD, Rea T, Swor RA, Bobrow BJ, Brennan EE, Terry M, Hemphill R, Gazmuri RJ, Hazinski MF, Travers AH.2017 American Heart Association Focused Update on Adult Basic Life Support and Cardiopulmonary Resuscitation Quality: An Update to the American Heart Association Guidelines for Cardiopulmonary Resuscitation and Emergency Cardiovascular Care.Circulation.2018;137:e7-e13. doi: 10.1161/CIR.0000000000000539
21. Nichol G, Leroux B, Wang H, Callaway CW, Sopko G, Weisfeldt M, Stiell I, Morrison LJ, Aufderheide TP, Cheskes S, Christenson J, Kudenchuk P, Vaillancourt C, Rea TD, Idris AH, Colella R, Isaacs M, Straight R, Stephens S, Richardson J, Condle J, Schmicker RH, Egan D, May S, Ornato JP; ROC Investigators.Trial of Continuous or Interrupted Chest Compressions during CPR.N Engl J Med.2015;373:2203-2214. doi: 10.1056/NEJMoa1509139
22. Vissers G, Soar J, Monsieurs KG.Ventilation rate in adults with a tracheal tube during cardiopulmonary resuscitation: A systematic review. Resuscitation.2017;119:5-12. doi: 10.1016/j.resuscitation.2017.07.018

除細動

「緒言」

VF または無脈性 VT（無脈性 VT）を原因とする突然の心停止が発生した場合は，CPR だけでなく迅速な除細動の実施も生存率を高めるために不可欠である[1,2]。除細動は，VF/VT の発症後できるだけ早期に実施し，発症からショックまでの間隔が非常に短い妥当な迅速性をもって処置を行った場合に最も成功率が高くなる。反対に，VF/VT が長引き，心臓のエネルギーが失われると，リズム解析の前に決められた期間の CPR を実施して補助しない限り，除細動の効果が損なわれる。ショック前後の CPR の中断を最小限に抑えることも，最優先で考える必要がある。

現在市販されている除細動器は，それぞれ独自のショック波形を使用しており，電気特性に違いを生み出している。これにより，同じプログラムエネルギーの設定であっても異なる最大電流が供給されることになるため，装置間でショックの有効性を比較することが困難になっている。電気ショックに対応するエネルギー設定の指定も除細動器ごとに異なる。特定の波形については，装置の製造業者の推奨エネルギー量を参照すること。

CPR の継続中に基礎的な心リズムを診断し，患者管理を円滑に進められる予後情報を心室波形から引き出す技術は，現在開発中である。このような技術をルーチン使用するためには，さらなるテストと検証が必要である。

除細動の適応，タイプ，エネルギーに関する 推奨事項		
COR	LOE	推奨事項
1	B-NR	1. ショックを必要とする頻脈性不整脈の治療には，除細動器（二相性波形または単相性波形を使用）が推奨される。
2a	B-R	2. 不整脈の停止に大きな成功を収めたことから，頻脈性不整脈の治療には，単相性除細動器よりも二相性波形を使用する除細動器が推奨される。
2a	B-NR	3. 心停止が目撃されていない状況での除細動については，連続ショックよりも1 回ショック法のほうが妥当である。
2a	C-LD	4. ショック抵抗性の不整脈と推定される状況で，2 回目以降のショックにおいて固定式エネルギーと漸増式エネルギーのどちらを選択するかは，その波形に対する製造業者の具体的な指示に従うことが妥当である。不明の場合は，最大量での除細動を考慮してもよい。
2b	B-R	5. ショック抵抗性不整脈と推定される状況で，エネルギー漸増が可能な除細動器を用いる場合，2 回目以降のショックにはより高いエネルギー量を考慮してもよい。
2b	C-LD	6. VF の停止において，ある二相性波形が他の二相性波形よりも優れているという決定的エビデンスはないため，初回ショックには製造業者の推奨エネルギー量を用いることが妥当である。不明の場合は，最大量での除細動を考慮してもよい。

「推奨事項の裏付けとなる解説」

1. VF/VT およびその他の頻脈性不整脈の消失において，緊急の電気的カルジオバージョンおよび除細動は効果が高い。一貫して高い ROSC または生存率を達成するショック波形は特定されていない。二相性波形と単相性波形の臨床的予後の有効性は，同等になる可能性が高い[3]。

2. ROSC または生存率の改善において，特定の波形が優位性を持つことは証明されていない。ただし，二相性除細動器（逆の極性のパルスを供給する）は，心房細動[4] および心室性の頻脈性不整脈の停止において，患者が曝される最大電流量を単相性（単極性）除細動器と比較してはるかに低く抑えながら，同等以上の有効性を提供する[5-10,13]。このような安全性および有効性の潜在的な差から，可能な場合は二相性除細動器の使用が推奨される。単相性除細動器は現在では製造されておらず，その大部分が二相性除細動器に置き換えられている。

3. 必要に応じて複数回の「連続した」ショックを与えた後ではなく，初回ショック後ただちにCPRを再開する1回ショック法を妥当とする根拠は，複数の考慮事項に基づいている。そのようなものとして，二相性波形による初回ショックの成功率の高さ（2回目以降のショックの必要性が低減される）や，初回ショックが奏効しなかった場合にただちに2回目および3回目のショックを実施しても成功率が低下すること[14]，連続ショックによりCPRを中断する時間が長くなることなどが挙げられる。1回ショック法ではCPRの中断時間が短くなるため，「連続」ショックと比較して，生存入院率および生存退院率が大幅に向上する（1年生存率はこの限りではない）[15-17]。目撃されモニタリングされた心停止（例については，「心臓手術後の心停止」セクションを参照）の状況において，連続ショックと1回ショックのどちらの方が有効性が高いのかは不明である。

4. 波形にかかわらず，除細動の成功には，VF/VTの停止に十分なエネルギーが必要である。初回のショックでVF/VTを停止できなかった場合は，同一または漸増したエネルギー設定で繰り返すことにより，2回目以降のショックが有効性を示す場合がある[18,19]。固定式か漸増式かにかかわらず，二相性除細動を試みる際の初回または2回目以降の最適なエネルギー量の設定は明確に特定されておらず，除細動器の製造業者の指定に基づいて選択できる。

5. 除細動において，ある二相性ショック波形が他の波形に対する優位性を持つという決定的エビデンスは存在しない[20]。電気特性は二相性波形ごとに異なるため，特定の装置に対するエネルギー設定は，製造業者によって指定されているものを使用するのが妥当である。製造業者によって指定された除細動のエネルギー設定が使用時に不明な場合は，その装置の最大エネルギー量の使用を検討してもよい。

6. 市販されている除細動器は，固定式のエネルギー設定，または漸増が可能なエネルギー設定のいずれかを提供するが，どちらのアプローチでもVF/VTの停止には高い有効性を示す[18]。固定式か漸増式かにかかわらず，二相性除細動を試みる際の初回または2回目以降の最適なエネルギー量の設定は明確に特定されておらず，除細動器の製造業者の指定に従うのが最適である。固定式の150J二相性除細動と，より高いショックエネルギー量（200-300-360 J）の漸増式を比較した無作為化試験では，初回ショック後に同様の除細動の成功率および規則的な心リズムへの転換率が認められた。ただし，全体的な生存率については2つの治療群で違いが見られなかったものの，複数回のショックを必要とし，ショックエネルギー量を漸増した患者群のほうが規則的な心リズムへの転換率が大幅に高かった[19]。VF/VTが初回のショックに抵抗性を示す場合は，初回と同等またはそれ以上のエネルギー設定を検討することができる。今のところ，除細動において，ある二相性ショック波形が他の波形に対する優位性を持つという決定的エビデンスは存在しない[20]。特定の装置に対するエネルギー設定は，製造業者によって指定されているものを使用するのが妥当である。製造業者によって指定された除細動のエネルギー設定が使用時に不明な場合は，その装置の最大エネルギー量の使用を検討してもよい。

推奨事項1，2，6は，直近で2015年に正式なエビデンスレビューを受けている[21]。推奨事項3，4，および5は，BLSに関する2020年のCoSTRで支持されている[22]。

除細動器のパッドに関する 推奨事項		
COR	LOE	推奨事項
2a	C-LD	1. 成人の場合，除細動器のパドルまたはパッドは，露出した胸の前-外側部または前後方向の位置に装着し，直径が8 cmを超えるパドルまたはパッドを使用するのが妥当である。

「推奨事項の裏付けとなる解説」

1. 前-外側部，前後方向，前-左肩甲骨下，前-右肩甲骨下への電極の装着は，上室不整脈および心室不整脈の治療に比較的有効である[24-28]。大きいサイズのパッド／パドル（直径8～12 cm）を使用することで，経胸壁インピーダンスが低下する[29,30]。臨床現場では，除細動パドルの大部分が粘着性のパッドに置き換えられている。パッドを貼る前に胸部のすべての衣服と装身具を取り除く必要がある。

この推奨事項は，2020年のILCORによるスコーピングレビューで支持されており，2010年の推奨事項を更新する新しい情報は認められていない[22,31]。

自動モードと手動モードの除細動に関する 推奨事項		
COR	LOE	推奨事項
2b	C-LD	1. オペレータの一連の手技に応じて，除細動器を自動モードではなく手動モードで使用することを妥当としてよい。

「推奨事項の裏付けとなる解説」

1. AEDは，ショック適応の不整脈を高い精度で検出するが，心リズムの自動解析のためにCPRを中断する必要がある[32,33]。迅速かつ信頼性を確保しながらリズムを解析できる十分なスキルを持つオペレータが使用する場合は，手動モードの除細動のほうがリズム確認のために胸骨圧迫を中断する時間が短縮される[34,35]。

この推奨事項は，2020年のILCORによるスコーピングレビューで支持されており[22]，2010年の推奨事項を更新する新しい情報は認められていない[31]。

除細動前のCPRに関する 推奨事項		
COR	LOE	推奨事項
1	C-LD	1. 除細動器またはAEDを装着するまでは，CPRの実施が推奨される。
2a	B-R	2. 心停止がモニタリングされていない状況では，除細動器を入手し，初回のリズム解析と除細動（適応の場合）を行う準備が整うまでの間，決められた短時間のCPRを実施するのが妥当である。
2a	C-LD	3. プロバイダーが目撃した状況またはモニタリングされている状況で，短時間のVF／無脈性VTが発生した場合は，除細動器がすでに取り付けられている，あるいはすぐに入手できる状況であれば，即時に除細動を実施するのが妥当である。

「推奨事項の裏付けとなる解説」

1. 心停止を起こした患者にとって，CPRは唯一の最も重要な介入であり，除細動器を装着するまでの間は，圧迫の中断を最小限に抑えるように実施する必要がある。
2. VF/VTが数分間持続した場合は，酸素およびその他のエネルギー基質による心筋の予備力が急速に低下する。ショック前にCPRを一定時間実施して補助することで，除細動の成功率が大幅に向上する[1,2,36,37]。初回のリズム解析の前に，CPRを短時間（通常は約30秒）実施した場合と長時間（最大3分）実施した場合を比較した研究では転帰に差が見られないため，心停止がモニタリングされていない状況では，除細動器を使用する準備を整えている間，短時間のCPRを実施すれば十分であると考えられる[38-40]。モニタリングされている心停止であっても，パッドを装着し，除細動器の電源を入れ，電気ショック実施のためにコンデンサがチャージされるまでには時間がかかるため，CPRを実施すべき十分な理由はあるといえる。
3. 除細動を早期に実施することで，心停止からの転帰が改善される[41-43]。VFの持続時間が短い場合，酸素およびその他のエネルギー基質による心筋の予備力は損なわれていない可能性が高い。このような早期の電気相では，除細動に対して心リズムが最も反応しやすい[44,45]。そのため，VFがモニタリング中または目撃された状況で発症した場合で，除細動器がすでに装着されている場合，またはすぐに入手できる場合は，できるだけ早くショックを実施するのが妥当である。除細動器の入手または使用準備に時間がかかる場合は，それまでの間はCPRを実施する必要がある。

推奨事項1および2は，BLSに関する2020年のCoSTRで支持されている[22]。推奨事項3は，直近で2010年に正式なエビデンスレビューを受けている[46]。

予測に基づく除細動器のチャージに関する 推奨事項		
COR	LOE	推奨事項
2b	C-EO	1. 予定されているリズム解析の前後に実施する胸骨圧迫中に手動式除細動器をチャージすることは妥当としてよい。

「推奨事項の裏付けとなる解説」

1. 蘇生中に手動式除細動器をチャージするアプローチはさまざまある。心リズム検知のために胸骨圧迫を中断し，除細動器をチャージして電気ショック実施に備えている間も中断し続けることは珍しくない。このアプローチでは，ショック前に胸骨圧迫を中断する時間が長くなる。胸骨圧迫を継続しながら除細動器を事前チャージすることで，除細動の実施前後に胸骨圧迫を中断する時間が短縮される。この方法を有害とするエビデンスは存在しない[47]。心停止の転帰に対する事前チャージの有効性を直接的に評価した研究は存在しないものの，このような方法による圧迫中断の短縮は，VFによる心停止からの生存率向上に関連付けられる[48]。妥当としてよいのは，心リズムのチェック前に充電器をチャージする方法，または心リズムのチェック後に除細動器をチャージする間，短時間でも胸骨圧迫を再開する方法のいずれか2種類のアプローチである。どちらのアプローチでも，血流停止時間を短縮できる[49,50]。

この推奨事項は，ALSに関する2020年のCoSTRで支持されている[51]。

ショック後のリズムチェックに関する 推奨事項		
COR	LOE	推奨事項
2b	C-LD	1. 心停止患者に対し，ショック後の心リズムチェックを実施するためにCPRを中断するのではなく，ショックの実施後ただちに胸骨圧迫を再開することを妥当としてよい。

「推奨事項の裏付けとなる解説」

1. ショック後ただちに胸骨圧迫を再開することで圧迫中断時間が短縮され，蘇生中の全体的な圧迫実施時間（胸骨圧迫の割合）が増加する。これは，VFによる心停止からの生存率向上に関連付けられている[16,48]。除細動が成功した場合であっても，多くの場合，その後は心停止または無脈性電気活動が発生し，その期間はさまざまである（場合によっては長引くことがある）。この間は，心リズムおよび脈拍が戻るまでCPRを実施することが推奨される。ショック後ただちにCPRを再開することでVF/VTを再誘発するかどうかについては，議論が分かれている[52-54]。この潜在的な懸念を裏付けるエビデンス（このような方法によって生存率が低下する）は，存在しない。ショック後の動脈波形やETCO$_2$の急上昇など，自己心拍再開の生理学的なエビデンスが存在する場合，確認の心リズム解析のために胸骨圧迫を短時間中断することは妥当である。

この推奨事項は，BLSに関する2020年のCoSTRで支持されている[22]。

補助的な除細動器技術に関する 推奨事項		
COR	LOE	推奨事項
2b	C-LD	1. 胸骨圧迫中に，心電図（ECG）リズムの解析にアーチファクトフィルタリングアルゴリズムを使用することの有用性は確立されていない。
2b	C-LD	2. 心停止を発症した成人の急性期管理の指針として VF 波形解析を使用することの有用性は確立されていない。

「推奨事項の裏付けとなる解説」

1. CPR を実施すると，胸骨圧迫によって ECG 上にアーチファクトが発生するため，基礎にある心リズムの解釈があいまいになる。これによりケアの次の手順を計画するのが困難になり，薬物療法の遅延につながる可能性があるだけでなく，場合によっては推定した（ただし実際には異なる）患者の基礎心リズムに基づいて経験的に（盲目的に）判断することで，誤った指示を出してしまう可能性もある。また，心リズム解析にかかる時間により，CPR が中断される。アーチファクトフィルタリングなど，CPR を継続しながら基礎にある心リズムを明からにする革新的な手法により，このような課題を克服し，より良い治療指示を導ける診断上の利点を提供しながら，胸骨圧迫の中断を最小限に抑えることができる[55-60]。理論的な利点はあるものの，このような技術をリアルタイムの臨床環境で評価した研究や，現行の蘇生法と比較した臨床的な有効性を検証した研究は存在しない。現在のところ，フィルタリングアルゴリズムの使用は視覚的な（手動の）心リズム解析に限られており，CPR の継続中に AED で自動的に行われる VF/VT リズム検知では使用されていない。これも潜在的な用途であるが，まだテストは行われていない。さらなる臨床研究の必要性を考慮し，2020 年の ILCOR システマティックレビューでは，現時点では CPR 実施中の心リズム解析にアーチファクトフィルタリングアルゴリズムを使用することを推奨していない[51]。執筆グループでも，このような技術を臨床現場で採用する前に，より詳しい調査と臨床的な検証が必要であることを支持している。

2. VF 波形の電気特性は，時間の経過とともに変化することがわかっている[61]。VF 波形の解析は，一連の蘇生措置の実施中に，除細動またはその他の治療法の成否を予測するうえで有用である可能性がある[62-64]。VF 波形によるリアルタイムの予後解析に基づいて治療法を判断する手法は，新たな研究対象として有望であり，開発の余地がある分野である。ただし，予測的解析に基づいてショックなどの治療法を促進したり控えたりするアプローチの妥当性，信頼性，臨床的有効性は，現在のところ不明である。標準的なショック優先のプロトコールと，波形解析を指針とするショックアルゴリズムを比較した唯一の前向き臨床試験では，転帰の差は認められていない[65]。現状では蘇生ケアの指針として波形解析をルーチン使用することを支持するエビデンスは不十分であるが，臨床的検証による詳細な調査が必要かつ推奨される分野であるというのが，執筆グループのコンセンサスである。推奨事項 1 は，ALS に関する 2020 年の CoSTR で支持されている[51]。推奨事項 2 は，2020 年の ILCOR エビデンス更新で支持されており[51]，2010 年の推奨事項を更新する新しい情報は認められていない[66]。

二重連続手動式電気ショックに関する 推奨事項		
COR	LOE	推奨事項
2b	C-LD	1. 治療抵抗性ショック適応のリズムに対する，二重連続手動式電気ショックの有用性は確立されていない。

「推奨事項の裏付けとなる解説」

1. 臨床現場での二重連続手動式電気ショックについて調べたエビデンスは限られている。二重連続手動式電気ショックを実施した患者の良好な転帰は，複数の症例報告で示されている。ただし，このような症例報告は出版バイアスの影響を受けやすく，その有効性を支持する目的で使用すべきではない[67]。また，少数の観察研究では，二重連続手動式電気ショックを使用した場合と標準的な除細動を比較した場合の転帰（ROSC，生存率，神経学的転帰）には差がないことが示されている[68-71]。二重連続手動式電気ショックの使用はプロトコール化されておらず，標準的な蘇生措置が失敗した後の遅い段階で使用されることが多いため，このような研究の解釈にもやはり注意が必要である。また，公開済みの報告では，二重連続手動式電気ショックの適用について，真にショック抵抗性の（絶え間ない）VF に適用した場合と，ショック成功後の CPR 期間中に再発した VF に適用した場合を区別していないが，臨床シナリオでは後者の方が一般的である[3,7]。2020 年の ILCOR によるシステマティックレビューでは，二重連続手動式電気ショックを支持するエビデンスは認められておらず，標準的な除細動との比較により，二重連続手動式電気ショックをルーチン使用することは推奨していない[51]。3 回以上ショックを実施しても VF が持続していた 152 人の患者を対象とした最近の予備的 RCT（システマティックレビューの対象とはなっていない）では，標準的な除細動と比較して，二重連続手動式電気ショックを使用した場合，または代替の除細動パッドを貼付した場合のほうが，VF 停止および ROSC に至る確率が高くなることが認められている。ただし，このような転帰に重点が置かれた試験ではなく，患者の生存率については報告されていない[72]。二重連続手動式電気ショックについては，ショック間のタイミングやパッドの配置，手法，エネルギーを増加した場合に有害となる可能性，除細動器の損傷など，複数の疑問が解消されていない[73,74]。エビデンスが不足していることから，二重連続手動式電気ショックをルーチンの臨床診療に組み込むのは時期尚早といえる。その有用性については，臨床試験によって検討する必要がある。このような疑問の一部は，進行中の

RCT（NCT04080986）によって答えが示される可能性がある。
この推奨事項は，ALSに関する2020年のCoSTRで支持されている[51]。

参考資料

1. Larsen MP, Eisenberg MS, Cummins RO, Hallstrom AP.Predicting survival from out-of-hospital cardiac arrest: a graphic model.Ann Emerg Med.1993;22:1652-1658. doi: 10.1016/s0196-0644 (05)81302-2
2. Swor RA, Jackson RE, Cynar M, Sadler E, Basse E, Boji B, Rivera-Rivera EJ, Maher A, Grubb W, Jacobson R. Bystander CPR, ventricular fibrillation, and survival in witnessed, unmonitored out-of-hospital cardiac arrest.Ann Emerg Med.1995;25:780-784. doi: 10.1016/s0196-0644 (95)70207-5
3. Kudenchuk PJ, Cobb LA, Copass MK, Olsufka M, Maynard C, Nichol G. Transthoracic incremental monophasic versus biphasic defibrillation by emergency responders (TIMBER): a randomized comparison of monophasic with biphasic waveform ascending energy defibrillation for the resuscitation of out-of-hospital cardiac arrest due to ventricular fibrillation.Circulation.2006;114:2010-2018. doi: 10.1161/CIRCULATIONAHA.106.636506
4. Inácio JF, da Rosa Mdos S, Shah J, Rosário J, Vissoci JR, Manica AL, Rodrigues CG.Monophasic and biphasic shock for transthoracic conversion of atrial fibrillation: systematic review and network meta-analysis. Resuscitation.2016;100:66-75. doi: 10.1016/j.resuscitation.2015.12.009
5. Higgins SL, O'Grady SG, Banville I, Chapman FW, Schmitt PW, Lank P, Walker RG, Ilina M. Efficacy of lower-energy biphasic shocks for transthoracic defibrillation: a follow-up clinical study.Prehosp Emerg Care.2004;8:262-267. doi: 10.1016/j.prehos.2004.02.002
6. Didon JP, Fontaine G, White RD, Jekova I, Schmid JJ, Cansell A. Clinical experience with a low-energy pulsed biphasic waveform in out-of-hospital cardiac arrest.Resuscitation.2008;76:350-353. doi: 10.1016/j.resuscitation.2007.08.010
7. van Alem AP, Chapman FW, Lank P, Hart AA, Koster RW.A prospective, randomised and blinded comparison of first shock success of monophasic and biphasic waveforms in out-of-hospital cardiac arrest. Resuscitation.2003;58:17-24. doi: 10.1016/s0300-9572 (03)00106-0
8. Morrison LJ, Dorian P, Long J, Vermeulen M, Schwartz B, Sawadsky B, Frank J, Cameron B, Burgess R, Shield J, Bagley P, Mausz V, Brewer JE, Lerman BB; Steering Committee, Central Validation Committee, Safety and Efficacy Committee.Out-of-hospital cardiac arrest rectilinear biphasic to monophasic damped sine defibrillation waveforms with advanced life support intervention trial (ORBIT).Resuscitation.2005;66:149-157. doi: 10.1016/j.resuscitation.2004.11.031
9. Schneider T, Martens PR, Paschen H, Kuisma M, Wolcke B, Gliner BE, Russell JK, Weaver WD, Bossaert L, Chamberlain D. Multicenter, randomized, controlled trial of 150-J biphasic shocks compared with 200- to 360-J monophasic shocks in the resuscitation of out-of-hospital cardiac arrest victims.Optimized Response to Cardiac Arrest (ORCA) Investigators. Circulation.2000;102:1780-1787. doi: 10.1161/01.cir.102.15.1780
10. White RD, Hankins DG, Bugliosi TF.Seven years' experience with early defibrillation by police and paramedics in an emergency medical services system.Resuscitation.1998;39:145-151. doi: 10.1016/s0300-9572 (98)00135-x
11. Deleted in proof.
12. Deleted in proof.
13. Leng CT, Paradis NA, Calkins H, Berger RD, Lardo AC, Rent KC, Halperin HR.Resuscitation after prolonged ventricular fibrillation with use of monophasic and biphasic waveform pulses for external defibrillation. Circulation.2000;101:2968-2974. doi: 10.1161/01.cir.101.25.2968
14. Koster RW, Walker RG, Chapman FW.Recurrent ventricular fibrillation during advanced life support care of patients with prehospital cardiac arrest. Resuscitation.2008;78:252-257. doi: 10.1016/j.resuscitation.2008.03.231
15. Bobrow BJ, Clark LL, Ewy GA, Chikani V, Sanders AB, Berg RA, Richman PB, Kern KB.Minimally interrupted cardiac resuscitation by emergency medical services for out-of-hospital cardiac arrest.JAMA.2008;299:1158-1165. doi: 10.1001/jama.299.10.1158
16. Rea TD, Helbock M, Perry S, Garcia M, Cloyd D, Becker L, Eisenberg M. Increasing use of cardiopulmonary resuscitation during out-of-hospital ventricular fibrillation arrest: survival implications of guideline changes.Circulation.2006;114:2760-2765. doi: 10.1161/CIRCULATIONAHA.106.654715
17. Jost D, Degrange H, Verret C, Hersan O, Banville IL, Chapman FW, Lank P, Petit JL, Fuilla C, Migliani R, et al; and the DEFI 2005 Work Group.DEFI 2005: a randomized controlled trial of the effect of automated external defibrillator cardiopulmonary resuscitation protocol on outcome from out-of-hospital cardiac arrest.Circulation.2010;121:1614-1622. doi: 10.1161/CIRCULATIONAHA.109.878389
18. Hess EP, Russell JK, Liu PY, White RD.A high peak current 150-J fixed-energy defibrillation protocol treats recurrent ventricular fibrillation (VF) as effectively as initial VF.Resuscitation.2008;79:28-33. doi: 10.1016/j.resuscitation.2008.04.028
19. Stiell IG, Walker RG, Nesbitt LP, Chapman FW, Cousineau D, Christenson J, Bradford P, Sookram S, Berringer R, Lank P, Wells GA. BIPHASIC Trial: a randomized comparison of fixed lower versus escalating higher energy levels for defibrillation in out-of-hospital cardiac arrest.Circulation.2007;115:1511-1517. doi: 10.1161/CIRCULATIONAHA.106.648204
20. Morrison LJ, Henry RM, Ku V, Nolan JP, Morley P, Deakin CD.Single-shock defibrillation success in adult cardiac arrest: a systematic review. Resuscitation.2013;84:1480-1486. doi: 10.1016/j.resuscitation.2013.07.008
21. Link MS, Berkow LC, Kudenchuk PJ, Halperin HR, Hess EP, Moitra VK, Neumar RW, O'Neil BJ, Paxton JH, Silvers SM, et al.Part 7: adult advanced cardiovascular life support: 2015 American Heart Association Guidelines Update for Cardiopulmonary Resuscitation and Emergency Cardiovascular Care.Circulation.2015;132 (suppl 2):S444-S464. doi: 10.1161/CIR.0000000000000261
22. Olasveengen TM, Mancini ME, Perkins GD, Avis S, Brooks S, Castrén M, Chung SP, Considine J, Couper K, Escalante R, et al; on behalf of the Adult Basic Life Support Collaborators.Adult basic life support: 2020 International Consensus on Cardiopulmonary Resuscitation and Emergency Cardiovascular Care Science With Treatment Recommendations.Circulation.2020;142 (suppl 1):S41-S91. doi: 10.1161/CIR.0000000000000892
23. Deleted in proof.
24. Boodhoo L, Mitchell AR, Bordoli G, Lloyd G, Patel N, Sulke N. DC cardioversion of persistent atrial fibrillation: a comparison of two protocols. Int J Cardiol.2007;114:16-21. doi: 10.1016/j.ijcard.2005.11.108
25. Brazdzionyte J, Babarskiene RM, Stanaitiene G. Anterior-posterior versus anterior-lateral electrode position for biphasic cardioversion of atrial fibrillation.Medicina (Kaunas).2006;42:994-998.
26. Chen CJ, Guo GB.External cardioversion in patients with persistent atrial fibrillation: a reappraisal of the effects of electrode pad position and transthoracic impedance on cardioversion success.Jpn Heart J. 2003;44:921-932. doi: 10.1536/jhj.44.921
27. Stanaitiene G, Babarskiene RM. [Impact of electrical shock waveform and paddle positions on efficacy of direct current cardioversion for atrial fibrillation].Medicina (Kaunas).2008;44:665-672.
28. Krasteva V, Matveev M, Mudrov N, Prokopova R. Transthoracic impedance study with large self-adhesive electrodes in two conventional positions for defibrillation.Physiol Meas.2006;27:1009-1022. doi: 10.1088/0967-3334/27/10/007
29. Kerber RE, Grayzel J, Hoyt R, Marcus M, Kennedy J. Transthoracic resistance in human defibrillation.Influence of body weight, chest size, serial shocks, paddle size and paddle contact pressure.Circulation.1981;63:676-682. doi: 10.1161/01.cir.63.3.676
30. Connell PN, Ewy GA, Dahl CF, Ewy MD.Transthoracic impedance to defibrillator discharge.Effect of electrode size and electrode-chest wall interface.J Electrocardiol.1973;6:313-31M. doi: 10.1016/s0022-0736 (73)80053-6
31. Jacobs I, Sunde K, Deakin CD, Hazinski MF, Kerber RE, Koster RW, Morrison LJ, Nolan JP, Sayre MR, Defibrillation Chapter C. Part 6: Defibrillation: 2010 International Consensus on Cardiopulmonary Resuscitation and Emergency Cardiovascular Care Science With Treatment Recommendations.Circulation.2010;122 (Suppl 2):S325-337. doi: 10.1161/CIRCULATIONAHA.110.971010
32. Loma-Osorio P, Nunez M, Aboal J, Bosch D, Batlle P, Ruiz de Morales E, Ramos R, Brugada J, Onaga H, Morales A, et al.The Girona Territori Cardioprotegit Project: performance evaluation of public defibrillators.Rev Esp Cardiol (Engl Ed).2018;71:79-85. doi: 10.1016/j.rec.2017.04.011
33. Zijlstra JA, Bekkers LE, Hulleman M, Beesems SG, Koster RW.Automated external defibrillator and operator performance in out-of-hospital cardiac arrest.Resuscitation.2017;118:140-146. doi: 10.1016/j.resuscitation.2017.05.017
34. Kramer-Johansen J, Edelson DP, Abella BS, Becker LB, Wik L, Steen PA.Pauses in chest compression and inappropriate shocks: a comparison of manual and semi-automatic defibrillation attempts.Resuscitation.2007;73:212-220. doi: 10.1016/j.resuscitation.2006.09.006
35. Cheskes S, Hillier M, Byers A, Verbeek PR, Drennan IR, Zhan C, Morrison LJ.The association between manual mode defibrillation, pre-shock pause duration and appropriate shock delivery when employed by

basic life support paramedics during out-of-hospital cardiac arrest. Resuscitation.2015;90:61-66. doi: 10.1016/j.resuscitation.2015.02.022
36. Eftestøl T, Wik L, Sunde K, Steen PA. Effects of cardiopulmonary resuscitation on predictors of ventricular fibrillation defibrillation success during out-of-hospital cardiac arrest.Circulation.2004;110:10-15. doi: 10.1161/01.CIR.0000133323.15565.75
37. Holmberg M, Holmberg S, Herlitz J. Incidence, duration and survival of ventricular fibrillation in out-of-hospital cardiac arrest patients in sweden. Resuscitation.2000;44:7-17. doi: 10.1016/s0300-9572 (99)00155-0
38. Baker PW, Conway J, Cotton C, Ashby DT, Smyth J, Woodman RJ, Grantham H; Clinical Investigators.Defibrillation or cardiopulmonary resuscitation first for patients with out-of-hospital cardiac arrests found by paramedics to be in ventricular fibrillation? A randomised control trial. Resuscitation.2008;79:424-431. doi: 10.1016/j.resuscitation.2008.07.017
39. Jacobs IG, Finn JC, Oxer HF, Jelinek GA.CPR before defibrillation in out-of-hospital cardiac arrest: a randomized trial.Emerg Med Australas.2005;17:39-45. doi: 10.1111/j.1742-6723.2005.00694.x
40. Stiell IG, Nichol G, Leroux BG, Rea TD, Ornato JP, Powell J, Christenson J, Callaway CW, Kudenchuk PJ, Aufderheide TP, Idris AH, Daya MR, Wang HE, Morrison LJ, Davis D, Andrusiek D, Stephens S, Cheskes S, Schmicker RH, Fowler R, Vaillancourt C, Hostler D, Zive D, Pirrallo RG, Vilke GM, Sopko G, Weisfeldt M; ROC Investigators.Early versus later rhythm analysis in patients with out-of-hospital cardiac arrest.N Engl J Med.2011;365:787-797. doi: 10.1056/NEJMoa1010076
41. Bircher NG, Chan PS, Xu Y; American Heart Association's Get With The Guidelines-Resuscitation Investigators.Delays in Cardiopulmonary Resuscitation, Defibrillation, and Epinephrine Administration All Decrease Survival in In-hospital Cardiac Arrest.Anesthesiology.2019;130:414-422. doi: 10.1097/ALN.0000000000002563
42. Valenzuela TD, Roe DJ, Nichol G, Clark LL, Spaite DW, Hardman RG.Outcomes of rapid defibrillation by security officers after cardiac arrest in casinos.N Engl J Med.2000;343:1206-1209. doi: 10.1056/NEJM200010263431701
43. White RD, Asplin BR, Bugliosi TF, Hankins DG.High discharge survival rate after out-of-hospital ventricular fibrillation with rapid defibrillation by police and paramedics.Ann Emerg Med.1996;28:480-485. doi: 10.1016/s0196-0644 (96)70109-9
44. Weisfeldt ML, Becker LB.Resuscitation after cardiac arrest: a 3-phase time-sensitive model.JAMA.2002;288:3035-3038. doi: 10.1001/jama.288.23.3035
45. Kern KB, Garewal HS, Sanders AB, Janas W, Nelson J, Sloan D, Tacker WA, Ewy GA.Depletion of myocardial adenosine triphosphate during prolonged untreated ventricular fibrillation: effect on defibrillation success. Resuscitation.1990;20:221-229. doi: 10.1016/0300-9572 (90)90005-y
46. Link MS, Atkins DL, Passman RS, Halperin HR, Samson RA, White RD, Cudnik MT, Berg MD, Kudenchuk PJ, Kerber RE.Part 6: electrical therapies: automated external defibrillators, defibrillation, cardioversion, and pacing: 2010 American Heart Association Guidelines for Cardiopulmonary Resuscitation and Emergency Cardiovascular Care.Circulation.2010;122 (suppl 3):S706-S719. doi: 10.1161/CIRCULATIONAHA.110.970954
47. Edelson DP, Robertson-Dick BJ, Yuen TC, Eilevstjønn J, Walsh D, Bareis CJ, Vanden Hoek TL, Abella BS.Safety and efficacy of defibrillator charging during ongoing chest compressions: a multi-center study. Resuscitation.2010;81:1521-1526. doi: 10.1016/j.resuscitation.2010.07.014
48. Cheskes S, Schmicker RH, Christenson J, Salcido DD, Rea T, Powell J, Edelson DP, Sell R, May S, Menegazzi JJ, Van Ottingham L, Olsufka M, Pennington S, Simonini J, Berg RA, Stiell I, Idris A, Bigham B, Morrison L; Resuscitation Outcomes Consortium (ROC) Investigators.Perishock pause: an independent predictor of survival from out-of-hospital shockable cardiac arrest.Circulation.2011;124:58-66. doi: 10.1161/CIRCULATIONAHA.110.010736
49. Hansen LK, Folkestad L, Brabrand M. Defibrillator charging before rhythm analysis significantly reduces hands-off time during resuscitation: a simulation study.Am J Emerg Med.2013;31:395-400. doi: 10.1016/j.ajem.2012.08.029
50. Kemper M, Zech A, Lazarovici M, Zwissler B, Prückner S, Meyer O. Defibrillator charging before rhythm analysis causes peri-shock pauses exceeding guideline recommended maximum 5 s: A randomized simulation trial. Anaesthesist.2019;68:546-554. doi: 10.1007/s00101-019-0623-x
51. Berg KM, Soar J, Andersen LW, Böttiger BW, Cacciola S, Callaway CW, Couper K, Cronberg T, D'Arrigo S, Deakin CD, et al; on behalf of the Adult Advanced Life Support Collaborators.Adult advanced life support: 2020 International Consensus on Cardiopulmonary Resuscitation and Emergency Cardiovascular Care Science With Treatment Recommendations.Circulation.2020;142 (suppl 1):S92-S139. doi: 10.1161/CIR.0000000000000893
52. Berdowski J, ten Haaf M, Tijssen JG, Chapman FW, Koster RW.Time in recurrent ventricular fibrillation and survival after out-of-hospital cardiac arrest.Circulation.2010;122:1101-1108. doi: 10.1161/CIRCULATIONAHA.110.958173
53. Hess EP, White RD.Ventricular fibrillation is not provoked by chest compression during post-shock organized rhythms in out-of-hospital cardiac arrest.Resuscitation.2005;66:7-11. doi: 10.1016/j.resuscitation.2005.01.011
54. Berdowski J, Tijssen JG, Koster RW.Chest compressions cause recurrence of ventricular fibrillation after the first successful conversion by defibrillation in out-of-hospital cardiac arrest.Circ Arrhythm Electrophysiol.2010;3:72-78. doi: 10.1161/CIRCEP.109.902114
55. Li Y, Bisera J, Tang W, Weil MH.Automated detection of ventricular fibrillation to guide cardiopulmonary resuscitation.Crit Pathw Cardiol.2007;6:131-134. doi: 10.1097/HPC.0b013e31813429b0
56. Tan Q, Freeman GA, Geheb F, Bisera J. Electrocardiographic analysis during uninterrupted cardiopulmonary resuscitation.Crit Care Med.2008;36 (11 Suppl):S409-S412. doi: 10.1097/ccm.0b013e31818a7fbf
57. Li Y, Bisera J, Weil MH, Tang W. An algorithm used for ventricular fibrillation detection without interrupting chest compression.IEEE Trans Biomed Eng. 2012;59:78-86. doi: 10.1109/TBME.2011.2118755
58. Babaeizadeh S, Firoozabadi R, Han C, Helfenbein ED.Analyzing cardiac rhythm in the presence of chest compression artifact for automated shock advisory.J Electrocardiol.2014;47:798-803. doi: 10.1016/j.jelectrocard.2014.07.021
59. Fumagalli F, Silver AE, Tan Q, Zaidi N, Ristagno G. Cardiac rhythm analysis during ongoing cardiopulmonary resuscitation using the Analysis During Compressions with Fast Reconfirmation technology.Heart Rhythm.2018;15:248-255. doi: 10.1016/j.hrthm.2017.09.003
60. Hu Y, Tang H, Liu C, Jing D, Zhu H, Zhang Y, Yu X, Zhang G, Xu J. The performance of a new shock advisory algorithm to reduce interruptions during CPR.Resuscitation.2019;143:1-9. doi: 10.1016/j.resuscitation.2019.07.026
61. Asano Y, Davidenko JM, Baxter WT, Gray RA, Jalife J. Optical mapping of drug-induced polymorphic arrhythmias and torsade de pointes in the isolated rabbit heart.J Am Coll Cardiol.1997;29:831-842. doi: 10.1016/s0735-1097 (96)00588-8
62. Callaway CW, Sherman LD, Mosesso VN Jr, Dietrich TJ, Holt E, Clarkson MC.Scaling exponent predicts defibrillation success for out-of-hospital ventricular fibrillation cardiac arrest. Circulation.2001;103:1656-1661. doi: 10.1161/01.cir.103.12.1656
63. Coult J, Blackwood J, Sherman L, Rea TD, Kudenchuk PJ, Kwok H. Ventricular Fibrillation Waveform Analysis During Chest Compressions to Predict Survival From Cardiac Arrest.Circ Arrhythm Electrophysiol.2019;12:e006924. doi: 10.1161/CIRCEP.118.006924
64. Coult J, Kwok H, Sherman L, Blackwood J, Kudenchuk PJ, Rea TD.Ventricular fibrillation waveform measures combined with prior shock outcome predict defibrillation success during cardiopulmonary resuscitation.J Electrocardiol.2018;51:99-106. doi: 10.1016/j.jelectrocard.2017.07.016
65. Freese JP, Jorgenson DB, Liu PY, Innes J, Matallana L, Nammi K, Donohoe RT, Whitbread M, Silverman RA, Prezant DJ.Waveform analysis-guided treatment versus a standard shock-first protocol for the treatment of out-of-hospital cardiac arrest presenting in ventricular fibrillation: results of an international randomized, controlled trial.Circulation.2013;128:995-1002. doi: 10.1161/CIRCULATIONAHA.113.003273
66. Neumar RW, Otto CW, Link MS, Kronick SL, Shuster M, Callaway CW, Kudenchuk PJ, Ornato JP, McNally B, Silvers SM, et al.Part 8: adult advanced cardiovascular life support: 2010 American Heart Association Guidelines for Cardiopulmonary Resuscitation and Emergency Cardiovascular Care.Circulation.2010;122:S729-S767. doi: 10.1161/CIRCULATIONAHA.110.970988
67. Clemency BM, Pastwik B, Gillen D. Double sequential defibrillation and the tyranny of the case study.Am J Emerg Med.2019;37:792-793. doi: 10.1016/j.ajem.2018.09.002
68. Beck LR, Ostermayer DG, Ponce JN, Srinivasan S, Wang HE.Effectiveness of Prehospital Dual Sequential Defibrillation for Refractory Ventricular Fibrillation and Ventricular Tachycardia Cardiac Arrest.Prehosp Emerg Care.2019;23:597-602. doi: 10.1080/10903127.2019.1584256
69. Mapp JG, Hans AJ, Darrington AM, Ross EM, Ho CC, Miramontes DA, Harper SA, Wampler DA; Prehospital Research and Innovation in Military and Expeditionary Environments (PRIME) Research Group.Prehospital Double Sequential Defibrillation: A Matched Case-Control Study.Acad Emerg Med.2019;26:994-1001. doi: 10.1111/acem.13672

70. Ross EM, Redman TT, Harper SA, Mapp JG, Wampler DA, Miramontes DA. Dual defibrillation in out-of-hospital cardiac arrest: A retrospective cohort analysis. Resuscitation.2016;106:14–17. doi: 10.1016/j.resuscitation.2016.06.011
71. Emmerson AC, Whitbread M, Fothergill RT.Double sequential defibrillation therapy for out-of-hospital cardiac arrests: The London experience. Resuscitation.2017;117:97–101. doi: 10.1016/j.resuscitation.2017.06.011
72. Cheskes S, Dorian P, Feldman M, McLeod S, Scales DC, Pinto R, Turner L, Morrison LJ, Drennan IR, Verbeek PR.Double sequential external defibrillation for refractory ventricular fibrillation: the DOSE VF pilot randomized controlled trial.Resuscitation.2020;150:178–184. doi: 10.1016/j.resuscitation.2020.02.010
73. Gerstein NS, McLean AR, Stecker EC, Schulman PM.External Defibrillator Damage Associated With Attempted Synchronized Dual-Dose Cardioversion.Ann Emerg Med.2018;71:109–112. doi: 10.1016/j.annemergmed.2017.04.005
74. Kudenchuk PJ.Shocking insights on double defibrillation: How, when and why not? Resuscitation.2019;140:209–210. doi: 10.1016/j.resuscitation.2019.05.022

心停止に対するその他の電気的または擬似電気的治療

「緒言」

心停止中に実施可能な治療オプションとしては，除細動に加え，複数のその他の電気的および擬似電気的治療が調査されてきた。徐脈性心静止リズムを伴う心停止については，経皮ペーシングが研究されている。理論的には，心臓が電気的な刺激に反応することで心筋収縮を起こし，順方向の血液の流れを生み出すが，臨床試験では，ペーシングによる患者転帰の改善は示されていない。

咳CPRや拳（連続叩打）によるペーシング，前胸部叩打法など，その他の擬似電気的治療は，すべて一時的な措置として説明されており，決定的治療をただちに実施できない場合に，心肺停止直前または心停止の目撃から最初の数秒以内（咳CPRについては意識を失う前）の限られた患者に対して実施するものとされている。前胸部叩打法では，固く握った拳の尺側を使って，胸骨中央部に鋭く高速な打撃（つまり「パンチ」）を1回だけ加える。前胸部叩打法は，ベースにある頻脈性不整脈の停止を期待して，衝撃によって低エネルギーショックと同様の電気エネルギーを心臓に伝えることを目的としている。

拳（連続叩打）ペーシングでは，握った拳を使って，連続した律動性のある比較的低速な衝撃を胸骨に与える[1]。拳ペーシングは，心筋の脱分極を起こすのに十分な電気刺激を与える試みとして実施する。咳CPRは，大動脈圧および心内圧を上昇させる試みとして，深い呼吸の直後に咳を数秒ごとに繰り返す行為とされており，意識を失う前に血行動態の一時的な補助を提供する。

電気ペーシングに関する 推奨事項		
COR	LOE	推奨事項
3：利益なし	B-R	1. 心停止が確定した場合，電気ペーシングのルーチン使用は推奨されない。

「推奨事項の裏付けとなる解説」

1. 観察研究およびRCTのデータを含め，既存のエビデンスでは，経皮的，経静脈的，または経心筋的なアプローチによるペーシングを行っても，心停止が確定してからのROSC率または生存率は向上しないことが示唆されている。これは，ペーシングを実施するタイミングや心停止を発症した場所（院内または院外），主要な心リズム（心停止，無脈性電気活動）を問わない[2-6]。ペーシングの成否を評価している間に胸骨圧迫の中断が長引いた場合も，生存率に悪影響を及ぼす可能性がある。ペーシングを開始するタイミングが成否に影響するかどうかは不明であり，その有用性は，目撃およびモニタリングされているケース（「心臓手術後の心停止」セクションを参照）の最初の数秒に限定される可能性がある。上記の特殊な環境に関連する心停止中にペーシングを試みる場合，プロバイダーは，特に電気的および機械的捕捉の評価時に，質の高いCPRを犠牲にするパフォーマンスを避けるように注意する必要がある。このトピックは，直近で2010年に正式なエビデンスレビューを受けている[7]。

前胸部叩打法に関する 推奨事項		
COR	LOE	推奨事項
2b	B-NR	1. 前胸部叩打法は，救助者によって目撃されモニタリングされた不安定な心室頻拍性不整脈の発症で，除細動器がただちに使用できない場合に検討できるが，CPRまたは電気ショックの実施を遅らせないようにする。
3：利益なし	C-LD	2. 心停止が確定している場合は，前胸部叩打法をルーチン使用しないこと。

「推奨事項の裏付けとなる解説」

1および2. 前胸部叩打法は，「拳で打つ」機械的な力を，（力の大きさに応じて）ペーシングの刺激または超低エネルギーのショックと同様の電気エネルギーとして心臓に伝えることを目的としている。このような仕組みは，電気機械変換と呼ばれる[1]。院外または院内環境でのルーチンの心停止ケアで前胸部叩打法を使用した場合に，ROSC率または生存退院率が向上するというエビデンスは存在しない[8-12]。有益な可能性があるのは，救助者によって目撃されモニタリングされているイベント，または管理下にある検査室環境など，不整脈が低エネルギーでも停止しやすいVT発症の超早期の段階のみであるが，そのような状況でさえ，あまり効果はない[13]。前胸部叩打が有害のエビデンスなしで成功したという症例報告も存在するが[9,14,15]，規則的な心リズムの中で電気的に脆弱な部分（T波）で実施してしまった場合，拳での打撃（非同期電気ショックと同様）により心リズムが速まる，またはVFへの転換が発生するリスク[16-19]（心臓振盪と同様）が高まる[20]。そのため，

拳での打撃が単回の短時間の介入として、特定の環境（心停止が救助者によって目撃され、モニターによって VF/VT が原因であることが確定的であり、除細動器をすぐに使用できない場合）において有用であると考えられる場合であっても、それによって CPR の実施や除細動器の使用を遅らせてはならない。

これらの推奨事項は、BLS に関する 2020 年の CoSTR で支持されている[21]。

COR	LOE	推奨事項
2b	C-LD	1. 目撃およびモニタリングされた病院内（心臓カテーテル室など）での心停止といった例外的な状況において、徐脈性心停止患者に対する拳（パーカッション）によるペーシングは、患者の意識消失前であり、その後遅滞なく決定的治療を行うのであれば、一時的な措置として考慮してもよい。

拳／パーカッションペーシングに関する 推奨事項

「推奨事項の裏付けとなる解説」

1. 拳（連続叩打）によるペーシングは、脱分極と心筋収縮を促し、脈拍を回復させるだけの十分な電気刺激を与えることを目的として実施される。多数の症例報告および症例収集研究によって、心停止事象または「生命を脅かす徐脈性」事象の発生時における拳ペーシングの使用が検証されている[1,22-25]。その結果良好な生存転帰が得られ[22]、ROSC が認められたことが確認されている[23]。ただし、これらのいずれも対照試験や比較試験ではなく、拳ペーシングの使用そのものが標準治療と比較して ROSC 率や生存率を向上させたかどうかは不明である。心停止患者に対し、拳ペーシングの果たし得る役割はない。

この推奨事項は、BLS に関する 2020 年の CoSTR で支持されている[21]。

咳 CPR に関する 推奨事項

COR	LOE	推奨事項
2b	C-LD	1. 「咳」CPR は、目撃およびモニタリングされた状況で発症した、血行動態に有意な影響を与える頻脈性不整脈または徐脈性不整脈において、患者の意識消失前であり、その後遅滞なく決定的治療を行うのであれば、一時的な措置として考慮してもよい。

「推奨事項の裏付けとなる解説」

1. 定義上、咳 CPR は意識のない患者には使用できないが、どのような状況においても、質の高い CPR を実施するための時間、労力、注意がそがれてしまうようなら、咳 CPR の実施は有害となりうることを強調することが重要である。咳 CPR は、患者が意識を失う前に、深吸気に続けて咳を数秒ごとに繰り返し行わせる手法と説明される。この手法は、意識のある協力的な患者（この実施方法について事前に指導を受けていることが望ましい）が血行動態に重大な影響を与える不整脈を発症した場合にのみ、決定的治療への橋渡しとして有効である。咳 CPR と標準的な蘇生処置とを比較した研究は行われていない。症例報告および症例収集研究から得られたエビデンスは限定的だが、意識のある患者が頻脈性不整脈または徐脈性不整脈を発症した際に咳 CPR を実施した場合に、大動脈圧および心内圧が一時的に上昇したことが示されている[10,26-28]。これらの試験の難点は、大きな選択バイアスがあり、比較群が存在せず、他の治療による交絡効果が制御されていないため、解釈が難しいことである。

この推奨事項は、BLS に関する 2020 年の CoSTR で支持されている[21]。

参考資料

1. Tucker KJ, Shaburihvili TS, Gedevanishvili AT.Manual external (fist) pacing during high-degree atrioventricular block: a lifesaving intervention.Am J Emerg Med.1995;13:53-54. doi: 10.1016/0735-6757(95)90243-0
2. Sherbino J, Verbeek PR, MacDonald RD, Sawadsky BV, McDonald AC, Morrison LJ.Prehospital transcutaneous cardiac pacing for symptomatic bradycardia or bradyasystolic cardiac arrest: a systematic review.Resuscitation.2006;70:193-200. doi: 10.1016/j.resuscitation.2005.11.019
3. White JD, Brown CG.Immediate transthoracic pacing for cardiac asystole in an emergency department setting.Am J Emerg Med.1985;3:125-128. doi: 10.1016/0735-6757(85)90034-8
4. Hedges JR, Syverud SA, Dalsey WC, Feero S, Easter R, Shultz B. Prehospital trial of emergency transcutaneous cardiac pacing.Circulation.1987;76:1337-1343. doi: 10.1161/01.cir.76.6.1337
5. Barthell E, Troiano P, Olson D, Stueven HA, Hendley G. Prehospital external cardiac pacing: a prospective, controlled clinical trial.Ann Emerg Med.1988;17:1221-1226. doi: 10.1016/s0196-0644(88)80074-x
6. Cummins RO, Graves JR, Larsen MP, Hallstrom AP, Hearne TR, Ciliberti J, Nicola RM, Horan S. Out-of-hospital transcutaneous pacing by emergency medical technicians in patients with asystolic cardiac arrest.N Engl J Med.1993;328:1377-1382. doi: 10.1056/NEJM199305133281903
7. Neumar RW, Otto CW, Link MS, Kronick SL, Shuster M, Callaway CW, Kudenchuk PJ, Ornato JP, McNally B, Silvers SM, et al.Part 8: adult advanced cardiovascular life support: 2010 American Heart Association Guidelines for Cardiopulmonary Resuscitation and Emergency Cardiovascular Care.Circulation.2010;122:S729-S767. doi: 10.1161/CIRCULATIONAHA.110.970988
8. Nehme Z, Andrew E, Bernard SA, Smith K. Treatment of monitored out-of-hospital ventricular fibrillation and pulseless ventricular tachycardia utilising the precordial thump.Resuscitation.2013;84:1691-1696. doi: 10.1016/j.resuscitation.2013.08.011
9. Pellis T, Kette F, Lovisa D, Franceschino E, Magagnin L, Mercante WP, Kohl P. Utility of pre-cordial thump for treatment of out of hospital cardiac arrest: a prospective study.Resuscitation.2009;80:17-23. doi: 10.1016/j.resuscitation.2008.10.018
10. Caldwell G, Millar G, Quinn E, Vincent R, Chamberlain DA.Simple mechanical methods for cardioversion: defence of the precordial thump and cough version.BMJ.(Clin Res Ed).1985;291:627-630. doi: 10.1136/bmj.291.6496.627
11. Gertsch M, Hottinger S, Hess T. Serial chest thumps for the treatment of ventricular tachycardia in patients with coronary artery disease.Clin Cardiol.1992;15:181-188. doi: 10.1002/clc.4960150309
12. Rajagopalan RS, Appu KS, Sultan SK, Jagannadhan TG, Nityanandan K, Sethuraman S. Precordial thump in ventricular tachycardia.J Assoc Physicians India.1971;19:725-729.
13. Haman L, Parizek P, Vojacek J. Precordial thump efficacy in termination of induced ventricular arrhythmias.Resuscitation.2009;80:14-16. doi: 10.1016/j.resuscitation.2008.07.022
14. Befeler B. Mechanical stimulation of the heart: its therapeutic value in tachyarrhythmias.Chest.1978;73:832-838. doi: 10.1378/chest.73.6.832
15. Volkmann H, Klumbies A, Kühnert H, Paliege R, Dannberg G, Siegert K. [Terminating ventricular tachycardias by mechanical heart stimulation with precordial thumps].Z Kardiol.1990;79:717-724.

16. Morgera T, Baldi N, Chersevani D, Medugno G, Camerini F. Chest thump and ventricular tachycardia.Pacing Clin Electrophysiol.1979;2:69-75. doi: 10.1111/j.1540-8159.1979.tb05178.x
17. Krijne R. Rate acceleration of ventricular tachycardia after a precordial chest thump.Am J Cardiol.1984;53:964-965. doi: 10.1016/0002-9149(84)90539-3
18. Sclarovsky S, Kracoff OH, Agmon J. Acceleration of ventricular tachycardia induced by a chest thump.Chest.1981;80:596-599. doi: 10.1378/chest.80.5.596
19. Yakaitis RW, Redding JS.Precordial thumping during cardiac resuscitation. Crit Care Med.1973;1:22-26. doi: 10.1097/00003246-197301000-00004
20. Link MS, Maron BJ, Wang PJ, VanderBrink BA, Zhu W, Estes NA III.Upper and lower limits of vulnerability to sudden arrhythmic death with chest-wall impact (commotio cordis).J Am Coll Cardiol.2003;41:99-104. doi: 10.1016/s0735-1097(02)02669-4
21. Olasveengen TM, Mancini ME, Perkins GD, Avis S, Brooks S, Castrén M, Chung SP, Considine J, Couper K, Escalante R, et al; on behalf of the Adult Basic Life Support Collaborators.Adult basic life support: 2020 International Consensus on Cardiopulmonary Resuscitation and Emergency Cardiovascular Care Science With Treatment Recommendations.Circulation.2020;142 (suppl 1):S41-S91. doi: 10.1161/CIR.0000000000000892
22. Klumbies A, Paliege R, Volkmann H. [Mechanical emergency stimulation in asystole and extreme bradycardia].Z Gesamte Inn Med.1988;43:348-352.
23. Iseri LT, Allen BJ, Baron K, Brodsky MA.Fist pacing, a forgotten procedure in bradyasystolic cardiac arrest.Am Heart J. 1987;113:1545-1550. doi: 10.1016/0002-8703(87)90697-1
24. Paliege R, Volkmann H, Klumbies A. The fist as a pacemaker for the heart—investigations about the mechanical stimulation of the heart in case of emergency.Deutsche Gesundheitswesen Zeitschrift für Klinische Medizin.1982;37:1094-1100.
25. Scherf D, Bornemann C. Thumping of the precordium in ventricular standstill. Am J Cardiol.1960;5:30-40. doi: 10.1016/0002-9149(60)90006-0
26. Petelenz T, Iwiński J, Chlebowczyk J, Czyz Z, Flak Z, Fiutowski L, Zaorski K, Petelenz T, Zeman S. Self-administered cough cardiopulmonary resuscitation (c-CPR) in patients threatened by MAS events of cardiovascular origin. Wiad Lek.1998;51:326-336.
27. Niemann JT, Rosborough J, Hausknecht M, Brown D, Criley JM.Cough-CPR: documentation of systemic perfusion in man and in an experimental model: a "window" to the mechanism of blood flow in external CPR.Crit Care Med.1980;8:141-146. doi: 10.1097/00003246-198003000-00011
28. Marozsán I, Albared JL, Szatmáry LJ.Life-threatening arrhythmias stopped by cough.Cor Vasa.1990;32:401-408.

血管確保

心停止管理での血管路確保に関する 推奨事項

COR	LOE	推奨事項
2a	B-NR	1. 心停止において，薬物投与のためにプロバイダーが最初に静脈路を確保することは妥当である。
2b	B-NR	2. 静脈路の確保が成功しないまたは可能でない場合，骨髄路の確保を考慮する。
2b	C-LD	3. 静脈路および骨髄路の確保が成功しないまたは可能でない場合，適切な訓練を受けたプロバイダーであれば，中心静脈路の確保を考慮する。
2b	C-LD	4. その他の投与経路が使用できない場合，気管内薬物投与を考慮する。

「概要」

緊急薬物療法を実施するための従来的なアプローチは，末梢静脈路を使用する手法である。しかし，緊急状態で静脈路を確保することは，患者の特性や術者の経験によっては困難であり，薬物投与の遅延を招きかねない。

緊急の薬物投与では，静脈路の代わりに骨髄路，中心静脈路，心臓内投与，気管内投与を使用できる。心臓内薬物投与は，『AHA 心肺蘇生と救急心血管治療のためのガイドライン 2000』では推奨していない。この措置にはきわめて専門的な一連の手技が必要とされ，合併症発生の可能性があり，利用できる投与経路が他にも存在するためである[1,2]。気管内薬物投与は血中濃度の低下につながり，予想外の薬理作用が生じるため，他の投与経路が利用できるなら非推奨となる場合が多い。中心静脈路は，必要な一連の手技を獲得および維持するには適切なトレーニングが必要とされることから，主に病院内で使用される。

骨髄路は比較的簡単かつ迅速に使用でき，静脈路確保より留置成功率が高く，施行の伴うリスクも比較的低いことから，広く使用されるようになりつつある。しかし，心停止において静脈路と骨髄路での薬物投与の有効性に差があるかどうかは，まだ十分に解明されていない。

「推奨事項の裏付けとなる解説」

1. 蘇生中に薬物および輸液を緊急投与する場合の血管確保では，末梢静脈路が従来的なアプローチとして使用されてきた。緊急薬物の薬物動態特性，急性効果，臨床有効性は，主に静脈内投与された場合に記録されたものである[3-6]。静脈路は優先的に使用され，通常は確保可能であり，薬物反応が予測でき，血管確保として妥当な初期アプローチである。

2. CPR 中の薬物骨髄内投与の有効性に関する情報が不足していると 2010 年に認識されたものの，これ以降，骨髄路の使用は一般的になりつつある。緊急時の血管確保において，骨髄路は第一選択の投与経路として使用されることが多くなっている。2020 年の ILCOR によるシステマティックレビュー[7] では，心停止における静脈路と骨髄路（主に脛骨前面からの穿刺）での薬物投与を比較しているが，5 件の後ろ向き試験で，静脈投与での臨床転帰が骨髄内投与より良好であったことが確認されている[8-12]。これらの試験には重大なバイアスがあり，特に骨髄路確保の必要性が，予後不良の危険因子となる患者の特性や心停止の特性と関連しているというバイアスがあった。このシステマティックレビューには，2 件の RCT に基づく静脈路と骨髄路を比較したサブグループ解析も含まれる。これらの解析では，投与経路による効果の違いには，統計的に有意な差は確認されなかった。静脈路のほうが有利であると推定されるが，PARAMEDIC2 試験での ROSC 率は例外で，いずれの投与経路でもアドレナリンの効果は類似していた[13,14]。これらの研究では，骨髄路はほぼ常に脛骨前面であった

ため，骨髄内投与においては部位特異性も問題となりうる。執筆グループはこのような結果を基に，末梢静脈路の確保は依然として妥当な初期アプローチであるが，静脈路の確保が成功しないか，または不可能な場合は骨髄路の確保を考慮すると結論付けた。薬物の静脈内投与の有効性を，骨髄内投与（脛骨および上腕骨）と比較して評価するには，さらなる研究が必要である。

3. 中心静脈路（内頸静脈または鎖骨下静脈）からの薬物投与は，末梢静脈内投与より最高血中濃度が高く，循環時間も速い[15-17]。しかし，この 2 つの投与経路による臨床転帰を比較したデータは，現時点ではまだ得られていない。中心経路は合併症発生率の上昇に関連付けられ，実施に時間がかかり，場合によってはCPRを中断しなければならないこともある。このアプローチは現在では主に病院内で使用され，静脈路および骨髄路の確保に失敗した場合，またはこれらを使用できない場合に，熟練したプロバイダーによる実施を考慮できる。

4. 薬物の気管内投与は，予測不可の（一般的には低い）薬物濃度[18-20] および低い ROSC 率[21]に関連付けられるため，最終手段としての薬物投与経路とみなされる。

推奨事項 1 および 2 は，ALS に関する 2020 年の CoSTR で支持されている[22]。推奨事項 3 および 4 は，直近で 2010 年に正式なエビデンスレビューを受けている[20]。

参考資料

1. The American Heart Association in collaboration with the International Liaison Committee on Resuscitation.Guidelines 2000 for Cardiopulmonary Resuscitation and Emergency Cardiovascular Care.Part 6: advanced cardiovascular life support: section 6: pharmacology II: agents to optimize cardiac output and blood pressure.Circulation.2000;102 (suppl):I129-I135.
2. Aitkenhead AR.Drug administration during CPR: what route? Resuscitation.1991;22:191-195. doi: 10.1016/0300-9572 (91)90011-m
3. Collinsworth KA, Kalman SM, Harrison DC.The clinical pharmacology of lidocaine as an antiarrhythmic drug.Circulation.1974;50:1217-1230. doi: 10.1161/01.cir.50.6.1217
4. Greenblatt DJ, Bolognini V, Koch-Weser J, Harmatz JS.Pharmacokinetic approach to the clinical use of lidocaine intravenously.JAMA.1976;236:273-277.
5. Riva E, Gerna M, Latini R, Giani P, Volpi A, Maggioni A. Pharmacokinetics of amiodarone in man.J Cardiovasc Pharmacol.1982;4:264-269. doi: 10.1097/00005344-198203000-00015
6. Orlowski JP, Porembka DT, Gallagher JM, Lockrem JD, VanLente F. Comparison study of intraosseous, central intravenous, and peripheral intravenous infusions of emergency drugs.Am J Dis Child.1990;144:112-117. doi: 10.1001/archpedi.1990.02150250124049
7. Granfeldt A, Avis SR, Lind PC, Holmberg MJ, Kleinman M, Maconochie I, Hsu CH, Fernanda de Almeida M, Wang TL, Neumar RW, AndersenLW.Intravenousvs.intraosseousadministrationofdrugsduringcardiac arrest: A systematic review.Resuscitation.2020;149:150-157. doi: 10.1016/j.resuscitation.2020.02.025
8. Feinstein BA, Stubbs BA, Rea T, Kudenchuk PJ.Intraosseous compared to intravenous drug resuscitation in out-of-hospital cardiac arrest.Resuscitation.2017;117:91-96. doi: 10.1016/j.resuscitation.2017.06.014
9. Kawano T, Grunau B, Scheuermeyer FX, Gibo K, Fordyce CB, Lin S, Stenstrom R, Schlamp R, Jenneson S, Christenson J. Intraosseous Vascular Access Is Associated With Lower Survival and Neurologic Recovery Among Patients With Out-of-Hospital Cardiac Arrest.Ann Emerg Med.2018;71:588-596. doi: 10.1016/j.annemergmed.2017.11.015
10. Clemency B, Tanaka K, May P, Innes J, Zagroba S, Blaszak J, Hostler D, Cooney D, McGee K, Lindstrom H. Intravenous vs. intraosseous access and return of spontaneous circulation during out of hospital cardiac arrest.Am J Emerg Med.2017;35:222-226. doi: 10.1016/j.ajem.2016.10.052
11. Nguyen L, Suarez S, Daniels J, Sanchez C, Landry K, Redfield C. Effect of Intravenous Versus Intraosseous Access in Prehospital Cardiac Arrest.Air Med J. 2019;38:147-149. doi: 10.1016/j.amj.2019.02.005
12. Mody P, Brown SP, Kudenchuk PJ, Chan PS, Khera R, Ayers C, Pandey A, Kern KB, de Lemos JA, Link MS, Idris AH.Intraosseous versus intravenous access in patients with out-of-hospital cardiac arrest: Insights from the resuscitation outcomes consortium continuous chest compression trial.Resuscitation.2019;134:69-75. doi: 10.1016/j.resuscitation.2018.10.031
13. Daya MR, Leroux BG, Dorian P, Rea TD, Newgard CD, Morrison LJ, Lupton JR, Menegazzi JJ, Ornato JP, Sopko G, Christenson J, Idris A, Mody P, Vilke GM, Herdeman C, Barbic D, Kudenchuk PJ; Resuscitation Outcomes Consortium Investigators.Survival After Intravenous Versus Intraosseous Amiodarone, Lidocaine, or Placebo in Out-of-Hospital Shock-Refractory Cardiac Arrest.Circulation.2020;141:188-198. doi: 10.1161/CIRCULATIONAHA.119.042240
14. Nolan JP, Deakin CD, Ji C, Gates S, Rosser A, Lall R, Perkins GD.Intraosseous versus intravenous administration of adrenaline in patients with out-of-hospital cardiac arrest: a secondary analysis of the PARAMEDIC2 placebo-controlled trial [published online January 30, 2020].Intensive Care Med.2020:Epub ahead of print. doi: 10.1007/s00134-019-05920-7
15. Barsan WG, Levy RC, Weir H. Lidocaine levels during CPR: differences after peripheral venous, central venous, and intracardiac injections.Ann Emerg Med.1981;10:73-78. doi: 10.1016/s0196-0644 (81)80339-3
16. Kuhn GJ, White BC, Swetnam RE, Mumey JF, Rydesky MF, Tintinalli JE, Krome RL, Hoehner PJ.Peripheral vs central circulation times during CPR: a pilot study.Ann Emerg Med.1981;10:417-419. doi: 10.1016/s0196-0644 (81)80308-3
17. Emerman CL, Pinchak AC, Hancock D, Hagen JF.Effect of injection site on circulation times during cardiac arrest.Crit Care Med.1988;16:1138-1141. doi: 10.1097/00003246-198811000-00011
18. Schüttler J, Bartsch A, Ebeling BJ, Hörnchen U, Kulka P, Sühling B, Stoeckel H. [Endobronchial administration of adrenaline in preclinical cardiopulmonary resuscitation] .Anasth Intensivther Notfallmed.1987;22:63-68.
19. Hörnchen U, Schüttler J, Stoeckel H, Eichelkraut W, Hahn N. Endobronchial instillation of epinephrine during cardiopulmonary resuscitation.Crit Care Med.1987;15:1037-1039. doi: 10.1097/00003246-198711000-00009
20. Neumar RW, Otto CW, Link MS, Kronick SL, Shuster M, Callaway CW, Kudenchuk PJ, Ornato JP, McNally B, Silvers SM, et al.Part 8: adult advanced cardiovascular life support: 2010 American Heart Association Guidelines for Cardiopulmonary Resuscitation and Emergency Cardiovascular Care.Circulation.2010;122:S729-S767. doi: 10.1161/CIRCULATIONAHA.110.970988
21. Niemann JT, Stratton SJ, Cruz B, Lewis RJ.Endotracheal drug administration during out-of-hospital resuscitation: where are the survivors? Resuscitation.2002;53:153-157. doi: 10.1016/s0300-9572 (02)00004-7
22. Berg KM, Soar J, Andersen LW, Böttiger BW, Cacciola S, Callaway CW, Couper K, Cronberg T, D'Arrigo S, Deakin CD, et al; on behalf of the Adult Advanced Life Support Collaborators.Adult advanced life support: 2020 International Consensus on Cardiopulmonary Resuscitation and Emergency Cardiovascular Care Science With Treatment Recommendations.Circulation.2020;142 (suppl 1):S92-S139. doi: 10.1161/CIR.0000000000000893

心停止中の血管収縮薬投与

COR	LOE	推奨事項
1	B-R	1. 心停止の患者にアドレナリンの投与を推奨する。
2a	B-R	2. 臨床試験で使用されたプロトコールに基づき，心停止の際はアドレナリンを3〜5分ごとに1mg投与することが妥当である。
2a	C-LD	3. 投与のタイミングに関しては，ショック不適応リズムを呈する心停止の場合，できるだけ速やかにアドレナリンを投与することが妥当である。
2b	C-LD	4. タイミングに関しては，ショック適応リズムでの心停止の場合，除細動が不成功後にアドレナリンを投与することは妥当としてよい。
2b	C-LD	5. バソプレシン単独投与，またはアドレナリンとバソプレシンの併用投与は心停止において考慮してもよいが，心停止でのアドレナリン単独投与に代わる利点はない。
3：利益なし	B-R	6. 心停止に対する高用量アドレナリンのルーチン使用は推奨しない。

「概要」

アドレナリンは心停止において有益な効果を発揮すると仮定されているが，その主な理由は，αアドレナリン作用によってCPR中に冠動脈灌流圧および脳灌流圧が上昇するためである。一方，βアドレナリン作用は心筋酸素需要量を増大させ，心内膜下の灌流を低下させ，催不整脈性となる可能性作用がある。2件の無作為化プラセボ対照比較試験において，8,500例以上の患者を対象とし，OHCA（院外心停止）に対するアドレナリンの有効性が評価された[1,2]。この2件，および他の試験に対するシステマティックレビューおよびメタアナリシスでは[3]，アドレナリンはROSC率および生存退院率を有意に上昇させると結論付けている。神経学的転帰が良好な場合も不良な場合も含め，アドレナリンは3か月生存率を上昇させることはなかったが，アドレナリン群ではいずれの転帰もわずかに頻度が高かった[2]。観察研究のデータは，アドレナリンの早期投与が良好な転帰につながることを示唆しており，検証可能な試験において，神経学的転帰は良好でありながら生存率が低いことについては，心停止からアドレナリン投与までの平均時間が21分であることが理由の1つである可能性を示している。この遅延時間は，OHCAの試験において一貫した問題である。一般的に，IHCA（院内心停止）では薬物投与までの時間がこれよりはるかに短いため，IHCA集団の転帰に対するアドレナリンの効果は異なる可能性がある。CPR中，標準用量のアドレナリンより高用量のアドレナリンまたは他の血管収縮薬が何らかの利益をもたらすことを認める試験は，現時点では存在しない。

「推奨事項の裏付けとなる解説」

1. システマティックレビューおよびメタアナリシス[3]に基づき，アドレナリン投与の提案は推奨事項へと強化された。このレビューおよびメタアナリシスには，OHCAでのアドレナリン投与を評価した2件の無作為化試験（このうち1件は8,000例の患者を対象とする）の結果が含まれ[1,2]，アドレナリン投与がROSC率および生存率の上昇につながることを示している。神経学的回復に関して最も有意と考えられた3か月間で，アドレナリン群において神経学的転帰が良好および不良の両群の生存者で，有意ではないが増加が示された[2]。ROSC率および生存率を上げる薬物を数分の心肺虚脱後に投与する場合，良好および不良の両方の神経学的転帰が増加する可能性がある。心停止の発症時点で，神経学的転帰が良好になるか，不良になるかを判断することは，現時点では不可能である。したがって，生存率を上げることが示される薬物投与を継続するとともに，すべての患者に対して薬物投与までの時間短縮により幅広い努力を注ぐことで，より多くの生存者が良好な神経学的転帰を得られるようにすることが，最も有効なアプローチであると思われる。
2. 既存の試験では，3〜5分ごとに1mgを投与するプロトコールが使用されていた。運用上は，初期投与の後，CPRサイクル2回ごとにアドレナリンを投与することも妥当としてよい。
3. 最近のシステマティックレビューにおける，タイミングに関する16件の観察研究のうちすべての研究で，ショック非適応リズム患者における，早期のアドレナリン投与とROSCとの関連が確認されているが，例外なく生存率の改善は認められていない[3]。
4. ショック適応のリズムに関しては，試験のプロトコールで，3回目のショック実施後にアドレナリンを投与するよう規定されている。最初に除細動およびCPRを優先し，CPRおよび除細動による初回処置が成功しない場合にアドレナリンを投与することが文献で支持されている[3]。
5. 最近のシステマティックレビュー[3]では，心停止に対するバソプレシン単独投与またはバソプレシンとアドレナリンの併用投与を，アドレナリン単独投与と比較した試験の結果，転帰に差異は見られなかったことが示されたが，これらの試験の検出力は低かった。
6. 多数のRCTにおいて，高用量と標準用量のアドレナリン投与を比較した結果，一部の試験は高用量アドレナリンが高いROSC率をもたらしたことを示していたが，生存退院率または何らかの長期的な転帰の改善を示すものはなかった[4-11]。

これらの推奨事項は，『2019 AHA Focused Update on Advanced Cardiovascular Life Support: Use of Advanced Airways, Vasopressors, and Extracorporeal CPR During Cardiac Arrest: An Update to the AHA Guidelines for CPR and Emergency Cardiovascular Care』によって支持されている[12]。

参考資料

1. Jacobs IG, Finn JC, Jelinek GA, Oxer HF, Thompson PL.Effect of adrenaline on survival in out-of-hospital cardiac arrest: a randomised double-blind placebo-controlled trial.Resuscitation.2011;82:1138-1143. doi: 10.1016/j.resuscitation.2011.06.029
2. Perkins GD, Ji C, Deakin CD, Quinn T, Nolan JP, Scomparin C, Regan S, Long J, Slowther A, Pocock H, Black JJM, Moore F, Fothergill RT, Rees N, O'Shea L, Docherty M, Gunson I, Han K, Charlton K, Finn J, Petrou S, Stallard N, Gates S, Lall R; PARAMEDIC2 Collaborators.A Randomized Trial of Epinephrine in Out-of-Hospital Cardiac Arrest.N Engl J Med.2018;379:711-721. doi: 10.1056/NEJMoa1806842
3. Holmberg MJ, Issa MS, Moskowitz A, Morley P, Welsford M, Neumar RW, Paiva EF, Coker A, Hansen CK, Andersen LW, Donnino MW, Berg KM; International Liaison Committee on Resuscitation Advanced Life Support Task Force Collaborators.Vasopressors during adult cardiac arrest: A systematic review and meta-analysis.Resuscitation.2019;139:106-121. doi: 10.1016/j.resuscitation.2019.04.008
4. Brown CG, Martin DR, Pepe PE, Stueven H, Cummins RO, Gonzalez E, Jastremski M. A comparison of standard-dose and high-dose epinephrine in cardiac arrest outside the hospital.The Multicenter High-Dose Epinephrine Study Group.N Engl J Med.1992;327:1051-1055. doi: 10.1056/NEJM199210083271503
5. Choux C, Gueugniaud PY, Barbieux A, Pham E, Lae C, Dubien PY, Petit P. Standard doses versus repeated high doses of epinephrine in cardiac arrest outside the hospital.Resuscitation.1995;29:3-9. doi: 10.1016/0300-9572(94)00810-3
6. Gueugniaud PY, Mols P, Goldstein P, Pham E, Dubien PY, Deweerdt C, Vergnion M, Petit P, Carli P. A comparison of repeated high doses and repeated standard doses of epinephrine for cardiac arrest outside the hospital.European Epinephrine Study Group.N Engl J Med.1998;339:1595-1601. doi: 10.1056/NEJM199811263392204
7. Lindner KH, Ahnefeld FW, Prengel AW.Comparison of standard and high-dose adrenaline in the resuscitation of asystole and electromechanical dissociation.Acta Anaesthesiol Scand.1991;35:253-256. doi: 10.1111/j.1399-6576.1991.tb03283.x
8. Lipman J, Wilson W, Kobilski S, Scribante J, Lee C, Kraus P, Cooper J, Barr J, Moyes D. High-dose adrenaline in adult in-hospital asystolic cardiopulmonary resuscitation: a double-blind randomised trial.Anaesth Intensive Care.1993;21:192-196. doi: 10.1177/0310057X9302100210
9. Sherman BW, Munger MA, Foulke GE, Rutherford WF, Panacek EA.High-dose versus standard-dose epinephrine treatment of cardiac arrest after failure of standard therapy.Pharmacotherapy.1997;17:242-247.
10. Stiell IG, Hebert PC, Weitzman BN, Wells GA, Raman S, Stark RM, Higginson LA, Ahuja J, Dickinson GE.High-dose epinephrine in adult cardiac arrest.N Engl J Med.1992;327:1045-1050. doi: 10.1056/NEJM199210083271502
11. Callaham M, Madsen CD, Barton CW, Saunders CE, Pointer J. A randomized clinical trial of high-dose epinephrine and norepinephrine vs standard-dose epinephrine in prehospital cardiac arrest.JAMA.1992;268:2667-2672.
12. Panchal AR, Berg KM, Hirsch KG, Kudenchuk PJ, Del Rios M, Cabañas JG, Link MS, Kurz MC, Chan PS, Morley PT, et al.2019 American Heart Association focused update on advanced cardiovascular life support: use of advanced airways, vasopressors, and extracorporeal cardiopulmonary resuscitation during cardiac arrest: an update to the American Heart Association guidelines for cardiopulmonary resuscitation and emergency cardiovascular care.Circulation.2019;140:e881-e894. doi: 10.1161/CIR.0000000000000732

心停止中の血管収縮薬以外の薬物投与

COR	LOE	推奨事項
2b	B-R	1. 除細動に反応しない VF／無脈性 VT に対して，アミオダロンまたはリドカインの使用を考慮してもよい。
2b	C-LD	2. OHCA 患者には，CPR 中のステロイド投与は利益が不確かである。
3：利益なし	B-NR	3. 心停止の治療にカルシウムをルーチン投与することは推奨されない。
3：利益なし	B-R	4. 心停止患者に対する炭酸水素ナトリウムのルーチン使用は推奨されない。
3：利益なし	B-R	5. 心停止に対するマグネシウムのルーチン使用は推奨されない。

「概要」

心停止に対する薬物投与は通常，除細動の試みがある場合もない場合も含め，CPR による ROSC の達成に失敗した場合に開始される。これには，アドレナリン（「心停止中の血管収縮薬投与」を参照）などの血管収縮薬の他，抗不整脈薬，マグネシウム，炭酸水素ナトリウム，ステロイドといった（後述），直接的な血行動態に効果のない薬物（非昇圧性薬物）が使用されることがある。理論上は魅力的であり，動物実験では一定の有益性も証明されているが，後者の薬物療法には，心停止後の全生存率の向上を明確に示すものはない。ただし，限定的な集団や特殊な状況下では，潜在的な有益性をもたらす可能性もある。

高カリウム血症による心停止の治療に関する推奨事項は，カルシウムおよび炭酸水素ナトリウムの使用も含め，「電解質異常」に記載した。トルサード・ド・ポワントの管理に関する推奨事項は，「トルサード・ド・ポワント」に記載した。

「推奨事項の裏付けとなる解説」

1. OHCA 患者へのアミオダロンまたはリドカインの投与は，直近で 2018 年に正式なレビューを受けている[1]。この療法による生存入院率の向上が立証されたが，全生存退院率の向上，または良好な神経学的転帰を伴う生存率の向上は認められなかった[1,2]。しかし，アミオダロンおよびリドカインはそれぞ

れ，バイスタンダーが心停止を目撃した患者の事前に規定されたサブグループでは，生存退院率を有意に向上させた。これは，時間依存的な有益性と，これらの薬物がより奏効しうる特定グループの存在を裏付けると考えられる。その他の抗不整脈薬については，最新のエビデンスレビューでは特に検討されておらず，今後のさらなる評価が期待される。その 1 つであるブレチリウムトシレートは，ただちに生命を脅かしうる心室不整脈の治療のために最近米国に再導入されたが，その有効性または安全性に関する新たな情報は得られていない[3]。ソタロールは緩徐投与を必要とするため，心停止の状況に使用することは現実的ではない[4]。同様の制約はプロカインアミドにも当てはまる。プロカインアミドは心停止の第二選択薬として急速投与されているが，有益性は明らかではない[5]。心停止に対して抗不整脈薬を併用投与する場合の有効性については，まだ系統的に検討されておらず，今後の課題である。除細動に成功して ROSC を達成した後に予防的に投与する抗不整脈薬の役割も，いまだ不明である。生存退院率の向上には関連付けられていないものの，リドカインは除細動に成功して ROSC を達成した後に予防的に投与した場合，VF／無脈性 VT の再発率を低下させた[6]。『2018 AHA Focused Update on Advanced Cardiovascular Life Support Use of Antiarrhythmic Drugs During and Immediately After Cardiac Arrest: An Update to the AHA Guidelines for CPR and Emergency Cardiovascular Care』[1] では，再発性 VF／無脈性 VT の治療に支障をきたす可能性がある場合，特定の状況下（EMS による搬送時など）ではリドカインの使用を検討できると結論付けている。このような特殊な適応に対する他の抗不整脈薬の使用についてのエビデンスはない。

2. 同一施設で行われた 2 件の無作為化試験では，心停止中，および心停止からの蘇生成功後にバソプレシンおよびアドレナリンと組み合わせてステロイドを投与した場合に生存率と神経学的転帰が向上したことが報告されている[7,8]。しかし，厳密に心停止中に副腎皮質ステロイドを投与し，さらに標準的な蘇生を行った場合の非無作為化試験では，一致した転帰は得られていない[9,10]。有益性を示唆した試験は薬剤投与の組み合わせが行われた単一施設で実施されたもののみであり，観察研究のデータからは相反する結果が得られていることから，心停止中のステロイドが有益であるかどうかは依然として不明である。ステロイドの有効性を示した Mentzelopoulos らの知見を検証するための，少なくとも 1 件の試験が現在進行中である（NCT03640949）。

3. 2010 年のガイドラインで最後に検討されて以来，2013 年のシステマティックレビューでは，原因未確定の心停止におけるカルシウムのルーチン使用を支持するエビデンスはほとんど得られなかった。臨床試験が行われておらず，治療抵抗性心停止の「最後の手段」となる薬物としてカルシウムが使用される傾向があるため，得られたエビデンスも非常に脆弱である[11]。高カリウム血症，カルシウム拮抗薬の過剰摂取といった特殊な状況におけるカルシウム投与については，「電解質異常」および「中毒：β アドレナリン遮断薬およびカルシウム拮抗薬」を参照されたい。

4. 2010 年のガイドライン以降の臨床試験および観察研究では，原因未確定の心停止の転帰が炭酸水素ナトリウムのルーチン投与によって改善されたことを示す新たなエビデンスはなく，エビデンスはむしろ，生存率および神経学的回復が悪化する可能性を示唆している[12-14]。高カリウム血症や薬物過剰摂取といった特殊な状況における炭酸水素ナトリウムの使用については，「電解質異常」および「中毒：三環系抗うつ薬を含むナトリウムチャネル遮断薬」を参照されたい。

5. マグネシウムの抗不整脈薬としての役割については，最後に 2018 年の二次救命処置（ACLS）に関する重点的アップデートで検討されている[1]。無作為化比較試験からは，心停止リズムの有無にかかわらず，抗不整脈薬としてのマグネシウムが ROSC，生存率，あるいは神経学的転帰を改善することはなく[15-18]，単形性 VT にも有益ではないことが示されている[19]。裏付けの乏しい症例報告，ならびに小規模な症例収集研究により，トルサード・ド・ポワントの治療においてマグネシウムが有効であることが証明されている（「トルサード・ド・ポワント」を参照）。

推奨事項 1 および 5 は，2018 年の ACLS ガイドラインに関する重点的アップデートで支持されている[1]。推奨事項 2 は，直近で 2015 年に正式な最新エビデンスレビューを受けている[20]。推奨事項 3 および 4 は，直近で 2010 年に正式なエビデンスレビューを受けている[21]。

参考資料

1. Panchal AR, Berg KM, Kudenchuk PJ, Del Rios M, Hirsch KG, Link MS, Kurz MC, Chan PS, Cabañas JG, Morley PT, Hazinski MF, Donnino MW.2018 American Heart Association Focused Update on Advanced Cardiovascular Life Support Use of Antiarrhythmic Drugs During and Immediately After Cardiac Arrest: An Update to the American Heart Association Guidelines for Cardiopulmonary Resuscitation and Emergency Cardiovascular Care. Circulation.2018;138:e740–e749. doi: 10.1161/CIR.0000000000000613
2. Kudenchuk PJ, Brown SP, Daya M, Rea T, Nichol G, Morrison LJ, Leroux B, Vaillancourt C, Wittwer L, Callaway CW, Christenson J, Egan D, Ornato JP, Weisfeldt ML, Stiell IG, Idris AH, Aufderheide TP, Dunford JV, Colella MR, Vilke GM, Brienza AM, Desvigne-Nickens P, Gray PC, Gray R, Seals N, Straight R, Dorian P; Resuscitation Outcomes Consortium Investigators. Amiodarone, Lidocaine, or Placebo in Out-of-Hospital Cardiac Arrest.N Engl J Med.2016;374:1711–1722. doi: 10.1056/NEJMoa1514204
3. Chowdhury A, Fernandes B, Melhuish TM, White LD.Antiarrhythmics in Cardiac Arrest: A Systematic Review and Meta-Analysis.Heart Lung Circ.2018;27:280–290. doi: 10.1016/j.hlc.2017.07.004
4. Batul SA, Gopinathannair R. Intravenous Sotalol – Reintroducing a Forgotten Agent to the Electrophysiology Therapeutic Arsenal.J Atr Fibrillation.2017;9:1499. doi: 10.4022/jafib.1499
5. Markel DT, Gold LS, Allen J, Fahrenbruch CE, Rea TD, Eisenberg MS, Kudenchuk PJ.Procainamide and survival in ventricular fibrillation out-of-hospital cardiac arrest.Acad Emerg Med.2010;17:617–623. doi: 10.1111/j.1553-2712.2010.00763.x
6. Kudenchuk PJ, Newell C, White L, Fahrenbruch C, Rea T, Eisenberg M. Prophylactic lidocaine for postresuscitation care of patients without-of-hospital

7. Mentzelopoulos SD, Zakynthinos SG, Tzoufi M, Katsios N, Papastylianou A, Gkisioti S, Stathopoulos A, Kollintza A, Stamataki E, Roussos C. Vasopressin, epinephrine, and corticosteroids for in-hospital cardiac arrest.Arch Intern Med.2009;169:15–24. doi: 10.1001/archinternmed.2008.509
8. Mentzelopoulos SD, Malachias S, Chamos C, Konstantopoulos D, Ntaidou T, Papastylianou A, Kolliantzaki I, Theodoridi M, Ischaki H, Makris D, Zakynthinos E, Zintzaras E, Sourlas S, Aloizos S, Zakynthinos SG.Vasopressin, steroids, and epinephrine and neurologically favorable survival after in-hospital cardiac arrest: a randomized clinical trial.JAMA.2013;310:270–279. doi: 10.1001/jama.2013.7832
9. Tsai MS, Chuang PY, Yu PH, Huang CH, Tang CH, Chang WT, Chen WJ.Glucocorticoid use during cardiopulmonary resuscitation may be beneficial for cardiac arrest.Int J Cardiol.2016;222:629–635. doi: 10.1016/j.ijcard.2016.08.017
10. Tsai MS, Huang CH, Chang WT, Chen WJ, Hsu CY, Hsieh CC, Yang CW, Chiang WC, Ma MH, Chen SC.The effect of hydrocortisone on the outcome of out-of-hospital cardiac arrest patients: a pilot study.Am J Emerg Med.2007;25:318–325. doi: 10.1016/j.ajem.2006.12.007
11. Kette F, Ghuman J, Parr M. Calcium administration during cardiac arrest: a systematic review.Eur J Emerg Med.2013;20:72–78. doi: 10.1097/MEJ.0b013e328358e336
12. Vukmir RB, Katz L; Sodium Bicarbonate Study Group.Sodium bicarbonate improves outcome in prolonged prehospital cardiac arrest.Am J Emerg Med.2006;24:156–161. doi: 10.1016/j.ajem.2005.08.016
13. Ahn S, Kim YJ, Sohn CH, Seo DW, Lim KS, Donnino MW, Kim WY.Sodium bicarbonate on severe metabolic acidosis during prolonged cardiopulmonary resuscitation: a double-blind, randomized, placebo-controlled pilot study.J Thorac Dis.2018;10:2295–2302. doi: 10.21037/jtd.2018.03.124
14. Kawano T, Grunau B, Scheuermeyer FX, Gibo K, Dick W, Fordyce CB, Dorian P, Stenstrom R, Straight R, Christenson J. Prehospital sodium bicarbonate use could worsen long term survival with favorable neurological recovery among patients with out-of-hospital cardiac arrest. Resuscitation.2017;119:63–69. doi: 10.1016/j.resuscitation.2017.08.008
15. Fatovich DM, Prentice DA, Dobb GJ.Magnesium in cardiac arrest (the magic trial).Resuscitation.1997;35:237–241. doi: 10.1016/s0300-9572(97)00062-2
16. Allegra J, Lavery R, Cody R, Birnbaum G, Brennan J, Hartman A, Horowitz M, Nashed A, Yablonski M. Magnesium sulfate in the treatment of refractory ventricular fibrillation in the prehospital setting. Resuscitation.2001;49:245–249. doi: 10.1016/s0300-9572(00)00375-0
17. Hassan TB, Jagger C, Barnett DB.A randomised trial to investigate the efficacy of magnesium sulphate for refractory ventricular fibrillation.Emerg Med J. 2002;19:57–62.
18. Thel MC, Armstrong AL, McNulty SE, Califf RM, O'Connor CM.Randomised trial of magnesium in in-hospital cardiac arrest.Duke Internal Medicine Housestaff.Lancet.1997;350:1272–1276. doi: 10.1016/s0140-6736(97)05048-4
19. Manz M, Jung W, Lüderitz B. Effect of magnesium on sustained ventricular tachycardia [in German].Herz.1997;22 (suppl 1):51–55. doi: 10.1007/bf03042655
20. Link MS, Berkow LC, Kudenchuk PJ, Halperin HR, Hess EP, Moitra VK, Neumar RW, O'Neil BJ, Paxton JH, Silvers SM, et al.Part 7: adult advanced cardiovascular life support: 2015 American Heart Association Guidelines Update for Cardiopulmonary Resuscitation and Emergency Cardiovascular Care.Circulation.2015;132 (suppl 2):S444–S464. doi: 10.1161/CIR.0000000000000261
21. Neumar RW, Otto CW, Link MS, Kronick SL, Shuster M, Callaway CW, Kudenchuk PJ, Ornato JP, McNally B, Silvers SM, et al.Part 8: adult advanced cardiovascular life support: 2010 American Heart Association Guidelines for Cardiopulmonary Resuscitation and Emergency Cardiovascular Care.Circulation.2010;122:S729–S767. doi: 10.1161/CIRCULATIONAHA.110.970988

CPRのための補助用具

COR	LOE	推奨事項
2b	C-LD	1. 経験豊富な超音波検査者が存在し，超音波検査の実施が標準的な心停止治療プロトコールの妨げにならないのであれば，超音波検査を標準的な患者評価の補助として考慮してもよい。ただし，その有用性はまだ十分に確立されていない。
2b	C-LD	2. 酸素投与が可能な場合，CPR中に利用可能な最大の吸入酸素濃度を用いることは妥当としてよい。
2b	C-LD	3. 呼気終末CO_2の急激な上昇は，圧迫中または心リズムのチェックによって適切なリズムの存在が明らかになった場合に，ROSCの検出に使用できる。
2b	C-EO	4. CPR中の動脈血ガスのルーチン測定では，確実な値が得られない。
2b	C-EO	5. 胸骨圧迫中，または心リズムのチェックによって適切なリズムの存在が明らかになった場合は，動脈ラインによる動脈圧モニタリングを利用してROSCを検出することもできる。

「概要」

心停止に関する試験の大多数はOHCAを対象に実施されているが，IHCAは米国で1年間に発生する心停止の約半数を占める。さらに，多くのOHCAの蘇生は救急部に引き継がれて続行される。IHCA患者は，中心静脈ラインや動脈ラインといった侵襲的モニタリングデバイスが留置されていることが多く，動脈血ガス分析やベッドサイドでの超音波検査などの高度な処置を実施するための担当者が同伴していることも多い。$ETCO_2$モニタリングなどの高度なモニタリングも普及しつつある。このような生理学的モニタリングまたは診断処置の有用性を判断することが重要である。質の高いCPR，必要に応じた除細動，血管収縮薬，抗不整脈薬，および気道管理が心停止の蘇生の基盤となることに変わりはないが，新たに得られたデータからは，蘇生に対するAHAのアプローチに患者固有の画像検査および生理学的データを組み込むことが，今後の期待につながると考えられる。CPR中の生理学的なモニタリングに関する推奨事項については，「質の高いCPRの指標」を参照のこと。この領域のさらなる研究が必要なことは明らかである。

「推奨事項の裏付けとなる解説」

1. ベッドサイドでの心臓超音波検査を行うことで，心タンポナーデ，または心停止の他の可逆的原因を特定し，無脈性電気活動に

おける心臓の動きを検出できる可能性がある[1,2]。ただし、心臓超音波検査の実施により、胸骨圧迫の中断が長引くことも予想される[3]。1 件の小規模な RCT では、CPR 中に心臓超音波検査を実施しても、転帰向上は認められなかった[4]。

2. 成人を対象として、CPR 中の吸入酸素濃度のレベルを直接比較した試験はない。少数の試験では、CPR 中の高い Pao_2 値が ROSC 率に関連付けられることを示しているが、これは患者または蘇生の質の違いが原因となっている可能性もある[5-7]。

3. いくつかの観察研究は、$ETCO_2$ の 10 mm Hg 超の上昇が ROSC を示す可能性があることを示しているが、ROSC を示す特定のカットオフ値は識別されていない[8]。

4. 動脈血 Po_2 および Pco_2 値は心拍出量と換気に依存するため、どちらも患者特性および CPR の質に左右される。1 件の小規模な試験では、CPR 中の混合静脈血と動脈血の血ガスの間に一定の関係がないことが確認され、蘇生中の動脈血サンプルは正確ではないと結論付けられている[9]。

5. 動脈ラインが留置されている場合は、拡張期圧の急激な上昇、または心リズムチェック中の適切なリズムを示す動脈波形の存在が認められれば、ROSC を示す可能性がある。

推奨事項 1、3、および 5 は、直近で 2015 年に正式なエビデンスレビューを受けている[10]。推奨事項 2 は、直近で 2015 年に正式なエビデンスレビューを受けているが[10]、2020 年にはこのエビデンスのアップデートが完了している[11]。推奨事項 4 は、直近で 2010 年に正式なエビデンスレビューを受けている[12]。

参考資料

1. Breitkreutz R, Price S, Steiger HV, Seeger FH, Ilper H, Ackermann H, Rudolph M, Uddin S, Weigand MA, Müller E, Walcher F; Emergency Ultrasound Working Group of the Johann Wolfgang Goethe-University Hospital, Frankfurt am Main.Focused echocardiographic evaluation in life support and peri-resuscitation of emergency patients: a prospective trial.Resuscitation.2010;81:1527–1533. doi: 10.1016/j.resuscitation.2010.07.013
2. Gaspari R, Weekes A, Adhikari S, Noble VE, Nomura JT, Theodoro D, Woo M, Atkinson P, Blehar D, Brown SM, Caffery T, Douglass E, Fraser J, Haines C, Lam S, Lanspa M, Lewis M, Liebmann O, Limkakeng A, Lopez F, Platz E, Mendoza M, Minnigan H, Moore C, Novik J, Rang L, Scruggs W, Raio C. Emergency department point-of-care ultrasound in out-of-hospital and in-ED cardiac arrest.Resuscitation.2016;109:33–39. doi: 10.1016/j.resuscitation.2016.09.018
3. Clattenburg EJ, Wroe P, Brown S, Gardner K, Losonczy L, Singh A, Nagdev A. Point-of-care ultrasound use in patients with cardiac arrest is associated prolonged cardiopulmonary resuscitation pauses: A prospective cohort study.Resuscitation.2018;122:65–68. doi: 10.1016/j.resuscitation.2017.11.056
4. Chardoli M, Heidari F, Rabiee H, Sharif-Alhoseini M, Shokoohi H, Rahimi-Movaghar V. Echocardiography integrated ACLS protocol versus conventional cardiopulmonary resuscitation in patients with pulseless electrical activity cardiac arrest.Chin J Traumatol. 2012;15:284-287.
5. Spindelboeck W, Schindler O, Moser A, Hausler F, Wallner S, Strasser C, Haas J, Gemes G, Prause G. Increasing arterial oxygen partial pressure during cardiopulmonary resuscitation is associated with improved rates of hospital admission.Resuscitation.2013;84:770–775. doi: 10.1016/j.resuscitation.2013.01.012
6. Spindelboeck W, Gemes G, Strasser C, Toescher K, Kores B, Metnitz P, Haas J, Prause G. Arterial blood gases during and their dynamic changes after cardiopulmonary resuscitation: A prospective clinical study.Resuscitation.2016;106:24–29. doi: 10.1016/j.resuscitation.2016.06.013
7. Patel JK, Schoenfeld E, Parikh PB, Parnia S. Association of Arterial Oxygen Tension During In-Hospital Cardiac Arrest With Return of Spontaneous Circulation and Survival.J Intensive Care Med.2018;33:407–414. doi: 10.1177/0885066616658420
8. Sandroni C, De Santis P, D'Arrigo S. Capnography during cardiac arrest. Resuscitation.2018;132:73–77. doi: 10.1016/j.resuscitation.2018.08.018
9. Weil MH, Rackow EC, Trevino R, Grundler W, Falk JL, Griffel MI.Difference in acid–base state between venous and arterial blood during cardiopulmonary resuscitation.N Engl J Med.1986;315:153–156. doi: 10.1056/NEJM198607173150303
10. Link MS, Berkow LC, Kudenchuk PJ, Halperin HR, Hess EP, Moitra VK, Neumar RW, O'Neil BJ, Paxton JH, Silvers SM, et al.Part 7: adult advanced cardiovascular life support: 2015 American Heart Association Guidelines Update for Cardiopulmonary Resuscitation and Emergency Cardiovascular Care.Circulation.2015;132(suppl 2):S444–S464. doi: 10.1161/CIR.0000000000000261
11. Berg KM, Soar J, Andersen LW, Böttiger BW, Cacciola S, Callaway CW, Couper K, Cronberg T, D'Arrigo S, Deakin CD, et al; on behalf of the Adult Advanced Life Support Collaborators.Adult advanced life support: 2020 International Consensus on Cardiopulmonary Resuscitation and Emergency Cardiovascular Care Science With Treatment Recommendations.Circulation.2020;142(suppl 1):S92–S139. doi: 10.1161/CIR.0000000000000893
12. Neumar RW, Otto CW, Link MS, Kronick SL, Shuster M, Callaway CW, Kudenchuk PJ, Ornato JP, McNally B, Silvers SM, et al.Part 8: adult advanced cardiovascular life support: 2010 American Heart Association Guidelines for Cardiopulmonary Resuscitation and Emergency Cardiovascular Care.Circulation.2010;122:S729–S767. doi: 10.1161/CIRCULATIONAHA.110.970988

蘇生終了

蘇生終了に関する 推奨事項

COR	LOE	推奨事項
1	B-NR	1. 蘇生終了（TOR）を考慮する際、ALS が施行できない、あるいは著しく遅れる可能性がある場合には、BLS EMS プロバイダーは BLS の蘇生終了ルールを実施すべきである。
2a	B-NR	2. 成人の OHCA 傷病者に対し、現場のプレホスピタル ALS プロバイダーが成人 ALS 蘇生終了ルールを使用して蘇生努力を終了することは妥当である。
2a	B-NR	3. 段階的な ALS および BLS プロバイダーシステムでは、BLS 蘇生終了ルールを利用することで、心停止の現場において診断精度を下げることなく混乱を回避できる。
2b	C-LD	4. 挿管患者において、ALS 蘇生の 20 分後に波形表示呼気 CO_2 モニターにより 10 mm Hg を超える呼気終末 CO_2 値を達成できないことは、蘇生努力を終了する時を決定する集学的アプローチの構成要素の 1 つとみなしてもよいが、それを単独で用いるべきでない。
3：利益なし	C-LD	5. CPR 中、ベッドサイドでの超音波検査を予後予測に使用することは控えるよう提案する。
3：有害	C-EO	6. 挿管されていない患者においては、CPR 中のいずれの時点においても特定の呼気終末 CO_2 カットオフ値を蘇生努力終了の指標として用いるべきではない。

「概要」

OHCA は多大な医療資源を必要とする状態であり、低い生存率に関連付けられることが多い。EMS プロバイダーにとって、蘇生の続行が無益である患者と、生存の可能性があり、蘇生の継続と病院への搬送を必要とする患者とを区別できることが重要となる。こうすることで、医療資源の有効活

用，および患者の生存可能性の最適化が促進される。妥当性が確認された蘇生終了（TOR）ルールの使用は，蘇生が無益な患者の正確な判定に役立つ（図5および6）。蘇生の無益性とは，1％未満の生存可能性と定義されることが多い[1]。これは，TORルールが有効であるためには，外部検証において99％超の下側信頼限界で無益性を予測できる高い精度を実証しなければならないことを示唆している。

「推奨事項の裏付けとなる解説」

1. BLS TORルールでは，患者を搬送するために救急車に収容する前に，以下の条件がすべて満たされている場合にはTORが推奨される。（1）EMSプロバイダーおよび第1救助者が心停止を目撃していない。（2）ROSC未達成。（3）ショックが実施されていない。7件の発表済みの研究（対象患者33,795例）に基づく最近のメタアナリシスでは，BLS蘇生終了条件を満たした患者の0.13％（95％CI，0.03％～0.58％）のみが生存退院を果たしていた[3]。

2. ALS TORルールでは，患者を搬送するために救急車に収容する前に，以下の条件がすべて満たされている場合にはTORが推奨される。（1）心停止が目撃されていない。（2）バイスタンダーによるCPRが実施されていない。（3）現場で完全なALSケアを行ってもROSCが認められない。（4）AEDでショックが実施されていない。2件の発表済みの研究（対象患者10,178例）に基づく最近のメタアナリシスでは，ALS蘇生終了条件を満たした患者の0.01％（95％CI，0.00％～0.07％）のみが生存退院を果たしていた[3]。

3. BLS TORルールは「ユニバーサルTORルール」とも呼ばれ（EMSプロバイダーによる心停止の目撃なし，ショック未実施，ROSC未達成），BLSおよびALSを組み合わせたシステムであらかじめ検証されている[4]。6分間の蘇生後では，このルールの十分な特異度は確認できなかったが（偽陽性率：2.1％），約15分間蘇生を試みた後では99％以上の特異度が得られ，搬送率の半減につながっている。1件の後ろ向き解析では，蘇生を20分間行った時点でユニバーサルTORを適用したところ，無益性を予測でき，99％以上の生存者および良好な神経学的転帰を示した患者が特定できた[5]。

4. 挿管患者の場合，$ETCO_2$の測定値が10mmHg未満だと，血流低下または血流なしの状態を意味する。いくつかの小規模な研究では，ALSの蘇生を20分間実施した後，$ETCO_2$が10mmHg未満であった場合は，完全ではないが強力に無益性を予測していることを示すエビデンスが認められた[6-9]。このような小規模な観察研究は，バイアスが高いことが難点である。代替となる$ETCO_2$の閾値と判断する時点が提唱されている。[2]患者転帰の予測における$ETCO_2$の単独使用については，大規模な前向き研究で検証する必要がある。

5. 最近のシステマティックレビューでは，心停止の蘇生を終了する唯一の基準なる臨床所見としては超音波検査所見は感度が高いとはいえないことが明らかにされている[10]。感度・特異度が高い範囲にあったことを示す所見も見られたが，ベッドサイドでの心停止超音波検査の使用を検証するいくつかの試験では，得られた結果に一貫性がなく，有意なバイアスが妨げとなっている。ベッドサイドでの超音波検査のタイミングと適用に関しては，試験ごとに大きな不均一性が見られ，心臓の動きに関する定義および用語にも不一致が認められた。さらに，心停止中の超音波検査の所見についても，その評価者間の信頼性を検証する研究はほとんど行われていない[11,12]。CPRの補助処置としての超音波検査については，「CPRのための補助用具」を参照されたい。

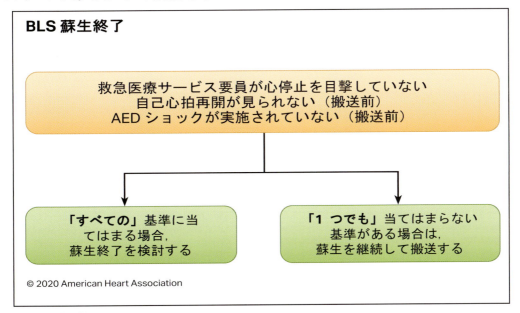

図5. 成人の一次救命処置の蘇生終了ルール。[2]
AED：自動体外式除細動器（automated external defibrillator），BLS：一次救命処置（basic life support）。

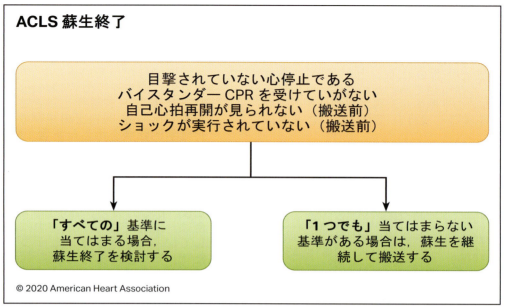

図6. 成人の二次救命処置の蘇生終了ルール。[2]
ACLS：二次救命処置（advanced cardiovascular life support），CPR：心肺蘇生（cardiopulmonary resuscitation）。

6. 高度な気道確保器具を留置していない心停止患者に対し，$ETCO_2$ の使用について具体的に検証した試験はない。バッグマスク換気実施中の $ETCO_2$ 値が，高度な気道確保器具が留置されている場合と同様の信頼性を持つかどうかは不明である。挿管されていない患者の TOR に関する決定に何らかの $ETCO_2$ カットオフ値を使用することは，エビデンスがないために支持されていない。

推奨事項 1，2，3，および 5 は，BLS および ALS に関する 2020 年の CoSTR で支持されている[13,14]。推奨事項 4 および 6 は，直近で 2015 年に正式なエビデンスレビューを受けている[15]。

参考資料

1. Schneiderman LJ.Defining Medical Futility and Improving Medical Care.J Bioeth Inq.2011;8:123-131. doi: 10.1007/s11673-011-9293-3
2. Morrison LJ, Kierzek G, Diekema DS, Sayre MR, Silvers SM, Idris AH, Mancini ME.Part 3: ethics: 2010 American Heart Association Guidelines for Cardiopulmonary Resuscitation and Emergency Cardiovascular Care.Circulation.2010;122 (suppl 3):S665-S675. doi: 10.1161/CIRCULATIONAHA.110.970905
3. Ebell MH, Vellinga A, Masterson S, Yun P. Meta-analysis of the accuracy of termination of resuscitation rules for out-of-hospital cardiac arrest.Emerg Med J. 2019;36:479-484. doi: 10.1136/emermed-2018-207833
4. Grunau B, Taylor J, Scheuermeyer FX, Stenstrom R, Dick W, Kawano T, Barbic D, Drennan I, Christenson J. External Validation of the Universal Termination of Resuscitation Rule for Out-of-Hospital Cardiac Arrest in British Columbia.Ann Emerg Med.2017;70:374-381.e1. doi: 10.1016/j.annemergmed.2017.01.030
5. Drennan IR, Case E, Verbeek PR, Reynolds JC, Goldberger ZD, Jasti J, Charleston M, Herren H, Idris AH, Leslie PR, Austin MA, Xiong Y, Schmicker RH, Morrison LJ; Resuscitation Outcomes Consortium Investigators.A comparison of the universal TOR Guideline to the absence of prehospital ROSC and duration of resuscitation in predicting futility from out-of-hospital cardiac arrest.Resuscitation.2017;111:96-102. doi: 10.1016/j.resuscitation.2016.11.021
6. Ahrens T, Schallom L, Bettorf K, Ellner S, Hurt G, O'Mara V, Ludwig J, George W, Marino T, Shannon W. End-tidal carbon dioxide measurements as a prognostic indicator of outcome in cardiac arrest.Am J Crit Care.2001;10:391-398.
7. Levine RL, Wayne MA, Miller CC.End-tidal carbon dioxide and outcome of out-of-hospital cardiac arrest.N Engl J Med.1997;337:301-306. doi: 10.1056/NEJM199707313370503
8. Wayne MA, Levine RL, Miller CC.Use of end-tidal carbon dioxide to predict outcome in prehospital cardiac arrest.Ann Emerg Med.1995;25:762-767. doi: 10.1016/s0196-0644 (95)70204-0
9. Akinci E, Ramadan H, Yuzbasioglu Y, Coskun F. Comparison of end-tidal carbon dioxide levels with cardiopulmonary resuscitation success presented to emergency department with cardiopulmonary arrest.Pak J Med Sci.2014;30:16-21. doi: 10.12669/pjms.301.4024
10. Reynolds JC, Mahmoud SI, Nicholson T, Drennan IR, Berg K, O'Neil BJ, Welsford M; on behalf of the Advanced Life Support Task Force of the International Liaison Committee on Resuscitation.Prognostication with point-of-care echocardiography during cardiac arrest: a systematic review. Resuscitation.2020: In press.
11. Flato UA, Paiva EF, Carballo MT, Buehler AM, Marco R, Timerman A. Echocardiography for prognostication during the resuscitation of intensive care unit patients with non-shockable rhythm cardiac arrest.Resuscitation.2015;92:1-6. doi: 10.1016/j.resuscitation.2015.03.024
12. Gaspari R, Weekes A, Adhikari S, Noble VE, Nomura JT, Theodoro D, Woo M, Atkinson P, Blehar D, Brown SM, Caffery T, Douglass E, Fraser J, Haines C, Lam S, Lanspa M, Lewis M, Liebmann O, Limkakeng A, Lopez F, Platz E, Mendoza M, Minnigan H, Moore C, Novik J, Rang L, Scruggs W, Raio C. Emergency department point-of-care ultrasound in out-of-hospital and in-ED cardiac arrest.Resuscitation.2016;109:33-39. doi: 10.1016/j.resuscitation.2016.09.018
13. Olasveengen TM, Mancini ME, Perkins GD, Avis S, Brooks S, Castrén M, Chung SP, Considine J, Couper K, Escalante R, et al; on behalf of the Adult Basic Life Support Collaborators.Adult basic life support: 2020 International Consensus on Cardiopulmonary Resuscitation and Emergency Cardiovascular Care Science With Treatment Recommendations.Circulation.2020;142 (suppl 1):S41-S91. doi: 10.1161/CIR.0000000000000892
14. Berg KM, Soar J, Andersen LW, Böttiger BW, Cacciola S, Callaway CW, Couper K, Cronberg T, D'Arrigo S, Deakin CD, et al; on behalf of the Adult Advanced Life Support Collaborators.Adult advanced life support: 2020 International Consensus on Cardiopulmonary Resuscitation and Emergency Cardiovascular Care Science With Treatment Recommendations.Circulation.2020;142 (suppl 1):S92-S139. doi: 10.1161/CIR.0000000000000893
15. Link MS, Berkow LC, Kudenchuk PJ, Halperin HR, Hess EP, Moitra VK, Neumar RW, O'Neil BJ, Paxton JH, Silvers SM, et al.Part 7: adult advanced cardiovascular life support: 2015 American Heart Association Guidelines Update for Cardiopulmonary Resuscitation and Emergency Cardiovascular Care.Circulation.2015;132 (suppl 2):S444-S464. doi: 10.1161/CIR.0000000000000261

蘇生のための高度な手技と器具
高度な気道確保器具の挿入
「緒言」

心停止中の気道確保は通常，バッグマスク換気などの基本的な手技から開始される。最初に選択した気道確保器具を使用できなかった場合のために，プロバイダーは高度な気道確保器具手技を習得しておき，さらに2番目（バックアップ）の方策を準備しておくとよい。高度な気道確保器具の挿入の際には，胸骨圧迫の中断，器具の位置ずれ，望ましくない過換気が生じる可能性があるため，プロバイダーはこれらのリスクに対し，高度な気道確保器具によって得られる可能性のある利点を十分に比較検討しなければならない。2019年のACLSガイドラインに関する重点的アップデートでは，心停止での高度な気道確保器具の使用について検証されており，どのような状況でも，成人心停止のCPR中にバッグマスク換気または高度な気道確保器具による方策を検討できるとしている[1]。高度な気道確保器具およびバッグマスク換気による介入の転帰は，プロバイダーの一連の手技と経験に大きく依存する（図7）。したがって，高度な気道確保器具の使用，種類，タイミングに関する最終決定には，患者およびプロバイダーの多くの特性を考慮する必要があるが，全体的推奨事項の中でこれを定義するのは容易ではない。

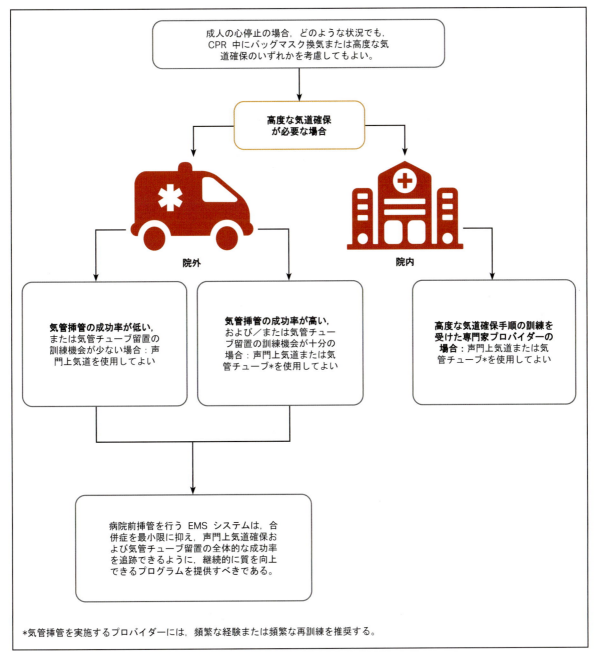

図7. CPR中に高度な気道確保器具を使用するためのALS推奨事項の模式図。
ALS：二次救命処置（advanced cardiovascular life support），CPR：心肺蘇生（cardiopulmonary resuscitation），EMS：救急医療サービス（emergency medical services）。

気道確保での合併症を最小限に留めるためにも，気道確保法を決定する際はプロバイダーの気道確保スキルおよび経験，プロバイダーの高頻度の再訓練，および継続的な技術の向上について考慮することが重要である。

心停止中の高度な気道確保器具による介入に関する 推奨事項		
COR	LOE	推奨事項
2b	B-R	1. 成人の心停止の場合はどのような状況でも，状況およびプロバイダーの一連の手技に応じて，CPR中にバッグマスク換気または高度な気道確保器具挿入のいずれかを考慮してもよい。

「推奨事項の裏付けとなる解説」
1. 医師ベースのEMSシステムでOHCA患者を対象にバッグマスク換気と気管挿管（ETI）を比較した，1件の大規模RCTでは，28日生存率または良好な神経学的転帰を伴う生存率において，どちらの手技によっても有意な有益性は得られなかった。[2] この試験でのETI成功率は98％であり，介入としてのETIを成功させる可能性のある比較的最適な状況を示唆している。急性期の気道確保における2つのアプローチの同等性または優越性を判断するには，さらなる研究が必要とされる。

これらの推奨事項は，ACLS ガイドラインに関する2019年の重点的アップデートで支持されている[1]。

高度な気道確保器具の挿入を考慮する際の に関する推奨事項：気管挿管と声門上気道確保の比較		
COR	LOE	推奨事項
2a	B-R	1. 高度な気道確保器具を使用する際，気管挿管の成功率が低い場合，または気管チューブ留置の訓練機会が少ない場合であれば，声門上気道確保器具を成人OHCA患者に使用してもよい。
2a	B-R	2. 高度な気道確保器具を使用する際，気管挿管の成功率が高い場合，または気管チューブ留置の最適な訓練機会がある場合であれば，声門上気道確保器具または気管挿管を成人OHCA患者に使用してもよい。
2a	B-R	3. これらの手順の訓練を受けた専門医が病院内で高度な気道確保を行う場合は，声門上気道確保（SGA）または気管チューブ留置を使用してもよい。

「推奨事項の裏付けとなる解説」
1, 2, および3 医師ベースではないEMSシステムで，OHCA患者を対象にSGA（iGelを使用）とETIを比較した1件のRCTでは（ETI成功率69％），生存率，または退院時に良好な神経学的転帰が得られた生存率に差は見られなかった[3]。医師ベースではないEMSシステムで，OHCA患者を対象にSGA（ラリンゲアルチューブを使用）とETIを比較した別のRCTでは（ETI成功率52％），生存退院率および良好な神経学的転帰を伴う生存退院率において，SGAによって管理された患者群がいずれも優れていた[4]。どちらの試験においても，臨床的判断に基づきプロバイダーがプロトコールを逸脱することを許容しているため，これらの結果を文脈付けることは困難である。さらに，既存の臨床試験に基づきガイダンスを規定することは可能であるが，気管挿管成功率の正確な上限閾値または下限閾値は特定されていない。したがって，特定の高度な気道確保器具を挿入するための判断基準となる，個人ごとの潜在的な利益（または有害性）を理解することは難しい。高度な気道確保器具を挿入するための判断には，患者およびプロバイダーの特性を考慮する必要があるが，全体的推奨事項の中でこれを定義するのは容易ではない。IHCA患者に対する高度な気道確保についての研究が不足していることから，IHCAに関する推奨事項はOHCAデータからの推定である。これらの問題を踏まえると，特に患者因子どうしのインタフェース，プロバイダーの経験，トレーニング，ツール，スキルの各分野において，さらなる研究が必要である。これらの理由により，ETIよりSGAを推奨することは時期尚早であると思われる。

これらの推奨事項は，ACLS ガイドラインに関する2019年の重点的アップデートで支持されている。[1]

高度な気道確保器具の挿入を考慮する際の 推奨事項		
COR	LOE	推奨事項
1	B-NR	1. 気管挿管を実施するプロバイダーには，頻繁な経験または頻繁な再訓練が推奨される。
1	C-LD	2. 高度な気道確保器具挿入によって胸骨圧迫が中断される場合，プロバイダーは患者が初期CPRおよび除細動の処置に応答しないか，またはROSCが得られるまで，気道確保器具の挿入を引き延ばすことを考慮できる。
1	C-LD	3. 気管チューブの正しい位置の確認と監視のための最も信頼できる手段として，臨床評価に加え，連続波形表示呼気CO_2モニターの使用が推奨される。
1	C-EO	4. 病院前挿管を行うEMSシステムは，合併症を最小限に抑え，声門上気道確保および気管チューブ留置の全体的な成功率を追跡するため，継続的に質を向上させるプログラムを提供すべきである。

「推奨事項の裏付けとなる解説」
1. 初回訓練を受けたプロバイダーのスキルを維持するため，再訓練を頻繁に実施することが重要である[5,6]。ただし，訓練の具体的な種類，量，頻度については，今後の研究によって検証する必要がある。
2. 高度な気道確保器具は胸骨圧迫を中断せずに挿入することができるが[7]，それでも中断は発生しうる。したがってプロバイダーは，高度な気道確保器具の挿入によって実現しうる利益と，高い胸部圧迫比を維持す

ることで得られる利益とを比較検討する必要がある[8-10]。
3. 1件の小規模な臨床試験および数件の観察研究では，心停止中に気管チューブの位置を確認する場合に，波形表示呼気 CO_2 モニターが 100％の特異度を示したことを認めている[11-13]。心停止時間が長引くと，波形表示呼気 CO_2 モニターの感度は低下する[11-13]。他の高度な気道確保器具（コンビチューブ，ラリンゲアルマスクエアウェイなど）の挿入を確認するための波形表示呼気 CO_2 モニターの使用については，まだ研究されていない。
4. ETI を実施するシステムの全体的な成功率を追跡することの根拠は，心停止患者に対し慣例的に ETI を使用するのか，SGA に移行するのか，あるいは単にバッグマスク換気を使用するのか，十分な情報に基づき意思決定を行えるようにすることである。特定のシステムにおける全体的な成功率に応じて，推奨事項も変化する。

これらの推奨事項は，ACLS ガイドラインに関する 2019 年の重点的アップデートで支持されている[1]。

参考資料

1. Panchal AR, Berg KM, Hirsch KG, Kudenchuk PJ, Del Rios M, Cabañas JG, Link MS, Kurz MC, Chan PS, Morley PT, et al. 2019 American Heart Association focused update on advanced cardiovascular life support: use of advanced airways, vasopressors, and extracorporeal cardiopulmonary resuscitation during cardiac arrest: an update to the American Heart Association guidelines for cardiopulmonary resuscitation and emergency cardiovascular care. Circulation. 2019;140:e881–e894. doi: 10.1161/CIR.0000000000000732
2. Jabre P, Penaloza A, Pinero D, Duchateau FX, Borron SW, Javaudin F, Richard O, de Longueville D, Bouilleau G, Devaud ML, Heidet M, Lejeune C, Fauroux S, Greingor JL, Manara A, Hubert JC, Guihard B, Vermylen O, Lievens P, Auffret Y, Maisondieu C, Huet S, Claessens B, Lapostolle F, Javaud N, Reuter PG, Baker E, Vicaut E, Adnet F. Effect of Bag-Mask Ventilation vs Endotracheal Intubation During Cardiopulmonary Resuscitation on Neurological Outcome After Out-of-Hospital Cardiorespiratory Arrest: A Randomized Clinical Trial. JAMA. 2018;319:779–787. doi: 10.1001/jama.2018.0156
3. Benger JR, Kirby K, Black S, Brett SJ, Clout M, Lazaroo MJ, Nolan JP, Reeves BC, Robinson M, Scott LJ, Smartt H, South A, Stokes EA, Taylor J, Thomas M, Voss S, Wordsworth S, Rogers CA. Effect of a Strategy of a Supraglottic Airway Device vs Tracheal Intubation During Out-of-Hospital Cardiac Arrest on Functional Outcome: The AIRWAYS-2 Randomized Clinical Trial. JAMA. 2018;320:779–791. doi: 10.1001/jama.2018.11597
4. Wang HE, Schmicker RH, Daya MR, Stephens SW, Idris AH, Carlson JN, Colella MR, Herren H, Hansen M, Richmond NJ, Puyana JCJ, Aufderheide TP, Gray RE, Gray PC, Verkest M, Owens PC, Brienza AM, Sternig KJ, May SJ, Sopko GR, Weisfeldt ML, Nichol G. Effect of a Strategy of Initial Laryngeal Tube Insertion vs Endotracheal Intubation on 72-Hour Survival in Adults With Out-of-Hospital Cardiac Arrest: A Randomized Clinical Trial. JAMA. 2018;320:769–778. doi: 10.1001/jama.2018.7044
5. Wong ML, Carey S, Mader TJ, Wang HE; American Heart Association National Registry of Cardiopulmonary Resuscitation Investigators. Time to invasive airway placement and resuscitation outcomes after inhospital cardiopulmonary arrest. Resuscitation. 2010;81:182–186. doi: 10.1016/j.resuscitation.2009.10.027
6. Warner KJ, Carlbom D, Cooke CR, Bulger EM, Copass MK, Sharar SR. Paramedic training for proficient prehospital endotracheal intubation. Prehosp Emerg Care. 2010;14:103–108. doi: 10.3109/10903120903144858
7. Gatward JJ, Thomas MJ, Nolan JP, Cook TM. Effect of chest compressions on the time taken to insert airway devices in a manikin. Br J Anaesth. 2008;100:351–356. doi: 10.1093/bja/aem364
8. Talikowska M, Tohira H, Finn J. Cardiopulmonary resuscitation quality and patient survival outcome in cardiac arrest: A systematic review and meta-analysis. Resuscitation. 2015;96:66–77. doi: 10.1016/j.resuscitation.2015.07.036
9. Vaillancourt C, Everson-Stewart S, Christenson J, Andrusiek D, Powell J, Nichol G, Cheskes S, Aufderheide TP, Berg R, Stiell IG; Resuscitation Outcomes Consortium Investigators. The impact of increased chest compression fraction on return of spontaneous circulation for out-of-hospital cardiac arrest patients not in ventricular fibrillation. Resuscitation. 2011;82:1501–1507. doi: 10.1016/j.resuscitation.2011.07.011
10. Christenson J, Andrusiek D, Everson-Stewart S, Kudenchuk P, Hostler D, Powell J, Callaway CW, Bishop D, Vaillancourt C, Davis D, Aufderheide TP, Idris A, Stouffer JA, Stiell I, Berg R; Resuscitation Outcomes Consortium Investigators. Chest compression fraction determines survival in patients with out-of-hospital ventricular fibrillation. Circulation. 2009;120:1241–1247. doi: 10.1161/CIRCULATIONAHA.109.852202
11. Grmec S. Comparison of three different methods to confirm tracheal tube placement in emergency intubation. Intensive Care Med. 2002;28:701–704. doi: 10.1007/s00134-002-1290-x
12. Takeda T, Tanigawa K, Tanaka H, Hayashi Y, Goto E, Tanaka K. The assessment of three methods to verify tracheal tube placement in the emergency setting. Resuscitation. 2003;56:153–157. doi: 10.1016/s0300-9572(02)00345-3
13. Tanigawa K, Takeda T, Goto E, Tanaka K. Accuracy and reliability of the self-inflating bulb to verify tracheal intubation in out-of-hospital cardiac arrest patients. Anesthesiology. 2000;93:1432–1436. doi: 10.1097/00000542-200012000-00015

代替の CPR 手技と器具

「緒言」

従来の CPR の代替手技や補助的器具は，これまでに多数開発されてきた。例えば，機械的 CPR，インピーダンス閾値器具（ITD），能動圧迫 − 減圧（ACD）CPR，間欠的腹部圧迫 CPR などである。そうした手技および器具の多くは，専門の器材や訓練を必要とする。

　機械的 CPR 器具は胸骨圧迫を自動的に実施し，用手的胸骨圧迫を不要にする。機械的 CPR 器具には 2 つの種類がある。胸郭全体を取り囲んで圧迫する負荷分布圧迫バンドと，胸部を前後方向に圧迫する空気式ピストン器具である。11 件の RCT（エビデンスの確実性は全体的に中等度から低度）に基づく最近のシステマティックレビューでは，用手的 CPR と比較した場合，OHCA と IHCA のどちらにおいても，機械的 CPR によって良好な神経学的転帰を伴う生存率が向上したことを示すエビデンスは認められなかった[1]。患者搬送中は人員や安全性に限界があり，これに関連して認識される後方支援的な利点により，機械的 CPR は一部のプロバイダーやシステム間で支持され続けている。

　ACD-CPR は吸引カップ付きの携帯式器具を使用して，カップを胸骨中線に吸着させた状態で実施する。減圧中は胸部を積極的に引き上げることで，胸郭の戻りによって生じる胸腔内の陰圧を増強し，次の胸骨圧迫中に静脈還流量および心拍出量を増大させる効果がある。ITD は高度な気道確保器具またはフェイスマスクに取り付ける圧感知弁である。CPR の減圧相中に肺に流入する空気を制限して，胸郭がもとに戻る際の

胸腔内陰圧を高めることにより，CPR 中の静脈還流量と心拍出量を増大させる。

多数の代替 CPR 手技が使用されているが，その多くは未検証である。例として，心停止に対する一連の治療に「ヘッドアップ」CPR を含めることについては，その使用を推奨できるだけの十分なエビデンスが得られていない[2]。この方法，およびその他の代替 CPR 手技に関する今後の研究については，正式な対照臨床研究の文脈で検討することが望ましい。

機械的 CPR 器具に関する 推奨事項

COR	LOE	推奨事項
2b	C-LD	1. プロバイダーにとって，質の高い用手的胸骨圧迫の実施が困難または危険と思われる特殊な状況では，救助者が器具の取り付け時と取り外し時の CPR の中断を厳しく制限することを条件に，機械的 CPR 器具の使用を考慮してもよい。
3：利益なし	B-R	2. 機械的 CPR 器具のルーチン使用は推奨されない。

「推奨事項の裏付けとなる解説」

1 および 2．機械的 CPR 器具に関する研究では，用手的 CPR と比較した場合の利点は実証されておらず，いくつかの研究では神経学的転帰の悪化が示唆されている。ASPIRE 試験（対象患者 1,071 例）では，用手的 CPR と比較した場合，自動荷重負荷バンド器具の使用は同様の生存退院率（調整後オッズ比［aOR］：0.56，CI：0.31〜1.00，P= 0.06）に関連付けられ，神経学的転帰が良好な生存率は低かった（3.1％対7.5％，P=0.006）[3]。CIRC 試験（n = 4,231）では，自動荷重不可バンド器具を使用した CPR は生存退院率（（aOR：1.06，CI：0.83〜1.37）および神経学的転帰が良好な生存率（aOR：0.80，CI：0.47〜1.37）のいずれにおいても，統計的に同等な値が得られた[4]。PARAMEDIC 試験（n = 4,470）では，機械的ピストン器具の使用を用手的 CPR と比較した結果，30 日生存率（aOR：0.86，CI：0.64〜1.15）は同様であったが，良好な神経学的転帰を伴う生存率は低かった（aOR：0.72，CI：0.52〜0.99）[5]。LINC 試験（n = 2,589）では，良好な神経学的転帰を伴う生存率は両群で同様であった（8.3 ％対7.8 ％，リスク差：0.55 ％，95 ％ CI：1.5 ％〜2.6 ％）[6]。

これらのデータを踏まえると，信頼性および質の高い用手的胸骨圧迫の実施が不可能であるか，あるいはプロバイダーに危険を及ぼしうる状況（人員数が限定的，走行中の救急車内，血管造影室内，長時間の蘇生，感染症への曝露の懸念など）では，訓練された救助者による機械的 CPR 器具の使用が有益である可能性がある。

このトピックは，直近で 2015 年に正式なエビデンスレビューを受けている[7]。

能動圧迫-減圧 CPR およびインピーダンス閾値器具に関する推奨事項

COR	LOE	推奨事項
2b	B-NR	1. 能動圧迫-減圧 CPR の有効性は不明である。プロバイダーが十分に訓練され，モニターされている場合は，能動圧迫-減圧 CPR の使用を考慮してもよい。
2b	C-LD	2. 器材の使用が可能で，適切に訓練された救助者がいる状況では，能動圧迫-減圧 CPR とインピーダンス閾値器具の併用は妥当としてよい。
3：利益なし	A	3. 従来的な CPR の実施中に，補助用具としてインピーダンス閾値器具をルーチン使用することは推奨されない。

「推奨事項の裏付けとなる解説」

1. 10 件の試験に基づき，ACD-CPR と標準的な CPR とを比較した 2013 年の Cochrane レビューでは，OHCA と IHCA のいずれの場合も，成人の死亡率および神経学的機能における差は認められなかった[8]。このモダリティで新たに出現した重要な考慮事項は，救助者の疲労増大であり，これによって CPR の全体的な質が損なわれる可能性がある。

2. ACD-CPR は，ITD と相乗的に作用して胸部減圧時の静脈還流量を増大させ，CPR 中の重要臓器への血流を改善する可能性がある。ResQ 試験では，ACD および ITD の併用と標準 CPR とを比較し，ACD および ITD の併用が，OHCA において良好な神経学的機能を維持した生存退院率の向上に関連付けられた。ただし，この試験には，盲検化されていない，両群間で CPR フィードバック要素が異なる（追加介入），CPR の質の評価をしていない，蘇生の早期中止といった限界がある[9,10]。『AHA CPR と ECC のためのガイドラインアップデート 2015』[7] ではこのトピックを評価し，質の低い 1 件の大規模 RCT がその使用による利益を実証しているものの，注記された試験の限界により，この結果を確認するにはさらなる試験が必要であると指摘している。したがって，AHA ガイドラインの旧版では，ACD-CPR および ITD の併用は推奨されていなかった。しかし，器材および訓練された救助者が揃っている状況では，ACD-CPR および ITD の併用が標準 CPR の代替手段となりうる。

3. PRIMED 試験（n = 8,178）では，OHCA 患者に対する ITD の使用（シャム器具との比較）は，生存退院率または良好な神経学的機能を維持した生存率のいずれをも有意に向上させることはなかった[11]。PRIMED 試験に対し，ITD を対象とした post hoc 解析が追加で実施されたが[12]，従来的な CPR 実施中の補助用具として ITD をルーチン使用することは推奨されない。

このトピックは，直近で2015年に正式なエビデンスレビューを受けている[7]。

COR	LOE	推奨事項
その他のCPR手技に関する推奨事項		
2b	B-NR	1. 間欠的腹部圧迫CPRは院内蘇生において，使用方法を十分に習熟した救助者がいる場合は考慮してもよい。

「推奨事項の裏付けとなる解説」

1. 間欠的腹部圧迫CPRは，従来の胸骨圧迫に，交互に行う腹部圧迫を組み合わせる，3名の救助者による手技である。腹部を手で圧迫する専任の救助者が，胸骨圧迫の減圧の間に剣状突起と臍部の中間を圧迫する。このトピックが最後にレビューされたのは2010年であり，2件の無作為化試験では，成人IHCA患者に対する従来的なCPRと比較して，訓練を受けた救助者による間欠的腹部圧迫CPRが短期生存率[13]および生存退院率[14]を向上させたことが認められている。成人OHCA患者を対象とした1件のRCT[15]では，間欠的腹部圧迫CPRによる生存率の向上は認められなかった。この手技のルーチン使用を詳細に定義するには，さらなる評価が必要である。

このトピックは，直近で2010年に正式なエビデンスレビューを受けている[16]。

参考資料

1. Wang PL, Brooks SC.Mechanical versus manual chest compressions for cardiac arrest.Cochrane Database Syst Rev. 2018;8:CD007260. doi: 10.1002/14651858.CD007260.pub4
2. Pepe PE, Scheppke KA, Antevy PM, Crowe RP, Millstone D, Coyle C, Prusansky C, Garay S, Ellis R, Fowler RL, Moore JC.Confirming the Clinical Safety and Feasibility of a Bundled Methodology to Improve Cardiopulmonary Resuscitation Involving a Head-Up/Torso-Up Chest Compression Technique.Crit Care Med.2019;47:449–455. doi: 10.1097/CCM.0000000000003608
3. Hallstrom A, Rea TD, Sayre MR, Christenson J, Anton AR, Mosesso VN Jr, Van Ottingham L, Olsufka M, Pennington S, White LJ, Yahn S, Husar J, Morris MF, Cobb LA.Manual chest compression vs use of an automated chest compression device during resuscitation following out-of-hospital cardiac arrest: a randomized trial.JAMA.2006;295:2620–2628. doi: 10.1001/jama.295.22.2620
4. Wik L, Olsen JA, Persse D, Sterz F, Lozano M Jr, Brouwer MA, Westfall M, Souders CM, Malzer R, van Grunsven PM, Travis DT, Whitehead A, Herken UR, Lerner EB.Manual vs. integrated automatic load-distributing band CPR with equal survival after out of hospital cardiac arrest.The randomized CIRC trial.Resuscitation.2014;85:741–748. doi: 10.1016/j.resuscitation.2014.03.005
5. Perkins GD, Lall R, Quinn T, Deakin CD, Cooke MW, Horton J, Lamb SE, Slowther AM, Woollard M, Carson A, Smyth M, Whitfield R, Williams A, Pocock H, Black JJ, Wright J, Han K, Gates S; PARAMEDIC trial collaborators.Mechanical versus manual chest compression for out-of-hospital cardiac arrest (PARAMEDIC): a pragmatic, cluster randomised controlled trial. Lancet.2015;385:947–955. doi: 10.1016/S0140-6736(14)61886-9
6. Rubertsson S, Lindgren E, Smekal D, Östlund O, Silfverstolpe J, Lichtveld RA, Boomars R, Ahlstedt B, Skoog G, Kastberg R, et al.Mechanical chest compressions and simultaneous defibrillation vs conventional cardiopulmonary resuscitation in out-of-hospital cardiac arrest: the LINC randomized trial. JAMA.2014;311:53–61. doi: 10.1001/jama.2013.282538
7. Brooks SC, Anderson ML, Bruder E, Daya MR, Gaffney A, Otto CW, Singer AJ, Thiagarajan RR, Travers AH.Part 6: alternative techniques and ancillary devices for cardiopulmonary resuscitation: 2015 American Heart Association Guidelines Update for Cardiopulmonary Resuscitation and Emergency Cardiovascular Care.Circulation.2015;132(suppl 2):S436–S443. doi: 10.1161/CIR.0000000000000260
8. Lafuente-Lafuente C, Melero-Bascones M. Active chest compression-decompression for cardiopulmonary resuscitation.Cochrane Database Syst Rev. 2013:CD002751. doi: 10.1002/14651858.CD002751.pub3
9. Aufderheide TP, Frascone RJ, Wayne MA, Mahoney BD, Swor RA, Domeier RM, Olinger ML, Holcomb RG, Tupper DE, Yannopoulos D, Lurie KG.Standard cardiopulmonary resuscitation versus active compression-decompression cardiopulmonary resuscitation with augmentation of negative intrathoracic pressure for out-of-hospital cardiac arrest: a randomised trial.Lancet.2011;377:301–311. doi: 10.1016/S0140-6736(10)62103-4
10. Frascone RJ, Wayne MA, Swor RA, Mahoney BD, Domeier RM, Olinger ML, Tupper DE, Setum CM, Burkhart N, Klann L, Salzman JG, Wewerka SS, Yannopoulos D, Lurie KG, O'Neil BJ, Holcomb RG, Aufderheide TP.Treatment of non-traumatic out-of-hospital cardiac arrest with active compression decompression cardiopulmonary resuscitation plus an impedance threshold device.Resuscitation.2013;84:1214–1222. doi: 10.1016/j.resuscitation.2013.05.002
11. Aufderheide TP, Nichol G, Rea TD, Brown SP, Leroux BG, Pepe PE, Kudenchuk PJ, Christenson J, Daya MR, Dorian P, Callaway CW, Idris AH, Andrusiek D, Stephens SW, Hostler D, Davis DP, Dunford JV, Pirrallo RG, Stiell IG, Clement CM, Craig A, Van Ottingham L, Schmidt TA, Wang HE, Weisfeldt ML, Ornato JP, Sopko G; Resuscitation Outcomes Consortium (ROC) Investigators.A trial of an impedance threshold device in out-of-hospital cardiac arrest.N Engl J Med.2011;365:798–806. doi: 10.1056/NEJMoa1010821
12. Sugiyama A, Duval S, Nakamura Y, Yoshihara K, Yannopoulos D. Impedance Threshold Device Combined With High-Quality Cardiopulmonary Resuscitation Improves Survival With Favorable Neurological Function After Witnessed Out-of-Hospital Cardiac Arrest.Circ J. 2016;80:2124–2132. doi: 10.1253/circj.CJ-16-0449
13. Sack JB, Kesselbrenner MB, Jarrad A. Interposed abdominal compression-cardiopulmonary resuscitation and resuscitation outcome during asystole and electromechanical dissociation.Circulation.1992;86:1692–1700. doi: 10.1161/01.cir.86.6.1692
14. Sack JB, Kesselbrenner MB, Bregman D. Survival from in-hospital cardiac arrest with interposed abdominal counterpulsation during cardiopulmonary resuscitation.JAMA.1992;267:379–385.
15. Mateer JR, Stueven HA, Thompson BM, Aprahamian C, Darin JC.Pre-hospital IAC-CPR versus standard CPR: paramedic resuscitation of cardiac arrests. Am J Emerg Med.1985;3:143–146. doi: 10.1016/0735-6757(85)90038-5
16. Cave DM, Gazmuri RJ, Otto CW, Nadkarni VM, Cheng A, Brooks SC, Daya M, Sutton RM, Branson R, Hazinski MF. Part 7: CPR techniques and devices: 2010 American Heart Association Guidelines for Cardiopulmonary Resuscitation and Emergency Cardiovascular Care.Circulation.2010;122:S720–728. doi: 10.1161/CIRCULATIONAHA.110.970970

体外循環式CPR

COR	LOE	推奨事項
体外循環式CPRに関する推奨事項		
2b	C-LD	1. 心停止患者に対する体外循環補助を用いたCPR（ECPR）のルーチン使用を推奨するには，エビデンスが不十分である。一部の心停止患者には（疑われる心停止の原因が機械的心肺補助中の限られた時間内で回復しうる場合），ECPRを考慮してもよい。

「概要」

「ECPR」という用語は，心停止患者の蘇生中に心肺バイパスを開始することを指す。ECPRは太い静脈と動脈へのカニューレ挿入，および静動脈体外膜型人工肺（ECMO）の開始を伴う（図8）。ECPRの目的は，治療可能と考えられる疾患に対処しながら，末端臓器への灌流をサポートすることである。ECPRは，高度に訓練されたチーム，専門器材，ヘルスケアシステムでの複数の専門分野にわたるサポートを必要とする複雑な介入である。ACLSガイドラインに関する2019年の重点的アップデート[1]では，心停止に対するECPRの使用について検討されており，心停止におけるECPRのルーチン使用を推

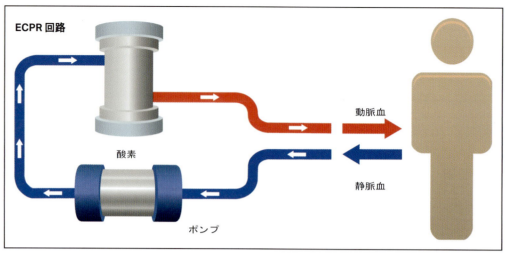

図8. ECPRに使用される体外膜型人工肺回路の構成部品の概略図。
構成部品には，静脈カニューレ，ポンプ，人工肺，および動脈カニューレが含まれる。ECPR：体外循環補助を用いたCPR（extracorporeal cardiopulmonary resuscitation）。

奨するエビデンスは十分に得られていないことが指摘されている。しかし，一時的な心肺補助の恩恵を享受しうる，治療可能と思われる病因のある心停止患者にはECPRを考慮してもよい。重要な考慮事項の1つは，ECPRを実施する患者の選択であり，この介入が最も有益とみられる患者の定義についてはさらなる研究が必要である。また，ECPRプログラムを開始し，維持するために必要なリソース使用量は，救命の連鎖内の他のリンクの強化という観点から検討する必要がある。蘇生におけるECPRのルーチン使用に関しては，費用対効果，リソースの分配，および倫理面を評価するためにさらなる研究が必要である。

「推奨事項の裏付けとなる解説」

1. OHCAまたはIHCAに対するECPRの使用を評価するRCTはない。OHCAに対しては15件の観察研究が確認されており，それぞれ適応基準，ECPR状況，試験デザインが異なるが，そのほとんどの試験では，ECPRに神経学的転帰の向上が関連付けられたことが報告されている[2]。病院内でのECPRの使用については，すべての試験がきわめて重大なバイアスのリスク（主に交絡によるもの）を包含していると評価され，すべての転帰に対し，エビデンスの全体的な確実性がきわめて低いと判定されている[2]。3件の試験において，ECPRには短期的または長期的な神経学的転帰に関する有益な効果が関連付けられなかったが[3-5]，1件の試験では[6]，短期的および長期的な神経学的転帰に関する利益との関連付けが報告されている。多くの試験でECPRの使用に対し良好な転帰が報告されているが，その大多数の試験は，適応基準や状況はさまざまだが単一施設で実施されたものであり，ECPRの実施は個々の事例に応じて決定されている。現在，「患者の選択基準」を明確に定義するためのエビデンスはないが，解析されたほとんどの試験には，併存疾患の少ない比較的若年の患者が含まれていた。無作為化試験など，より質の高い方法論による試験のデータが必要なことは明らかである。

これらの推奨事項は，ACLSガイドラインに関する2019年の重点的アップデートで支持されている[1]。

参考資料

1. Panchal AR, Berg KM, Hirsch KG, Kudenchuk PJ, Del Rios M, Cabañas JG, Link MS, Kurz MC, Chan PS, Morley PT, et al.2019 American Heart Association focused update on advanced cardiovascular life support: use of advanced airways, vasopressors, and extracorporeal cardiopulmonary resuscitation during cardiac arrest: an update to the American Heart Association guidelines for cardiopulmonary resuscitation and emergency cardiovascular care.Circulation.2019;140:e881-e894. doi: 10.1161/CIR.0000000000000732
2. Holmberg MJ, Geri G, Wiberg S, Guerguerian AM, Donnino MW, Nolan JP, Deakin CD, Andersen LW; International Liaison Committee on Resuscitation's (ILCOR) Advanced Life Support and Pediatric Task Forces.Extracorporeal cardiopulmonary resuscitation for cardiac arrest: A systematic review. Resuscitation.2018;131:91-100. doi: 10.1016/j.resuscitation.2018.07.029
3. Blumenstein J, Leick J, Liebetrau C, Kempfert J, Gaede L, Groß S, Krug M, Berkowitsch A, Nef H, Rolf A, Arlt M, Walther T, Hamm CW, Möllmann H. Extracorporeal life support in cardiovascular patients with observed refractory in-hospital cardiac arrest is associated with favourable short and long-term outcomes: A propensity-matched analysis.Eur Heart J Acute Cardiovasc Care.2016;5:13-22. doi: 10.1177/2048872615612454
4. Chen YS, Lin JW, Yu HY, Ko WJ, Jerng JS, Chang WT, Chen WJ, Huang SC, Chi NH, Wang CH, Chen LC, Tsai PR, Wang SS, Hwang JJ, Lin FY.Cardiopulmonary resuscitation with assisted extracorporeal life-support versus conventional cardiopulmonary resuscitation in adults with in-hospital cardiac arrest: an observational study and propensity analysis. Lancet.2008;372:554-561. doi: 10.1016/S0140-6736(08)60958-7
5. Lin JW, Wang MJ, Yu HY, Wang CH, Chang WT, Jerng JS, Huang SC, Chou NK, Chi NH, Ko WJ, Wang YC, Wang SS, Hwang JJ, Lin FY, Chen YS.Comparing the survival between extracorporeal rescue and conventional resuscitation in adult in-hospital cardiac arrests: propensity analysis of three-year data. Resuscitation.2010;81:796-803. doi: 10.1016/j.resuscitation.2010.03.002
6. Shin TG, Choi JH, Jo IJ, Sim MS, Song HG, Jeong YK, Song YB, Hahn JY, Choi SH, Gwon HC, Jeon ES, Sung K, Kim WS, Lee YT.Extracorporeal cardiopulmonary resuscitation in patients with inhospital cardiac arrest: A comparison with conventional cardiopulmonary resuscitation.Crit Care Med.2011;39:1-7. doi: 10.1097/CCM.0b013e3181feb339

特定の不整脈管理
広いQRS幅の頻拍

COR	LOE	推奨事項
2b	B-NR	1. 血行動態が安定している患者に対しては，規則的で単形性の心リズムの原因を判定できない場合，治療および心リズム診断の補助にアデノシンの静注を考慮してもよい。
2b	B-R	2. 広いQRS幅の頻拍の治療には，アミオダロン，プロカインアミド，またはソタロールの静注を考慮してもよい。
3：有害	B-NR	3. 広いQRS幅の頻拍を呈すどのような病態にも，ベラパミルは投与すべきではない。ただし，上室起源であることが確認され，副伝導路からの伝導が生じていない場合は除く。
3：有害	C-LD	4. 血行動態が不安定で，不規則な不整または多形性の広いQRS幅の頻拍患者には，アデノシンを投与すべきではない。

血行動態が安定している広いQRS幅の頻拍の薬理学的管理に関する推奨事項

「概要」

広いQRS幅の頻拍は，QRS時間が0.12秒以上の頻拍（不整脈に起因する場合は通常150回/分以上）として定義される。何らかの伝導異常をきたした上室性頻拍（SVT）の総称であり，房室（AV）リエントリーによって生じる発作性SVT，伝導異常による心房細動，心房粗動，異所性心房性頻拍が含まれる。広いQRS幅の頻拍は，副伝導路からの伝導によってこれらの上室性不整脈が発症した場合にも起こり得る（「早期興奮性不整脈」とも呼ぶ）。一方，ペースメーカーを装着している患者では，VTあるいは速い心室ペーシングによって広いQRS幅の頻拍が生じることもある。

広いQRS幅の頻拍の初期管理では，患者の血行動態の安定化を迅速に評価することが必要となる。血行動態の不安定な患者には，緊急電気ショックが必要である。血行動態が安定している場合は，12誘導心電図を取得して頻拍の特徴を評価することで，心リズムの推定診断を試みる。このとき，P波，およびP波とQRS波との関係を識別し，ペースメーカー装着患者の場合はQRS幅に先行するペーシングスパイクを識別する。

広いQRS幅の頻拍は，規則的である場合と規則性のない不整である場合とがあり，QRS波形が心拍ごとに単一形態であるもの（単形性）と，形態が変化するもの（多形性）とがある。こうした特徴の1つ1つが，心リズムの推定診断を下す場合に有効になる。規則性のない不整を呈する，単形性のQRS波形を示す広いQRS幅の頻拍は，変行伝導を伴う心房細動を示唆している。一方，心拍ごとにQRS幅の形態が変化する場合は，早期興奮性の心房細動または多形性VTである可能性がある。規則的な広いQRS幅の頻拍は，単形性VT，伝導障害をきたしたリエントリー性発作性SVT，異所性心房性頻拍，または心房粗動である可能性がある。心リズムのこれらの病因を区別することが，治療に適した薬物を選択するうえで重要となる。血行動態の安定した心リズムの場合は，評価し，薬物投与する時間的余裕があるが，これらの処置に無反応であることが判明した不整脈の場合，または急速な代償不全が生じている場合には，緊急電気ショックの必要性を予測する必要がある。心リズム管理に対する詳細なアプローチについては，関連文献を参照のこと[1-3]。

「推奨事項の裏付けとなる解説」

1. 経験に基づく薬物療法を開始する前に，可能であれば12誘導心電図を取得しておくか，診断に関して専門家に相談することが奨励される。規則的で広いQRS幅の頻拍が発作性SVTであると疑われる場合は，薬物療法を開始する前に，迷走神経刺激を検討できる（「規則的で狭いQRS幅の頻拍」を参照）。アデノシンは超短時間作用型の薬物であり，AVリエントリーによって生じた規則的な頻拍の停止に奏効する。アデノシンは通常は心房性不整脈（心房粗動，心房性頻拍など）を停止する効果はないが，房室結節を介したP波の伝導を遮断することで心室レートを一時的に遅くし，認識を可能にするため，心リズムの診断の確立に役立つ。アデノシンには心室性不整脈を停止する効果はないものの，血圧への作用は比較的短時間しか持続しないため，血行動態が安定していた患者の単形性VTを不安定化する可能性は低い。このような特徴から，種類が不明であっても，血行動態の安定した，規則的で単形性の広いQRS幅の頻拍の治療においてアデノシンは比較的安全である[4]。さらに心リズムの診断の補助にも使用できるが，その使用にまったくリスクが伴わないわけではない[5,6]。

2. 広いQRS幅の頻拍を有する安定した患者には，特にVTが疑われる場合やアデノシンが奏効しなかった場合，抗不整脈薬の静注を考慮してもよい。抗不整脈薬は作用持続時間が長いため，広いQRS幅の頻拍の再発防止にも有効となる可能性がある。診断未確定の広いQRS幅の頻拍に対し，リドカインは治療オプションに含まれていない。これは，リドカインが比較的「狭域性」の薬剤であり，SVTには奏効しないためであるが，これは恐らく，血行動態的に耐えられる心拍数でのVTに対し，アミオダロン，プロカインアミド，またはソタロールと比較してリドカインのその動態学的特性はのため，効果が弱いためと考えられる[7-10]。一方，アミオダロン，プロカインアミド，ソタロールはリドカインより「広域性」の抗不整脈薬であり，SVTとVTのいずれの治療にも効果があるが，低血圧を生じさせる可能性もある。2010年のガイドライン以降，アミオダロンと生物学的同等性を持つ新ブランドの製剤が静注投与可能となり，

その降圧効果もこれまでのジェネリック製剤より低い[11]。アミオダロン，プロカインアミド，ソタロールそれぞれの有効性が直接比較されることは，これまでにほとんどなかった[12]。執筆グループはこのため，これらの薬剤の中からどれが優れているかを判断するには根拠に乏しいと考える。ただし，QT時間延長の認められる患者にこれらの薬剤を使用する場合，早期興奮性不整脈に対してアミオダロンを使用する場合，ならびに，事前に専門家に相談することなくこれらの薬剤を組み合わせて投与する場合には注意が必要であることを警告する。このいずれかの薬剤の使用により，広いQRS幅の頻拍が悪化する可能性もある。拍動がさらに速く，血行動態が不安定化した，またはより悪性化した不整脈に変化する場合に備え，これらの薬剤を投与する際は除細動器を用意しておくことが奨励される[13]。

3. ベラパミルはカルシウム拮抗薬であり，房室結節伝導を遅らせ，副伝導路の不応期を短縮し，陰性変力作用薬および血管拡張薬として作用する。その効果はアデノシンとは異なる機序によって作用し，作用持続時間もアデノシンより長い。上室起源であることが確認され，副伝導路からの伝導が関与していない場合にはベラパミルは奏効するが，その陰性変力作用と降圧効果はVTを不安定化させる場合があり[14]，早期興奮性の心房細動および心房粗動を悪化させ，加速させる可能性がある[15]。同様の懸念が，ジルチアゼムやβアドレナリン遮断薬といった，SVTの治療に一般的に使用される他の薬剤にも当てはまるが，これについては推奨事項に取り上げられておらず，エビデンスレビューが必要である。

4. アデノシンの持続時間の短い房室結節伝導遅延効果，心筋および副伝導路における不応期の短縮，および降圧効果が組み合わさると，血行動態的に不安定な患者には適さず，不規則な不整，および多形性で広いQRS幅の頻拍の治療にも適さない。アデノシンは心房細動などの不規則な不整リズムを一時的に遅らせるだけなので，これらの病態の管理には適さない。アデノシンの降圧効果，および組織不応期の短縮効果は，多形性VTの心室レートを加速させる場合があり，副伝導路を介して心房細動または心房粗動が伝導した場合にVFへと悪化させるリスクがある[16]。したがって，血行動態的に不安定な患者や，不規則な不整または多形性で広いQRS幅の頻拍の治療には，この薬剤は推奨されない。

このトピックは，直近で2010年に正式なエビデンスレビューを受けている[17]。

血行動態的に安定した広いQRS幅の頻拍の電気的管理に関する推奨事項

COR	LOE	推奨事項
2a	C-LD	1. 血行動態的に安定した広いQRS幅の頻拍に対し，薬物療法が奏効しなかった場合は，電気ショックの実施，または専門家への緊急相談が妥当である。

「推奨事項の裏付けとなる解説」

1. 治療抵抗性の広いQRS幅の頻拍を診断および管理するうえで，可能であれば専門家に相談することは有用である。電気ショックは第一選択の治療法としても，リエントリー性の心リズムに起因する，薬物治療抵抗性の広いQRS幅の頻拍（心房細動，心房粗動，AVリエントリー，VTなど）にも有用である。しかし，電気ショックは自動性頻拍（異所性心房性頻拍など）には奏効しない場合があり，鎮静に関連するリスクを伴い，広いQRS幅の頻拍の再発を阻止するものではない。特に，QRS幅波形の形態が一様である場合は，ショックをQRSに同期させることが奨励される。心周期（T波）の受攻期中において，タイミングがずれたショックによりVFが発生するリスクを最小限に抑えられるためである[18]。これとは対照的に，多形性の広いQRS幅の頻拍では，各QRS幅波形の特性にばらつきがあるため信頼性の高い同期を行うことができず，高エネルギーの除細動が必要となる[19]。

このトピックは，直近で2010年に正式なエビデンスレビューを受けている[17]。

参考資料

1. Al-Khatib SM, Stevenson WG, Ackerman MJ, Bryant WJ, Callans DJ, Curtis AB, Deal BJ, Dickfeld T, Field ME, Fonarow GC, et al.2017 AHA/ACC/HRS guideline for management of patients with ventricular arrhythmias and the prevention of sudden cardiac death: A report of the American College of Cardiology/American Heart Association Task Force on Clinical Practice Guidelines and the Heart Rhythm Society.Circulation.2018;138:e272-e391. doi: 10.1161/CIR.0000000000000549

2. Page RL, Joglar JA, Caldwell MA, Calkins H, Conti JB, Deal BJ, Estes NA III, Field ME, Goldberger ZD, Hammill SC, Indik JH, Lindsay BD, Olshansky B, Russo AM, Shen WK, Tracy CM, Al-Khatib SM; Evidence Review Committee Chair ǂ.2015 ACC/AHA/HRS Guideline for the Management of Adult Patients With Supraventricular Tachycardia: A Report of the American College of Cardiology/American Heart Association Task Force on Practice Guidelines Circulation.2016;133:e506-e574. doi: 10.1161/CIR.0000000000000311

3. January CT, Wann LS, Calkins H, Chen LY, Cigarroa JE, Cleveland JC Jr, Ellinor PT, Ezekowitz MD, Field ME, Furie KL, Heidenreich PA, Murray KT, Shea JB, Tracy CM, Yancy CW.2019 AHA/ACC/HRS Focused Update of the 2014 AHA/ACC/HRS Guideline for the Management of Patients With Atrial Fibrillation: A Report of the American College of Cardiology/American Heart Association Task Force on Clinical Practice Guidelines and the Heart Rhythm Society in Collaboration With the Society of Thoracic Surgeons. Circulation.2019;140:e125-e151. doi: 10.1161/CIR.0000000000000665

4. Marill KA, Wolfram S, Desouza IS, Nishijima DK, Kay D, Setnik GS, Stair TO, Ellinor PT.Adenosine for wide-complex tachycardia: efficacy and safety.Crit Care Med.2009;37:2512-2518. doi: 10.1097/CCM.0b013e3181a93661

5. Shah CP, Gupta AK, Thakur RK, Hayes OW, Mehrotra A, Lokhandwala YY.Adenosine-induced ventricular fibrillation.Indian Heart J. 2001;53:208-210.
6. Parham WA, Mehdirad AA, Biermann KM, Fredman CS.Case report: adenosine induced ventricular fibrillation in a patient with stable ventricular tachycardia.J Interv Card Electrophysiol.2001;5:71-74. doi: 10.1023/a:1009810025584
7. Josephson ME.Lidocaine and sustained monomorphic ventricular tachycardia: fact or fiction.Am J Cardiol.1996;78:82-83. doi: 10.1016/s0002-9149(96)00271-8
8. Somberg JC, Bailin SJ, Haffajee CI, Paladino WP, Kerin NZ, Bridges D, Timar S, Molnar J; Amio-Aqueous Investigators.Intravenous lidocaine versus intravenous amiodarone (in a new aqueous formulation) for incessant ventricular tachycardia.Am J Cardiol.2002;90:853-859. doi: 10.1016/s0002-9149(02)02707-8
9. Gorgels AP, van den Dool A, Hofs A, Mulleneers R, Smeets JL, Vos MA, Wellens HJ.Comparison of procainamide and lidocaine in terminating sustained monomorphic ventricular tachycardia.Am J Cardiol.1996;78:43-46. doi: 10.1016/s0002-9149(96)00224-x
10. Ho DS, Zecchin RP, Richards DA, Uther JB, Ross DL.Double-blind trial of lignocaine versus sotalol for acute termination of spontaneous sustained ventricular tachycardia.Lancet.1994;344:18-23. doi: 10.1016/s0140-6736(94)91048-0
11. Cushing DJ, Cooper WD, Gralinski MR, Lipicky RJ.The hypotensive effect of intravenous amiodarone is sustained throughout the maintenance infusion period.Clin Exp Pharmacol Physiol.2010;37:358-361. doi: 10.1111/j.1440-1681.2009.05303.x
12. Ortiz M, Martín A, Arribas F, Coll-Vinent B, Del Arco C, Peinado R, Almendral J; PROCAMIO Study Investigators.Randomized comparison of intravenous procainamide vs. intravenous amiodarone for the acute treatment of tolerated wide QRS tachycardia: the PROCAMIO study.Eur Heart J. 2017;38:1329-1335. doi: 10.1093/eurheartj/ehw230
13. Friedman PL, Stevenson WG.Proarrhythmia.Am J Cardiol.1998;82:50N-58N. doi: 10.1016/s0002-9149(98)00586-4
14. Buxton AE, Marchlinski FE, Doherty JU, Flores B, Josephson ME.Hazards of intravenous verapamil for sustained ventricular tachycardia.Am J Cardiol.1987;59:1107-1110. doi: 10.1016/0002-9149(87)90857-5
15. Gulamhusein S, Ko P, Carruthers SG, Klein GJ.Acceleration of the ventricular response during atrial fibrillation in the Wolff-Parkinson-White syndrome after verapamil.Circulation.1982;65:348-354. doi: 10.1161/01.cir.65.2.348
16. Gupta AK, Shah CP, Maheshwari A, Thakur RK, Hayes OW, Lokhandwala YY.Adenosine induced ventricular fibrillation in Wolff-Parkinson-White syndrome.Pacing Clin Electrophysiol.2002;25(4 Pt 1):477-480. doi: 10.1046/j.1460-9592.2002.00477.x
17. Neumar RW, Otto CW, Link MS, Kronick SL, Shuster M, Callaway CW, Kudenchuk PJ, Ornato JP, McNally B, Silvers SM, et al.Part 8: adult advanced cardiovascular life support: 2010 American Heart Association Guidelines for Cardiopulmonary Resuscitation and Emergency Cardiovascular Care.Circulation.2010;122:S729-S767. doi: 10.1161/CIRCULATIONAHA.110.970988
18. Trohman RG, Parrillo JE.Direct current cardioversion: indications, techniques, and recent advances.Crit Care Med.2000;28(suppl):N170-N173. doi: 10.1097/00003246-200010001-00010
19. Dell'Orfano JT, Naccarelli GV.Update on external cardioversion and defibrillation.Curr Opin Cardiol.2001;16:54-57. doi: 10.1097/00001573-200101000-00008

トルサード・ド・ポワント
「概要」

多形性 VT とは，心室を起源とする広い QRS 幅の頻拍であり，心拍ごとに QRS 幅波の形態が変化する。しかし，多形性 VT の診断および治療において最も重要な特徴ポイントは，心リズムの形態ではなく，患者の QT 時間異常の背景に何があるか（または何が疑われているか）である。トルサード・ド・ポワントは多形性 VT の一種であり，心リズムは正常で VT でない場合心拍数で補正した QT 時間延長に関連付けられる。トルサード・ド・ポワントを発症するリスクは，補正 QT 時間が 500 ミリ秒を超え，徐脈を伴う場合に増大する[1]。トルサード・ド・ポワントは遺伝性の遺伝子異常に起因する場合もあるが[2]，QT 時間延長を引き起こす薬剤および電解質異常によって発症することもある[3]。

逆に QT 延長と関連していない多形性 VT は，大半が急性心筋虚血によるものである[4,5]。その他の潜在原因には，QT 延長を伴わず，運動や感情によって多形性 VT が発生する遺伝的異常の一種である，カテコラミン誘発性多形性 VT[6]，「QT 時間短縮」症候群と呼ばれる，非常に短い QT 時間（330〜370ミリ秒を下回る補正 QT 時間）と関連する多形性 VT の一種[7,8]，ならびに交互に出現する QRS 幅波形の軸が交互に180°移変動する，ジギタリス中毒で認められる2方向性 VT が含まれる[9]。多形性 VT（補正 QT 時間延長の有無を問わない）に対する薬物による急性期治療を支持するデータは，RCT が存在しないため，症例報告と症例集積研究に大きく依存している。

多形性 VT の電気的治療に関する推奨事項		
COR	LOE	推奨事項
1	B-NR	1. 即時の除細動は，持続的で，血行動態が不安定な多形性 VT に対して推奨されている。

「推奨事項の裏付けとなる解説」

1. QT 時間の異常の有無にかかわらず，あらゆる種類の多形性 VT は，血行動態的にも電気的にも不安定である傾向が強い。これらは繰り返し再発する場合もあれば，自然に寛解したり，持続性となったり，あるいは電気ショックが必要となることがある VF に進行する場合もある。VT の QRS 幅波の形態が一様である場合は，QRS に同期させた電気ショックを実行することで，心周期の受攻期（T波）中の不適切なタイミングでのショックにより VF が発生するリスクを最小限に抑える[10]。これとは対照的に多形性 VT では，各 QRS 幅の特性にばらつきがあるため信頼性の高い同期を行うことができず，高エネルギーの非同期除細動が必要となる[11]。電気ショックは，多形性 VT を停止させる際には有効であるが，その再発を防止することはできない。このような VT の多くは薬物治療が必要となり，次の推奨事項において最重要視されている。

このトピックは，直近で 2010 年に正式なエビデンスレビューを受けている[12]。

QT 時間延長（トルサード・ド・ポワントと関連している多形性 VT の薬物治療に関する 推奨事項		
COR	LOE	推奨事項
2b	C-LD	1. マグネシウムは，QT 時間延長（トルサード・ド・ポワントと関連している多形性 VT の治療薬として検討できる場合がある。

「推奨事項の裏付けとなる解説」

1. トルサード・ド・ポワントは，典型的には，自然停止する血行動態的に不安定な多形性VTの反復様式をとり，既知または疑いのあるQT時間延長異常と関連し，しばしば徐脈を伴う。トルサード・ド・ポワントが持続するか，またはVFに進行した場合，即時の除細動は最も推奨される治療である。ただしショックによりトルサード・ド・ポワントが収束しても，再発を防止することはできず，この場合は追加の処置が必要となる。小規模の症例集積研究では，トルサード・ド・ポワントの抑制と再発防止に，マグネシウムの静脈内投与が有効であるとされている[13-16]。マグネシウムは，トルサード・ド・ポワントにおいて見られるVT連発を引き起こすおそれがある心筋活動電位の変動である，早期後脱分極を抑制する効果があると考えられている[17]。あらゆる電解質異常（特に低カリウム血症）の是正も推奨されている。トルサーデポアンは，抗不整脈薬により治療することはできない。抗不整脈薬自体がQT時間を延長し，不整脈を促進させてしまうことがあるからである。急激に投与すると，βアドレナリン遮断薬も徐脈を発生または悪化させることで，トルサード・ド・ポワントを促進させてしまう場合がある。徐脈または休止により引き起こされたトルサード・ド・ポワントの患者では，必要に応じて専門家との相談により，オーバードライブペーシングまたはイソプロテレノールなどの追加処置を仰ぐことが最も好ましい[18-20]。トルサード・ド・ポワントに対するマグネシウムの使用は2010年のガイドラインで言及されているうえに，2018年に発表されたACLSガイドラインの重点的アップデートにおいて内容が更新されており[21]，過去の推奨事項の変更が必要になる新しい情報は発見されなかったとする中間エビデンスレビューが掲載されている。

このトピックは，直近で2010年に正式なエビデンスレビューを受けている[12]。

QT時間延長（トルサード・ド・ポワントと関連していない多形性VTの薬物治療に関する 推奨事項）

COR	LOE	推奨事項
2b	C-LD	1. QT時間延長を伴わない多形性VTの治療に，リドカイン静注，アミオダロン，および心筋虚血の治療手段を検討することが可能である。
3：利益なし	C-LD	2. QT時間が正常な多形性VTに対する通常の治療として，マグネシウムを使用することを推奨していない。

「推奨事項の裏付けとなる解説」

1. QT時間延長と関連していない多形性VTは，急性心筋虚血および梗塞により引き起こされる場合が多く[4,5]，このようなVTの多くは急速にVFに進行し，他の心室不整脈（VTおよびVF）と同様に治療が行われる。ただし，除細動により多形性VTを収束させても，その再発は防止できないことがあり，そのような場合は追加の処置が必要となる。薬物による多形性VTの管理に最適な方法を確認するRCTは実施されていない。ただし不整脈が持続する場合，心筋虚血を治療する方法（βアドレナリン遮断薬または緊急冠動脈インターベンション）ならびにリドカインおよびアミオダロンを，除細動と組み合わせて使用すると[22-29]，有効となることがある。βアドレナリン遮断薬も，急性冠症候群における心室不整脈の発生率を減少させることが証明されている[30,31]。βアドレナリン遮断薬および抗不整脈薬も有効となる可能性がある。他のVTの原因が疑われる場合は，専門家への相談が推奨されている[6,32]。このトピックが最後に言及されたのは2010年のガイドラインで，過去の推奨事項の変更が必要となる新しい情報は発見されなかったとする中間エビデンスレビューが掲載されている。多形性VTを引き起こす，より新しく定義された診断要素は，今後のエビデンス評価に役立つ。

2. QT時間延長が認められない場合，マグネシウムは多形性VTの治療における有効性が確認されておらず[13]，また他の心室頻脈性不整脈の急性期管理において利益をもたらす効果も証明されていない[16]。

これらの推奨事項は，ACLSガイドラインに関する2018年の重点的アップデートで支持されている[21]。

参考資料

1. Chan A, Isbister GK, Kirkpatrick CM, Dufful SB.Drug-induced QT prolongation and torsades de pointes: evaluation of a QT nomogram. QJM.2007;100:609–615. doi: 10.1093/qjmed/hcm072
2. Saprungruang A, Khongphatthanayothin A, Mauleekoonphairoj J, Wandee P, Kanjanauthai S, Bhuiyan ZA, Wilde AAM, Poovorawan Y. Genotype and clinical characteristics of congenital long QT syndrome in Thailand.Indian Pacing Electrophysiol J. 2018;18:165-171. doi: 10.1016/j.ipej.2018.07.007
3. Drew BJ, Ackerman MJ, Funk M, Gibler WB, Kligfield P, Menon V, Philippides GJ, Roden DM, Zareba W; American Heart Association Acute Cardiac Care Committee of the Council on Clinical Cardiology; Council on Cardiovascular Nursing; American College of Cardiology Foundation. Prevention of torsade de pointes in hospital settings: a scientific statement from the American Heart Association and the American College of Cardiology Foundation.J Am Coll Cardiol.2010;55:934–947. doi: 10.1016/j.jacc.2010.01.001
4. Pogwizd SM, Corr PB.Electrophysiologic mechanisms underlying arrhythmias due to reperfusion of ischemic myocardium.Circulation.1987;76:404-426. doi: 10.1161/01.cir.76.2.404
5. Wolfe CL, Nibley C, Bhandari A, Chatterjee K, Scheinman M. Polymorphous ventricular tachycardia associated with acute myocardial infarction.Circulation.1991;84:1543–1551. doi: 10.1161/01.cir.84.4.1543
6. Liu N, Ruan Y, Priori SG.Catecholaminergic polymorphic ventricular tachycardia.Prog Cardiovasc Dis..2008;51:23–30. doi: 10.1016/j.pcad.2007.10.005
7. Cross B, Homoud M, Link M, Foote C, Garlitski AC, Weinstock J, Estes NA III.The short QT syndrome.J Interv Card Electrophysiol.2011;31:25–31. doi: 10.1007/s10840-011-9566-0
8. Gollob MH, Redpath CJ, Roberts JD.The short QT syndrome: proposed diagnostic criteria.J Am Coll Cardiol.2011;57:802–812. doi: 10.1016/j.jacc.2010.09.048
9. Chapman M, Hargreaves M, Schneider H, Royle M. Bidirectional ventricular tachycardia associated with digoxin toxicity and with normal digoxin levels.Heart Rhythm.2014;11:1222–1225. doi: 10.1016/j.hrthm.2014.03.050
10. Trohman RG, Parrillo JE.Direct current cardioversion: indications, techniques, and recent advances.Crit Care Med.2000;28(suppl):N170-N173. doi: 10.1097/00003246-200001001-00010
11. Dell'Orfano JT, Naccarelli GV.Update on external cardioversion and defibrillation.Curr Opin Cardiol.2001;16:54-57. doi: 10.1097/00001573-200101000-00008

12. Neumar RW, Otto CW, Link MS, Kronick SL, Shuster M, Callaway CW, Kudenchuk PJ, Ornato JP, McNally B, Silvers SM, et al. Part 8: adult advanced cardiovascular life support: 2010 American Heart Association Guidelines for Cardiopulmonary Resuscitation and Emergency Cardiovascular Care. Circulation. 2010;122:S729-S767. doi: 10.1161/CIRCULATIONAHA.110.970988
13. Tzivoni D, Banai S, Schuger C, Benhorin J, Keren A, Gottlieb S, Stern S. Treatment of torsade de pointes with magnesium sulfate. Circulation. 1988;77:392-397. doi: 10.1161/01.cir.77.2.392
14. Tzivoni D, Keren A, Cohen AM, Loebel H, Zahavi I, Chenzbraun A, Stern S. Magnesium therapy for torsades de pointes. Am J Cardiol. 1984;53:528-530. doi: 10.1016/0002-9149(84)90025-0
15. Hoshino K, Ogawa K, Hishitani T, Isobe T, Etoh Y. Successful uses of magnesium sulfate for torsades de pointes in children with long QT syndrome. Pediatr Int. 2006;48:112-117. doi: 10.1111/j.1442-200X.2006.02177.x
16. Manz M, Jung W, Lüderitz B. Effect of magnesium on sustained ventricular tachycardia [in German]. Herz. 1997;22(suppl 1):51-55. doi: 10.1007/bf03042655
17. Baker WL. Treating arrhythmias with adjunctive magnesium: identifying future research directions. Eur Heart J Cardiovasc Pharmacother. 2017;3:108-117. doi: 10.1093/ehjcvp/pvw028
18. DiSegni E, Klein HO, David D, Libhaber C, Kaplinsky E. Overdrive pacing in quinidine syncope and other long QT-interval syndromes. Arch Intern Med. 1980;140:1036-1040.
19. Damiano BP, Rosen MR. Effects of pacing on triggered activity induced by early afterdepolarizations. Circulation. 1984;69:1013-1025. doi: 10.1161/01.cir.69.5.1013
20. Suarez K, Mack R, Hardegree EL, Chiles C, Banchs JE, Gonzalez MD. Isoproterenol suppresses recurrent torsades de pointes in a patient with long QT syndrome type 2. HeartRhythm Case Rep. 2018;4:576-579. doi: 10.1016/j.hrcr.2018.08.013
21. Panchal AR, Berg KM, Kudenchuk PJ, Del Rios M, Hirsch KG, Link MS, Kurz MC, Chan PS, Cabañas JG, Morley PT, Hazinski MF, Donnino MW. 2018 American Heart Association Focused Update on Advanced Cardiovascular Life Support Use of Antiarrhythmic Drugs During and Immediately After Cardiac Arrest: An Update to the American Heart Association Guidelines for Cardiopulmonary Resuscitation and Emergency Cardiovascular Care. Circulation. 2018;138:e740-e749. doi: 10.1161/CIR.0000000000000613
22. Vrana M, Pokorny J, Marcian P, Fejfar Z. Class I and III antiarrhythmic drugs for prevention of sudden cardiac death and management of postmyocardial infarction arrhythmias. A review. Biomed Pap Med Fac Univ Palacky Olomouc Czech Repub. 2013;157:114-124. doi: 10.5507/bp.2013.030
23. Nalliah CJ, Zaman S, Narayan A, Sullivan J, Kovoor P. Coronary artery reperfusion for ST elevation myocardial infarction is associated with shorter cycle length ventricular tachycardia and fewer spontaneous arrhythmias. Europace. 2014;16:1053-1060. doi: 10.1093/europace/eut307
24. Brady W, Meldon S, DeBehnke D. Comparison of prehospital monomorphic and polymorphic ventricular tachycardia: prevalence, response to therapy, and outcome. Ann Emerg Med. 1995;25:64-70. doi: 10.1016/s0196-0644(95)70357-8
25. Brady WJ, DeBehnke DJ, Laundrie D. Prevalence, therapeutic response, and outcome of ventricular tachycardia in the out-of-hospital setting: a comparison of monomorphic ventricular tachycardia, polymorphic ventricular tachycardia, and torsades de pointes. Acad Emerg Med. 1999;6:609-617. doi: 10.1111/j.1553-2712.1999.tb00414.x
26. Luqman N, Sung RJ, Wang CL, Kuo CT. Myocardial ischemia and ventricular fibrillation: pathophysiology and clinical implications. Int J Cardiol. 2007;119:283-290. doi: 10.1016/j.ijcard.2006.09.016
27. Gorenek B, Lundqvist CB, Terradellas JB, Camm AJ, Hindricks G, Huber K, Kirchhof P, Kuck KH, Kudaiberdieva G, Lin T, Raviele A, Santini M, Tilz RR, Valgimigli M, Vos MA, Vrints C, Zeymer U. Cardiac arrhythmias in acute coronary syndromes: position paper from the joint EHRA, ACCA, and EAPCI task force. Eur Heart J Acute Cardiovasc Care. 2015;4:386. doi: 10.1177/2048872614550583
28. Carmeliet E. Cardiac ionic currents and acute ischemia: from channels to arrhythmias. Physiol Rev. 1999;79:917-1017. doi: 10.1152/physrev.1999.79.3.917
29. Steg PG, James SK, Atar D, Badano LP, Blömstrom-Lundqvist C, Borger MA, Di Mario C, Dickstein K, Ducrocq G, Fernandez-Aviles F, et al; and the Task Force on the management of ST-segment elevation acute myocardial infarction of the European Society of Cardiology. ESC Guidelines for the management of acute myocardial infarction in patients presenting with ST-segment elevation. Eur Heart J. 2012;33:2569-2619. doi: 10.1093/eurheartj/ehs215
30. Al-Khatib SM, Stevenson WG, Ackerman MJ, Bryant WJ, Callans DJ, Curtis AB, Deal BJ, Dickfeld T, Field ME, Fonarow GC, et al. 2017 AHA/ACC/HRS guideline for management of patients with ventricular arrhythmias and the prevention of sudden cardiac death: A report of the American College of Cardiology/American Heart Association Task Force on Clinical Practice Guidelines and the Heart Rhythm Society. Circulation. 2018;138:e272-e391. doi: 10.1161/CIR.0000000000000549
31. Chatterjee S, Chaudhuri D, Vedanthan R, Fuster V, Ibanez B, Bangalore S, Mukherjee D. Early intravenous beta-blockers in patients with acute coronary syndrome—a meta-analysis of randomized trials. Int J Cardiol. 2013;168:915-921. doi: 10.1016/j.ijcard.2012.10.050
32. Van Houzen NE, Alsheikh-Ali AA, Garlitski AC, Homoud MK, Weinstock J, Link MS, Estes NA III. Short QT syndrome review. J Interv Card Electrophysiol. 2008;23:1-5. doi: 10.1007/s10840-008-9201-x

規則的で狭いQRS幅の頻拍

「緒言」

SVTの管理は，AHA，American College of Cardiology，およびHeart Rhythm Societyから発表された最近の合同治療ガイドラインにおける主題である[1]。

QRS幅の狭い頻拍とは，心房または房室結節における回路またはフォーカスから発生したさまざまな頻脈性不整脈を表す病態である。臨床医は，頻拍がQRS幅の狭い頻拍か，または広い頻拍かに加えて，リズムが規則的か，または不規則であるかを判断する必要がある。洞性頻脈（心拍数が100/分超，P波）の患者の場合では，特別な薬物治療は不要で，臨床医は頻拍の基礎原因（発熱，脱水，疼痛）の特定と治療に集中するべきである。患者にSVTが認められる場合，血行動態が不安定（虚血性胸痛，意識障害，ショック，低血圧，急性心不全）か，または不整脈による症状を伴う患者の特定と治療を迅速に行うことが，治療の第一目標となる。不安定型または症候性の規則的でQRS幅の狭い頻拍のコントロールに，同期電気ショックまたは薬剤，あるいはこれらの両方を使用することができる。入手可能なエビデンスでは，奏効率または主要な有害事象発生率に関して，カルシウム拮抗薬とアデノシンとの間に大きな差はないことが示唆されている[2]。

これまでに説明した方法が奏効しないQRS幅の狭い頻拍の患者では，場合によっては専門家への相談が推奨される，より複雑なリズム障害が発生している可能性がある。

規則的で狭いQRS幅の頻拍の電気的治療に関する推奨事項

COR	LOE	推奨事項
1	B-NR	1. 同期電気ショックは，血行動態が不安定なSVT患者に対する急性期治療として推奨されている。
1	B-NR	2. 同期電気ショックは，迷走神経刺激および薬物療法が有効でないか，または禁忌で，血行動態が安定したSVT患者に対する急性期治療として推奨されている。

「推奨事項の裏付けとなる解説」

1 および 2. 血行動態が不安定な SVT 患者の管理では、最初に電気ショックを実施して洞調律の回復を行う必要がある。プレホスピタル環境において、迷走神経刺激および薬物の静脈内投与が奏効しなかった、血行動態が不安定な SVT 患者に対して、電気ショックは安全かつ有効であることが証明されている[3]。電気ショックは、低血圧、急性意識障害、ショック徴候、胸痛、または急性心不全が認められる患者に対して実施することが推奨されている。まれに、安定型の SVT 患者にも電気ショックが必要となることがある。大半の安定型 SVT 患者では、内科的管理（アデノシン、ジルチアゼム）により、80 %から 98 %という高い確率で洞調律が回復する[4,5]。ただし、薬物により洞調律が回復しなかった場合、十分な鎮静薬と麻酔を使用した安定型患者に対する電気ショックは安全かつ有効である。

これらの推奨事項は、「2015 ACC/AHA/HRS Guideline for the Management of Adult Patients With SVT: A Report of the American College of Cardiology/AHA Task Force on Clinical Practice Guidelines and the Heart Rhythm Society」により支持されている[6]。

規則的で QRS 幅の狭い頻拍の薬物治療に関する 推奨事項

COR	LOE	推奨事項
1	B-R	1. 迷走神経刺激は、心拍数が規則的な SVT 患者に対する急性期治療として推奨されている。
1	B-R	2. アデノシンは、心拍数が規則的な SVT 患者に対する急性期治療として推奨されている。
2a	B-R	3. ベラパミルまたはジルチアゼム静注は、心拍数が規則的で、血行動態が安定した SVT 患者に対する急性期治療に有効となる場合がある。
2a	C-LD	4. β アドレナリン遮断薬静注は、心拍数が規則的で、血行動態が安定した SVT 患者に対する合理的な急性期治療である。

「推奨事項の裏付けとなる解説」

1. 迷走神経刺激による SVT 停止の奏効率は、19 %から 54 %である[7]。受動的下肢挙上による迷走神経刺激の補助は、より有効である[8]。高齢患者に対して頸動脈のマッサージを行う際は、血栓塞栓症のリスクを考慮し、注意する。

2. 2015 年に発表された American College of Cardiology、AHA、および Heart Rhythm Society のガイドラインでは、規則的な SVT の第一選択治療としてアデノシンを評価し、有効性、非常に短い半減期、および優れた副作用プロファイルを理由に、これを推奨している[6]。7 件の RCT（患者 622 例）のコクランシステマティックレビューでは、アデノシンとカルシウム拮抗薬の間には、洞調律回復率に関して大きな差はなく（90 %対 93 %）、低血圧についても有意差はないことが確認されている[2]。アデノシンは、心臓移植後の患者に対して重大な影響を及ぼす可能性があり、また喘息患者に対しては重度の気管支けいれんを発生させるおそれがある。

3. 血行動態が安定している患者に対して、ベラパミルまたはジルチアゼム静注による治療を実施することで、64 %から 98 %の患者において SVT が正常な洞調律に回復することが証明されている[4,9-11]。これらの薬剤は、特に β アドレナリン遮断薬を許容できないか、またはアデノシンによる治療後に SVT を再発した患者に対して有用である。これらの薬剤は、徐々に投与することで低血圧のリスクを減少させるよう注意する[11]。収縮期心不全が疑われる状況では、ジルチアゼムとベラパミルは適切ではない[6]。

4. SVT 停止における β アドレナリン遮断薬の有効性を示すエビデンスは限られている。エスモロールとジルチアゼムを比較した試験では、ジルチアゼムは SVT の停止に関してエスモロールよりも有効であった[5]。しかし、一般的に β アドレナリン遮断薬は安全であるため、血行動態が安定している患者の SVT 停止にこれらを使用することは妥当である[6]。

これらの推奨事項は、成人 SVT 患者の管理に関する、American College of Cardiology、AHA、および Heart Rhythm Society による 2015 年のガイドラインにより支持されている[6]。

参考資料

1. Page RL, Joglar JA, Caldwell MA, Calkins H, Conti JB, Deal BJ, Estes NAM 3rd, Field ME, Goldberger ZD, Hammill SC, Indik JH, Lindsay BD, Olshansky B, Russo AM, Shen WK, Tracy CM, Al-Khatib SM.2015 ACC/AHA/HRS Guideline for the Management of Adult Patients With Supraventricular Tachycardia: A Report of the American College of Cardiology/American Heart Association Task Force on Clinical Practice Guidelines and the Heart Rhythm Society. J Am Coll Cardiol.2016;67: e27-e115. doi: 10.1016/j.jacc.2015.08.856

2. Alabed S, Sabouni A, Providencia R, Atallah E, Qintar M, Chico TJ.Adenosine versus intravenous calcium channel antagonists for supraventricular tachycardia.Cochrane Database Syst Rev. 2017;10:CD005154. doi: 10.1002/14651858.CD005154.pub4

3. Roth A, Elkayam I, Shapira I, Sander J, Malov N, Kehati M, Golovner M. Effectiveness of prehospital synchronous direct-current cardioversion for supraventricular tachyarrhythmias causing unstable hemodynamic states. Am J Cardiol.2003;91:489-491. doi: 10.1016/s0002-9149(02)03257-5

4. Brady WJ Jr, DeBehnke DJ, Wickman LL, Lindbeck G. Treatment of out-of-hospital supraventricular tachycardia: adenosine vs verapamil.Acad Emerg Med.1996;3:574-585. doi: 10.1111/j.1553-2712.1996.tb03467.x

5. Gupta A, Naik A, Vora A, Lokhandwala Y. Comparison of efficacy of intravenous diltiazem and esmolol in terminating supraventricular tachycardia.J Assoc Physicians India.1999;47:969-972.

6. Page RL, Joglar JA, Caldwell MA, Calkins H, Conti JB, Deal BJ, Estes NA III, Field ME, Goldberger ZD, Hammill SC, Indik JH, Lindsay BD, Olshansky B, Russo AM, Shen WK, Tracy CM, Al-Khatib SM; Evidence Review Committee Chair ‡.2015 ACC/AHA/HRS Guideline for the Management of Adult Patients With Supraventricular Tachycardia: A Report of the American College of Cardiology/American Heart Association Task Force on Practice Guidelines Circulation.2016;133:e506-e574. doi: 10.1161/CIR.0000000000000311

7. Smith GD, Fry MM, Taylor D, Morgans A, Cantwell K. Effectiveness of the Valsalva Manoeuvre for reversion of supraventricular tachycardia. Cochrane Database Syst Rev. 2015:Cd009502. doi: 10.1002/14651858.CD009502.pub3

8. Appelboam A, Reuben A, Mann C, Gagg J, Ewings P, Barton A, Lobban T, Dayer M, Vickery J, Benger J; REVERT trial collaborators.Postural modification to the standard Valsalva manoeuvre for emergency treatment of supraventricular tachycardias (REVERT): a randomised controlled trial.Lancet.2015;386:1747–1753. doi: 10.1016/S0140-6736(15)61485-4
9. Lim SH, Anantharaman V, Teo WS, Chan YH.Slow infusion of calcium channel blockers compared with intravenous adenosine in the emergency treatment of supraventricular tachycardia.Resuscitation.2009;80:523–528. doi: 10.1016/j.resuscitation.2009.01.017
10. Madsen CD, Pointer JE, Lynch TG.A comparison of adenosine and verapamil for the treatment of supraventricular tachycardia in the prehospital setting.Ann Emerg Med.1995;25:649–655. doi: 10.1016/s0196-0644(95)70179-6
11. Lim SH, Anantharaman V, Teo WS.Slow-infusion of calcium channel blockers in the emergency management of supraventricular tachycardia.Resuscitation.2002;52:167–174. doi: 10.1016/s0300-9572(01)00459-2

速い心室応答を伴う心房細動または粗動

「緒言」

心房細動とは，心房の不規則な電気伝導と，乱れた心房収縮で構成された SVT である。心房粗動とは，心房伝導が速くなる一方で，間欠的な心室応答をもたらすマクロリエントリ回路を伴う SVT である。これらの不整脈は，頻度が高く，併存する場合も多いうえに，治療上の推奨事項も似ている。

心房細動／粗動の治療は，患者の血行動態の安定性ならびに不整脈の既往，併存疾患，および薬剤に対する反応により異なる。血行動態が不安定な患者および心拍数に関連した虚血が認められる患者は，緊急電気ショックの実施が必要となる。血行動態が安定している患者は，心拍数コントロールまたは心リズムコントロールを行う治療戦略による治療が可能である。救急環境では，非ジヒドロピリジン系カルシウム拮抗薬（ジルチアゼム，ベラパミルなど）または β アドレナリン遮断薬（メトプロロール，エスモロールなど）の静脈内投与を行う心拍数コントロールが，より頻繁に実施される。アミオダロンは，一般的にリズムコントロール薬と考えられているが，β アドレナリン拮抗薬を許容できず，非ジヒドロピリジン系カルシウム拮抗薬が禁忌であるうっ血性心不全患者に対しては，これを使用することで心室レートを効果的に減少できる場合がある。CHA_2DS_2-VASc スコアに基づいて血栓塞栓イベントのリスクが高いと考えられる患者に対しては，長期的抗凝固療法が必要となることがある。抗凝固療法の選択は，これらのガイドラインの対象範囲外である。

リズムコントロール戦略（「化学的カルディオバージョン」と呼ばれることもある）では，リズムを洞調律に調整したり，心房細動／粗動（表 3）を予防することを目的とした抗不整脈薬の投与などを行う）。リズムコントロールを受けている患者に対する患者の選別，評価，タイミング，薬剤の選択，および抗凝固療法は，これらのガイドラインの対象範囲外であるため，ここでは紹介されていない[1,2]。

早期興奮症候群（別名Wolff-Parkinson-White症候群）患者の管理は，「QRS 幅の広い頻拍」のセクションに記載されている。

心房細動／粗動の電気的治療に関する 推奨事項		
COR	LOE	推奨事項
1	C-LD	1. 血行動態が不安定で，心室応答が速い心房粗動または心房細動の患者は，電気ショックを行う必要がある。
1	C-LD	2. 急性冠症候群環境における，心房細動の新規発症に対する緊急の直流電気ショックは，血行動態障害，虚血，または不十分な心拍数コントロールが認められる患者に対して推奨されている。
2a	C-LD	3. 二相性エネルギーを使用した心房細動に対する同期電気ショックの場合では，使用する二相性除細動器の種類に従って，初回エネルギーを 120～200 J とすることが合理的である。
2b	C-LD	4. 心房粗動に対する二相性エネルギーを使用した同期電気ショックの場合では，使用する二相性除細動器の種類に従って，初回エネルギーを 50～100 J とすることが合理的である。

「推奨事項の裏付けとなる解説」

1 および 2. コントロール不良の頻拍は，心筋の酸素需要が増加する一方で，心室充満，心拍出量，および冠動脈灌流に障害をもたらす場合がある。特定の場合では迅速な投薬や輸液が適切である一方で，不安定型患者または心虚血が発生している心房細動もしくは心房粗動の患者では，迅速な電気ショックが必要となる[1-3]。電気ショックの要否を判断する際には，不整脈が頻拍の原因であるかどうかも考慮する必要がある。二次的原因（敗血症など）により，速い心室応答が増悪する可能性を考慮する必要があり，これに基づいて初回の血行動態安定化を薬物療法で行うことがある。血行動態が不安定な患者に対するこれらの戦略に言及したデータは少ない。ただし，電気ショックの成功による血行動態面での利益を証明した研究は発表されている[4,5]。さらに，血圧が正常な患者であっても，陰性変力作用薬の使用により低血圧および低灌流が発生するリスクが証明されている[6-8]。血行動態が不安定な患者および心虚血が発生している患者では，洞調律への復帰による血行動態の改善ならびに代替薬物療法に起因する低血圧の回避により利益を得られる可能性が高い。臨床シナリオによっては，48 時間以上に及ぶ心房細動または心房粗動に対して電気ショックを行った患者は，抗凝固療法の候補患者となる。抗凝固療法の選択に関する詳細はここでは言及しない[2]。

表3. 心房細動時および心房粗動時における急性期レートコントロールに一般的に使用される静注薬剤[18]

薬物	ボーラス投与	注入速度	注意
非ジヒドロピリジン系カルシウム拮抗薬			
ジルチアゼム	0.25 mg/kgを2分かけてボーラス静注	5〜10 mg/時	低血圧, 心不全, 心筋症, および急性冠症候群の発症時は避ける
ベラパミル	0.075〜0.15 mg/kgを2分かけてボーラス静注。反応がない場合は, 30分後に追加投与してよい	0.005 mg/kg/分	低血圧, 心不全, 心筋症, および急性冠症候群の発症時は避ける
βアドレナリン遮断薬			
メトプロロール	2.5〜5 mgを2分かけて静注, 最大投与回数3回		非代償性心不全の場合は避ける
エスモロール	500 µg/kgを1分かけて静注	50〜300 µg/kg/分	作用持続時間が短い。非代償性心不全の場合は避ける
プロプラノロール	1 mgを1分かけて静注, 最大投与回数3回		非代償性心不全の場合は避ける
その他の薬物			
アミオダロン	300 mgを1時間かけて静注	10〜50 mg/時（24時間）	アミオダロンについては複数の投与方式が存在する
ジゴキシン	0.25 mgを静注。24時間かけて最大投与量1.5 mgまで繰り返す		通常, 上記の静注の補完療法として使用する。腎機能障害患者の場合は注意する

IV：静脈内（intravenous）。

3および4. 心房細動または心房粗動患者に対して, 電気ショックを実施して洞調律を回復させるために必要な電気エネルギーはさまざまで, 不整脈の新規発症患者や痩せ型の患者の場合, および二相性波形ショックを実施する場合では, 一般的に必要エネルギーが少なくなる[9-15]。肥満体型の患者では, より大きなエネルギーが必要となる場合がある[16]。初回電気ショックが成功しなかった場合は, その後の試行でエネルギーを増加する。一般的に, 心房粗動の場合では, 心房細動の場合よりも必要エネルギーが小さい[11]。200 J以上の高いエネルギーは, 初回ショック成功率の改善および合計使用エネルギー量の減少と関連している。さらに, ある後ろ向き解析では, 低エネルギーによるショックが電気ショック誘発型VFのリスク上昇と関連していることが確認されている[17]。過去のガイドラインでは, 単相および二相性波形の比較が記載されていた。本推奨事項では, 主に二相性波形に注目している。推奨されているエネルギーレベルは, 機器の種類により異なり, 一般的な推奨事項の妥当性は低下する。このトピックでは, 最新の機器による最適な電気エネルギー量をより深く理解するにあたって, 包括的なシステマティックレビューによる詳細な研究を必要としている。C-LDとしてのLOEの執筆グループ評価の内容は, 現在の機器とエネルギー波形を使用した, 限られたエビデンスをもとにしている。

これらの推奨事項は,「2014 AHA/ACC/HRS Guideline for the Management of Patients With Atrial Fibrillation: A Report of the American College of Cardiology/AHA Task Force on Practice Guidelines and the Heart Rhythm Society」[18], ならびに2019年に発表されたこれらのガイドラインの重点的アップデートで支持されている[2]。

心房細動／粗動の薬物療法に関する 推奨事項

COR	LOE	推奨事項
1	B-NR	1. 非ジヒドロピリジン系カルシウム拮抗薬またはβアドレナリン遮断薬の静脈内投与は, 早期興奮を伴わず, 心室応答が速い, 急性期の心房細動または心房粗動患者の心拍数を減少させる場合に推奨されている。
2a	B-NR	2. アミオダロンの静脈内投与は, 早期興奮を伴わず, 心室応答が速い心房細動が認められる重篤患者の心拍数コントロールに有用となることがある。
3：有害	C-LD	3. 早期興奮が認められる心房細動および心房粗動の患者に対しては, ジゴキシン, 非ジヒドロピリジン系カルシウム拮抗薬, βアドレナリン遮断薬, および静脈内アミオダロンを投与すると, 心室応答が増加し, VFにつながる場合があるため, これらの投与は避けるべきである。
3：有害	C-EO	4. 非ジヒドロピリジン系カルシウム拮抗薬および静脈内βアドレナリン遮断薬は, 左室収縮機能障害および非代償性心不全が認められる患者に使用すると, 血行動態障害を省く可能性があるため, これらの投与は避けるべきである。

「推奨事項の裏付けとなる解説」

1および2. 臨床試験のエビデンスにより, 非ジヒドロピリジン系カルシウム拮抗薬（ジルチアゼム, ベラパミルなど）, βアドレナリン遮断薬（エスモロール, プロプラノロールなど）, アミオダロン, およびジゴキシンは, いずれも心房細動/粗動患者の心拍数コントロールに有効であることが証明されている[6-8,19-23]。カルシウム拮抗薬は, アミオダロンよりも有効な場合がある反面, 低血圧がより多く引き起こされる[6]。ジゴキシンは, 作用が発現するまでに時間がかかるため, 急性期に使用されることはまれである[1,2]。

3. 限られた症例報告と小規模の症例集積に基づいて，早期興奮と心房細動または心房粗動が同時に発生している患者では，ジゴキシン，非ジヒドロピリジン系カルシウム拮抗薬，βアドレナリン遮断薬，または静脈内アミオダロンなどの房室結節伝導抑制薬の投与による心室応答上昇の結果，VF が発生する可能性があるとの懸念が存在する[24-27]。このような状況では，最も適切な管理方法として電気ショックが推奨されている。

4. 非ジヒドロピリジン系カルシウム拮抗薬（ジルチアゼム，ベラパミルなど）には陰性変力作用があるため，左室収縮機能障害および症候性心不全が認められる患者の代償不全が増悪する可能性がある。これらは駆出率が保たれている心不全患者には使用できる。βアドレナリン遮断薬は，機能が代償されている心筋症患者に使用できるが，使用の際には注意が必要であったり，非代償性心不全患者には使用を避けなければならない。本推奨事項は，専門家のコンセンサスと病態生理学的根拠に基づいている[2,18,28]。βアドレナリン遮断薬は，複数の研究において有害作用がないことが証明されているため，慢性閉塞性肺疾患患者に使用できる[29]。

これらの推奨事項は，「2014 AHA, American College of Cardiology, and Heart Rhythm Society Guideline for the Management of Patients With Atrial Fibrillation」[18] ならびに 2019 年に発表されたこれらのガイドラインの重点的アップデートで支持されている[2]。

参考資料

1. January CT, Wann LS, Alpert JS, Calkins H, Cigarroa JE, Cleveland JC Jr, Conti JB, Ellinor PT, Ezekowitz MD, Field ME, Murray KT, Sacco RL, Stevenson WG, Tchou PJ, Tracy CM, Yancy CW; ACC/AHA Task Force Members.2014 AHA/ACC/HRS guideline for the management of patients with atrial fibrillation: executive summary: a report of the American College of Cardiology/American Heart Association Task Force on practice guidelines and the Heart Rhythm Society.Circulation.2014;130:2071-2104. doi: 10.1161/CIR.0000000000000040

2. January CT, Wann LS, Calkins H, Chen LY, Cigarroa JE, Cleveland JC Jr, Ellinor PT, Ezekowitz MD, Field ME, Furie KL, Heidenreich PA, Murray KT, Shea JB, Tracy CM, Yancy CW.2019 AHA/ACC/HRS Focused Update of the 2014 AHA/ACC/HRS Guideline for the Management of Patients With Atrial Fibrillation: A Report of the American College of Cardiology/American Heart Association Task Force on Clinical Practice Guidelines and the Heart Rhythm Society in Collaboration With the Society of Thoracic Surgeons. Circulation.2019;140:e125-e151. doi: 10.1161/CIR.0000000000000665

3. McMurray J, Køber L, Robertson M, Dargie H, Colucci W, Lopez-Sendon J, Remme W, Sharpe DN, Ford I. Antiarrhythmic effect of carvedilol after acute myocardial infarction: results of the Carvedilol Post-Infarct Survival Control in Left Ventricular Dysfunction (CAPRICORN) trial.J Am Coll Cardiol.2005;45:525-530. doi: 10.1016/j.jacc.2004.09.076

4. DeMaria AN, Lies JE, King JF, Miller RR, Amsterdam EA, Mason DT.Echographic assessment of atrial transport, mitral movement, and ventricular performance following electroversion of supraventricular arrhythmias.Circulation.1975;51:273-282. doi: 10.1161/01.cir.51.2.273

5. Raymond RJ, Lee AJ, Messineo FC, Manning WJ, Silverman DI.Cardiac performance early after cardioversion from atrial fibrillation.Am Heart J. 1998;136:435-442. doi: 10.1016/s0002-8703(98)70217-0

6. Delle Karth G, Geppert A, Neunteufl T, Priglinger U, Haumer M, Gschwandtner M, Siostrzonek P, Heinz G. Amiodarone versus diltiazem for rate control in critically ill patients with atrial tachyarrhythmias.Crit Care Med.2001;29:1149-1153. doi: 10.1097/00003246-200106000-00011

7. Platia EV, Michelson EL, Porterfield JK, Das G. Esmolol versus verapamil in the acute treatment of atrial fibrillation or atrial flutter.Am J Cardiol.1989;63:925-929. doi: 10.1016/0002-9149(89)90141-0

8. Ellenbogen KA, Dias VC, Plumb VJ, Heywood JT, Mirvis DM.A placebo-controlled trial of continuous intravenous diltiazem infusion for 24-hour heart rate control during atrial fibrillation and atrial flutter: a multicenter study.J Am Coll Cardiol.1991;18:891-897. doi: 10.1016/0735-1097(91)90743-s

9. Glover BM, Walsh SJ, McCann CJ, Moore MJ, Manoharan G, Dalzell GW, McAllister A, McClements B, McEneaney DJ, Trouton TG, Mathew TP, Adgey AA.Biphasic energy selection for transthoracic cardioversion of atrial fibrillation.The BEST AF Trial.Heart.2008;94:884-887. doi: 10.1136/hrt.2007.120782

10. Inácio JF, da Rosa Mdos S, Shah J, Rosário J, Vissoci JR, Manica AL, Rodrigues CG.Monophasic and biphasic shock for transthoracic conversion of atrial fibrillation: systematic review and network meta-analysis.Resuscitation.2016;100:66-75. doi: 10.1016/j.resuscitation.2015.12.009

11. Gallagher MM, Guo XH, Poloniecki JD, Guan Yap Y, Ward D, Camm AJ.Initial energy setting, outcome and efficiency in direct current cardioversion of atrial fibrillation and flutter.J Am Coll Cardiol.2001;38:1498-1504. doi: 10.1016/s0735-1097(01)01540-6

12. Scholten M, Szili-Torok T, Klootwijk P, Jordaens L. Comparison of monophasic and biphasic shocks for transthoracic cardioversion of atrial fibrillation.Heart.2003;89:1032-1034. doi: 10.1136/heart.89.9.1032

13. Page RL, Kerber RE, Russell JK, Trouton T, Waktare J, Gallik D, Olgin JE, Ricard P, Dalzell GW, Reddy R, Lazzara R, Lee K, Carlson M, Halperin B, Bardy GH; BiCard Investigators.Biphasic versus monophasic shock waveform for conversion of atrial fibrillation: the results of an international randomized, double-blind multicenter trial.J Am Coll Cardiol.2002;39:1956-1963. doi: 10.1016/s0735-1097(02)01898-3

14. Reisinger J, Gstrein C, Winter T, Zeindlhofer E, Höllinger K, Mori M, Schiller A, Winter A, Geiger H, Siostrzonek P. Optimization of initial energy for cardioversion of atrial tachyarrhythmias with biphasic shocks.Am J Emerg Med.2010;28:159-165. doi: 10.1016/j.ajem.2008.10.028

15. Alatawi F, Gurevitz O, White RD, Ammash NM, Malouf JF, Bruce CJ, Moon BS, Rosales AG, Hodge D, Hammill SC, Gersh BJ, Friedman PA.Prospective, randomized comparison of two biphasic waveforms for the efficacy and safety of transthoracic biphasic cardioversion of atrial fibrillation.Heart Rhythm.2005;2:382-387. doi: 10.1016/j.hrthm.2004.12.024

16. Voskoboinik A, Moskovitch J, Plunkett G, Bloom J, Wong G, Nalliah C, Prabhu S, Sugumar H, Paramasweran R, McLellan A, et al.Cardioversion of atrial fibrillation in obese patients: Results from the Cardioversion-BMI randomized controlled trial.J Cardiovasc Electrophysiol.2019;30:155-161. doi: 10.1111/jce.13786

17. Gallagher MM, Yap YG, Padula M, Ward DE, Rowland E, Camm AJ.Arrhythmic complications of electrical cardioversion: relationship to shock energy.Int J Cardiol.2008;123:307-312. doi: 10.1016/j.ijcard.2006.12.014

18. January CT, Wann LS, Alpert JS, Calkins H, Cigarroa JE, Cleveland JC Jr, Conti JB, Ellinor PT, Ezekowitz MD, Field ME, et al.2014 AHA/ACC/HRS guideline for the management of patients with atrial fibrillation: a report of the American College of Cardiology/American Heart Association Task Force on practice guidelines and the Heart Rhythm Society. Circulation.2014;130:e199-e267. doi: 10.1161/CIR.0000000000000041

19. Abrams J, Allen J, Allin D, Anderson J, Anderson S, Blanski L, Chadda K, DiBianco R, Favrot L, Gonzalez J. Efficacy and safety of esmolol vs propranolol in the treatment of supraventricular tachyarrhythmias: a multicenter double-blind clinical trial.Am Heart J. 1985;110:913-922. doi: 10.1016/0002-8703(85)90185-1

20. Siu CW, Lau CP, Lee WL, Lam KF, Tse HF.Intravenous diltiazem is superior to intravenous amiodarone or digoxin for achieving ventricular rate control in patients with acute uncomplicated atrial fibrillation.Crit Care Med.2009;37:2174-9; quiz 2180. doi: 10.1097/CCM.0b013e3181a02f56

21. Clemo HF, Wood MA, Gilligan DM, Ellenbogen KA.Intravenous amiodarone for acute heart rate control in the critically ill patient with atrial tachyarrhythmias.Am J Cardiol.1998;81:594-598. doi: 10.1016/s0002-9149(97)00962-4

22. Hou ZY, Chang MS, Chen CY, Tu MS, Lin SL, Chiang HT, Woosley RL.Acute treatment of recent-onset atrial fibrillation and flutter with a tailored dosing regimen of intravenous amiodarone.A randomized, digoxin-controlled study.Eur Heart J. 1995;16:521-528. doi: 10.1093/oxfordjournals.eurheartj.a060945

23. Salerno DM, Dias VC, Kleiger RE, Tschida VH, Sung RJ, Sami M, Giorgi LV. Efficacy and safety of intravenous diltiazem for treatment of atrial fibrillation and atrial flutter. The Diltiazem-Atrial Fibrillation/Flutter Study Group. Am J Cardiol. 1989;63:1046–1051. doi: 10.1016/0002-9149(89)90076-3
24. Gulamhusein S, Ko P, Carruthers SG, Klein GJ. Acceleration of the ventricular response during atrial fibrillation in the Wolff-Parkinson-White syndrome after verapamil. Circulation. 1982;65:348–354. doi: 10.1161/01.cir.65.2.348
25. Jacob AS, Nielsen DH, Gianelly RE. Fatal ventricular fibrillation following verapamil in Wolff-Parkinson-White syndrome with atrial fibrillation. Ann Emerg Med. 1985;14:159–160. doi: 10.1016/s0196-0644(85)81080-5
26. Boriani G, Biffi M, Frabetti L, Azzolini U, Sabbatani P, Bronzetti G, Capucci A, Magnani B. Ventricular fibrillation after intravenous amiodarone in Wolff-Parkinson-White syndrome with atrial fibrillation. Am Heart J. 1996;131:1214–1216. doi: 10.1016/s0002-8703(96)90098-8
27. Kim RJ, Gerling BR, Kono AT, Greenberg ML. Precipitation of ventricular fibrillation by intravenous diltiazem and metoprolol in a young patient with occult Wolff-Parkinson-White syndrome. Pacing Clin Electrophysiol. 2008;31:776–779. doi: 10.1111/j.1540-8159.2008.01086.x
28. Yancy CW, Jessup M, Bozkurt B, Butler J, Casey DE Jr, Drazner MH, Fonarow GC, Geraci SA, Horwich T, Januzzi JL, et al; on behalf of the American College of Cardiology Foundation/American Heart Association Task Force on Practice Guidelines. 2013 ACCF/AHA guideline for the management of heart failure: a report of the American College of Cardiology Foundation/American Heart Association Task Force on practice guidelines. Circulation. 2013;128:e240–e327. doi: 10.1161/CIR.0b013e31829e8776
29. Salpeter S, Ormiston T, Salpeter E. Cardioselective beta-blockers for chronic obstructive pulmonary disease. Cochrane Database Syst Rev. 2005:CD003566. doi: 10.1002/14651858.CD003566.pub2

徐脈

「緒言」

徐脈は，一般的には60/分を下回る心拍数と定義されている。特に運動選手または睡眠中の場合，徐脈は正常な所見となることがある。徐脈が病理学的原因に伴って発生した場合，低血圧および組織灌流低下をもたらす，心拍出量の減少につながる可能性がある。徐脈の臨床症状は，無症状から症候性徐脈（急性意識障害，虚血性胸部不快感，急性心不全，低血圧，または十分な気道と呼吸にもかかわらず持続するその他のショック徴候に関連する徐脈）にまで及ぶ。徐脈の原因により，症状の重症度が変化することがある。例えば，重度の低酸素症および切迫した呼吸不全の患者では，迅速に対処しなければ，心停止につながる重度の徐脈が突発することがある。これとは対照的に，3度心房ブロックが発生したものの，他の部分は十分に代償機能が働いている患者では，かなりの低血圧が認められる以外は安定した状態となる場合がある。このため，徐脈の管理は，基礎疾患と臨床症状の重症度の両方に基づいて行う。2018年に，AHA，American College of Cardiology，および Heart Rhythm Society は，安定型および不安定型徐脈の評価および管理に関する広範なガイドラインを発表した[2]。このガイドラインでは，ACLS環境における症候性徐脈のみを重点的に扱っており，2018年のガイドラインとの整合性が維持されている。

徐脈の初期管理に関する 推奨事項

COR	LOE	推奨事項
1	C-EO	1. 急性症候性徐脈が発生した患者では，可逆性原因の評価および治療が推奨されている。
2a	B-NR	2. 血行動態障害と関連する急性徐脈の患者では，アトロピンの投与による心拍数の増加が妥当である。
2b	C-LD	3. 徐脈がアトロピンに反応しない場合は，必要に応じて，患者に対する緊急の一時的な経静脈ペーシングを準備する間，心拍の加速効果があるアドレナリン作動薬（アドレナリンなど）の静注，または経皮ペーシングを行うと有効な場合がある。
2b	C-EO	4. 高度房室ブロックを伴う不安定患者で，静脈路/骨髄路が確保できない場合には，即時のペーシングを考慮してもよい。

「推奨事項の裏付けとなる解説」

1. 症候性徐脈は，器質性心疾患，迷走神経緊張の亢進，低酸素血症，心筋虚血，または投薬などのさまざまな可逆的または治療可能な原因により発生することがある[2]。徐脈は，基礎疾患を治療しなければ寛解が難しいため，緊急治療による安定化と並行して，基礎疾患を評価することが不可欠である。
2. 観察研究と1件の限定的なRCTにおいて，アトロピンが症候性徐脈の治療に有効であることが証明されている[3-7]。
3. アトロピンが有効でない場合は，心拍数と血圧を上昇させる代替薬剤か，または経皮ペーシングが合理的な次の処置となる。心停止前後の患者の内科的管理では，急性徐脈および低血圧に対して，静注および「プッシュドーズ」投与などにより，アドレナリンを使用する例が増加している。徐脈に対するプッシュドーズアドレナリンに関する研究は不足しているが，限られたデータにより低血圧への使用が支持されている[8]。プッシュドーズ血管収縮薬を使用する場合は，正しく投与できるように細心の注意が必要である。副作用につながる投薬過誤が報告されている[9]。ドパミン注入も，心拍数を上昇させることが可能である[10]。徐脈の治療に関して，薬物療法と経皮ペーシングを比較した研究は少ない。アトロピンが奏効しない患者を対象とした，ある無作為化実用性試験において，ドパミンと経皮ペーシングが比較されており，生存退院率に差がないことが確認されている[10]。このため，経皮ペーシング，アドレナリン，ドパミン，またはその他の血管作動薬のいずれを使用するかは，臨床医の経験と利用可能なリソースによって決まる可能性が高いと考えられる。
4. ショックを引き起こす重度の症候性徐脈に関しては，静脈路も骨髄路も利用できない場合，投与経路の確保を実施しながら

早急な経皮ペーシングを行うことが可能である。プレホスピタル環境における症候性徐脈および徐脈性心停止に対する経皮ペーシングに関する 7 件の研究を対象とした 2006 年のシステマティックレビューでは，利益の点でペーシングが標準的な ACLS を上回ることは確認されなかったが，1 件の試験のサブグループ解析では，症候性徐脈患者において利益が得られる可能性が示唆されていた[11]。

これらの推奨事項は，「2018 ACC/AHA/HRS Guideline on the Evaluation and Management of Patients With Bradycardia and Cardiac Conduction Delay: A Report of the American College of Cardiology/AHA Task Force on Clinical Practice Guidelines and the Heart Rhythm Society」により支持されている[2]。

徐脈に対する経静脈ペーシングに関する 推奨事項		
COR	LOE	推奨事項
2a	C-LD	1. 内科療法が奏効せず，不安定な血行動態が持続する徐脈患者に対しては，一時的な経静脈ペーシングによる心拍数の増加と症状の改善が妥当である。

「推奨事項の裏付けとなる解説」

1. 徐脈に対する内科的管理が奏効せず，重度の症状が発生した場合，一時的なペーシングカテーテルの留置による経静脈ペーシングが次の合理的な処置となる。このようなインターベンションを支持する限られたエビデンスは，観察研究が大きな割合を占めており，その多くは適応および相当高い合併症（特に血流感染および気胸）発生率に重点を置いている[12-14]。ただし，投薬により心拍数が改善せず，ショックが持続する場合では，より決定的な治療（基礎疾患の是正またはペースメーカーの永久的な植え込み）が実施されるまでの間，経静脈ペーシングにより心拍数と症状が改善することがある。

これらの推奨事項は，「2018 American College of Cardiology, AHA, and Heart Rhythm Society guideline on the evaluation and management of patients with bradycardia and cardiac conduction delay」により支持されている[2]。

参考資料

1. Deleted in proof.
2. Kusumoto FM, Schoenfeld MH, Barrett C, Edgerton JR, Ellenbogen KA, Gold MR, Goldschlager NF, Hamilton RM, Joglar JA, Kim RJ, Lee R, Marine JE, McLeod CJ, Oken KR, Patton KK, Pellegrini CN, Selzman KA, Thompson A, Varosy PD.2018 ACC/AHA/HRS Guideline on the Evaluation and Management of Patients With Bradycardia and Cardiac Conduction Delay: A Report of the American College of Cardiology/American Heart Association Task Force on Practice Guidelines Circulation.2019;140:e382-e482. doi: 10.1161/CIR.0000000000000628
3. Smith I, Monk TG, White PF.Comparison of transesophageal atrial pacing with anticholinergic drugs for the treatment of intraoperative bradycardia.Anesth Analg.1994;78:245-252. doi: 10.1213/00000539-199402000-00009
4. Brady WJ, Swart G, DeBehnke DJ, Ma OJ, Aufderheide TP.The efficacy of atropine in the treatment of hemodynamically unstable bradycardia and atrioventricular block: prehospital and emergency department considerations. Resuscitation.1999;41:47-55. doi: 10.1016/s0300-9572(99)00032-5
5. Chadda KD, Lichstein E, Gupta PK, Kourtesis P. Effects of atropine in patients with bradyarrhythmia complicating myocardial infarction.Usefulness of an optimum dose for overdrive.Am J Med.1977;63:503-510. doi: 10.1016/0002-9343(77)90194-2
6. Swart G, Brady WJ Jr, DeBehnke DJ, MA OJ, Aufderheide TP.Acute myocardial infarction complicated by hemodynamically unstable bradyarrhythmia: prehospital and ED treatment with atropine.Am J Emerg Med.1999;17:647-652. doi: 10.1016/s0735-6757(99)90151-1
7. Chadda KD, Lichstein E, Gupta PK, Choy R. Bradycardia-hypotension syndrome in acute myocardial infarction.Reappraisal of the overdrive effects of atropine.Am J Med.1975;59:158-164. doi: 10.1016/0002-9343(75)90349-6
8. Nawrocki PS, Poremba M, Lawner BJ.Push Dose Epinephrine Use in the Management of Hypotension During Critical Care Transport.Prehosp Emerg Care.2020;24:188-195. doi: 10.1080/10903127.2019.1588443
9. Cole JB, Knack SK, Karl ER, Horton GB, Satpathy R, Driver BE.Human Errors and Adverse Hemodynamic Events Related to "Push Dose Pressors" in the Emergency Department.J Med Toxicol.2019;15:276-286. doi: 10.1007/s13181-019-00716-z
10. Morrison LJ, Long J, Vermeulen M, Schwartz B, Sawadsky B, Frank J, Cameron B, Burgess R, Shield J, Bagley P, Mausz V, Brewer JE, Dorian P. A randomized controlled feasibility trial comparing safety and effectiveness of prehospital pacing versus conventional treatment: 'PrePACE'.Resuscitation.2008;76:341-349. doi: 10.1016/j.resuscitation.2007.08.008
11. Sherbino J, Verbeek PR, MacDonald RD, Sawadsky BV, McDonald AC, Morrison LJ.Prehospital transcutaneous cardiac pacing for symptomatic bradycardia or bradyasystolic cardiac arrest: a systematic review.Resuscitation.2006;70:193-200. doi: 10.1016/j.resuscitation.2005.11.019
12. Ferguson JD, Banning AP, Bashir Y. Randomised trial of temporary cardiac pacing with semirigid and balloon-flotation electrode catheters.Lancet.1997;349:1883. doi: 10.1016/S0140-6736(97)24026-2
13. McCann P. A review of temporary cardiac pacing wires.Indian Pacing Electrophysiol J. 2007;7:40-49.
14. Jou YL, Hsu HP, Tuan TC, Wang KL, Lin YJ, Lo LW, Hu YF, Kong CW, Chang SL, Chen SA.Trends of temporary pacemaker implant and underlying disease substrate.Pacing Clin Electrophysiol.2010;33:1475-1484. doi: 10.1111/j.1540-8159.2010.02893.x

ROSC 後のケア
蘇生後管理
「緒言」

心停止後ケアは，救命の連鎖において重要な要素である。心停止後の ROSC 患者に対する最適な病院ケアを定義する基準は，完全には把握されていないが，転帰を改善できる可能性が高い診療の特定と最適化に対する関心が高まっている。心停止とその後の蘇生に起因する虚血-再灌流により，全身への影響が認められる場合では，心停止後ケアを実施して，影響を受けた複数の臓器系を同時にサポートすることが必要である。初期の安定化後は，血行動態，機械的換気，体温管理，基礎疾患の診断および治療，けいれん発作の診断および治療，感染症に対する警戒と治療，ならびに患者の重篤状態の管理に基づいて心停止後の重篤患者のケアを行う。初期イベント時に死亡しなかった心停止患者の多くは，神経損傷環境において，生命維持治療の中止により終的に死亡する。このような死因は，特に OHCA 患者だけでなく，IHCA 後の患者にも頻繁に見られる[1,2]。

したがって、心拍再開後の治療では、脳の損傷を緩和することが重視されている。このような目標に寄与しうる因子として、脳灌流圧の最適化、酸素および二酸化炭素の濃度管理、深部体温のコントロール、ならびにけいれん発作の検出および治療などが挙げられる（図9）。心停止は、さまざまな種類の損傷をもたらすため、多臓器不全またはショックにより死亡に至ることもある。心拍再開後の患者の複雑性を考慮すると、心停止ケアの専門知識に優れた集学的治療チームが望ましい。また集学的プロトコルの作成は、生存率および神経転帰の最適化において重要である。

蘇生後ケアにおける主なトピックについては、このセクションでは言及していないが、目標体温管理（TTM）、心停止における経皮的冠動脈インターベンション（PCI）、神経学的予後予測、および回復を中心に後で扱うこととする。

COR	LOE	推奨事項
		蘇生後早期に考慮すべき事項に関する 推奨事項
1	B-NR	1. 心拍再開後患者の治療には、包括的、体系的、かつ複数の専門分野にわたるケアのシステムが一貫した方法で実施されるべきである。
1	B-NR	2. 12誘導心電図を、ROSC後可能な限り早急に記録して、急激なST上昇の有無を確認する。
2a	C-EO	3. 心停止直後にROSCが認められた成人患者における低酸素症を回避するため、信頼性の高い動脈血酸素飽和度または動脈酸素分圧の測定が可能になるまで、利用可能な最高酸素濃度を用いることは妥当である。

「推奨事項の裏付けとなる解説」
1. 心停止患者受入れ施設の能力を評価する観察研究では、強力なケアシステムは、蘇生の成功と最終的な生存率を論理的かつ臨床的に関連付けるものである可能性が示唆されている[3]。データは限られているものの、地域化アプローチから、外傷、脳卒中、およびST上昇型急性心筋梗塞などの他の救急処置までの経験を総合すると、一貫したケアシステムの導入により心停止患者を管理することで、転帰が改善する可能性がある。
2. 12誘導心電図によりST上昇型心筋梗塞（STEMI）が確認された患者に対しては、冠動脈血管造影によりPCIの要否を判断する必要があり、診断を目的としたECG記録の重要性が強調されている[4]。ただし複数の研究において、ST上昇の非存在は、介入可能な冠動脈病変を除外するものではないことが報告されている[5-7]。
3. 数件のRCTにおいて、調整アプローチによる酸素投与と、ROSC後1～2時間に100％酸素を投与するアプローチが比較されている[8-10]。これらはすべてプレホスピタル環境で実施されている。ただしこれらの試験は、パルスオキシメータで酸素飽和度を測定できる条件下でのみ酸素を調整している。血中の酸素飽和度（パルスオキシメータで測定）も酸素分圧（動脈血ガスで測定）も測定できない患者に対する酸素の調整を調査する研究は行われていない。したがって、このバイタルサインが測定可能となるまで100％酸素を投与することを支持する推奨事項は、終末臓器の損傷をもたらすおそれがある低酸素症を防止するべきであるという専門家の意見と生理学に基づいている。

推奨事項1は、2019年のACLSガイドラインの重点的アップデートにより支持されている[3]。推奨事項2は、直近で2015年に正式な最新エビデンスレビューを受けている[4]。推奨事項3は、ALSに関する2020年のCoSTRで支持されている[11]。

COR	LOE	推奨事項
		ROSC後の血圧管理に関する 推奨事項
2a	B-NR	1. 蘇生後において、収縮期血圧を90 mm Hg以上、平均動脈圧を65 mm Hg以上に維持して、低血圧を防止することが望ましい。

「推奨事項の裏付けとなる解説」
1. 心停止後の低血圧により、組織への酸素供給が減少して、脳およびその他の臓器損傷が悪化する場合がある。ただしROSC後の最適な平均動脈圧目標は不明である。このトピックは、2015年にILCORによりレビューされており[12]、2020年にAustralia and New Zealand Council of ResuscitationがILCORに代わって詳細な最新エビデンスを発表している[11]。数件の観察研究において、蘇生後の低血圧が生存率と神経学的転帰の悪化と関連していることが確認されている[13-19]。1件の研究では、TTM治療中の平均動脈圧の上昇と転帰との間に関連はないが、入院時のショックは不良転帰と関連していることが確認されている[20]。「低血圧」の定義は研究によって異なっているが、収縮期血圧は90 mm Hg、平均動脈圧は65 mm Hgがそれぞれカットオフ値として利用されている場合が多い。2015年以降に実施された2件のRCTでは、低い目標血圧値（1件の研究で標準的治療法、すなわち平均動脈圧65 mm Hg超、他方の研究では平均動脈圧65～75 mm Hg）と、高い目標値（1件の研究で平均動脈圧85～100 mm Hg、他方の研究では平均動脈圧80～100 mm Hg）が比較されている[21,22]。いずれの研究においても、生存率および良好な神経学的転帰を伴う生存率に関して差は検出されなかったが、いずれの研究もこれらの転帰について検出能が十分ではなかった。1件の試験では、平均動脈圧の上昇に伴って脳への酸素供給が改善することが確認されており[21]、低酸素性虚血性脳症において、平均動脈圧の上昇により有益な効果をもたらす仕組みとして提案

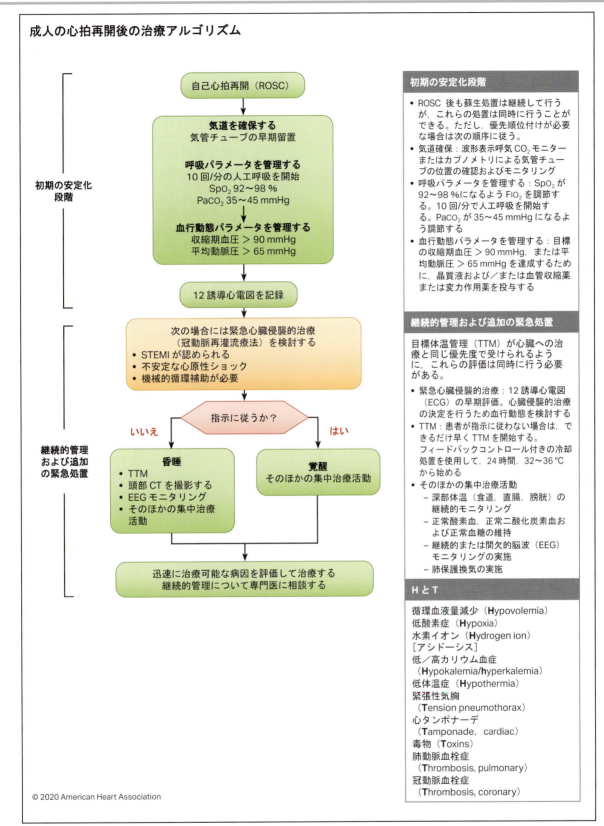

図9. 成人の心拍再開後の治療アルゴリズム。
CT：コンピュータ断層撮影（computed tomography），ROSC：自己心拍再開（return of spontaneous circulation），STEMI：ST上昇型心筋梗塞（ST-segment elevation myocardial infarction）。

されている。平均動脈圧が70〜90 mm Hgの患者の転帰と，平均動脈圧が90 mm Hgを超える患者の転帰を比較した最近の観察研究においても，平均動脈圧の上昇が神経学的転帰の改善と関連していることが確認されている[23]。これらのデータの中には，心停止後の神経損傷のリスクが高い患者に対して，平均動脈圧の目標値を80 mm Hg以上とすることが有益であると示唆するものもあるが，まだ証明されていない。

これらの推奨事項は，2015年のガイドラインアップデート[24]，および2020年のエビデンスアップデートにより支持されている[11]。

COR	LOE	推奨事項
1	B-NR	1. ROSC後に昏睡状態が継続しているすべての患者に対して，低酸素血症の防止を推奨している。
2b	B-R	2. 信頼性の高い末梢血酸素飽和度測定が実施できるようになったら，ROSC後も昏睡状態が続いている患者に対して，吸入酸素濃度を調整し，酸素飽和度の目標を92%から98%とすることにより高酸素血症を防ぐことは妥当かもしれない。
2b	B-R	3. 動脈血二酸化炭素分圧（$Paco_2$）を，生理学的に正常な範囲内（一般的には35〜45 mm Hg）に維持することは，ROSC後も昏睡状態が継続している患者に対して妥当かもしれない。

ROSC後の酸素供給および換気に関する推奨事項

「推奨事項固有の裏付けテキスト」

1. 2020年のILCORシステマティックレビューでは[11]，1件の観察研究において，心拍再開後の低酸素血症が転帰の悪化と関連していることが報告されている[25]。これは他の研究には見られなかったもので[26-28]，すべての研究はバイアスのリスクが高かった。このためこの推奨事項は，主に低酸素症により終末臓器損傷のリスクが上昇するという生理学的根拠と，低酸素血症が，低酸素症の利用可能な最適代理疾患であるという事実に基づいている。

2. 心拍再開後患者では高酸素血症が炎症の増加と脳損傷の増悪につながるという，生理学的根拠と前臨床データがいくつか存在する[29]。2020年のILCORによるシステマティックレビュー[11]では，心拍再開後の患者を対象として，酸素投与量の調整または減少を行う戦略と，通常のケアまたはより高い酸素投与を行う戦略を比較した5件のRCT（3件がプレホスピタル環境，2件がICU環境）が検討された[8-10,30,31]。全てのRCTにおいて，臨床転帰における差は確認されなかったが，いずれの試験もこれらの転帰に関して検出能が不足していた。ある最近の大規模RCTでは，機械的換気を受けている重篤状態患者を対象として，通常のケアと積極的な高酸素血症予防との比較が行われ，コホート全体において群間差は認められなかったが，164例の心拍再開後患者で構成されたサブグループの介入群では，生存率が上昇していた[32]。観察研究データは一貫性を欠くうえに，交絡により非常に限定的である[11]。このトピックに関して3件のRCTが現在進行中である（NCT03138005, NCT03653325, NCT03141099）。提案されている範囲（92%から98%）は，正常範囲を実用的に近似させる意図に基づいている。

3. 2件のRCTでは，高〜正常$Paco_2$（44〜46 mm Hg）を目標とした戦略と，低〜正常$Paco_2$（33〜35 mm Hg）[31]を目標とした戦略の比較と，中等度高炭酸ガス血症（$Paco_2$ 50〜55 mm Hg）を目標とした戦略と正常な炭酸状態（$Paco_2$ 35〜45 mm Hg）を目標とした戦略の比較が行われている[33]。いずれの試験でも，臨床転帰に差は認められなかった。6件の観察研究の結果は一貫しておらず，どの研究もバイアスのリスクが有意に高かったため，限定的であった[25,34-38]。この疑問を調査する1件の大規模RCTが現在進行中である（NCT03114033）。

これらの推奨事項は，ALSに関する2020年のCoSTRで支持されている[11]。

COR	LOE	推奨事項
1	C-LD	1. 心停止後の成人生存患者に対して，臨床的に明白なけいれん発作の治療を行うことを推奨している。
1	C-LD	2. ROSC後の昏睡状態患者すべてに対して，脳波検査（EEG）を迅速に行って判読することにより，けいれん発作の診断を行うことを推奨している。
2b	C-LD	3. 非けいれん性てんかん発作（EEGのみにより診断）も，場合によっては治療を検討してもよい。
2b	C-LD	4. 心停止後に検出されたけいれん発作に対しても，他の病因により発生したけいれん発作の治療と同じ抗けいれん薬のレジメンを検討できる。
3：利益なし	B-R	5. 心停止蘇生後の成人患者に対しては，けいれん発作予防は推奨されない。

けいれん発作の診断および管理に関する推奨事項

「推奨事項の裏付けとなる解説」

1. 2020年のILCORによるシステマティックレビュー[11]では，このような集団に対してけいれん発作の治療を実施した場合と，しなかった場合とを比較した対照研究は確認されなかった。エビデンスが不足しているにもかかわらず，臨床的に明白なけいれん発作を治療しなかった場合では，脳に悪影響が及ぶ可能性があると考えられており，他の環境ではけいれん発作の治療が推奨されているが[39]，心停止後の場合でも必要となる可能性が高い。

2. 執筆グループでは，非けいれん性てんかん発作を検出するEEGにより，転帰が改善することを示す直接的なエビデンスは存在しないことを認めている。この推奨事項は，非けいれん性てんかん発作は心拍再開後患者において好発すること，ならびにけいれん発作の存在は予後に重要な影響を及ぼす可能性があるという事実に基づいているが，このような環境での非けいれん性てんかん発作の治療が転帰に影響するかどうかは不明である。2020年に実施されたILCORのシステマティックレビューでは，心拍再開後に反応がない状態が継続する患者に対するEEG録取のタイミングと方法については特に記述がなかった。EEGの継続的録取と断続的録取による利益の比較に関

するデータは限られている。1 件の研究では，3 ヵ月の時点での神経学的転帰が良好な生存率に関して，通常のモニタリングを行った患者（24 時間で 20 分間の EEG を 1～2 回実施）と継続的に EEG モニタリングを行った患者（18～24 時間）との間に差は認められなかった[40]。

3. 非けいれん性てんかん発作は，心停止後に好発する。臨床的に明白なけいれん発作と関連していない，EEG で確認された非けいれん性発作の治療が，転帰に影響するかどうかは現時点では不明である。この疑問を調査する 1 件の無作為化試験が現在進行中である（NCT02056236）。

4. 2020 年版 CoSTR では，心拍再開後患者においてけいれん発作が診断された場合，治療を推奨している[11]。具体的な薬剤は推奨されていない。ただし CoSTR では，バルプロエート，レベチラセタム，およびホスフェニトインのすべてが有効である可能性を示唆する 2 件の後ろ向き研究について説明している。このうち 1 件の研究では，ホスフェニトインが低血圧の増加と関連していることが確認されている[41,42]。プロポフォールおよびミダゾラムなどの一般的な鎮静薬も，心停止後におけるけいれん発作の抑制に有効であることが確認されている[43-45]。

5. 2020 年の ILCOR によるシステマティックレビュー[11]では，2 件の RCT において，心拍再開後の昏睡状態患者を対象として，けいれん発作予防を実施した場合と実施しなかった場合の比較が行われていたことが確認されている[46,47]。いずれの研究でも，けいれん発作の発生率および良好な神経学的転帰を伴う生存率に関して，群間差は確認されなかった。

これらの推奨事項は，ALS に関する 2020 年の CoSTR で支持されている[11]。

そのほかの蘇生後のケアに関する推奨事項

COR	LOE	推奨事項
2b	B-R	1. 心停止後に ROSC を達成した成人患者において，特定の目標範囲を設けた血糖管理の効果は不明である。
2b	B-R	2. 心拍再開後患者について，予防的抗生物質のルーチン使用の効果は不明である。
2b	B-R	3. ROSC 後に昏睡状態が続く患者について，神経損傷を緩和するために薬剤が有効であるかどうかは不明である。
2b	B-R	4. ROSC 後にショックが起こった患者について，ステロイドのルーチン使用の効果は不明である。

「推奨事項の裏付けとなる解説」

1. 2007 年に実施された 1 件の小規模 RCT では[48]，厳格な血糖コントロールと中等度血糖コントロールとの間に生存率の差はないことが確認されている。心停止に固有のその他のエビデンスは存在せず，心拍再開後患者に対しては，一般的な重篤状態患者の場合と同じアプローチ（すなわち必要に応じてインスリン療法により，血糖値を 150～180 mg/dL に維持）で，血糖値を管理することが妥当であると考えられる[49]。

2. 2020 年版 ILCOR システマティックレビューでは，2 件の RCT と小規模観察研究において，心拍再開後患者の転帰に対する予防的抗生物質の効果が評価されていることが確認されている[11,50]。これらの RCT では，生存率または神経学的転帰に差は認められなかった[51,52]。1 件の RCT[51] では，予防的抗生物質の投与を受けた患者において，早期肺炎の発生率が減少することが確認されているが，これは他の転帰の差につながるものではなかった。これら 2 件の RCT のデータを統合したところ，感染に関して全体的に差は認められなかった[51,52]。

3. 神経保護薬のトピックは，直近で 2010 年に詳細なレビューが発表されている。マグネシウム，コエンザイム Q10（ユビキノール），エキセナチド，キセノンガス，メチルフェニデート，アマンタジンなどの複数の薬剤は，神経損傷の緩和または患者覚醒の促進の候補治療薬として検討されてきた。この研究の多くは観察研究であるが[53-57]，コエンザイム Q10，キセノンガス，およびエキセナチドを対象とした無作為化試験が実施されている[58-60]。コエンザイム Q10 の効果に関する小規模試験では，コエンザイム Q10 を投与した患者において生存率が改善したことが報告されているが，良好な神経学的転帰については有意差は存在せず，これらの結果の妥当性もまだ検証されていない[58]。もう 1 件のコエンザイム Q10 に関する試験が最近完了したが，結果はまだ発表されていない（NCT02934555）。確認された他のどの研究も，研究対象薬の使用による臨床転帰の差を証明できていない。

4. 直近で 2015 年にこのトピックの詳細なアップデートが発表されて以来，ショックおよびその他の ROSC 後の転帰に対するステロイドの効果に関して，2 件以上の無作為化試験が完了しており，これまでに 1 件のみが公開されている[61]。この研究では，ショックの回復およびその他の転帰に関して群間差は認められなかった。1 件の大規模な後ろ向き観察研究では，心停止後のステロイド使用が生存率と関連することが確認されている[62]。敗血症性ショックに対するステロイドの使用は，広範な評価が実施されており，1200 例を超える患者を対象とした最近の試験では，ステロイドを使用した治療を行った患者では生存率が改善したという結

果が出ている[63]。患者3800例が参加した1件の試験では，死亡率に関して利益は認められなかったが，ステロイド群ではICUから退院するまでの時間およびショックの回復までの時間の両方が短縮されていた[64]。総合すると，ROSC後のステロイドによる利益を示す確実なエビデンスは存在しない。ただし敗血症のデータは，重度のショックが発生した患者の一部では，ステロイドによる利益が得られる場合があること，ならびに敗血症と心停止の併発は検討すべき重大事項であることを示唆している。

推奨事項1は，直近で2010年に正式なエビデンスレビューを受けており，またSociety for Critical Care Medicineから発表された「Guidelines for the Use of an Insulin Infusion for the Management of Hyperglycemia in Critically Ill Patients」により支持されている[49]。推奨事項2は，ALSに関する2020年のCoSTRで支持されている[11]。推奨事項3および4は，直近で2015年に正式なエビデンスレビューを受けている[24]。

参考資料

1. Witten L, Gardner R, Holmberg MJ, Wiberg S, Moskowitz A, Mehta S, Grossestreuer AV, Yankama T, Donnino MW, Berg KM.Reasons for death in patients successfully resuscitated from out-of-hospital and in-hospital cardiac arrest.Resuscitation.2019;136:93–99. doi: 10.1016/j.resuscitation.2019.01.031
2. Laver S, Farrow C, Turner D, Nolan J. Mode of death after admission to an intensive care unit following cardiac arrest.Intensive Care Med.2004;30:2126–2128. doi: 10.1007/s00134-004-2425-z
3. Panchal AR, Berg KM, Cabanas JG, Kurz MC, Link MS, Del Rios M, Hirsch KG, Chan PS, Hazinski MF, Morley PT, et al.2019 American Heart Association focused update on systems of care: dispatcher-assisted cardiopulmonary resuscitation and cardiac arrest centers: an update to the American Heart Association Guidelines for Cardiopulmonary Resuscitation and Emergency Cardiovascular Care.Circulation.2019;140:e895–e903. doi: 10.1161/CIR.0000000000000733
4. Levine GN, Bates ER, Blankenship JC, Bailey SR, Bittl JA, Cercek B, Chambers CE, Ellis SG, Guyton RA, Hollenberg SM, Khot UN, Lange RA, Mauri L, Mehran R, Moussa ID, Mukherjee D, Ting HH, O'Gara PT, Kushner FG, Ascheim DD, Brindis RG, Casey DE Jr, Chung MK, de Lemos JA, Diercks DB, Fang JC, Franklin BA, Granger CB, Krumholz HM, Linderbaum JA, Morrow DA, Newby LK, Ornato JP, Ou N, Radford MJ, Tamis-Holland JE, Tommaso CL, Tracy CM, Woo YJ, Zhao DX.2015 ACC/AHA/SCAI Focused Update on Primary Percutaneous Coronary Intervention for Patients With ST-Elevation Myocardial Infarction: An Update of the 2011 ACCF/AHA/SCAI Guideline for Percutaneous Coronary Intervention and the 2013 ACCF/AHA Guideline for the Management of ST-Elevation Myocardial Infarction.Circulation.2016;133:1135–1147. doi: 10.1161/CIR.0000000000000336
5. Stær-Jensen H, Nakstad ER, Fossum E, Mangschau A, Eritsland J, Draegni T, Jacobsen D, Sunde K, Andersen GO.Post-resuscitation ECG for selection of patients for immediate coronary angiography in out-of-hospital cardiac arrest.Circ Cardiovasc Interv.2015;8 doi: 10.1161/CIRCINTERVENTIONS.115.002784
6. Zanuttini D, Armellini I, Nucifora G, Grillo MT, Morocutti G, Carchietti E, Trillò G, Spedicato L, Bernardi G, Proclemer A. Predictive value of electrocardiogram in diagnosing acute coronary artery lesions among patients with out-of-hospital-cardiac-arrest.Resuscitation.2013;84:1250–1254. doi: 10.1016/j.resuscitation.2013.04.023
7. Sideris G, Voicu S, Dillinger JG, Stratiev V, Logeart D, Broche C, Vivien B, Brun PY, Deye N, Capan D, Aout M, Megarbane B, Baud FJ, Henry P. Value of post-resuscitation electrocardiogram in the diagnosis of acute myocardial infarction in out-of-hospital cardiac arrest patients.Resuscitation.2011;82:1148–1153. doi: 10.1016/j.resuscitation.2011.04.023
8. Kuisma M, Boyd J, Voipio V, Alaspää A, Roine RO, Rosenberg P. Comparison of 30 and the 100% inspired oxygen concentrations during early post-resuscitation period: a randomised controlled pilot study.Resuscitation.2006;69:199–206. doi: 10.1016/j.resuscitation.2005.08.010
9. Bray JE, Hein C, Smith K, Stephenson M, Grantham H, Finn J, Stub D, Cameron P, Bernard S; EXACT Investigators.Oxygen titration after resuscitation from out-of-hospital cardiac arrest: A multi-centre, randomised controlled pilot study (the EXACT pilot trial).Resuscitation.2018;128:211–215. doi: 10.1016/j.resuscitation.2018.04.019
10. Thomas M, Voss S, Benger J, Kirby K, Nolan JP.Cluster randomised comparison of the effectiveness of 100% oxygen versus titrated oxygen in patients with a sustained return of spontaneous circulation following out of hospital cardiac arrest: a feasibility study.PROXY: post ROSC OXYgenation study. BMC Emerg Med.2019;19:16. doi: 10.1186/s12873-018-0214-1
11. Berg KM, Soar J, Andersen LW, Böttiger BW, Cacciola S, Callaway CW, Couper K, Cronberg T, D'Arrigo S, Deakin CD, et al; on behalf of the Adult Advanced Life Support Collaborators.Adult advanced life support: 2020 International Consensus on Cardiopulmonary Resuscitation and Emergency Cardiovascular Care Science With Treatment Recommendations.Circulation.2020;142 (suppl 1):S92–S139. doi: 10.1161/CIR.0000000000000893
12. Soar J, Nolan JP, Böttiger BW, Perkins GD, Lott C, Carli P, Pellis T, Sandroni C, Skrifvars MB, Smith GB, Sunde K, Deakin CD; Adult advanced life support section Collaborators.European Resuscitation Council Guidelines for Resuscitation 2015: Section 3.Adult advanced life support.Resuscitation.2015;95:100–147. doi: 10.1016/j.resuscitation.2015.07.016
13. Trzeciak S, Jones AE, Kilgannon JH, Milcarek B, Hunter K, Shapiro NI, Hollenberg SM, Dellinger P, Parrillo JE.Significance of arterial hypotension after resuscitation from cardiac arrest.Crit Care Med.2009;37:2895–903; quiz 2904. doi: 10.1097/ccm.0b013e3181b01d8c
14. Chiu YK, Lui CT, Tsui KL.Impact of hypotension after return of spontaneous circulation on survival in patients of out-of-hospital cardiac arrest.Am J Emerg Med.2018;36:79–83. doi: 10.1016/j.ajem.2017.07.019
15. Bray JE, Bernard S, Cantwell K, Stephenson M, Smith K; and the VACAR Steering Committee.The association between systolic blood pressure on arrival at hospital and outcome in adults surviving from out-of-hospital cardiac arrests of presumed cardiac aetiology.Resuscitation.2014;85:509–515. doi: 10.1016/j.resuscitation.2013.12.005
16. Russo JJ, Di Santo P, Simard T, James TE, Hibbert B, Couture E, Marbach J, Osborne C, Ramirez FD, Wells GA, Labinaz M, Le May MR; from the CAPITAL study group.Optimal mean arterial pressure in comatose survivors of out-of-hospital cardiac arrest: An analysis of area below blood pressure thresholds.Resuscitation.2018;128:175–180. doi: 10.1016/j.resuscitation.2018.04.028
17. Laurikkala J, Wilkman E, Pettilä V, Kurola J, Reinikainen M, Hoppu S, Ala-Kokko T, Tallgren M, Tiainen M, Vaahersalo J, Varpula T, Skrifvars MB; FINNRESUSCI Study Group.Mean arterial pressure and vasopressor load after out-of-hospital cardiac arrest: Associations with one-year neurologic outcome.Resuscitation.2016;105:116–122. doi: 10.1016/j.resuscitation.2016.05.026
18. Annoni F, Dell'Anna AM, Franchi F, Creteur J, Scolletta S, Vincent JL, Taccone FS.The impact of diastolic blood pressure values on the neurological outcome of cardiac arrest patients.Resuscitation.2018;130:167–173. doi: 10.1016/j.resuscitation.2018.07.017
19. Janiczek JA, Winger DG, Coppler P, Sabedra AR, Murray H, Pinsky MR, Rittenberger JC, Reynolds JC, Dezfulian C. Hemodynamic Resuscitation Characteristics Associated with Improved Survival and Shock Resolution After Cardiac Arrest.Shock.2016;45:613–619. doi: 10.1097/SHK.0000000000000554
20. Young MN, Hollenbeck RD, Pollock JS, Giuseffi JL, Wang L, Harrell FE, McPherson JA.Higher achieved mean arterial pressure during therapeutic hypothermia is not associated with neurologically intact survival following cardiac arrest.Resuscitation.2015;88:158–164. doi: 10.1016/j.resuscitation.2014.12.008
21. Ameloot K, De Deyne C, Eertmans W, Ferdinande B, Dupont M, Palmers PJ, Petit T, Nuyens P, Maeremans J, Vundelinckx J, Vanhaverbeke M, Belmans A, Peeters R, Demaerel P, Lemmens R, Dens J, Janssens S. Early goal-directed haemodynamic optimization of cerebral oxygenation in comatose survivors after cardiac arrest: the Neuroprotect post-cardiac arrest trial.Eur Heart J. 2019;40:1804-1814. doi: 10.1093/eurheartj/ehz120
22. Jakkula P, Pettilä V, Skrifvars MB, Hästbacka J, Loisa P, Tiainen M, Wilkman E, Toppila J, Koskue T, Bendel S, Birkelund T, Laru-Sompa R, Valkonen M, Reinikainen M; COMACARE study group.Targeting low-normal or high-normal mean arterial pressure after cardiac arrest and resuscitation: a randomised pilot trial.Intensive Care Med.2018;44:2091–2101. doi: 10.1007/s00134-018-5446-8
23. Roberts BW, Kilgannon JH, Hunter BR, Puskarich MA, Shea L, Donnino M, Jones C, Fuller BM, Kline JA, Jones AE, Shapiro NI, Abella BS, Trzeciak S. Association Between Elevated Mean Arterial Blood Pressure and Neurologic Outcome After Resuscitation From Cardiac Arrest: Results From a Multicenter Prospective Cohort Study.Crit Care Med.2019;47:93–100. doi: 10.1097/CCM.0000000000003474

24. Callaway CW, Donnino MW, Fink EL, Geocadin RG, Golan E, Kern KB, Leary M, Meurer WJ, Peberdy MA, Thompson TM, et al.Part 8: post-cardiac arrest care: 2015 American Heart Association Guidelines Update for Cardiopulmonary Resuscitation and Emergency Cardiovascular Care.Circulation.2015;132 (suppl 2):S465-482. doi: 10.1161/cir.0000000000000262
25. Wang HE, Prince DK, Drennan IR, Grunau B, Carlbom DJ, Johnson N, Hansen M, Elmer J, Christenson J, Kudenchuk P, Aufderheide T, Weisfeldt M, Idris A, Trzeciak S, Kurz M, Rittenberger JC, Griffiths D, Jasti J, May S; Resuscitation Outcomes Consortium (ROC) Investigators.Post-resuscitation arterial oxygen and carbon dioxide and outcomes after out-of-hospital cardiac arrest.Resuscitation.2017;120:113-118. doi: 10.1016/j.resuscitation.2017.08.244
26. Ebner F, Ullén S, Åneman A, Cronberg T, Mattsson N, Friberg H, Hassager C, Kjærgaard J, Kuiper M, Pelosi P, Undén J, Wise MP, Wetterslev J, Nielsen N. Associations between partial pressure of oxygen and neurological outcome in out-of-hospital cardiac arrest patients: an explorative analysis of a randomized trial.Crit Care.2019;23:30. doi: 10.1186/s13054-019-2322-z
27. Humaloja J, Litonius E, Efendijev I, Folger D, Raj R, Pekkarinen PT, Skrifvars MB.Early hyperoxemia is not associated with cardiac arrest outcome.Resuscitation.2019;140:185-193. doi: 10.1016/j.resuscitation.2019.04.035
28. Johnson NJ, Dodampahala K, Rosselot B, Perman SM, Mikkelsen ME, Goyal M, Gaieski DF, Grossestreuer AV.The Association Between Arterial Oxygen Tension and Neurological Outcome After Cardiac Arrest.Ther Hypothermia Temp Manag.2017;7:36-41. doi: 10.1089/ther.2016.0015
29. Pilcher J, Weatherall M, Shirtcliffe P, Bellomo R, Young P, Beasley R. The effect of hyperoxia following cardiac arrest – A systematic review and meta-analysis of animal trials.Resuscitation.2012;83:417-422. doi: 10.1016/j.resuscitation.2011.12.021
30. Young P, Bailey M, Bellomo R, Bernard S, Dicker B, Freebairn R, Henderson S, Mackle D, McArthur C, McGuinness S, Smith T, Swain A, Weatherall M, Beasley R. HyperOxic Therapy OR NormOxic Therapy after out-of-hospital cardiac arrest (HOT OR NOT): a randomised controlled feasibility trial.Resuscitation.2014;85:1686-1691. doi: 10.1016/j.resuscitation.2014.09.011
31. Jakkula P, Reinikainen M, Hästbacka J, Loisa P, Tiainen M, Pettilä V, Toppila J, Lähde M, Bäcklund M, Okkonen M, et al; and the COMACARE study group. Targeting two different levels of both arterial carbon dioxide and arterial oxygen after cardiac arrest and resuscitation: a randomised pilot trial.Intensive Care Med.2018;44:2112-2121. doi: 10.1007/s00134-018-5453-9
32. Mackle D, Bellomo R, Bailey M, Beasley R, Deane A, Eastwood G, Finfer S, Freebairn R, King V, Linke N, et al; and the ICU-ROX Investigators the Australian New Zealand Intensive Care Society Clinical Trials Group.Conservative oxygen therapy during mechanical ventilation in the ICU.N Engl J Med.2020;382:989-998. doi: 10.1056/NEJMoa1903297
33. Eastwood GM, Schneider AG, Suzuki S, Peck L, Young H, Tanaka A, Mårtensson J, Warrillow S, McGuinness S, Parke R, Gilder E, Mccarthy L, Galt P, Taori G, Eliott S, Lamac T, Bailey M, Harley N, Barge D, Hodgson CL, Morganti-Kossmann MC, Pébay A, Conquest A, Archer JS, Bernard S, Stub D, Hart GK, Bellomo R. Targeted therapeutic mild hypercapnia after cardiac arrest: A phase II multi-centre randomised controlled trial (the CCC trial).Resuscitation.2016;104:83-90. doi: 10.1016/j.resuscitation.2016.03.023
34. Vaahersalo J, Bendel S, Reinikainen M, Kurola J, Tiainen M, Raj R, Pettilä V, Varpula T, Skrifvars MB; FINNRESUSCI Study Group.Arterial blood gas tensions after resuscitation from out-of-hospital cardiac arrest: associations with long-term neurologic outcome.Crit Care Med.2014;42:1463-1470. doi: 10.1097/CCM.0000000000000228
35. Hope Kilgannon J, Hunter BR, Puskarich MA, Shea L, Fuller BM, Jones C, Donnino M, Kline JA, Jones AE, Shapiro NI, Abella BS, Trzeciak S, Roberts BW.Partial pressure of arterial carbon dioxide after resuscitation from cardiac arrest and neurological outcome: A prospective multi-center protocol-directed cohort study.Resuscitation.2019;135:212-220. doi: 10.1016/j.resuscitation.2018.11.015
36. Roberts BW, Kilgannon JH, Chansky ME, Mittal N, Wooden J, Trzeciak S. Association between postresuscitation partial pressure of arterial carbon dioxide and neurological outcome in patients with post-cardiac arrest syndrome.Circulation.2013;127:2107-2113. doi: 10.1161/CIRCULATIONAHA.112.000168
37. von Auenmueller KI, Christ M, Sasko BM, Trappe HJ.The Value of Arterial Blood Gas Parameters for Prediction of Mortality in Survivors of Out-of-hospital Cardiac Arrest.J Emerg Trauma Shock.2017;10:134-139. doi: 10.4103/JETS.JETS_146_16
38. Ebner F, Harmon MBA, Aneman A, Cronberg T, Friberg H, Hassager C, Juffermans N, Kjærgaard J, Kuiper M, Mattsson N, Pelosi P, Ullén S, Undén J, Wise MP, Nielsen N. Carbon dioxide dynamics in relation to neurological outcome in resuscitated out-of-hospital cardiac arrest patients: an exploratory Target Temperature Management Trial substudy.Crit Care.2018;22:196. doi: 10.1186/s13054-018-2119-5
39. Glauser T, Shinnar S, Gloss D, Alldredge B, Arya R, Bainbridge J, Bare M, Bleck T, Dodson WE, Garrity L, Jagoda A, Lowenstein D, Pellock J, Riviello J, Sloan E, Treiman DM.Evidence-Based Guideline: Treatment of Convulsive Status Epilepticus in Children and Adults: Report of the Guideline Committee of the American Epilepsy Society.Epilepsy Curr.2016;16:48-61. doi: 10.5698/1535-7597-16.1.48
40. Fatuzzo D, Beuchat I, Alvarez V, Novy J, Oddo M, Rossetti AO.Does continuous EEG influence prognosis in patients after cardiac arrest? Resuscitation.2018;132:29-32. doi: 10.1016/j.resuscitation.2018.08.023
41. Solanki P, Coppler PJ, Kvaløy JT, Baldwin MA, Callaway CW, Elmer J; Pittsburgh Post-Cardiac Arrest Service.Association of antiepileptic drugs with resolution of epileptiform activity after cardiac arrest.Resuscitation.2019;142:82-90. doi: 10.1016/j.resuscitation.2019.07.007
42. Kapur J, Elm J, Chamberlain JM, Barsan W, Cloyd J, Lowenstein D, Shinnar S, Conwit R, Meinzer C, Cock H, Fountain N, Connor JT, Silbergleit R; NETT and PECARN Investigators.Randomized Trial of Three Anticonvulsant Medications for Status Epilepticus.N Engl J Med.2019;381:2103-2113. doi: 10.1056/NEJMoa1905795
43. Thömke F, Weilemann SL.Poor prognosis despite successful treatment of postanoxic generalized myoclonus.Neurology.2010;74:1392-1394. doi: 10.1212/WNL.0b013e3181dad5b9
44. Aicua RI, Rapun I, Novy J, Solari D, Oddo M, Rossetti AO.Early Lance-Adams syndrome after cardiac arrest: prevalence, time to return to awareness, and outcome in a large cohort.Resuscitation.2017;115:169-172. doi: 10.1016/j.resuscitation.2017.03.020
45. Koutroumanidis M, Sakellariou D. Low frequency nonevolving generalized periodic epileptiform discharges and the borderland of hypoxic nonconvulsive status epilepticus in comatose patients after cardiac arrest.Epilepsy Behav.2015;49:255-262. doi: 10.1016/j.yebeh.2015.04.060
46. Brain Resuscitation Clinical Trial I Study Group.Randomized clinical study of thiopental loading in comatose survivors of cardiac arrest.N Engl J Med.1986;314:397-403. doi: 10.1056/nejm198602133140701
47. Longstreth WT Jr, Fahrenbruch CE, Olsufka M, Walsh TR, Copass MK, Cobb LA.Randomized clinical trial of magnesium, diazepam, or both after out-of-hospital cardiac arrest.Neurology.2002;59:506-514. doi: 10.1212/wnl.59.4.506
48. Oksanen T, Skrifvars MB, Varpula T, Kuitunen A, Pettilä V, Nurmi J, Castrén M. Strict versus moderate glucose control after resuscitation from ventricular fibrillation.Intensive Care Med.2007;33:2093-2100. doi: 10.1007/s00134-007-0876-8
49. Jacobi J, Bircher N, Krinsley J, Agus M, Braithwaite SS, Deutschman C, Freire AX, Geehan D, Kohl B, Nasraway SA, Rigby M, Sands K, Schallom L, Taylor B, Umpierrez G, Mazuski J, Schunemann H. Guidelines for the use of an insulin infusion for the management of hyperglycemia in critically ill patients.Crit Care Med.2012;40:3251-3276. doi: 10.1097/CCM.0b013e3182653269
50. Couper K, Laloo R, Field R, Perkins GD, Thomas M, Yeung J. Prophylactic antibiotic use following cardiac arrest: A systematic review and meta-analysis.Resuscitation.2019;141:166-173. doi: 10.1016/j.resuscitation.2019.04.047
51. François B, Cariou A, Clere-Jehl R, Dequin PF, Renon-Carron F, Daix T, Guitton C, Deye N, Legriel S, Plantefève G, Quenot JP, Desachy A, Kamel T, Bedon-Carte S, Diehl JL, Chudeau N, Karam E, Durand-Zaleski I, Giraudeau B, Vignon P, Le Gouge A; CRICS-TRIGGERSEP Network and the ANTHARTIC Study Group.Prevention of Early Ventilator-Associated Pneumonia after Cardiac Arrest.N Engl J Med.2019;381:1831-1842. doi: 10.1056/NEJMoa1812379
52. Ribaric SF, Turel M, Knafelj R, Gorjup V, Stanic R, Gradisek P, Cerovic O, Mirkovic T, Noc M. Prophylactic versus clinically-driven antibiotics in comatose survivors of out-of-hospital cardiac arrest–A randomized pilot study.Resuscitation.2017;111:103-109. doi: 10.1016/j.resuscitation.2016.11.025
53. Pearce A, Lockwood C, van den Heuvel C, Pearce J. The use of therapeutic magnesium for neuroprotection during global cerebral ischemia associated with cardiac arrest and cardiac surgery in adults: a systematic review.JBI Database System Rev Implement Rep.2017;15:86-118. doi: 10.11124/JBISRIR-2016-003236
54. Perucki WH, Hiendlmayr B, O'Sullivan DM, Gunaseelan AC, Fayas F, Fernandez AB.Magnesium Levels and Neurologic Outcomes in Patients Undergoing Therapeutic Hypothermia After Cardiac Arrest.Ther Hypothermia Temp Manag.2018;8:14-17. doi: 10.1089/ther.2017.0016
55. Suzuki M, Hatakeyama T, Nakamura R, Saiki T, Kamisasanuki T, Sugiki D, Matsushima H. Serum Magnesium Levels and Neurological Outcomes in Patients Undergoing Targeted Temperature Management After Cardiac Arrest.J Emerg Nurs.2020;46:59-65. doi: 10.1016/j.jen.2019.10.006
56. Cocchi MN, Giberson B, Berg K, Salciccioli JD, Naini A, Buettner C, Akuthota P, Gautam S, Donnino MW.Coenzyme Q10 levels are low and associated with increased mortality in post-cardiac arrest patients.Resuscitation.2012;83:991-995. doi: 10.1016/j.resuscitation.2012.03.023

57. Reynolds JC, Rittenberger JC, Callaway CW.Methylphenidate and amantadine to stimulate reawakening in comatose patients resuscitated from cardiac arrest.Resuscitation.2013;84:818–824. doi: 10.1016/j.resuscitation.2012.11.014
58. Damian MS, Ellenberg D, Gildemeister R, Lauermann J, Simonis G, Sauter W, Georgi C. Coenzyme Q10 combined with mild hypothermia after cardiac arrest: a preliminary study.Circulation.2004;110:3011–3016. doi: 10.1161/01.CIR.0000146894.45533.C2
59. Laitio R, Hynninen M, Arola O, Virtanen S, Parkkola R, Saunavaara J, Roine RO, Grönlund J, Ylikoski E, Wennervirta J, Bäcklund M, Silvasti P, Nukarinen E, Tiainen M, Saraste A, Pietilä M, Airaksinen J, Valanne L, Martola J, Silvennoinen H, Scheinin H, Harjola VP, Niiranen J, Korpi K, Varpula M, Inkinen O, Olkkola KT, Maze M, Vahlberg T, Laitio T. Effect of Inhaled Xenon on Cerebral White Matter Damage in Comatose Survivors of Out-of-Hospital Cardiac Arrest: A Randomized Clinical Trial.JAMA.2016;315:1120–1128. doi: 10.1001/jama.2016.1933
60. Wiberg S, Hassager C, Schmidt H, Thomsen JH, Frydland M, Lindholm MG, Høfsten DE, Engstrøm T, Køber L, Møller JE, Kjaergaard J. Neuroprotective Effects of the Glucagon-Like Peptide-1 Analog Exenatide After Out-of-Hospital Cardiac Arrest: A Randomized Controlled Trial.Circulation.2016;134:2115–2124. doi: 10.1161/CIRCULATIONAHA.116.024088
61. Donnino MW, Andersen LW, Berg KM, Chase M, Sherwin R, Smithline H, Carney E, Ngo L, Patel PV, Liu X, Cutlip D, Zimetbaum P, Cocchi MN; Collaborating Authors from the Beth Israel Deaconess Medical Center's Center for Resuscitation Science Research Group.Corticosteroid therapy in refractory shock following cardiac arrest: a randomized, double-blind, placebo-controlled, trial.Crit Care.2016;20:82. doi: 10.1186/s13054-016-1257-x
62. Tsai MS, Chuang PY, Huang CH, Tang CH, Yu PH, Chang WT, Chen WJ.Postarrest Steroid Use May Improve Outcomes of Cardiac Arrest Survivors.Crit Care Med.2019;47:167–175. doi: 10.1097/CCM.0000000000003468
63. Annane D, Renault A, Brun-Buisson C, Megarbane B, Quenot JP, Siami S, Cariou A, Forceville X, Schwebel C, Martin C, Timsit JF, Misset B, Ali Benali M, Colin G, Souweine B, Asehnoune K, Mercier E, Chimot L, Charpentier C, François B, Boulain T, Petitpas F, Constantin JM, Dhonneur G, Baudin F, Combes A, Bohé J, Loriferne JF, Amathieu R, Cook F, Slama M, Leroy O, Capellier G, Dargent A, Hissem T, Maxime V, Bellissant E; CRICS-TRIGGERSEP Network.Hydrocortisone plus Fludrocortisone for Adults with Septic Shock.N Engl J Med.2018;378:809–818. doi: 10.1056/NEJMoa1705716
64. Venkatesh B, Finfer S, Cohen J, Rajbhandari D, Arabi Y, Bellomo R, Billot L, Correa M, Glass P, Harward M, et al; on behalf of the ADRENAL Trial Investigators and the Australian-New Zealand Intensive Care Society Clinical Trials Group.Adjunctive glucocorticoid therapy in patients with septic shock.N Engl J Med.2018;378:797–808. doi: 10.1056/NEJMoa1705835

目標体温管理

「緒言」

現在のところ，OHCAとIHCAの両方のすべての心リズムに対して，TTMを32°C〜36°Cの間で24時間以上実施することが推奨されている。さまざまな領域のTTMにおいて複数の無作為化試験が実施され，2015年に公表されたシステマティックレビューで要約されている[1]。2015年の推奨事項に続き，追加の無作為化試験によってショック非適応リズムおよびTTMの時間に対してTTMが評価された。これらの多くは，ASLに関する2020年のCOSTRで実施されたエビデンスアップデートにおいて確認された[2]。患者の特性に基づいて温度を変更するべきかどうか，TTMの継続時間，開始すべきタイミングなど，TTMのトピック内には多くの不確実性が残されている。現在進行中の臨床試験の完了後，この重要なトピックのいくつかの側面についてシステマティックレビューのアップデートが必要となる。

\multicolumn{3}{l	}{TTMの適応に関する 推奨事項}
COR	LOE	推奨事項
1	B-R	1. いずれの初期心リズムを伴うOHCAからのROSC後に指示に従わない成人には，TTMが推奨される。
1	B-R	2. 初期のショック非適応リズムを伴うIHCAからのROSC後に指示に従わない成人には，TTMが推奨される。
1	B-NR	3. 初期のショック適応リズムを伴うIHCAからのROSC後に指示に従わない成人には，TTMが推奨される。

「推奨事項の裏付けとなる解説」

1. 2002年に公表された，初期のショック適応のリズムを伴うOHCA患者の2つのRCTでは，体温管理を行わない場合と比較して，軽度の低体温の有益性が報告されている[1,3,4]。初期のショック非適応リズムを伴う患者（IHCAおよびOHCA）について33°C〜37°Cの目標体温を比較した，より最近の試験でも，33°Cの温度で治療を受けた患者において転帰が改善した[5]。正常体温と比較してTTMをテストする大規模な試験が，現在進行中である（NCT03114033）。

2. 2019年に公表されたRCTでは，初期のショック非適応リズムを伴う心停止からのROSC後に指示に従わなかった患者について，33°Cと37°CでのTTMが比較された。良好な神経学的転帰（脳機能カテゴリー1-2）を伴う生存率は，33°Cで治療を受けたグループで高かった[5]。この試験にはOHCAとIHCAの両方が組み込まれており，心停止後のTTMに対し，IHCA患者を対象に実施された最初の無作為化試験である。サブグループの解析において，IHCA/OHCAサブグループごとにTTMの利益に有意差は認められなかった。

3. TTMのRCTには，初期のショック適応リズムを伴うIHCA患者を対象としたものがないため，この推奨事項は主にOHCA試験，および初期のショック非適応リズムを伴う患者の試験（IHCA患者を含む）からの推定に基づく。ショック適応非適応いずれの初期心リズムでも，IHCAのTTMに対する観察研究の結果はさまざまである。AHA Get With The Guidelines-Resuscitation Registryに登録された患者を対象とした2つの試験では，TTMによって利益が得られないか，または転帰が不良となることが報告されている[6,7]。両者とも，登録内で全般的にTTMの使用が少なく，昏睡状態の有無に関するデータがないという制約により，TTMが特定のIHCA患者に適応となるかどうかを判断するのは難しい。

このトピックは，直近で2015年に正式なエビデンスレビューを受けている[8]。また，ALSに関する2020年のCoSTRでエビデンスアップデートが実施された[2]。

TTMのパフォーマンスに関する 推奨事項

COR	LOE	推奨事項
1	B-R	1. TTM 中は 32°C〜36°C の一定温度を選択して維持することが推奨される。
2a	B-NR	2. 目標体温に達したら、少なくとも 24 時間 TTM を維持することは妥当である。
2b	C-LD	3. TTM 後に昏睡状態にある患者に対して、積極的な発熱予防を行うことは妥当としてよい。
3：利益なし	A	4. ROSC 後の患者の入院前冷却のために、冷却静脈内輸液の急速注入をルーチン使用することは推奨されない。

「推奨事項の裏付けとなる解説」

1. 2013 年、900 人を超える患者の試験において、何らかの初期心リズムを伴う OHCA 患者（目撃者のいない心静止を除く）に対して 33°C と 36°C での TTM が比較された。その結果、33°C は 36°C に対して優位ではいことが判明した[9]。より最近の試験では、初期のショック非適応リズム後に ROSC が見られた患者について、33°C と 37°C での治療が比較された。その結果、33°C で治療を受けたグループで神経学的転帰が良好となり、生存率が改善した[5]。近年、TTM の利用が減少していることが報告されている。1 つの仮説として、一部の臨床医が 36°C の適応を正常体温と同等の目標体温、または厳密な温度管理なしと解釈している[10]。どの目標体温が最も有益かという問いに対して、更新済みのシステマティックレビューが必要である。ただし、現在のエビデンスに基づき、32°C〜36°C の TTM は引き続きクラス 1 の推奨事項となっている。

2. 355 人の患者を対象としたある RCT では、24 時間と 48 時間の TTM に転帰の差異は認められなかった[11]。この試験は、臨床転帰の差異を特定するには検討不足であった可能性がある。初期の 2002 年の試験では、患者の体が 12 時間[3] および 24 時間[4] 冷却された。一方、2013 年の試験では 28 時間冷却された[9]。登録されたすべての患者に対して 33°C の目標体温を使用し、さまざまな時間長（6〜72 時間）の低体温を調査する、より大規模な適応臨床試験が現在進行中である（NCT04217551）。2013 年の試験では毎時 0.5°C というプロトコルに従っていたものの、TTM の復温について明白な最良のアプローチは存在しない[9]。復温の最適な速度、具体的には低速の方が有益であるかどうかは今後の課題であり、少なくとも 1 件の試験が進行中である（NCT02555254）。

3. ROSC 後の発熱は、TTM を施行されていない患者での神経学的転帰不良と関連付けられる。一方、TTM を施行された患者では、この所見は必ずしも報告されていない[12-20]。発熱の治療が転帰の改善と関連付けられるかどうかは立証されていないが、発熱の治療または予防は妥当なアプローチとされる。

4. 2015 年のシステマティックレビューでは、冷却静脈内輸液の急速注入という特定の方法による入院前冷却が、肺水腫の増加および再心停止の高いリスクと関連付けられることが示された[1]。このレビュー以降、入院前冷却について多数の RCT が実施された。ある試験では、何らかの方法（氷の袋や冷却静脈内輸液など）による低体温の入院前導入が、入院前冷却なしの場合と比較され、早期に冷却が開始された患者において院内 TTM の施行率が高かったことが示された。この試験では、入院前冷却を施行された患者において有害事象の増加は認められなかった[21]。入院前冷却のその他の方法（食道内や鼻内の機器など）も検討された。これらが転帰に影響を与えるかどうかは、今後の課題である。

このトピックは、直近で 2015 年に正式なエビデンスレビューを受けている[8]。また、ALS に関する 2020 年の CoSTR でエビデンスアップデートが実施された[2]。

参考資料

1. Donnino MW, Andersen LW, Berg KM, Reynolds JC, Nolan JP, Morley PT, Lang E, Cocchi MN, Xanthos T, Callaway CW, Soar J; ILCOR ALS Task Force. Temperature Management After Cardiac Arrest: An Advisory Statement by the Advanced Life Support Task Force of the International Liaison Committee on Resuscitation and the American Heart Association Emergency Cardiovascular Care Committee and the Council on Cardiopulmonary, Critical Care, Perioperative and Resuscitation.Circulation.2015;132:2448–2456. doi: 10.1161/CIR.0000000000000313

2. Berg KM, Soar J, Andersen LW, Böttiger BW, Cacciola S, Callaway CW, Couper K, Cronberg T, D'Arrigo S, Deakin CD, et al; on behalf of the Adult Advanced Life Support Collaborators.Adult advanced life support: 2020 International Consensus on Cardiopulmonary Resuscitation and Emergency Cardiovascular Care Science With Treatment Recommendations.Circulation.2020;142(suppl 1):S92–S139. doi: 10.1161/CIR.0000000000000893

3. Bernard SA, Gray TW, Buist MD, Jones BM, Silvester W, Gutteridge G, Smith K. Treatment of comatose survivors of out-of-hospital cardiac arrest with induced hypothermia.N Engl J Med.2002;346:557–563. doi: 10.1056/NEJMoa003289

4. Hypothermia after Cardiac Arrest Study Group.Mild therapeutic hypothermia to improve the neurologic outcome after cardiac arrest.N Engl J Med.2002;346:549–556. doi: 10.1056/NEJMoa012689

5. Lascarrou JB, Merdji H, Le Gouge A, Colin G, Grillet G, Girardie P, Coupez E, Dequin PF, Cariou A, Boulain T, Brule N, Frat JP, Asfar P, Pichon N, Landais M, Plantefeve G, Quenot JP, Chakarian JC, Sirodot M, Legriel S, Letheulle J, Thevenin D, Desachy A, Delahaye A, Botoc V, Vimeux S, Martino F, Giraudeau B, Reignier J; CRICS-TRIGGERSEP Group.Targeted Temperature Management for Cardiac Arrest with Nonshockable Rhythm.N Engl J Med.2019;381:2327–2337. doi: 10.1056/NEJMoa1906661

6. Nichol G, Huszti E, Kim F, Fly D, Parnia S, Donnino M, Sorenson T, Callaway CW; American Heart Association Get With the Guideline–Resuscitation Investigators.Does induction of hypothermia improve outcomes after in-hospital cardiac arrest? Resuscitation.2013;84:620–625. doi: 10.1016/j.resuscitation.2012.12.009

7. Chan PS, Berg RA, Tang Y, Curtis LH, Spertus JA; American Heart Association's Get With the Guidelines-Resuscitation Investigators.Association Between Therapeutic Hypothermia and Survival After In-Hospital Cardiac Arrest.JAMA.2016;316:1375–1382. doi: 10.1001/jama.2016.14380

8. Callaway CW, Donnino MW, Fink EL, Geocadin RG, Golan E, Kern KB, Leary M, Meurer WJ, Peberdy MA, Thompson TM, et al.Part 8: post-cardiac arrest care: 2015 American Heart Association Guidelines Update for Cardiopulmonary Resuscitation and Emergency Cardiovascular Care.Circulation.2015;132 (suppl 2):S465-482. doi: 10.1161/cir.0000000000000262
9. Nielsen N, Wettersley J, Cronberg T, Erlinge D, Gasche Y, Hassager C, Horn J, Hovdenes J, Kjaergaard J, Kuiper M, Pellis T, Stammet P, Wanscher M, Wise MP, Åneman A, Al-Subaie N, Boesgaard S, Bro-Jeppesen J, Brunetti I, Bugge JF, Hingston CD, Juffermans NP, Koopmans M, Køber L, Langørgen J, Lilja G, Møller JE, Rundgren M, Rylander C, Smid O, Werer C, Winkel P, Friberg H; TTM Trial Investigators.Targeted temperature management at 33°C versus 36°C after cardiac arrest.N Engl J Med.2013;369:2197-2206. doi: 10.1056/NEJMoa1310519
10. Khera R, Humbert A, Leroux B, Nichol G, Kudenchuk P, Scales D, Baker A, Austin M, Newgard CD, Radecki R, Vilke GM, Sawyer KN, Sopko G, Idris AH, Wang H, Chan PS, Kurz MC.Hospital Variation in the Utilization and Implementation of Targeted Temperature Management in Out-of-Hospital Cardiac Arrest.Circ Cardiovasc Qual Outcomes.2018;11:e004829. doi: 10.1161/CIRCOUTCOMES.118.004829
11. Kirkegaard H, Søreide E, de Haas I, Pettilä V, Taccone FS, Arus U, Storm C, Hassager C, Nielsen JF, Sørensen CA, Ilkjær S, Jeppesen AN, Grejs AM, Duez CHV, Hjort J, Larsen AI, Toome V, Tiainen M, Hästbacka J, Laitio T, Skrifvars MB.Targeted Temperature Management for 48 vs 24 Hours and Neurologic Outcome After Out-of-Hospital Cardiac Arrest: A Randomized Clinical Trial.JAMA.2017;318:341-350. doi: 10.1001/jama.2017.8978
12. Nolan JP, Laver SR, Welch CA, Harrison DA, Gupta V, Rowan K. Outcome following admission to UK intensive care units after cardiac arrest: a secondary analysis of the ICNARC Case Mix Programme Database.Anaesthesia.2007;62:1207-1216. doi: 10.1111/j.1365-2044.2007.05232.x
13. Langhelle A, Tyvold SS, Lexow K, Hapnes SA, Sunde K, Steen PA.In-hospital factors associated with improved outcome after out-of-hospital cardiac arrest.A comparison between four regions in Norway.Resuscitation.2003;56:247-263. doi: 10.1016/s0300-9572(02)00409-4
14. Suffoletto B, Peberdy MA, van der Hoek T, Callaway C. Body temperature changes are associated with outcomes following in-hospital cardiac arrest and return of spontaneous circulation.Resuscitation.2009;80:1365-1370. doi: 10.1016/j.resuscitation.2009.08.020
15. Gebhardt K, Guyette FX, Doshi AA, Callaway CW, Rittenberger JC; Post Cardiac Arrest Service.Prevalence and effect of fever on outcome following resuscitation from cardiac arrest.Resuscitation.2013;84:1062-1067. doi: 10.1016/j.resuscitation.2013.03.038
16. Benz-Woerner J, Delodder F, Benz R, Cueni-Villoz N, Feihl F, Rossetti AO, Liaudet L, Oddo M. Body temperature regulation and outcome after cardiac arrest and therapeutic hypothermia.Resuscitation.2012;83:338-342. doi: 10.1016/j.resuscitation.2011.10.026
17. Leary M, Grossestreuer AV, Iannacone S, Gonzalez M, Shofer FS, Povey C, Wendell G, Archer SE, Gaieski DF, Abella BS.Pyrexia and neurologic outcomes after therapeutic hypothermia for cardiac arrest.Resuscitation.2013;84:1056-1061. doi: 10.1016/j.resuscitation.2012.11.003
18. Cocchi MN, Boone MD, Giberson B, Giberson T, Farrell E, Salciccioli JD, Talmor D, Williams D, Donnino MW.Fever after rewarming: incidence of pyrexia in postcardiac arrest patients who have undergone mild therapeutic hypothermia.J Intensive Care Med.2014;29:365-369. doi: 10.1177/0885066613491932
19. Bro-Jeppesen J, Hassager C, Wanscher M, Søholm H, Thomsen JH, Lippert FK, Møller JE, Køber L, Kjaergaard J. Post-hypothermia fever is associated with increased mortality after out-of-hospital cardiac arrest.Resuscitation.2013;84:1734-1740. doi: 10.1016/j.resuscitation.2013.07.023
20. Winters SA, Wolf KH, Kettinger SA, Seif EK, Jones JS, Bacon-Baguley T. Assessment of risk factors for post-rewarming "rebound hyperthermia" in cardiac arrest patients undergoing therapeutic hypothermia.Resuscitation.2013;84:1245-1249. doi: 10.1016/j.resuscitation.2013.03.027
21. Scales DC, Cheskes S, Verbeek PR, Pinto R, Austin D, Brooks SC, Dainty KN, Goncharenko K, Mamdani M, Thorpe KE, Morrison LJ; Strategies for Post-Arrest Care SPARC Network.Prehospital cooling to improve successful targeted temperature management after cardiac arrest: A randomized controlled trial.Resuscitation.2017;121:187-194. doi: 10.1016/j.resuscitation.2017.10.002

心停止後のPCI

心停止後のPCIに関する 推奨事項

COR	LOE	推奨事項
1	B-NR	1. 心原性心停止が疑われ，ECGでST上昇が認められるすべての心停止患者に対して，直ちに冠動脈造影を実施する必要がある。
2a	B-NR	2. 心原性が疑われるがECGでST上昇が認められないOHCA後の昏睡状態にある一部の成人患者（電気的に不安定または血行動態が不安定である）に対して，緊急冠動脈造影を実施することは妥当である。
2a	C-LD	3. 患者の意識状態に関係なく，それ以外の点は冠動脈造影が適応となるすべての心拍再開後の患者において冠動脈造影は妥当である。

「概要」

心停止では，冠動脈疾患（CAD）が高頻度で確認される[1-4]。ショック適応リズムによる心停止患者では，重度のCADの発症率が特に高い。蘇生後のECGにおいてSTEMI患者の最大96％[2,5]，ST上昇が認められない患者の最大42％[2,5-7]，治療抵抗性の院外VF/VT心停止患者の85％で重度のCADが確認されている[8]。ショック非適応リズムを伴う心停止におけるCADの役割は不明である。

ROSC後の冠動脈造影中に有意なCADが観察された場合，ほとんどのケースで血行再建術を安全に実施できる[5,7,9]。また，複数の観察研究において，PCIの成功は生存率の改善と関連付けられている[2,6,7,10,11]。さらに心臓カテーテル検査を行う利益として，冠動脈異常起始症の発見，左心室機能と血行動態の評価の機会，一時的な機械的循環補助装置の挿入の可能性などがある。

2015年のガイドラインアップデートでは，ROSC後のECGでST上昇が認められる患者に対して緊急冠動脈造影が推奨されている。緊急冠動脈造影とPCIは，ROSCからの蘇生後のECGでSTEMIが認められない患者における神経学的転帰の改善とも関連付けられている[4,12]。ただし，ある大規模な無作為化試験では，初期のショック適応リズムを伴うOHCAから蘇生した，ST上昇またはショックの徴候が認められない患者において，生存率の改善は示されなかった[13]。複数のRCTが進行中である。ショックの徴候が認められる患者にとって緊急冠動脈造影とPCIが有益であるかどうかについては，さらなる検証が必要である。

「推奨事項の裏付けとなる解説」

1. 複数の観察研究により，STEMI が認められる心停止患者において，早期の冠動脈造影に引き続いてのPCIが実施された場合，神経学的に良好な状態での生存率の改善が示されている[5,14-17]。これは，2015 年のガイドラインアップデートでクラス 1 の推奨事項となり，最近の他のいずれの試験によっても反論されていない。この推奨事項は，すべての STEMI 患者に対する全体的推奨事項と一致する。

2. 複数の観察研究により，緊急冠動脈造影とPCI は，ST 上昇が認められない患者における神経学的転帰の改善と関連づけられている[5,7,14,15,18]。ST 上昇が認められない患者における早期の冠動脈造影の使用は，メタアナリシスによっても支持されている[19]。ただし，ある大規模な無作為化試験では，初期のショック適応リズムを伴う OHCA から蘇生した，ST 上昇またはショックの徴候が認められない患者において，生存率の改善は示されなかった[20]。また，冠動脈造影を施行された患者の 65 %で冠動脈疾患が見つかったが，急性血栓性冠動脈閉塞を発症した患者はわずか 5 %であった。複数の RCT が進行中である。ただし，ST 上昇は認められないがショックの徴候が認められる患者における緊急冠動脈造影と PCI の役割については，さらなる検査証が必要である。血行動態または電気的に不安定な患者における緊急冠動脈造影の使用は，NSTEMI 患者に対するガイドラインと一致する[21-23]。血行動態または電気的に安定した，ST 上昇が認められない患者の最適な治療法は，不明のままである。この領域が最後にレビューされたのは 2015 年であり，現在進行中の試験（NCT03119571，NCT02309151，NCT02387398，NCT02641626，NCT02750462，NCT02876458）の完了後に追加のシステマティックレビューが必要である。

3. エビデンスにより，ROSC 後に昏睡状態にある患者にとって，覚醒している患者と同様に侵襲性血管造影が適応のある場合には有益である（適応のある場合）ことが示唆されている[4,14,18]。したがって，侵襲性冠動脈造影は神経症候に関係なく妥当である。

このトピックは，直近で 2015 年に正式なエビデンスレビューを受けている[24]。

参考資料

1. Spaulding CM, Joly LM, Rosenberg A, Monchi M, Weber SN, Dhainaut JF, Carli P. Immediate coronary angiography in survivors of out-of-hospital cardiac arrest.N Engl J Med.1997;336:1629–1633. doi: 10.1056/NEJM199706053362302
2. Dumas F, Cariou A, Manzo-Silberman S, Grimaldi D, Vivien B, Rosencher J, Empana JP, Carli P, Mira JP, Jouven X, Spaulding C. Immediate percutaneous coronary intervention is associated with better survival after out-of-hospital cardiac arrest: insights from the PROCAT (Parisian Region Out of hospital Cardiac ArresT) registry.Circ Cardiovasc Interv.2010;3:200–207. doi: 10.1161/CIRCINTERVENTIONS.109.913665
3. Davies MJ.Anatomic features in victims of sudden coronary death.Coronary artery pathology.Circulation.1992;85（1 Suppl):I19-I24.
4. Yannopoulos D, Bartos JA, Aufderheide TP, Callaway CW, Deo R, Garcia S, Halperin HR, Kern KB, Kudenchuk PJ, Neumar RW, Raveendran G; American Heart Association Emergency Cardiovascular Care Committee.The Evolving Role of the Cardiac Catheterization Laboratory in the Management of Patients With Out-of-Hospital Cardiac Arrest: A Scientific Statement From the American Heart Association.Circulation.2019;139:e530-e552. doi: 10.1161/CIR.0000000000000630
5. Kern KB, Lotun K, Patel N, Mooney MR, Hollenbeck RD, McPherson JA, McMullan PW, Unger B, Hsu CH, Seder DB; INTCAR-Cardiology Registry.Outcomes of Comatose Cardiac Arrest Survivors With and Without ST-Segment Elevation Myocardial Infarction: Importance of Coronary Angiography.J AM COLL CARDIOL.Cardiovasc Interv.2015;8:1031–1040. doi: 10.1016/j.jcin.2015.02.021
6. Dumas F, Bougouin W, Geri G, Lamhaut L, Rosencher J, Pène F, Chiche JD, Varenne O, Carli P, Jouven X, Mira JP, Spaulding C, Cariou A. Emergency Percutaneous Coronary Intervention in Post-Cardiac Arrest Patients Without ST-Segment Elevation Pattern: Insights From the PROCAT II Registry.J AM COLL CARDIOL.Cardiovasc Interv.2016;9:1011–1018. doi: 10.1016/j.jcin.2016.02.001
7. Garcia S, Drexel T, Bekwelem W, Raveendran G, Caldwell E, Hodgson L, Wang Q, Adabag S, Mahoney B, Frascone R, et al.Early access to the cardiac catheterization laboratory for patients resuscitated from cardiac arrest due to a shockable rhythm: the Minnesota Resuscitation Consortium Twin Cities Unified Protocol.J Am Heart Assoc.2016;5:e002670. doi: 10.1161/JAHA.115.002670
8. Yannopoulos D, Bartos JA, Raveendran G, Conterato M, Frascone RJ, Trembley A, John R, Connett J, Benditt DG, Lurie KG, Wilson RF, Aufderheide TP.Coronary Artery Disease in Patients With Out-of-Hospital Refractory Ventricular Fibrillation Cardiac Arrest.J Am Coll Cardiol.2017;70:1109–1117. doi: 10.1016/j.jacc.2017.06.059
9. Sideris G, Voicu S, Yannopoulos D, Dillinger JG, Adjedj J, Deye N, Gueye P, Manzo-Silberman S, Malissin I, Logeart D, Magkoutis N, Capan DD, Makhloufi S, Megarbane B, Vivien B, Cohen-Solal A, Payen D, Baud FJ, Henry P. Favourable 5-year postdischarge survival of comatose patients resuscitated from out-of-hospital cardiac arrest, managed with immediate coronary angiogram on admission.Eur Heart J Acute Cardiovasc Care.2014;3:183–191. doi: 10.1177/2048872614523348
10. Geri G, Dumas F, Bougouin W, Varenne O, Daviaud F, Pene F, Lamhaut L, Chiche JD, Spaulding C, Mira JP, et al.Immediate percutaneous coronary intervention is associated with improved short- and long-term survival after out-of-hospital cardiac arrest.Circ Cardiovasc Interv.2015;8 doi: 10.1161/circinterventions.114.002303
11. Zanuttini D, Armellini I, Nucifora G, Carchietti E, Trillò G, Spedicato L, Bernardi G, Proclemer A. Impact of emergency coronary angiography on in-hospital outcome of unconscious survivors after out-of-hospital cardiac arrest.Am J Cardiol.2012;110:1723–1728. doi: 10.1016/j.amjcard.2012.08.006
12. Patel N, Patel NJ, Macon CJ, Thakkar B, Desai M, Rengifo-Moreno P, Alfonso CE, Myerburg RJ, Bhatt DL, Cohen MG.Trends and Outcomes of Coronary Angiography and Percutaneous Coronary Intervention After Out-of-Hospital Cardiac Arrest Associated With Ventricular Fibrillation or Pulseless Ventricular Tachycardia.JAMA Cardiol.2016;1:890–899. doi: 10.1001/jamacardio.2016.2860
13. Lemkes JS, Janssens GN, van der Hoeven NW, Jewbali LSD, Dubois EA, Meuwissen M, Rijpstra TA, Bosker HA, Blans MJ, Bleeker GB, Baak R, Vlachojannis GJ, Eikemans BJW, van der Harst P, van der Horst ICC, Voskuil M, van der Heijden JJ, Beishuizen A, Stoel M, Camaro C, van der Hoeven H, Henriques JP, Vlaar APJ, Vink MA, van den Bogaard B, Heestermans TACM, de Ruijter W, Delnoij TSR, Crijns HJGM, Jessurun GAJ, Oemrawsingh PV, Gosselink MTM, Plomp K, Magro M, Elbers PWG, van de Ven PM, Oudemans-van Straaten HM, van Royen N. Coronary Angiography after Cardiac Arrest without ST-Segment Elevation.N Engl J Med.2019;380:1397–1407. doi: 10.1056/NEJMoa1816897
14. Bro-Jeppesen J, Kjaergaard J, Wanscher M, Pedersen F, Holmvang L, Lippert FK, Møller JE, Køber L, Hassager C. Emergency coronary angiography in comatose cardiac arrest patients: do real-life experiences support the guidelines? Eur Heart J Acute Cardiovasc Care.2012;1:291–301. doi: 10.1177/2048872612465588
15. Vyas A, Chan PS, Cram P, Nallamothu BK, McNally B, Girotra S. Early coronary angiography and survival after out-of-hospital cardiac arrest.Circ Cardiovasc Interv.2015;8:e002321. doi: 10.1161/CIRCINTERVENTIONS.114.002321
16. Waldo SW, Armstrong EJ, Kulkarni A, Hoffmayer K, Kinlay S, Hsue P, Ganz P, McCabe JM.Comparison of clinical characteristics and outcomes of

cardiac arrest survivors having versus not having coronary angiography. Am J Cardiol.2013;111:1253-1258. doi: 10.1016/j.amjcard.2013.01.267

17. Hosmane VR, Mustafa NG, Reddy VK, Reese CL IV, DiSabatino A, Kolm P, Hopkins JT, Weintraub WS, Rahman E. Survival and neurologic recovery in patients with ST-segment elevation myocardial infarction resuscitated from cardiac arrest.J Am Coll Cardiol.2009;53:409-415. doi: 10.1016/j.jacc.2008.08.076

18. Hollenbeck RD, McPherson JA, Mooney MR, Unger BT, Patel NC, McMullan PW Jr, Hsu CH, Seder DB, Kern KB.Early cardiac catheterization is associated with improved survival in comatose survivors of cardiac arrest without STEMI.Resuscitation.2014;85:88-95. doi: 10.1016/j.resuscitation.2013.07.027

19. Khan MS, Shah SMM, Mubashir A, Khan AR, Fatima K, Schenone AL, Khosa F, Samady H, Menon V. Early coronary angiography in patients resuscitated from out of hospital cardiac arrest without ST-segment elevation: A systematic review and meta-analysis.Resuscitation.2017;121:127-134. doi: 10.1016/j.resuscitation.2017.10.019

20. Lemkes JS, Janssens GN, van Royen N. Coronary Angiography after Cardiac Arrest without ST-Segment Elevation.Reply.N Engl J Med.2019;381:189-190. doi: 10.1056/NEJMc1906523

21. Amsterdam EA, Wenger NK, Brindis RG, Casey DE Jr, Ganiats TG, Holmes DR Jr, Jaffe AS, Jneid H, Kelly RF, Kontos MC, Levine GN, Liebson PR, Mukherjee D, Peterson ED, Sabatine MS, Smalling RW, Zieman SJ; ACC/AHA Task Force Members; Society for Cardiovascular Angiography and Interventions and the Society of Thoracic Surgeons.2014 AHA/ACC guideline for the management of patients with non-ST-elevation acute coronary syndromes: executive summary: a report of the American College of Cardiology/American Heart Association Task Force on Practice Guidelines. Circulation.2014;130:2354-2394. doi: 10.1161/CIR.0000000000000133

22. Lee L, Bates ER, Pitt B, Walton JA, Laufer N, O'Neill WW.Percutaneous transluminal coronary angioplasty improves survival in acute myocardial infarction complicated by cardiogenic shock.Circulation.1988;78:1345-1351. doi: 10.1161/01.cir.78.6.1345

23. Hochman JS, Sleeper LA, Webb JG, Sanborn TA, White HD, Talley JD, Buller CE, Jacobs AK, Slater JN, Col J, McKinlay SM, LeJemtel TH.Early revascularization in acute myocardial infarction complicated by cardiogenic shock.SHOCK Investigators.Should We Emergently Revascularize Occluded Coronaries for Cardiogenic Shock.N Engl J Med.1999;341:625-634. doi: 10.1056/NEJM199908263410901

24. Callaway CW, Donnino MW, Fink EL, Geocadin RG, Golan E, Kern KB, Leary M, Meurer WJ, Peberdy MA, Thompson TM, et al.Part 8: postcardiac arrest care: 2015 American Heart Association Guidelines Update for Cardiopulmonary Resuscitation and Emergency Cardiovascular Care.Circulation.2015;132(suppl 2):S465-482. doi: 10.1161/cir.0000000000000262

神経学的予後予測

「神経学的予後予測の一般的な考慮事項」
「緒言」

低酸素虚血性の脳損傷は，OHCAの生存者における合併症および死亡の主要な原因であり，IHCAからの蘇生後の転帰不良においては，比較的少ないが重大な部分を占める[1,2]。心停止後脳損傷に起因する死亡の大部分は，神経

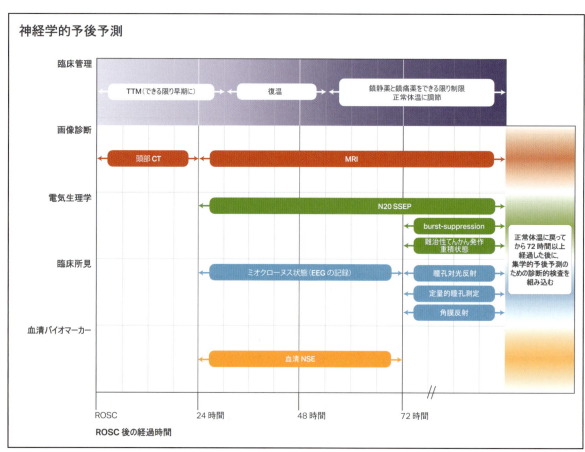

図 10. 集学的な神経学的予後予測への推奨アプローチ。
神経学的予後予測では，複数の診断的検査を使用して，正常体温の回復後 72 時間以上経過し，鎮静および鎮痛を可能な限り制限した状態で集学的な総合評価を行う。個々の診断的検査に潜在的なエラーソースが存在することを認識して見込むことが重要である。集学的診断の推奨タイミングをこの図に示す。CT：コンピュータ断層撮影（computed tomography），EEG：脳波図（electroencephalogram），MRI：磁気共鳴画像法（magnetic resonance imaging），NSE：ニューロン特異的エノラーゼ（neuron-specific enolase），ROSC：自己心拍再開（return of spontaneous circulation），SSEP：体性感覚誘発電位（somatosensory evoked potential），TTM：目標体温管理（targeted temperature management）。

学的転帰不良の予測に基づく生命維持治療の能動的な中止によるものである。有意の神経学的回復の可能性がある患者における生命維持治療の不適切な中止を回避するとともに，転帰不良が避けられない場合に効果のない治療を回避するには，正確な神経学的予後予測が重要となる（図 10）[3]。

COR	LOE	推奨事項
1	B-NR	1. 心停止後に昏睡状態が続く患者では，神経学的予後予測に集学的アプローチを採用することが推奨され，単一の所見に基づいてはならない。
1	B-NR	2. 心停止後に昏睡状態が続く患者では，薬物投与効果または一時的な所見不良による交絡を防止するために，適度な時間が経過するまで神経学的予後予測を遅らせることが推奨される。
1	C-EO	3. 昏睡状態にある心停止からの生存者を治療するチームは，神経学的予後予測の想定経時変化および不確実性について，患者の代理人との間で透明性の高い集多職種による会話を定期的に行うことが推奨される。
2a	B-NR	4. 心停止後に昏睡状態が続く患者については，個別の予後検査を早期に実施できる場合でも，正常体温に戻ってから 72 時間以上経過した後に集学的な神経学的予後予測を実施することが妥当である。

「概要」

神経学的予後予測は，診断的検査結果の解釈，およびこれらの結果と転帰との相関関係に依存する。神経学的転帰不良の偽陽性試験は，回復の可能性がある患者における生命維持の不適切な中止につながるおそれがあるため，試験の最も重要な特徴は特異度である。試験の多くは，薬物投与の効果，臓器機能障害，および体温に起因するエラーの影響を受ける。さらに，多くの研究試験には，サンプルサイズが小さい，単一施設デザインである，盲検化されていない，自己実現的な予測である，最大の回復に関連する時点（通常は心停止後 3～6 か月）ではなく退院時の転帰を使用しているなど，方法論的な限界がある[3]。

神経学的予後予測のいずれの方法にも，エラー発生率が内在しており，交絡の影響を受ける可能性があるため，意思決定の精度を高めるために複数の方法を組み合わせる必要がある。

「推奨事項の裏付けとなる解説」

1. 試験の内的信頼性を損なうバイアスと，外的信頼性を損なう一般化の問題により，神経学的予後予測試験のエビデンスにおける全般的な確実性は低い。したがって，実施された診断的検査の予後予測における信頼性も低い。集学的検査を使用する神経学的予後予測は，単一の検査の結果に依存して予後不良を予測する場合よりも，転帰の予測において優れていると考えられる[3,4]。
2. 心拍再開後の患者では，鎮静薬および筋弛緩薬の代謝にさらに時間がかかるおそれがあり，損傷した脳はさまざまな薬物の抑制作用への感受性が高い可能性がある。残存する鎮静薬や筋弛緩薬は，臨床所見の精度に影響することがある[5]。
3. 神経学的回復の予後予測は複雑で，ほとんどのケースで不確実性による制約を受ける。臨床医と家族／代理人との間で治療の目標が一致しないケースが，重篤な患者の 25 ％以上で報告されている[6]。コミュニケーション不足が重要な要因の 1 つであり，多職種による会話を定期的に行うことで改善できると考えられる。
4. TTM を施行された患者に対する予後予測のタイミングは，通常は ROSC から少なくとも 5 日後（正常体温に戻ってから約 72 時間後）であり，鎮静性投薬の交絡効果を最小限に抑える条件下で実施する必要がある。個々の検査モダリティはそれより早く得ることができ，その結果は，正常体温に戻ってから 72 時間以上経過した時点で行われる集学的評価へと統合される。場合によっては，非神経系疾患，脳ヘルニア，患者の目標と意志，または明らかに生存不可能な状況により，予後予測と救命処置の中止を適切な方法でそれより早く実施してよい。

これらの推奨事項は，ALS に関する 2020 年の CoSTR で支持されている[4]。これは，2015 年に最後に実施されたこのトピックの包括的なレビューを補足するものである[7]。

「神経学的予後予測での臨床所見の使用」

神経学的予後予測での臨床所見に関する 推奨事項

COR	LOE	推奨事項
2b	B-NR	1. 他の予後検査と併せて実施する場合，心停止から 72 時間以上経過した後の両側性の対光反射消失を考慮して，昏睡状態が続く患者の神経学的転帰不良の予後を支持することは妥当としてよい。
2b	B-NR	2. 他の予後検査と併せて実施する場合，心停止から 72 時間以上経過した後の定量的瞳孔測定を考慮して，昏睡状態が続く患者の神経学的転帰不良の予後を支持することは妥当としてよい。
2b	B-NR	3. 他の予後検査と併せて実施する場合，心停止から 72 時間以上経過した後の両側性の角膜反射消失を考慮して，昏睡状態が続く患者の神経学的転帰不良の予後を支持することは妥当としてよい。
2b.	B-NR	4. 他のの予後検査と併せて実施する場合，心停止から 72 時間以内に発生したミオクローヌス状態を考慮して，神経学的転帰不良の予後を支持することは妥当としてよい。
2b	B-NR	5. ミオクローヌスが見られる場合に EEG を記録して，関連する脳の相関が見られるかどうかを判断することが推奨される。
3：有害	B-NR	6. 鑑別診断が行われていない，心停止後のミオクローヌスの動きが見られることだけを考慮して，神経学的予後不良を支持するべきではない。
3：有害	B-NR	7. 上肢の最良の運動反応の所見が，存在しないかまたは伸筋の動きであることだけを考慮して，心停止後に昏睡状態が続く患者における神経学的転帰不良を予測することは推奨されない。

「概要」

臨床所見は転帰不良と相関するが，TTM および投薬による交絡の影響も受ける。また，過去の試験には方法論的な限界があった。意識レベルの評価と基本的な神経学的診察の実施に加えて，臨床所見の要素には，瞳孔対光反射，瞳孔測定，角膜反射，ミオクローヌス，心停止から 1 週間以内に評価されたミオクローヌス状態などがある。ILCOR システマティックレビューには，TTM 施行の有無を問わない試験が含まれ，所見は，さまざまな時点（退院時～心停止後 12 か月）での神経学的転帰と相関していた[4]。定量的瞳孔測定は，自動化された瞳孔反応の評価であり，神経学的瞳孔指数として報告される瞳孔の大きさの縮小率および反応の程度によって測定される。この方法は，標準的で再現性のある評価であることを利点とする。ミオクローヌス状態 は一般的に，心停止から 24 時間以内のほぼ終日，顔と四肢の両方で不定期に反復する，自発性または音誘発性の短発作として定義される[8]。ミオクローヌス状態は，ミオクローヌスてんかん重積症とは異なる。ミオクローヌスてんかん重積症 は，持続的なミオクローヌスの動きの身体的発現を伴うてんかん重積症として定義され，これらのガイドラインではてんかん重積症のサブタイプと見なされる。

「推奨事項の裏付けとなる解説」

1. 17 件の試験で[9-25]，ROSC の直後から心停止後最大 7 日までの瞳孔対光反射の欠如は 48 %～100 % の特異度で神経学的転帰不良が予測された。タイミングによって特異度が有意に異なり，停止後 72 時間またはそれ以上の場合に最大の特異度が認められた。

2. 心停止後 24～72 時間に 3 件の試験で定量的瞳孔対光反射[15,26,27]を評価し，3 件の試験で神経学的瞳孔指標[15,28,29] を評価した。定量的瞳孔測定によって評価された瞳孔対光反射の消失（定量的瞳孔対光反射 =0 %）は客観的所見であり，271 人の患者を対象とする 1 つの試験では，心停止後 72 時間時点で評価された時に転帰不良に対して高い特異度がであった[15]。神経学的瞳孔指標は非特異的であり，薬物の影響を受けることがある。したがって，絶対的な神経学的瞳孔指標カットオフや予後不良を予測する特定の閾値は知られていない[15,28,29]。

3. 11 件の観察研究[9-11,14,16,17,19,21,22,30,31] で，ROSC の直後から心停止後 7 日の時点までの角膜反射の欠如を評価した。転帰不良に対する特異度は 25 %～100 %で，停止後 72 時間以上経過した時点での角膜反射を評価する試験では増加した（89 %～100 %）。他の検査所見と同様に，角膜反射は薬物による交絡を受けやすく，残存薬物効果の可能性を特に評価した試験は殆どない。

4. 347 例の患者を対象とする 2 つの試験では[21,32] 72 時間以内のミオクローヌス状態の存在によって退院から 6 カ月までの神経学的転帰不良が予測され，特異度は 97 %～100 % だった。

5. ミオクローヌス状態で EEG を得ることは，基礎にある発作活動を除外するために重要である。また，ミオクローヌス状態には明らかに発作ではないが予後的意味のある EEG 相関が存在する可能性があり，これらのパターンを詳細に叙述するにはさらなる研究が必要である。ミオクローヌス状態の一部の EEG 相関パターンには予後不良が存在する可能性があるが，EEG 相関のあるミオクローヌス状態の良性サブタイプのほうが多い可能性もある[33,34]。

6. 6件の観察研究[16,19,30,35-37]が，77.8％～97.4％の転帰不良に対する特異度で停止後96時間以内にミオクローヌスの存在を評価した。すべての試験において方法論的な限界があった。例えば，標準的な定義が欠如している，盲検化されていない，EEG相関についてのデータが不完全，ミオクローヌスのサブタイプを区別できないなどである。文献に詳細が記載されていないため，鑑別不能なミオクローヌスが予後マーカーとして使用されている場合に有害となる可能性がある。

7. 歴史的には，伸筋または移動の消失が転帰不良と相関する上肢の最良運動検査が予後予測ツールとして使用されてきた。先の文献は，TTMおよび薬物の作用の制御が不十分であることや自己実現的な予測であることなど，方法論上の問題による制限があり，許容できない偽陽性率（10％～15％）が存在した[7]。運動検査の成果は2020年のILCORシステマティックレビューで評価されなかった。2015年推奨事項に行われたアップデートは，運動検査が交絡を受ける可能性があって容認できないほど高い偽陽性率があり，したがって，予後ツールとして，または以降の検査のスクリーニングとして使用すべきではないという問題に基づいたものである。

これらの推奨事項は，ALSに関する2020年のCoSTRで支持されている[4]。これは，2015年に最後に実施されたこのトピックの包括的なレビューを補足するものである[7]。

「神経学的予後予測のための血清バイオマーカーの使用」

COR	LOE	推奨事項
2b	B-NR	1. 他の予後検査と組み合わせて実施される場合，昏睡状態が続く患者の神経学的転帰不良の予後を補助するために心停止後72時間以内にニューロン特異的エノラーゼ（neuron-specific enolase, NSE）の高血清値を考慮することは妥当としてよい。
2b	C-LD	2. 神経学的予後予測におけるS100カルシウム結合蛋白（calcium-binding protein, S100B），タウ，ニューロフィラメントL鎖，グリア線維酸性蛋白の有用性は不明である。

「概要」

血清バイオマーカーは，中枢神経系（central nervous system, CNS）に通常認められる蛋白の濃度を測定する血液ベースの検査である。これらの蛋白は神経損傷時に血液に吸収され，その血清レベルは脳損傷の程度を反映する。これらの予後における有用性に対する制限には，施設や検査室による検査方法のばらつき，検査室間のレベルの非一貫性，溶血による不確実性増加の影響，脳外からの蛋白の影響可能性がある。NSEとS100Bは研究で使用される最も一般的な2つのマーカーであるが，このレビューではその他のマーカーも取り上げられている。2020年のILCORシステマティックレビューでは，停止後最初の7日以内に血清バイオマーカーを採取して血清バイオマーカー濃度を神経学的転帰との相関を見る試験を評価した。他の血清バイオマーカーは，停止後の経時的な検査も含めて，評価されなかった。これらの血清バイオマーカーと他の新しい血清バイオマーカーとについて予後バイオマーカーとしての有用性を調査する大規模な観察コホート研究は，臨床的に重要性が高い。

「推奨事項の裏付けとなる解説」

1. 12件の経過観察で，停止後72時間以内に採取されたNSEを評価した[10,13,21,23,38-45]。転帰不良と相関する最大レベルは，33～120μg/Lであり、転帰不良の特異度は75％～100％であった。盲検化されていないこと，検査室間の非一貫性，100％の特異度を実現するために必要な閾値の広範さ，検査精度によって，エビデンスは制限される。そのため，統合された予後予測の一部としてNSE値が非常に高値であることが使用されることがあるが，予後不良を予測するNSEの絶対値カットオフは不明である。1つの絶対値を使用する代わりに，停止後最初の数日の連続測定を予後ツールとして評価することについて研究的関心が存在する[10,46]。

2. 3件の観察研究[40,47,48]が，停止後最初の72時間以内のS100Bレベルを評価した。転帰不良と相関する最大レベルは，試験と停止後測定されたタイミングによって大きく変動した。100％の特異度を実現すると報告された値で，検査感度は2.8％～77.6％であった。試験数の少なさと100％の特異度を実現するために必要となる試験全体の閾値の広範さによって，エビデンスは制限される。ILCORレビューでも，グリア線維酸性蛋白[44]とタウ[49]をそれぞれ評価する1件の試験と，ニューロフィラメントL鎖を評価する2件の試験を評価した[50,51]。試験数の少なさを考慮すれば，LOEが低く，これらの血清バイオマーカーは臨床診療には推奨できない。

これらの推奨事項は，ALSに関する2020年のCoSTRで支持されている[4]。これは，2015年に最後に実施されたこのトピックの包括的なレビューを補足するものである[7]。

「神経学的予後予測のための電気生理学的検査の使用」

神経学的予後予測のための電気生理学に関する 推奨事項

COR	LOE	推奨事項
2b	B-NR	1. 他の予後検査で評価される場合、心停止後に昏睡状態のままの患者のけいれん発作の予後値は不明である。
2b	B-NR	2. 他の予後検査で実施された場合、神経学的転帰不良の予後を補助するために心停止後 72 時間以上の持続性てんかん重積状態を考慮することは妥当としてよい。
2b	B-NR	3. 他の予後検査で実施された場合、神経学的転帰不良の予後を補助するために停止後 72 時間以上の鎮静性投薬の欠如において EEG のバーストサプレッションを考慮することは妥当としてよい。
2b	B-NR	4. 他の予後検査で実施された場合、神経学的転帰不良の予後を補助するために心停止後 24 時間以上の両側性の N20 体性感覚誘発電位（somatosensory evoked potential, SSEP）波消失を考慮することは妥当としてよい。
2b	B-NR	5. 停止後に他の予後検査で評価された場合、神経学的転帰不良の予後を補助するための律動性／周期性放電の有用性は不明である。
3：利益なし	B-NR	6. 停止後 72 時間以内の EEG 反応の欠如は神経学的予後不良を補助するために単独で使用されないことを推奨する。

「概要」

脳波は、大脳皮質脳活動を評価してけいれん発作を診断するために臨床診療において広く使われている。神経学的予後予測ツールとしてのその検査は有望である。しかし、文献はいくつかの要因によって制限される。すなわち、標準化された用語や定義の欠如、サンプルサイズの相対的な小ささ、単一施設試験設計、盲検化されていないこと、解釈の主観性、薬物の影響を排除できないことである。特定の所見やパターンの記述に使用される定義も一貫性に欠けている。2020 年の ILCOR システマティックレビューで評価された EEG パターンには、非反応性 EEG、てんかん様放電、けいれん発作、てんかん重積状態、バーストサプレッション、「極めて悪性の」EEG がある。残念ながら、様々な試験で極めて悪性の EEG を別々かつ不正確に定義しているので、この所見が役に立たなくなっている。

SSEP は、正中神経を刺激して皮質 N20 波の存在を評価することによって得られる。両側性 N20 SSEP 波消失は予後不良と相関しているが、筋アーチファクトや ICU 環境からの電気的干渉を避けるために適切なオペレータスキルと治療が必要となることによって、このモダリティの信頼性は制限される。SSEP の利点の 1 つは、他のモダリティより薬物から受ける干渉が少ないことである。

「推奨事項の裏付けとなる解説」

1. 5 件の観察研究[35,52-55]が、脳波上発作および／またはけいれん性発作の神経学的予後予測における役割を評価した。これらの試験は、けいれん性発作も対象にした試験もあったものの、脳波上けいれん発作に重点が置かれた。ILCOR システマティックレビューに含まれる試験のけいれん発作の特異度は 100 %であったが、この所見の感度は不良であった（0.6 %～26.8 %）。また、レビューには含まれていない他の試験では良好な転帰を示した患者で心拍再開後のけいれん発作を有する患者が報告されている[36,56,57]。その他の方法論的な問題としては、EEG モニタリングを行う患者に対する選択バイアスやけいれん発作の定義の一貫性のなさがある。けいれん発作という用語は、1 回の短い脳波上けいれん発作から難治性てんかん重積状態まで広範な病理を対象とし、予後が異なることが多い。この不正確さによって、推奨事項のさらなる制限が妥当とされた。

2. 6 件の観察研究[21,55,58-61]が、停止後 5 日以内のてんかん重積状態を評価し、退院から停止後 6 カ月間までの複数の時点で転帰を評価した。転帰不良に対するてんかん重積状態の特異度は 82.6 %～100 %であった。興味深いことに、てんかん重積状態はけいれん発作の重篤な形態であるにもかかわらず、転帰不良に対するてんかん重積状態の特異性度は（上記のように）けいれん発作全体的を調べた試験で報告された特異度よりも少なかった。その他の問題としては、てんかん重積状態の定義が一貫しないこと、盲検化されていないこと、自己実現的な予測の可能性につながる生命維持治療中止の正当化がある。

3. 6 件の研究[21,35,54,59,62,63]が、停止後 120 時間以内のバーストサプレッションを評価した。1 件の追加研究[64]では、バーストサプレッションを同期パターンと不均一なパターンに細分化させた。バーストサプレッションの定義は多様であり、明記されていなかった。特異度は 90.7 %～100 %であり、感度は 1.1 %～51 %であった。特異度が全体的に高いにもかかわらず、標準化された定義の欠如、自己実現的な予測である可能性、薬物効果の制御の欠如によって、より強力な推奨事項は制限された。（1 件の試験において極めて特異的に見えた）同期サブタイプなどのバーストサプレッションのサブタイプの特定にさらに重点を置くこと

について詳しい調査が望まれる。バーストサプレッションは薬物に起因することがあるため，この予後ツールにおける薬物の潜在的作用についての知識が医療従事者にあることは特に重要である。

4. 14件の観察研究[9,13,15-17,23,59,64-70]が，停止後96日以内の両側性N20 SSEP波消失を評価し，退院から停止後6ヵ月間までの複数の時点での転帰の所見を評価した。特異度は50％〜100％であった。3件の試験で特異度は100％未満であった。その他の方法論的な制限には，盲検化されていないことや自己実現的な予測の可能性がある。試験は停止直後からの任意の時点で得られたSSEPを評価したが，停止後の早期に交絡要因が存在する可能性があり，SSEPは停止後24時間以上経過してから取得することが推奨される。

5. EEGの放電は，律動性／周期性放電と非律動周期性放電の2種類に分かれた。9件の観察研究が，律動性／周期性放電を評価した[16,45,52-54,61,63,66,69]。律動性／周期性放電の特異度は66.7％〜100％であり，感度は不良であった（2.4％〜50.8％）。律動性／周期性放電を評価する試験は，放電の定義において一貫性がなかった。殆どの試験では薬物の効果を説明しておらず，一部の試験では容認できないほど低い特異度が見られた。ただし，心停止からの時間が増加するにつれて，転帰不良に対する律動性／周期性放電の特異度は向上した。このEEG所見は予後ツールとして発展させる余地がある。5件の観察研究[52,53,64,66,69]が，非律動性／周期性放電を評価した。試験で評価された心拍再開後の全期間にわたって転帰不良に対する特異度は低かった。

6. 10件の観察研究[16,30,53-55,62,65,71-73]が，非反応性EEGの予後値について報告した。特異度は41.7％〜100％であり，大部分の試験では90％以下であった。EEG反応性の定義やそれに使用される刺激に一貫性がなかった。試験では，温度と薬物の効果も説明されていなかった。したがって，エビデンスの全体的な確実性は非常に低いと評価された。

これらの推奨事項は，ALSに関する2020年のCoSTRで支持されている[4]。これは，2015年に最後に実施されたこのトピックの包括的なレビューを補足するものである[7]。

神経学的予後予測に対する神経画像検査の使用

神経学的予後予測に対する神経画像検査に関する 推奨事項

COR	LOE	推奨事項
2b	B-NR	1. 他の予後検査と組み合わせて実施される場合，昏睡状態が続く患者の神経学的転帰不良の予後を補助するために心停止後の脳コンピュータ断層撮影上での灰白質/白質比（gray-white ratio, GWR）の減少を考慮することは妥当としてよい。
2b	B-NR	2. 他の予後検査と組み合わせて実施される場合，昏睡状態が続く患者の神経学的転帰不良の予後を補助するために心停止後2〜7日に脳MRI上で広範な拡散制限を考慮することは妥当としてよい。
2b	B-NR	3. 他の予後検査と組み合わせて実施される場合，昏睡状態が続く患者の神経学的転帰不良の予後を補助するために心停止後2〜7日に脳MRI上で広範な見かけ上の拡散係数（apparent diffusion coefficient, ADC）低下を考慮することは妥当としてよい。

「概要」

停止後の神経画像検査は，器質的脳損傷の検出と定量化に役に立つ可能性がある。CTおよびMRIは，最も一般的な2つのモダリティである。CTでは，脳浮腫をGWRとして定量化できる。これは，灰白質と白質の密度（ハウンズフィールド単位として測定）の間の比率と定義される。通常の脳のGWRは約1.3である。この数は浮腫によって減少する。MRIでは，細胞毒性損傷を拡散強調画像（diffusion-weighted imaging, DWI）として測定でき，ADCによって定量化できる。DWI／ADCは損傷の高感度測定である。正常値は700〜800×10^{-6} mm^2/sであり，値は損傷によって減少する。脳損傷のCTおよびMRIの所見は，停止後最初の数日間で増加する。したがって，対象の画像検査のタイミングは極めて重要である。予後にかかわるからである。

「推奨事項の裏付けとなる解説」

1. 12件の観察研究[23,24,31,38,66,74-79]が，頭部CTのGWRを評価した。全脳GWR（GWR平均）と特定の領域のGWRが評価された。特異度は85％〜100％であった。1件の試験だけ100％の特異度ではなかった。一部の試験は停止後72時間以内に得られた頭部CTを対象にしていたが，試験の多くは停止後最初の24時間以内に得られた頭部CTを評価した。方法論的な制限が存在した。例えば，選択バイアス，多重比較のリスク，解剖学的部位や計算方法など測定技術の不均一性である。したがって，100％の特異度で予後不良を予測する特定のGWR閾値は不

明である。さらに，GWR を予後ツールとして最適化するための停止後の頭部 CT を撮像する最適なタイミングは不明である。

2. 5 件の観察研究[11,23,74,80,81]が，停止後 5 日以内に MRI で DWI 変化を調査した。試験は「高信号」および「陽性所見」について定性的に MRI を評価したが，陽性所見の定義は 試験によって異なり，一部の試験では特定の領域のみを調べた。特異度は 55.7 %～100 %であった。一部の試験では，不正確な定義と短期的な転帰によって，予後不良を予測するために DWI MRI を使用する方法に大幅な不確実性が生じた。正しい状況下では，DWI MRI での有意な異常所見または特定の関心領域における DWI MRI 所見は予後不良と相関する可能性があるが，まだ一般的に推奨することはできない。

3. 3 件の観察研究[82-84]が，停止後 7 日以内に MRI 上の ADC を調査した。それらの試験は 100％の特異度を得るための閾値を決定するようデザインされていたが，その特異度を達成するための ADC と脳容積の閾値は試験によって大きく異なっていた。定量的 ADC 測定は有望なツールではあるが，それを広く活用できるかは，実施可能か否かによって制限される。また，試験数が比較的少なく，他の画像機能のように部位や計算方法など測定技術の不均一性が存在した。予後不良を予測する特定の ADC 閾値は不明である。

これらの推奨事項は，ALS に関する 2020 年の CoSTR で支持されている[4]。これは，2015 年に最後に実施されたこのトピックの包括的なレビューを補足するものである[7]。

参考資料

1. Laver S, Farrow C, Turner D, Nolan J. Mode of death after admission to an intensive care unit following cardiac arrest.Intensive Care Med.2004;30:2126-2128. doi: 10.1007/s00134-004-2425-z
2. Witten L, Gardner R, Holmberg MJ, Wiberg S, Moskowitz A, Mehta S, Grossestreuer AV, Yankama T, Donnino MW, Berg KM.Reasons for death in patients successfully resuscitated from out-of-hospital and in-hospital cardiac arrest.Resuscitation.2019;136:93-99. doi: 10.1016/j.resuscitation.2019.01.031
3. Geocadin RG, Callaway CW, Fink EL, Golan E, Greer DM, Ko NU, Lang E, Licht DJ, Marino BS, McNair ND, Peberdy MA, Perman SM, Sims DB, Soar J, Sandroni C; American Heart Association Emergency Cardiovascular Care Committee.Standards for Studies of Neurological Prognostication in Comatose Survivors of Cardiac Arrest: A Scientific Statement From the American Heart Association.Circulation.2019;140:e517-e542. doi: 10.1161/CIR.0000000000000702
4. Berg KM, Soar J, Andersen LW, Böttiger BW, Cacciola S, Callaway CW, Couper K, Cronberg T, D'Arrigo S, Deakin CD, et al; on behalf of the Adult Advanced Life Support Collaborators.Adult advanced life support: 2020 International Consensus on Cardiopulmonary Resuscitation and Emergency Cardiovascular Care Science With Treatment Recommendations.Circulation.2020;142(suppl 1):S92-S139. doi: 10.1161/CIR.0000000000000893
5. Samaniego EA, Mlynash M, Caulfield AF, Eyngorn I, Wijman CA.Sedation confounds outcome prediction in cardiac arrest survivors treated with hypothermia.Neurocrit Care.2011;15:113-119. doi: 10.1007/s12028-010-9412-8
6. Wilson ME, Dobler CC, Zubek L, Gajic O, Talmor D, Curtis JR, Hinds RF, Banner-Goodspeed VM, Mueller A, Rickett DM, Elo G, Filipe M, Szucs O, Novotny PJ, Piers RD, Benoit DD.Prevalence of Disagreement About Appropriateness of Treatment Between ICU Patients/Surrogates and Clinicians. Chest.2019;155:1140-1147. doi: 10.1016/j.chest.2019.02.404
7. Callaway CW, Donnino MW, Fink EL, Geocadin RG, Golan E, Kern KB, Leary M, Meurer WJ, Peberdy MA, Thompson TM, et al.Part 8: post-cardiac arrest care: 2015 American Heart Association Guidelines Update for Cardiopulmonary Resuscitation and Emergency Cardiovascular Care.Circulation.2015;132(suppl 2):S465-482. doi: 10.1161/cir.0000000000000262
8. Wijdicks EF, Parisi JE, Sharbrough FW.Prognostic value of myoclonus status in comatose survivors of cardiac arrest.Ann Neurol.1994;35:239-243. doi: 10.1002/ana.410350219
9. Choi SP, Park KN, Wee JH, Park JH, Youn CS, Kim HJ, Oh SH, Oh YS, Kim SH, Oh JS.Can somatosensory and visual evoked potentials predict neurological outcome during targeted temperature management in post cardiac arrest patients? Resuscitation.2017;119:70-75. doi: 10.1016/j.resuscitation.2017.06.022
10. Chung-Esaki HM, Mui G, Mlynash M, Eyngorn I, Catabay K, Hirsch KG.The neuron specific enolase (NSE) ratio offers benefits over absolute value thresholds in post-cardiac arrest coma prognosis.J Clin Neurosci.2018;57:99-104. doi: 10.1016/j.jocn.2018.08.020
11. Ryoo SM, Jeon SB, Sohn CH, Ahn S, Han C, Lee BK, Lee DH, Kim SH, Donnino MW, Kim WY; Korean Hypothermia Network Investigators.Predicting Outcome With Diffusion-Weighted Imaging in Cardiac Arrest Patients Receiving Hypothermia Therapy: Multicenter Retrospective Cohort Study.Crit Care Med.2015;43:2370-2377. doi: 10.1097/CCM.0000000000001263
12. Javaudin F, Leclere B, Segard J, Le Bastard Q, Pes P, Penverne Y, Le Conte P, Jenvrin J, Hubert H, Escutnaire J, Batard E, Montassier E, Gr-RéAC.Prognostic performance of early absence of pupillary light reaction after recovery of out of hospital cardiac arrest.Resuscitation.2018;127:8-13. doi: 10.1016/j.resuscitation.2018.03.020
13. Dhakal LP, Sen A, Stanko CM, Rawal B, Heckman MG, Hoyne JB, Dimberg EL, Freeman ML, Ng LK, Rabinstein AA, Freeman WD.Early Absent Pupillary Light Reflexes After Cardiac Arrest in Patients Treated with Therapeutic Hypothermia.Ther Hypothermia Temp Manag.2016;6:116-121. doi: 10.1089/ther.2015.0035
14. Matthews EA, Magid-Bernstein J, Sobczak E, Velazquez A, Falo CM, Park S, Claassen J, Agarwal S. Prognostic Value of the Neurological Examination in Cardiac Arrest Patients After Therapeutic Hypothermia.Neurohospitalist.2018;8:66-73. doi: 10.1177/1941874417733217
15. Oddo M, Sandroni C, Citerio G, Miroz JP, Horn J, Rundgren M, Cariou A, Payen JF, Storm C, Stammet P, Taccone FS.Quantitative versus standard pupillary light reflex for early prognostication in comatose cardiac arrest patients: an international prospective multicenter double-blinded study.Intensive Care Med.2018;44:2102-2111. doi: 10.1007/s00134-018-5448-6
16. Fatuzzo D, Beuchat I, Alvarez V, Novy J, Oddo M, Rossetti AO.Does continuous EEG influence prognosis in patients after cardiac arrest? Resuscitation.2018;132:29-32. doi: 10.1016/j.resuscitation.2018.08.023
17. Dragancea I, Horn J, Kuiper M, Friberg H, Ullén S, Wetterslev J, Cranshaw J, Hassager C, Nielsen N, Cronberg T; TTM Trial Investigators.Neurological prognostication after cardiac arrest and targeted temperature management 33°C versus 36°C: Results from a randomised controlled clinical trial.Resuscitation.2015;93:164-170. doi: 10.1016/j.resuscitation.2015.04.013
18. Hofmeijer J, Beernink TM, Bosch FH, Beishuizen A, Tjepkema-Cloostermans MC, van Putten MJ.Early EEG contributes to multimodal outcome prediction of postanoxic coma.Neurology.2015;85:137-143. doi: 10.1212/WNL.0000000000001742
19. Kongpolprom N, Cholkraisuwat J. Neurological Prognostications for the Therapeutic Hypothermia among Comatose Survivors of Cardiac Arrest.Indian J Crit Care Med.2018;22:509-518. doi: 10.4103/ijccm.IJCCM_500_17
20. Roger C, Palmier L, Louart B, Molinari N, Claret PG, de la Coussaye JE, Lefrant JY, Muller L. Neuron specific enolase and Glasgow motor score remain useful tools for assessing neurological prognosis after out-of-hospital cardiac arrest treated with therapeutic hypothermia.Anaesth Crit Care Pain Med.2015;34:231-237. doi: 10.1016/j.accpm.2015.05.004
21. Zhou SE, Maciel CB, Ormseth CH, Beekman R, Gilmore EJ, Greer DM.Distinct predictive values of current neuroprognostic guidelines in post-cardiac arrest patients.Resuscitation.2019;139:343-350. doi: 10.1016/j.resuscitation.2019.03.035

22. Greer DM, Yang J, Scripko PD, Sims JR, Cash S, Wu O, Hafler JP, Schoenfeld DA, Furie KL.Clinical examination for prognostication in comatose cardiac arrest patients.Resuscitation.2013;84:1546-1551. doi: 10.1016/j.resuscitation.2013.07.028
23. Kim JH, Kim MJ, You JS, Lee HS, Park YS, Park I, Chung SP.Multimodal approach for neurologic prognostication of out-of-hospital cardiac arrest patients undergoing targeted temperature management.Resuscitation.2019;134:33-40. doi: 10.1016/j.resuscitation.2018.11.007
24. Lee KS, Lee SE, Choi JY, Gho YR, Chae MK, Park EJ, Choi MH, Hong JM.Useful Computed Tomography Score for Estimation of Early Neurologic Outcome in Post-Cardiac Arrest Patients With Therapeutic Hypothermia. Circ J. 2017;81:1628-1635. doi: 10.1253/circj.CJ-16-1327
25. Scarpino M, Carrai R, Lolli F, Lanzo G, Spalletti M, Valzania F, Lombardi M, Audenino D, Contardi S, Celani MG, et al; on behalf of the ProNeCA Study Group.Neurophysiology for predicting good and poor neurological outcome at 12 and 72 h after cardiac arrest: the ProNeCA multicentre prospective study.Resuscitation.2020;147:95-103. doi: 10.1016/j.resuscitation.2019.11.014
26. Heimburger D, Durand M, Gaide-Chevronnay L, Dessertaine G, Moury PH, Bouzat P, Albaladejo P, Payen JF.Quantitative pupillometry and transcranial Doppler measurements in patients treated with hypothermia after cardiac arrest.Resuscitation.2016;103:88-93. doi: 10.1016/j.resuscitation.2016.02.026
27. Solari D, Rossetti AO, Carteron L, Miroz JP, Novy J, Eckert P, Oddo M. Early prediction of coma recovery after cardiac arrest with blinded pupillometry. Ann Neurol.2017;81:804-810. doi: 10.1002/ana.24943
28. Riker RR, Sawyer ME, Fischman VG, May T, Lord C, Eldridge A, Seder DB.Neurological Pupil Index and Pupillary Light Reflex by Pupillometry Predict Outcome Early After Cardiac Arrest.Neurocrit Care.2020;32:152-161. doi: 10.1007/s12028-019-00717-4
29. Obling L, Hassager C, Illum C, Grand J, Wiberg S, Lindholm MG, Winther-Jensen M, Kondziella D, Kjaergaard J. Prognostic value of automated pupillometry: an unselected cohort from a cardiac intensive care unit.Eur Heart J Acute Cardiovasc Care. 2019:2048872619842004. doi: 10.1177/2048872619842004
30. Sivaraju A, Gilmore EJ, Wira CR, Stevens A, Rampal N, Moeller JJ, Greer DM, Hirsch LJ, Gaspard N. Prognostication of post-cardiac arrest coma: early clinical and electroencephalographic predictors of outcome.Intensive Care Med.2015;41:1264-1272. doi: 10.1007/s00134-015-3834-x
31. Kim SH, Choi SP, Park KN, Youn CS, Oh SH, Choi SM.Early brain computed tomography findings are associated with outcome in patients treated with therapeutic hypothermia after out-of-hospital cardiac arrest.Scand J Trauma.2013;21:57. doi: 10.1186/1757-7241-21-57
32. Ruknuddeen MI, Ramadoss R, Rajajee V, Grzeskowiak LE, Rajagopalan RE.Early clinical prediction of neurological outcome following out of hospital cardiac arrest managed with therapeutic hypothermia.Indian J Crit Care Med.2015;19:304-310. doi: 10.4103/0972-5229.158256
33. Elmer J, Rittenberger JC, Faro J, Molyneaux BJ, Popescu A, Callaway CW, Baldwin M; Pittsburgh Post-Cardiac Arrest Service.Clinically distinct electroencephalographic phenotypes of early myoclonus after cardiac arrest. Ann Neurol.2016;80:175-184. doi: 10.1002/ana.24697
34. Aicua RI, Rapun I, Novy J, Solari D, Oddo M, Rossetti AO.Early Lance-Adams syndrome after cardiac arrest: prevalence, time to return to awareness, and outcome in a large cohort.Resuscitation.2017;115:169-172. doi: 10.1016/j.resuscitation.2017.03.020
35. Sadaka F, Doerr D, Hindia J, Lee KP, Logan W. Continuous Electroencephalogram in Comatose Postcardiac Arrest Syndrome Patients Treated With Therapeutic Hypothermia: Outcome Prediction Study.J Intensive Care Med.2015;30:292-296. doi: 10.1177/0885066613517214
36. Lybeck A, Friberg H, Aneman A, Hassager C, Horn J, Kjærgaard J, Kuiper M, Nielsen N, Ullén S, Wise MP, Westhall E, Cronberg T; TTM-trial Investigators.Prognostic significance of clinical seizures after cardiac arrest and target temperature management.Resuscitation.2017;114:146-151. doi: 10.1016/j.resuscitation.2017.01.017
37. Reynolds AS, Rohaut B, Holmes MG, Robinson D, Roth W, Velazquez A, Couch CK, Presciutti A, Brodie D, Moitra VK, Rabbani LE, Agarwal S, Park S, Roh DJ, Claassen J. Early myoclonus following anoxic brain injury.Neurol Clin Pract.2018;8:249-256. doi: 10.1212/CPJ.0000000000000466
38. Lee BK, Jeung KW, Lee HY, Jung YH, Lee DH.Combining brain computed tomography and serum neuron specific enolase improves the prognostic performance compared to either alone in comatose cardiac arrest survivors treated with therapeutic hypothermia.Resuscitation.2013;84:1387-1392. doi: 10.1016/j.resuscitation.2013.05.026
39. Vondrakova D, Kruger A, Janotka M, Malek F, Dudkova V, Neuzil P, Ostadal P. Association of neuron-specific enolase values with outcomes in cardiac arrest survivors is dependent on the time of sample collection.Crit Care.2017;21:172. doi: 10.1186/s13054-017-1766-2
40. Duez CHV, Grejs AM, Jeppesen AN, Schrøder AD, Søreide E, Nielsen JF, Kirkegaard H. Neuron-specific enolase and S-100b in prolonged targeted temperature management after cardiac arrest: A randomised study.Resuscitation.2018;122:79-86. doi: 10.1016/j.resuscitation.2017.11.052
41. Stammet P, Collignon O, Hassager C, Wise MP, Hovdenes J, Åneman A, Horn J, Devaux Y, Erlinge D, Kjaergaard J, Gasche Y, Wanscher M, Cronberg T, Friberg H, Wetterslev J, Pellis T, Kuiper M, Gilson G, Nielsen N; TTM-Trial Investigators.Neuron-Specific Enolase as a Predictor of Death or Poor Neurological Outcome After Out-of-Hospital Cardiac Arrest and Targeted Temperature Management at 33°C and 36°C. J Am Coll Cardiol.2015;65:2104-2114. doi: 10.1016/j.jacc.2015.03.538
42. Zellner T, Gärtner R, Schopohl J, Angstwurm M. NSE and S-100B are not sufficiently predictive of neurologic outcome after therapeutic hypothermia for cardiac arrest.Resuscitation.2013;84:1382-1386. doi: 10.1016/j.resuscitation.2013.03.021
43. Tsetsou S, Novy J, Pfeiffer C, Oddo M, Rossetti AO.Multimodal Outcome Prognostication After Cardiac Arrest and Targeted Temperature Management: Analysis at 36 °C. Neurocrit Care.2018;28:104-109. doi: 10.1007/s12028-017-0393-8
44. Helwig K, Seeger F, Hölschermann H, Lischke V, Gerriets T, Niessner M, Foerch C. Elevated Serum Glial Fibrillary Acidic Protein (GFAP) is Associated with Poor Functional Outcome After Cardiopulmonary Resuscitation. Neurocrit Care.2017;27:68-74. doi: 10.1007/s12028-016-0371-6
45. Rossetti AO, Tovar Quiroga DF, Juan E, Novy J, White RD, Ben-Hamouda N, Britton JW, Oddo M, Rabinstein AA.Electroencephalography predicts poor and good outcomes after cardiac arrest: a two-center study.Crit Care Med.2017;45:e674-e682. doi: 10.1097/CCM.0000000000002337
46. Wiberg S, Hassager C, Stammet P, Winther-Jensen M, Thomsen JH, Erlinge D, Wanscher M, Nielsen N, Pellis T, Åneman A, Friberg H, Hovdenes J, Horn J, Wetterslev J, Bro-Jeppesen J, Wise MP, Kuiper M, Cronberg T, Gasche Y, Devaux Y, Kjaergaard J. Single versus Serial Measurements of Neuron-Specific Enolase and Prediction of Poor Neurological Outcome in Persistently Unconscious Patients after Out-Of-Hospital Cardiac Arrest – A TTM-Trial Substudy.PLoS One.2017;12:e0168894. doi: 10.1371/journal.pone.0168894
47. Jang JH, Park WB, Lim YS, Choi JY, Cho JS, Woo JH, Choi WS, Yang HJ, Hyun SY.Combination of S100B and procalcitonin improves prognostic performance compared to either alone in patients with cardiac arrest: a prospective observational study.Medicine (Baltimore).2019;98:e14496. doi: 10.1097/MD.0000000000014496
48. Stammet P, Dankiewicz J, Nielsen N, Fays F, Collignon O, Hassager C, Wanscher M, Undèn J, Wetterslev J, Pellis T, Aneman A, Hovdenes J, Wise MP, Gilson G, Erlinge D, Horn J, Cronberg T, Kuiper M, Kjaergaard J, Gasche Y, Devaux Y, Friberg H; Target Temperature Management after Out-of-Hospital Cardiac Arrest (TTM) trial investigators.Protein S100 as outcome predictor after out-of-hospital cardiac arrest and targeted temperature management at 33°C and 36°C. Crit Care.2017;21:153. doi: 10.1186/s13054-017-1729-7
49. Mattsson N, Zetterberg H, Nielsen N, Blennow K, Dankiewicz J, Friberg H, Lilja G, Insel PS, Rylander C, Stammet P, Aneman A, Hassager C, Kjaergaard J, Kuiper M, Pellis T, Wetterslev J, Wise M, Cronberg T. Serum tau and neurological outcome in cardiac arrest.Ann Neurol.2017;82:665-675. doi: 10.1002/ana.25067
50. Moseby-Knappe M, Mattsson N, Nielsen N, Zetterberg H, Blennow K, Dankiewicz J, Dragancea I, Friberg H, Lilja G, Insel PS, Rylander C, Westhall E, Kjaergaard J, Wise MP, Hassager C, Kuiper MA, Stammet P, Wanscher MCJ, Wetterslev J, Erlinge D, Horn J, Pellis T, Cronberg T. Serum Neurofilament Light Chain for Prognosis of Outcome After Cardiac Arrest.JAMA Neurol.2019;76:64-71. doi: 10.1001/jamaneurol.2018.3223
51. Rana OR, Schröder JW, Baukloh JK, Saygili E, Mischke K, Schiefer J, Weis J, Marx N, Rassaf T, Kelm M, Shin DI, Meyer C, Saygili E. Neurofilament light chain as an early and sensitive predictor of long-term neurological outcome in patients after cardiac arrest.Int J Cardiol.2013;168:1322-1327. doi: 10.1016/j.ijcard.2012.12.016
52. Lamartine Monteiro M, Taccone FS, Depondt C, Lamanna I, Gaspard N, Ligot N, Mavroudakis N, Naeije G, Vincent JL, Legros B. The Prognostic Value of 48-h Continuous EEG During Therapeutic Hypothermia After Cardiac Arrest.Neurocrit Care.2016;24:153-162. doi: 10.1007/s12028-015-0215-9
53. Benarous L, Gavaret M, Soda Diop M, Tobarias J, de Ghaisne de Bourmont S, Allez C, Bouzana F, Gainnier M, Trebuchon A. Sources of interrater variability and prognostic value of standardized EEG features in post-anoxic coma after resuscitated cardiac arrest.Clin Neurophysiol Pract.2019;4:20-26. doi: 10.1016/j.cnp.2018.12.001

54. Westhall E, Rossetti AO, van Rootselaar AF, Wesenberg Kjaer T, Horn J, Ullén S, Friberg H, Nielsen N, Rosén I, Åneman A, Erlinge D, Gasche Y, Hassager C, Hovdenes J, Kjaergaard J, Kuiper M, Pellis T, Stammet P, Wanscher M, Wettersley J, Wise MP, Cronberg T; TTM-trial investigators.Standardized EEG interpretation accurately predicts prognosis after cardiac arrest.Neurology.2016;86:1482–1490. doi: 10.1212/WNL.0000000000002462

55. Amorim E, Rittenberger JC, Zheng JJ, Westover MB, Baldwin ME, Callaway CW, Popescu A; Post Cardiac Arrest Service.Continuous EEG monitoring enhances multimodal outcome prediction in hypoxic-ischemic brain injury.Resuscitation.2016;109:121–126. doi: 10.1016/j.resuscitation.2016.08.012

56. Rundgren M, Westhall E, Cronberg T, Rosén I, Friberg H. Continuous amplitude-integrated electroencephalogram predicts outcome in hypothermia-treated cardiac arrest patients.Crit Care Med.2010;38:1838–1844. doi: 10.1097/CCM.0b013e3181eaa1e7

57. Legriel S, Hilly-Ginoux J, Resche-Rigon M, Merceron S, Pinoteau J, Henry-Lagarrigue M, Bruneel F, Nguyen A, Guezennec P, Troché G, Richard O, Pico F, Bédos JP.Prognostic value of electrographic postanoxic status epilepticus in comatose cardiac-arrest survivors in the therapeutic hypothermia era.Resuscitation.2013;84:343–350. doi: 10.1016/j.resuscitation.2012.11.001

58. Oh SH, Park KN, Shon YM, Kim YM, Kim HJ, Youn CS, Kim SH, Choi SP, Kim SC.Continuous Amplitude-Integrated Electroencephalographic Monitoring Is a Useful Prognostic Tool for Hypothermia-Treated Cardiac Arrest Patients.Circulation.2015;132:1094–1103. doi: 10.1161/CIRCULATIONAHA.115.015754

59. Leão RN, Ávila P, Cavaco R, Germano N, Bento L. Therapeutic hypothermia after cardiac arrest: outcome predictors.Rev Bras Ter Intensiva.2015;27:322–332. doi: 10.5935/0103-507X.20150056

60. Dragancea I, Backman S, Westhall E, Rundgren M, Friberg H, Cronberg T. Outcome following postanoxic status epilepticus in patients with targeted temperature management after cardiac arrest.Epilepsy Behav.2015;49:173–177. doi: 10.1016/j.yebeh.2015.04.043

61. Beretta S, Coppo A, Bianchi E, Zanchi C, Carone D, Stabile A, Padovano G, Sulmina E, Grassi A, Bogliun G, Foti G, Ferrarese C, Pesenti A, Beghi E, Avalli L. Neurological outcome of postanoxic refractory status epilepticus after aggressive treatment.Epilepsy Behav.2019;101 (Pt B):106374. doi: 10.1016/j.yebeh.2019.06.018

62. Alvarez V, Reinsberger C, Scirica B, O'Brien MH, Avery KR, Henderson G, Lee JW.Continuous electrodermal activity as a potential novel neurophysiological biomarker of prognosis after cardiac arrest-A pilot study.Resuscitation.2015;93:128–135. doi: 10.1016/j.resuscitation.2015.06.006

63. Backman S, Cronberg T, Friberg H, Ullén S, Horn J, Kjaergaard J, Hassager C, Wanscher M, Nielsen N, Westhall E. Highly malignant routine EEG predicts poor prognosis after cardiac arrest in the Target Temperature Management trial.Resuscitation.2018;131:24–28. doi: 10.1016/j.resuscitation.2018.07.024

64. Ruijter BJ, Tjepkema-Cloostermans MC, Tromp SC, van den Bergh WM, Foudraine NA, Kornips FHM, Drost G, Scholten E, Bosch FH, Beishuizen A, van Putten MJAM, Hofmeijer J. Early electroencephalography for outcome prediction of postanoxic coma: A prospective cohort study.Ann Neurol.2019;86:203–214. doi: 10.1002/ana.25518

65. Grippo A, Carrai R, Scarpino M, Spalletti M, Lanzo G, Cossu C, Peris A, Valente S, Amantini A. Neurophysiological prediction of neurological good and poor outcome in post-anoxic coma.Acta Neurol Scand.2017;135:641–648. doi: 10.1111/ane.12659

66. Scarpino M, Lolli F, Lanzo G, Carrai R, Spalletti M, Valzania F, Lombardi M, Audenino D, Celani MG, Marrelli A, Contardi S, Peris A, Amantini A, Sandroni C, Grippo A; ProNeCAStudy Group.Neurophysiological and neuroradiological test for early poor outcome (Cerebral Performance Categories 3–5) prediction after cardiac arrest: Prospective multicentre prognostication data.Data Brief.2019;27:104755. doi: 10.1016/j.dib.2019.104755

67. De Santis P, Lamanna I, Mavroudakis N, Legros B, Vincent JL, Creteur J, Taccone FS.The potential role of auditory evoked potentials to assess prognosis in comatose survivors from cardiac arrest.Resuscitation.2017;120:119–124. doi: 10.1016/j.resuscitation.2017.09.013

68. Kim SW, Oh JS, Park J, Jeong HH, Kim JH, Wee JH, Oh SH, Choi SP, Park KN; Cerebral Resuscitation and Outcome evaluation Within catholic Network (CROWN) Investigators.Short-Latency Positive Peak Following N20 Somatosensory Evoked Potential Is Superior to N20 in Predicting Neurologic Outcome After Out-of-Hospital Cardiac Arrest.Crit Care Med.2018;46:e545–e551. doi: 10.1097/CCM.0000000000003083

69. Scarpino M, Carrai R, Lolli F, Lanzo G, Spalletti M, Valzania F, Lombardi M, Audenino D, Contardi S, Celani MG, Marrelli A, Mecarelli O, Minardi C, Minicucci F, Politini L, Vitelli E, Peris A, Amantini A, Sandroni C, Grippo A; ProNeCA study group.Neurophysiology for predicting good and poor neurological outcome at 12 and 72 h after cardiac arrest: The ProNeCA multicentre prospective study.Resuscitation.2020;147:95–103. doi: 10.1016/j.resuscitation.2019.11.014

70. Maciel CB, Morawo AO, Tsao CY, Youn TS, Labar DR, Rubens EO, Greer DM.SSEP in Therapeutic Hypothermia Era.J Clin Neurophysiol.2017;34:469–475. doi: 10.1097/WNP.0000000000000392

71. Admiraal MM, van Rootselaar AF, Hofmeijer J, Hoedemaekers CWE, van Kaam CR, Keijzer HM, van Putten MJAM, Schultz MJ, Horn J. Electroencephalographic reactivity as predictor of neurological outcome in postanoxic coma: A multicenter prospective cohort study.Ann Neurol.2019;86:17–27. doi: 10.1002/ana.25507

72. Duez CHV, Johnsen B, Ebbesen MQ, Kvaløy MB, Grejs AM, Jeppesen AN, Søreide E, Nielsen JF, Kirkegaard H. Post resuscitation prognostication by EEG in 24 vs 48 h of targeted temperature management.Resuscitation.2019;135:145–152. doi: 10.1016/j.resuscitation.2018.10.035

73. Liu G, Su Y, Liu Y, Jiang M, Zhang Y, Zhang Y, Gao D. Predicting Outcome in Comatose Patients: The Role of EEG Reactivity to Quantifiable Electrical Stimuli.Evid Based Complement Alternat Med.2016;2016:8273716. doi: 10.1155/2016/8273716

74. Jeon CH, Park JS, Lee JH, Kim H, Kim SC, Park KH, Yi KS, Kim SM, Youn CS, Kim YM, Lee BK.Comparison of brain computed tomography and diffusion-weighted magnetic resonance imaging to predict early neurologic outcome before target temperature management comatose cardiac arrest survivors.Resuscitation.2017;118:21–26. doi: 10.1016/j.resuscitation.2017.06.021

75. Kim Y, Ho LJ, Kun HC, Won CK, Hoon YJ, Ju KM, Weon KY, Yul LK, Joo KJ, Youn HS.Feasibility of optic nerve sheath diameter measured on initial brain computed tomography as an early neurologic outcome predictor after cardiac arrest Academic Emergency Medicine 2014;21:1121-1128.

76. Lee DH, Lee BK, Jeung KW, Jung YH, Cho YS, Cho IS, Youn CS, Kim JW, Park JS, Min YI.Relationship between ventricular characteristics on brain computed tomography and 6-month neurologic outcome in cardiac arrest survivors who underwent targeted temperature management.Resuscitation.2018;129:37–42. doi: 10.1016/j.resuscitation.2018.06.008

77. Scarpino M, Lanzo G, Lolli F, Carrai R, Moretti M, Spalletti M, Cozzolino M, Peris A, Amantini A, Grippo A. Neurophysiological and neuroradiological multimodal approach for early poor outcome prediction after cardiac arrest.Resuscitation.2018;129:114–120. doi: 10.1016/j.resuscitation.2018.04.016

78. Wang GN, Chen XF, Lv JR, Sun NN, Xu XQ, Zhang JS.The prognostic value of gray-white matter ratio on brain computed tomography in adult comatose cardiac arrest survivors.J Chin Med Assoc.2018;81:599–604. doi: 10.1016/j.jcma.2018.03.003

79. Youn CS, Callaway CW, Rittenberger JC; Post Cardiac Arrest Service.Combination of initial neurologic examination, quantitative brain imaging and electroencephalography to predict outcome after cardiac arrest.Resuscitation.2017;110:120–125. doi: 10.1016/j.resuscitation.2016.10.024

80. Greer DM, Scripko PD, Wu O, Edlow BL, Bartscher J, Sims JR, Camargo EE, Singhal AB, Furie KL.Hippocampal magnetic resonance imaging abnormalities in cardiac arrest are associated with poor outcome.J Stroke.Cerebrovasc Dis.2013;22:899–905. doi: 10.1016/j.jstrokecerebrovasdis.2012.08.006

81. Jang J, Oh SH, Nam Y, Lee K, Choi HS, Jung SL, Ahn KJ, Park KN, Kim BS.Prognostic value of phase information of 2D T2*-weighted gradient echo brain imaging in cardiac arrest survivors: A preliminary study.Resuscitation.2019;140:142–149. doi: 10.1016/j.resuscitation.2019.05.026

82. Moon HK, Jang J, Park KN, Kim SH, Lee BK, Oh SH, Jeung KW, Choi SP, Cho IS, Youn CS.Quantitative analysis of relative volume of low apparent diffusion coefficient value can predict neurologic outcome after cardiac arrest.Resuscitation.2018;126:36–42. doi: 10.1016/j.resuscitation.2018.02.020

83. Kim J, Kim K, Hong S, Kwon B, Yun ID, Choi BS, Jung C, Lee JH, Jo YH, Kim T, et al. Low apparent diffusion coefficient cluster-based analysis of diffusion-weighted MRI for prognostication of out-of-hospital cardiac arrest survivors.Resuscitation.2013;84:1393–1399. doi: 10.1016/j.resuscitation.2013.04.011

84. Hirsch KG, Fischbein N, Mlynash M, Kemp S, Bammer R, Eyngorn I, Tong J, Moseley M, Venkatasubramanian C, Caulfield AF, Albers G. Prognostic value of diffusion-weighted MRI for post-cardiac arrest coma.Neurology.2020;94:e1684–e1692. doi: 10.1212/WNL.0000000000009289

回復
心停止後の回復と生存

COR	LOE	推奨事項
1	B-NR	1. 心停止からの生存者およびその介護者の不安，うつ状態，心的外傷後ストレス障害，および疲労についての体系的な評価が推奨される。
1	C-LD	2. 心停止からの生存者は，退院前に身体，神経，心肺，および認知機能障害に関して，複数のリハビリ評価と治療を受けることが推奨される。
1	C-LD	3. 心停止からの生存者およびその介護者に，医療およびリハビリ治療の推奨事項を採り入れて，求める活動／仕事に復帰するための，包括的かつ集学的な退院計画を提供することが推奨される。
2b	C-LD	4. 心停止イベント後の市民救助者，EMSプロバイダー，および病院の医療従事者に対する精神的支援をフォローアップするため，デブリーフィングと紹介が有用な可能性がある。

「概要」
心停止からの生存者は，重症疾患の生存者の多くと同様に，身体的，神経的，認知的，感情的，あるいは社会的な問題をしばしば経験する。その一部は退院まで明らかにならない可能性がある。心停止後の生存はリハビリテーションと回復の道のりであり，患者，家族，医療のパートナー，地域社会にとって遥か彼方の目標である（図11）[1-3]。

心停止の治療システムアプローチには，心停止に対する地域社会と医療の対応も含まれる。しかし，心停止からの生存者が増えることで，退院計画と長期的なリハビリテーションケアリソースを整えることが必要になる。治療，監視，およびリハビリテーションについて説明した生存者への存計画を退院時に提供し，外来での治療への転換を最適化する必要がある。これらの計画とリソースは，多くの患者や家族にとって心停止後の生活の質を改善するうえでの最重要となりうる。生存者への計画は患者，介護者，一次診療医に役立ち，経過の要約，推奨される外来予約，退院後の回復目標が含まれる（図12）。

心停止からの生存者，その家族，および非生存者の家族は，心停止と患者中心の転帰に対する地域社会の対応を強力に擁護することがある。心停止後の生存と回復を改善するには，脳卒中，がん，およびその他の重症疾患の生存患者に対する治療の推奨事項と連携した系統的な優先順位付けが必要である[3-5]。

「推奨事項の裏付けとなる解説」
1. 心停止生存者の約3分の1は，不安，うつ状態，心的外傷後ストレス障害を経験する[6-9]。疲労も頻繁に見られ，身体的，認知的，感情的な障害にいたる可能性がある。家族や介護者が大きなストレスを経験することもあり，治療によって改善する[10-17]。

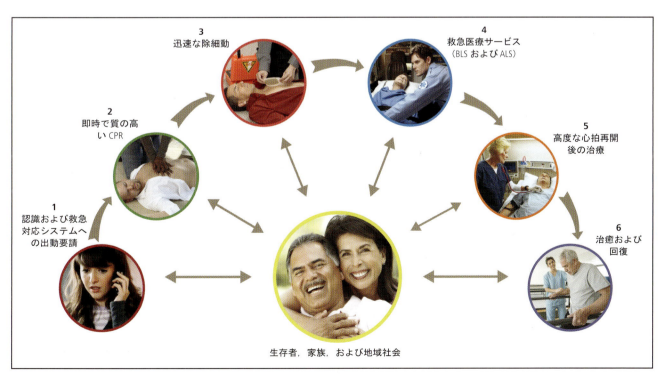

図11. 心停止からの生存を中心に据えた治療体系。[3]
CPR＝心肺蘇生。

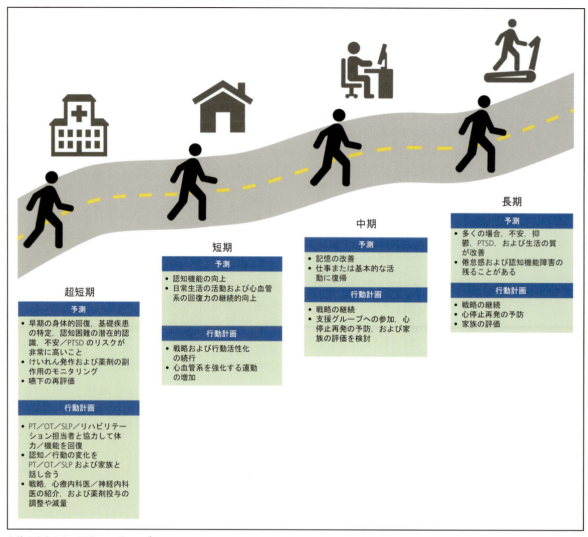

図12. 心停止生存からの回復ロードマップ。[3]
OT：作業療法（occupational therapy），PT：理学療法（physical therapy），PTSD：外傷後ストレス障害（posttraumatic stress disorder），SLP：言語病理学者（speech-language pathologist）。

2. 心停止の後の認知機能障害には，記憶，注意，遂行機能の障害も含まれる[18-22]。身体的，神経学的，心肺的な障害も多く見られる[3]。心臓リハビリテーションと理学療法，作業療法，言語療法の早期評価は，障害の回復，克服，適応の戦略を立てるのに役立つ可能性がある[3,23-25]。

3. 地域社会復帰と職場復帰などの活動には時間がかかることがあり，社会のサポートと社会との関係に依存する[26-29]。運転を始める時期や親密な交流を再開する時期についての指導が患者に必要となる[30,31]。

4. 救助者は，BLSを実施するまたは実施しないことに関する不安や心的外傷後ストレス障害を経験する可能性がある[23,32]。病院の医療従事者も，心停止患者のケアにおいて，情動的または精神的な影響を受ける可能性がある[34]。チームデブリーフィングにより，チームパフォーマンス（教育や品質改善），および終末期患者のケアに関連する特定のストレス要因の認識が可能となる[35]。

これらの各種推奨事項は，『Sudden Cardiac Arrest Survivorship: a Scientific Statement From the AHA』によって裏付けられている[3]。

参考資料

1. Iwashyna TJ.Survivorship will be the defining challenge of critical care in the 21st century.Ann Intern Med.2010;153:204-205. doi: 10.7326/0003-4819-153-3-201008030-00013
2. Hope AA, Munro CL.Understanding and Improving Critical Care Survivorship.Am J Crit Care.2019;28:410-412. doi: 10.4037/ajcc2019442
3. Sawyer KN, Camp-Rogers TR, Kotini-Shah P, Del Rios M, Gossip MR, Moitra VK, Haywood KL, Dougherty CM, Lubitz SA, Rabinstein AA, Rittenberger JC, Callaway CW, Abella BS, Geocadin RG, Kurz MC; American Heart Association Emergency Cardiovascular Care Committee; Council on Cardiovascular and Stroke Nursing; Council on Genomic and Precision Medicine; Council on Quality of Care and Outcomes Research; and Stroke Council.Sudden Cardiac Arrest Survivorship: A Scientific Statement From the American Heart Association.Circulation.2020;141:e654-e685. doi: 10.1161/CIR.0000000000000747

4. Nekhlyudov L, O'Malley D M, Hudson SV.Integrating primary care providers in the care of cancer survivors: gaps in evidence and future opportunities. Lancet Oncol.2017;18:e30-e38. doi: 10.1016/S1470-2045(16)30570-8
5. Committee on Cancer Survivorship: Improving Care and Quality of life. From Cancer Patient to Cancer Survivor—Lost in Transition.Washington, DC: Institute of Medicine and National Research Council of the National Academies of Sciences; 2006.
6. Wilder Schaaf KP, Artman LK, Peberdy MA, Walker WC, Ornato JP, Gossip MR, Kreutzer JS; Virginia Commonwealth University ARCTIC Investigators. Anxiety, depression, and PTSD following cardiac arrest: a systematic review of the literature.Resuscitation.2013;84:873-877. doi: 10.1016/j.resuscitation.2012.11.021
7. Presciutti A, Verma J, Pavol M, Anbarasan D, Falo C, Brodie D, Rabbani LE, Roh DJ, Park S, Claassen J, Agarwal S. Posttraumatic stress and depressive symptoms characterize cardiac arrest survivors' perceived recovery at hospital discharge.Gen Hosp Psychiatry.2018;53:108-113. doi: 10.1016/j.genhosppsych.2018.02.006
8. Presciutti A, Sobczak E, Sumner JA, Roh DJ, Park S, Claassen J, Kronish I, Agarwal S. The impact of psychological distress on long-term recovery perceptions in survivors of cardiac arrest.J Crit Care.2019;50:227-233. doi: 10.1016/j.jcrc.2018.12.011
9. Lilja G, Nilsson G, Nielsen N, Friberg H, Hassager C, Koopmans M, Kuiper M, Martini A, Mellinghoff J, Pelosi P, Wanscher M, Wise MP, Östman I, Cronberg T. Anxiety and depression among out-of-hospital cardiac arrest survivors.Resuscitation.2015;97:68-75. doi: 10.1016/j.resuscitation.2015.09.389
10. Doolittle ND, Sauvé MJ.Impact of aborted sudden cardiac death on survivors and their spouses: the phenomenon of different reference points.Am J Crit Care.1995;4:389-396.
11. Pusswald G, Fertl E, Faltl M, Auff E. Neurological rehabilitation of severely disabled cardiac arrest survivors.Part II.Life situation of patients and families after treatment.Resuscitation.2000;47:241-248. doi: 10.1016/s0300-9572(00)00240-9
12. Löf S, Sandström A, Engström A. Patients treated with therapeutic hypothermia after cardiac arrest: relatives' experiences.J Adv Nurs.2010;66:1760-1768. doi: 10.1111/j.1365-2648.2010.05352.x
13. Weslien M, Nilstun T, Lundqvist A, Fridlund B. When the unreal becomes real: family members' experiences of cardiac arrest.Nurs Crit Care.2005;10:15-22. doi: 10.1111/j.1362-1017.2005.00094.x
14. Wallin E, Larsson IM, Rubertsson S, Kristoferzon ML.Relatives' experiences of everyday life six months after hypothermia treatment of a significant other's cardiac arrest.J Clin Nurs.2013;22:1639-1646. doi: 10.1111/jocn.12112
15. Larsson IM, Wallin E, Rubertsson S, Kristoferzon ML.Relatives' experiences during the next of kin's hospital stay after surviving cardiac arrest and therapeutic hypothermia.Eur J Cardiovasc Nurs.2013;12:353-359. doi: 10.1177/1474515112459618
16. Dougherty CM.Longitudinal recovery following sudden cardiac arrest and internal cardioverter defibrillator implantation: survivors and their families. Am J Crit Care.1994;3:145-154.
17. Dougherty CM.Family-focused interventions for survivors of sudden cardiac arrest.J Cardiovasc Nurs.1997;12:45-58. doi: 10.1097/00005082-199710000-00006
18. Lilja G, Nielsen N, Friberg H, Horn J, Kjaergaard J, Nilsson F, Pellis T, Wetterslev J, Wise MP, Bosch F, Bro-Jeppesen J, Brunetti I, Buratti AF, Hassager C, Hofgren C, Insorsi A, Kuiper M, Martini A, Palmer N, Rundgren M, Rylander C, van der Veen A, Wanscher M, Watkins H, Cronberg T. Cognitive function in survivors of out-of-hospital cardiac arrest after target temperature management at 33°C versus 36°C. Circulation.2015;131:1340-1349. doi: 10.1161/CIRCULATIONAHA.114.014414
19. Tiainen M, Poutiainen E, Oksanen T, Kaukonen KM, Pettilä V, Skrifvars M, Varpula T, Castrén M. Functional outcome, cognition and quality of life after out-of-hospital cardiac arrest and therapeutic hypothermia: data from a randomized controlled trial.Scand J Trauma Resusc Emerg Med.2015;23:12. doi: 10.1186/s13049-014-0084-9
20. Buanes EA, Gramstad A, Søvig KK, Hufthammer KO, Flaatten H, Husby T, Langørgen J, Heltne JK.Cognitive function and health-related quality of life four years after cardiac arrest.Resuscitation.2015;89:13-18. doi: 10.1016/j.resuscitation.2014.12.021
21. Mateen FJ, Josephs KA, Trenerry MR, Felmlee-Devine MD, Weaver AL, Carone M, White RD.Long-term cognitive outcomes following out-of-hospital cardiac arrest: a population-based study.Neurology.2011;77:1438-1445. doi: 10.1212/WNL.0b013e318232ab33
22. Steinbusch CVM, van Heugten CM, Rasquin SMC, Verbunt JA, Moulaert VRM.Cognitive impairments and subjective cognitive complaints after survival of cardiac arrest: A prospective longitudinal cohort study.Resuscitation.2017;120:132-137. doi: 10.1016/j.resuscitation.2017.08.007
23. Nolan JP, Soar J, Cariou A, Cronberg T, Moulaert VR, Deakin CD, Bottiger BW, Friberg H, Sunde K, Sandroni C. European Resuscitation Council and European Society of Intensive Care Medicine 2015 guidelines for post-resuscitation care.Intensive Care Med.2015;41:2039-2056. doi: 10.1007/s00134-015-4051-3
24. Moulaert VR, Verbunt JA, Bakx WG, Gorgels AP, de Krom MC, Heuts PH, Wade DT, van Heugten CM. 'Stand still., and move on', a new early intervention service for cardiac arrest survivors and their caregivers: rationale and description of the intervention.Clin Rehabil.2011;25:867-879. doi: 10.1177/0269215511399937
25. Cowan MJ, Pike KC, Budzynski HK.Psychosocial nursing therapy following sudden cardiac arrest: impact on two-year survival.Nurs Res.2001;50:68-76. doi: 10.1097/00006199-200103000-00002
26. Lundgren-Nilsson A, Rosén H, Hofgren C, Sunnerhagen KS.The first year after successful cardiac resuscitation: function, activity, participation and quality of life.Resuscitation.2005;66:285-289. doi: 10.1016/j.resuscitation.2005.04.001
27. Middelkamp W, Moulaert VR, Verbunt JA, van Heugten CM, Bakx WG, Wade DT.Life after survival: long-term daily life functioning and quality of life of patients with hypoxic brain injury as a result of a cardiac arrest.Clin Rehabil.2007;21:425-431. doi: 10.1177/0269215507075307
28. Kragholm K, Wissenberg M, Mortensen RN, Fonager K, Jensen SE, Rajan S, Lippert FK, Christensen EF, Hansen PA, Lang-Jensen T, Hendriksen OM, Kober L, Gislason G, Torp-Pedersen C, Rasmussen BS.Return to Work in Out-of-Hospital Cardiac Arrest Survivors: A Nationwide Register-Based Follow-Up Study.Circulation.2015;131:1682-1690. doi: 10.1161/CIRCULATIONAHA.114.011366
29. Lilja G, Nielsen N, Bro-Jeppesen J, Dunford H, Friberg H, Hofgren C, Horn J, Insorsi A, Kjaergaard J, Nilsson F, Pelosi P, Winters T, Wise MP, Cronberg T. Return to Work and Participation in Society After Out-of-Hospital Cardiac Arrest.Circ Cardiovasc Qual Outcomes.2018;11:e003566. doi: 10.1161/CIRCOUTCOMES.117.003566
30. Dougherty CM, Benoliel JQ, Bellin C. Domains of nursing intervention after sudden cardiac arrest and automatic internal cardioverter defibrillator implantation.Heart Lung.2000;29:79-86.
31. Forslund AS, Lundblad D, Jansson JH, Zingmark K, Söderberg S. Risk factors among people surviving out-of-hospital cardiac arrest and their thoughts about what lifestyle means to them: a mixed methods study.BMC Cardiovasc Disord.2013;13:62. doi: 10.1186/1471-2261-13-62
32. Møller TP, Hansen CM, Fjordholt M, Pedersen BD, Østergaard D, Lippert FK.Debriefing bystanders of out-of-hospital cardiac arrest is valuable.Resuscitation.2014;85:1504-1511. doi: 10.1016/j.resuscitation.2014.08.006
33. Deleted in proof.
34. Clark R, McLean C. The professional and personal debriefing needs of ward based nurses after involvement in a cardiac arrest: An explorative qualitative pilot study.Intensive Crit Care Nurs.2018;47:78-84. doi: 10.1016/j.iccn.2018.03.009
35. Ireland S, Gilchrist J, Maconochie I. Debriefing after failed paediatric resuscitation: a survey of current UK practice.Emerg Med J. 2008;25:328-330. doi: 10.1136/emj.2007.048942

特殊な蘇生の状況
偶発性低体温症

COR	LOE	推奨事項
1	C-LD	1. 生存の可能性を低くする特徴がなく、かつ明らかな致死的外傷の特徴のないすべての偶発性低体温症者について、使用可能であれば体外復温を含む完全な蘇生法が推奨される。
1	C-EO	2. 偶発性低体温症者は、明らかな死の徴候がない限り、復温を行う前に死亡しているとみなすべきではない。
2b	C-LD	3. 復温方法とともに標準的BLSアルゴリズムに従って除細動を試みることが妥当であろう。
2b	C-LD	4. 復温法とともに標準的なACLSアルゴリズムに従い、心停止中のアドレナリン投与を考慮することが妥当である。

「概要」

環境による重篤な偶然性低体温（体温が30℃［86°F］未満）によって、心拍数と呼吸数が著しく減少し、患者が本当に心停止しているかどうかの判断が困難な場合ある。傷病者は、極めて低い体温の影響で臨床的に死亡したように見える可能性がある。したがって、患者が明らかに死亡している場合（死体硬直や生存不可能な外傷がある場合）を除き、復温するまで標準的BLSやACLSなどの救命処置を続けることは重要である。侵襲的手法を含む積極的な復温が必要な可能性があり、他のOHCA状況の場合よりも迅速な病院への輸送が必要となる場合がある[1]。雪崩の被災者である患者特有の治療はこれらのガイドラインには含まれていないが、他の箇所から参照できる[2]。

「推奨事項の裏付けとなる解説」

1. 偶発性低体温症患者は、しばしば顕著なCNSと心血管系の抑制および死または死に近い外見を示す。したがって、明らかな死の徴候がない限り、完全な蘇生法を迅速に実施する必要がある。標準的BLSおよびALS治療を施すとともに、次の手順として、濡れた衣服を脱がし、それ以上の環境への暴露から患者を保護することにより、さらに蒸発性の放熱が起こるのを防ぐことが挙げられる。灌流リズムの見られる重篤な低体温症患者（30℃未満）には、内加温法がしばしば使用される。手法としては、加温加湿酸素、加温した輸液静注、胸腔内または腹腔内温水投与による洗浄がある[3-5]。重篤な低体温症と心停止が認められる患者には、可能であれば、最も迅速な復温が可能な体外復温を実施する[6-11]。重篤な高カリウム血症の場合で深部体温が極めて低い場合も、蘇生が無効なことが予測される場合がある[12,13]。

2. 傷病者が低体温の場合、脈および呼吸数は遅い、または検出が難しい可能性があり[13,14]、心電図上で心静止が示される場合さえある。したがって、患者が復温するか明らかな死亡にいたるまで救命処置を実施することが重要になる。重度の低体温では、他の障害（例えば、薬物過量投与、飲酒、外傷）が先行する場合が多いため、低体温の治療と同時に、これらの基礎にある状態を探し、それを治療することが推奨される。

3. 低体温の心臓は、心血管治療薬、ペーシング装置による刺激、除細動に反応しないことがある。しかし、これを支持するデータは本質的に理論的なものである[15]。VTまたはVFが1回のショック後に持続する場合、次の除細動を目標体温が達成されるまで引き延ばすことの価値は不確かである。除細動に対する標準的BLSプロトコルから外れることによる利益を示すエビデンスはない。

4. 低体温状況の心停止中の昇圧薬またはその他の薬物による人間に対する効果のエビデンスは、症例報告のみに限られる[11,16,17]。複数の動物実験のシステマティックレビューでは、低体温性心停止中の昇圧薬の使用がROSCを増加させたと結論付けている[18]。過去のレビューの時点で、低体温性心停止中の昇圧薬などの標準的ACLSに従うことによる害についてのエビデンスは見出されなかった。

このトピックは、直近で2010年に正式なエビデンスレビューを受けている[1]。

参考資料

1. Vanden Hoek TL, Morrison LJ, Shuster M, Donnino M, Sinz E, Lavonas EJ, Jeejeebhoy FM, Gabrielli A. Part 12: cardiac arrest in special situations: 2010 American Heart Association Guidelines for Cardiopulmonary Resuscitation and Emergency Cardiovascular Care.Circulation.2010;122(suppl 3):S829-S861. doi: 10.1161/CIRCULATIONAHA.110.971069
2. Brugger H, Durrer B, Elsensohn F, Paal P, Strapazzon G, Winterberger E, Zafren K, Boyd J. Resuscitation of avalanche victims: Evidence-based guidelines of the international commission for mountain emergency medicine (ICAR MEDCOM): intended for physicians and other advanced life support personnel.Resuscitation.2013;84:539-546. doi: 10.1016/j.resuscitation.2012.10.020
3. Kangas E, Niemelä H, Kojo N. Treatment of hypothermic circulatory arrest with thoracotomy and pleural lavage.Ann Chir Gynaecol.1994;83:258-260.
4. Walters DT.Closed thoracic cavity lavage for hypothermia with cardiac arrest.Ann Emerg Med.1991;20:439-440. doi: 10.1016/s0196-0644(05)81687-7
5. Plaisier BR.Thoracic lavage in accidental hypothermia with cardiac arrest-report of a case and review of the literature.Resuscitation.2005;66:99-104. doi: 10.1016/j.resuscitation.2004.12.024

6. Farstad M, Andersen KS, Koller ME, Grong K, Segadal L, Husby P. Rewarming from accidental hypothermia by extracorporeal circulation.A retrospective study.Eur J Cardiothorac Surg.2001;20:58-64. doi: 10.1016/s1010-7940(01)00713-8
7. Sheridan RL, Goldstein MA, Stoddard FJ Jr, Walker TG.Case records of the Massachusetts General Hospital.Case 41-2009.A 16-year-old boy with hypothermia and frostbite.N Engl J Med.2009;361:2654-2662. doi: 10.1056/NEJMcpc0910088
8. Gilbert M, Busund R, Skagseth A, Nilsen PA, Solbø JP.Resuscitation from accidental hypothermia of 13.7 degrees C with circulatory arrest.Lancet.2000;355:375-376. doi: 10.1016/S0140-6736 (00)01021-7
9. Coleman E, Doddakula K, Meeke R, Marshall C, Jahangir S, Hinchion J. An atypical case of successful resuscitation of an accidental profound hypothermia patient, occurring in a temperate climate.Perfusion.2010;25:103-106. doi: 10.1177/0267659110366066
10. Althaus U, Aeberhard P, Schüpbach P, Nachbur BH, Mühlemann W. Management of profound accidental hypothermia with cardiorespiratory arrest.Ann Surg.1982;195:492-495. doi: 10.1097/00000658-198204000-00018
11. Dobson JA, Burgess JJ.Resuscitation of severe hypothermia by extracorporeal rewarming in a child.J Trauma.1996;40:483-485. doi: 10.1097/00005373-199603000-00032
12. Brugger H, Bouzat P, Pasquier M, Mair P, Fieler J, Darocha T, Blancher M, de Riedmatten M, Falk M, Paal P, Strapazzon G, Zafren K, Brodmann Maeder M. Cut-off values of serum potassium and core temperature at hospital admission for extracorporeal rewarming of avalanche victims in cardiac arrest: A retrospective multi-centre study.Resuscitation.2019;139:222-229. doi: 10.1016/j.resuscitation.2019.04.025
13. Paal P, Gordon L, Strapazzon G, Brodmann Maeder M, Putzer G, Walpoth B, Wanscher M, Brown D, Holzer M, Broessner G, Brugger H. Accidental hypothermia-an update: The content of this review is endorsed by the International Commission for Mountain Emergency Medicine (ICAR MEDCOM).Scand J Trauma Resusc Emerg Med.2016;24:111. doi: 10.1186/s13049-016-0303-7
14. Danzl DF, Pozos RS.Accidental hypothermia.N Engl J Med.1994;331:1756-1760. doi: 10.1056/NEJM199412293312607
15. Clift J, Munro-Davies L. Best evidence topic report.Is defibrillation effective in accidental severe hypothermia in adults? Emerg Med J. 2007;24:50-51. doi: 10.1136/emj.2006.044404
16. Winegard C. Successful treatment of severe hypothermia and prolonged cardiac arrest with closed thoracic cavity lavage.J Emerg Med.1997;15:629-632. doi: 10.1016/s0736-4679(97)00139-x
17. Lienhart HG, John W, Wenzel V. Cardiopulmonary resuscitation of a near-drowned child with a combination of epinephrine and vasopressin.Pediatr Crit Care Med.2005;6:486-488. doi: 10.1097/01.PCC.0000163673.40424.E7
18. Wira CR, Becker JU, Martin G, Donnino MW.Anti-arrhythmic and vasopressor medications for the treatment of ventricular fibrillation in severe hypothermia: a systematic review of the literature.Resuscitation.2008;78:21-29. doi: 10.1016/j.resuscitation.2008.01.025

アナフィラキシー

「緒言」

アナフィラキシーの経験がある米国の成人は 1.6％〜5.1％である[1]。毎年，約 200 人の米国人がアナフィラキシーで死亡する。その殆どは薬物の副作用による[2]。アナフィラキシーは多臓器疾患であるが，致命的な症状は，多くの場合，気道（浮腫，気管支けいれん）および／または循環系（血管拡張性ショック）に関するものである。アドレナリンは，アナフィラキシーに対する治療の要である[3-5]。

COR	LOE	推奨事項
アナフィラキシーによる心停止 に関する推奨事項		
1	C-LD	1. アナフィラキシーに続発する心停止では，標準的な蘇生法とアドレナリンの迅速な投与が優先される。

「推奨事項の裏付けとなる解説」

1. アナフィラキシーによる心停止のための代替的な治療アルゴリズムを評価した RCT はない。エビデンスは症例報告および非致死的症例に基づく推測や，病態生理学の解釈，統一見解に限られている。アナフィラキシー反応の疑いがある場合，気道，呼吸，循環を早急に補助することが重要であることを認識しなければならない。エビデンスが限られているため，アナフィラキシーに続発する心停止管理の基礎は，標準的 BLS および ACLS（気道確保と早期アドレナリン投与を含む）である。アナフィラキシーによって誘発された心停止中に，抗ヒスタミン薬，吸入 β 作動薬副腎皮質ステロイド薬を使用することによる利益は証明されていない。

COR	LOE	推奨事項
心停止のないアナフィラキシーに関する 推奨事項		
1	C-LD	1. アドレナリンは全身性のアレルギー反応の兆候，特に低血圧，気道の腫脹，または呼吸困難のある患者全員に，早期に筋注（または自動注射器）により投与されるべきである。
1	C-LD	2. アナフィラキシーにおけるアドレナリンの推奨用量は 0.2〜0.5 mg（1,000 倍希釈）の筋注であり，必要に応じて 5〜15 分ごとに繰り返す。
1	C-LD	3. アナフィラキシーショックの患者では，緊密な血行動態モニタリングが推薦される。
1	C-LD	4. 口腔咽頭または喉頭浮腫の急速な発生の可能性を考慮すると，外科的な気道確保を含む高度な気道確保器具挿入の専門知識を持つ医療従事者に直ちに照会することが推奨される。
2a	C-LD	5. 静注ラインが取り付けられている場合，アナフィラキシーショックにおいて 0.05〜0.1 mg（0.1 mg/ml，すなわち 10,000 倍希釈液）のアドレナリンの静注投与を検討することが妥当である。
2a	C-LD	6. アドレナリンの静注は，心停止患者のアナフィラキシー治療において静注ボーラスに代わる妥当な方法である。
2b	C-LD	7. アドレナリンの静注は，アナフィラキシー患者の心拍再開後のショックに対して考慮してもよい。

「推奨事項固有の裏付けテキスト」

1. アナフィラキシーのエビデンスを有するすべての患者は，アドレナリンによる早期処置を必要とする。重度のアナフィラキシーでは，気道の完全な閉塞と血管原性ショックによる心血管虚脱が起こる可能性がある。アドレナリンの投与が救命につながる可能性がある[6]。投与の容易さ，効果，安全性を考えると，初期の投与としては筋注が望ましい[7]。
2. 大腿の外側面のアドレナリン注射は，急速なピーク血漿アドレナリン濃度をもたらす[7]。成人用アドレナリン筋肉内自動注

入器は 0.3 mg のアドレナリンを投与し，小児用アドレナリン筋肉内自動注入器は 0.15 mg のアドレナリンを投与する。多くの患者は 5～15 分後に症状の再発が報告され，追加投与が必要となる[8]。

3. アナフィラキシーショックの患者は非常に重篤であり，心血管と呼吸の状態が急速に変化するため，緊密なモニタリングが避けられない[9]。

4. アナフィラキシーから閉塞性気道浮腫が見られる場合は，高度な気道確保を早急に実施することが重要である。場合によっては，緊急輪状甲状靭帯切開または気管切開が必要になる[10,11]。

5. 静注アドレナリンは，静脈路が確保されている場合の，アナフィラキシーショックにおける筋内投与に代わる適切な方法である。0.05～0.1 mg（心停止で通常使用されるアドレナリン用量の 5 %～10 %）の静脈内投与はアナフィラキシーショックに使用され，奏効している[9]。アナフィラキシーにおける骨髄内投与は特に研究されていないが，骨髄内投与も同様の用量で効果があると考えられる。

6. アナフィラキシーショックのイヌを用いたモデルでは，血圧低下の治療において，アドレナリンの持続点滴は治療しない場合やボーラスアドレナリン治療よりも効果的であった[12]。初期治療の後でショックが繰り返される場合は，静注（5～15 μg/分）も慎重な滴定とアドレナリン過剰投与の回避により役立つ可能性がある。

7. アナフィラキシーによる心停止後に ROSC を達成した患者特有のデータは特定されなかったが，アナフィラキシーショックの観察研究は，アドレナリンの静注（5～15 μg/分）が，輸液蘇生などの他の蘇生との併用で，アナフィラキシーショックの治療を成功させる可能性があることを示唆している[13]。アナフィラキシーの治療における役割を考慮すると，アドレナリンはこの状況における心拍再開後のショックの治療に対する理に適った選択である。

このトピックは，直近で 2010 年に正式なエビデンスレビューを受けている[14]。

参考資料

1. Wood RA, Camargo CA Jr, Lieberman P, Sampson HA, Schwartz LB, Zitt M, Collins C, Tringale M, Wilkinson M, Boyle J, et al.Anaphylaxis in America: the prevalence and characteristics of anaphylaxis in the United States.J Allergy Clin Immunol.2014;133:461–467. doi: 10.1016/j.jaci.2013.08.016
2. Jerschow E, Lin RY, Scaperotti MM, McGinn AP.Fatal anaphylaxis in the United States, 1999-2010: temporal patterns and demographic associations.J Allergy Clin Immunol.2014;134:1318.e7-1328.e7. doi: 10.1016/j.jaci.2014.08.018
3. Dhami S, Panesar SS, Roberts G, Muraro A, Worm M, Bilò MB, Cardona V, Dubois AE, DunnGalvin A, Eigenmann P, Fernandez-Rivas M, Halken S, Lack G, Niggemann B, Rueff F, Santos AF, Vlieg-Boerstra B, Zolkipli ZQ, Sheikh A; EAACI Food Allergy and Anaphylaxis Guidelines Group.Management of anaphylaxis: a systematic review.Allergy.2014;69:168–175. doi: 10.1111/all.12318
4. Sheikh A, Simons FE, Barbour V, Worth A. Adrenaline auto-injectors for the treatment of anaphylaxis with and without cardiovascular collapse in the community.Cochrane Database Syst Rev. 2012:CD008935. doi: 10.1002/14651858.CD008935.pub2
5. Shaker MS, Wallace DV, Golden DBK, Oppenheimer J, Bernstein JA, Campbell RL, Dinakar C, Ellis A, Greenhawt M, Khan DA, Lang DM, Lang ES, Lieberman JA, Portnoy J, Rank MA, Stukus DR, Wang J, Riblet N, Bobrownicki AMP, Bontrager T, Dusin J, Foley J, Frederick B, Fregene E, Hellerstedt S, Hassan F, Hess K, Horner C, Huntington K, Kasireddy P, Keeler D, Kim B, Lieberman P, Lindhorst E, McEnany F, Milbank J, Murphy H, Pando O, Patel AK, Ratliff N, Rhodes R, Robertson K, Scott H, Snell A, Sullivan R, Trivedi V, Wickham A, Shaker MS, Wallace DV, Shaker MS, Wallace DV, Bernstein JA, Campbell RL, Dinakar C, Ellis A, Golden DBK, Greenhawt M, Lieberman JA, Rank MA, Stukus DR, Wang J, Shaker MS, Wallace DV, Golden DBK, Bernstein JA, Dinakar C, Ellis A, Greenhawt M, Horner C, Khan DA, Lieberman JA, Oppenheimer J, Rank MA, Shaker MS, Stukus DR, Wang J; Collaborators; Chief Editors; Workgroup Contributors; Joint Task Force on Practice Parameters Reviewers.Anaphylaxis-a 2020 practice parameter update, systematic review, and Grading of Recommendations, Assessment, Development and Evaluation (GRADE) analysis.J Allergy Clin Immunol.2020;145:1082–1123. doi: 10.1016/j.jaci.2020.01.017
6. Sheikh A, Shehata YA, Brown SG, Simons FE.Adrenaline (epinephrine) for the treatment of anaphylaxis with and without shock.Cochrane Database Syst Rev. 2008:CD006312. doi: 10.1002/14651858.CD006312.pub2
7. Simons FE, Gu X, Simons KJ.Epinephrine absorption in adults: intramuscular versus subcutaneous injection.J Allergy Clin Immunol.2001;108:871–873. doi: 10.1067/mai.2001.119409
8. Korenblat P, Lundie MJ, Dankner RE, Day JH.A retrospective study of epinephrine administration for anaphylaxis: how many doses are needed? Allergy Asthma Proc.1999;20:383–386. doi: 10.2500/108854199778251834
9. Bochner BS, Lichtenstein LM.Anaphylaxis.N Engl J Med.1991;324:1785–1790. doi: 10.1056/NEJM199106203242506
10. Yilmaz R, Yuksekbas O, Erkol Z, Bulut ER, Arslan MN.Postmortem findings after anaphylactic reactions to drugs in Turkey.Am J Forensic Med Pathol.2009;30:346–349. doi: 10.1097/PAF.0b013e3181c0e7bb
11. Yunginger JW, Sweeney KG, Sturner WQ, Giannandrea LA, Teigland JD, Bray M, Benson PA, York JA, Biedrzycki L, Squillace DL.Fatal food-induced anaphylaxis.JAMA.1988;260:1450–1452.
12. Mink SN, Simons FE, Simons KJ, Becker AB, Duke K. Constant infusion of epinephrine, but not bolus treatment, improves haemodynamic recovery in anaphylactic shock in dogs.Clin Exp Allergy.2004;34:1776–1783. doi: 10.1111/j.1365-2222.2004.02106.x
13. Brown SG, Blackman KE, Stenlake V, Heddle RJ.Insect sting anaphylaxis; prospective evaluation of treatment with intravenous adrenaline and volume resuscitation.Emerg Med J. 2004;21:149–154. doi: 10.1136/emj.2003.009449
14. Vanden Hoek TL, Morrison LJ, Shuster M, Donnino M, Sinz E, Lavonas EJ, Jeejeebhoy FM, Gabrielli A. Part 12: cardiac arrest in special situations: 2010 American Heart Association Guidelines for Cardiopulmonary Resuscitation and Emergency Cardiovascular Care.Circulation.2010;122(suppl 3):S829–S861. doi: 10.1161/CIRCULATIONAHA.110.971069

喘息による心停止

喘息による心停止の管理に関する 推奨事項

COR	LOE	推奨事項
1	C-LD	1. 心停止を有する喘息患者，最大吸気圧の突然の上昇がある喘息患者，人工呼吸が困難な喘息患者については，緊張性気胸の評価を早急に実施しなければならない。
2a	C-LD	2. 内因性呼気終末陽圧（intrinsic positive end-expiratory pressure，auto-PEEP）の潜在的作用と心停止喘息患者の圧外傷のリスクがあるため，呼吸数と 1 回換気量の少ない人工呼吸の方法が妥当である。
2a	C-LD	3. 心停止前後の状態で換気補助を受けている喘息患者に auto-PEEP の増加や血圧の急減が見られる場合は，短時間バッグマスクまたは人工呼吸器から外し，胸壁を圧迫してエアトラッピングを緩和することが効果的となりうる。

「概要」

喘息発作の重症化は，重度の呼吸不全，二酸化炭素の滞留，エアトラッピングを招き，急性呼吸性アシドーシスと胸腔内圧の上昇につながる可能性がある。米国では急性喘息による死亡は減少しているが，喘息は 1 年に 3,500 人以上の成人の深刻な死因になっている[1,2]。喘息による呼吸停止患者は，致命的な急性呼吸性アシドーシスを発症する[3]。重大なアシドーシスも，胸腔内圧が上昇して心臓への静脈還流が減少することも，いずれも喘息における心停止の原因になりうる。

喘息の急性増悪の状況における心停止患者の治療は，必ず，標準的 BLS から始まる。心停止の根本原因に呼吸がある可能性があれば気道確保と人工呼吸の重要性が増加するが，喘息からの心停止患者に対する ACLS も特別な変更はない。緊急喘息の処置は，2010 年のガイドラインでレビューされている[4]。2020 年では，執筆グループは，心停止直後の喘息患者に特有の ACLS に関する追加の考慮事項に着目した。

「推奨事項の裏付けとなる解説」

1. 緊張性気胸は，喘息のまれな致命的合併症であり，心停止の可逆的原因である[5]。通常は機械的換気を受けている患者で起こることだが，自発呼吸がある患者の事例も報告されてきた[5-7]。陽圧人工呼吸から生じる最大気道内圧の上昇は，気胸につながることがある。瀕死の状態の喘息患者は過膨張と胸腔内圧の上昇によって人工呼吸が困難な場合が多いが，緊張気胸の評価が重要であることは変わらない。
2. 喘息患者の心停止を促進することのある急性呼吸不全は，エアトラッピングにつながる重度閉塞によって特徴づけられる。呼気の制限のため，呼吸数上昇時に大量の 1 回換気量を提供することはエアトラッピングの進行性悪化と有効換気量の減少につながることがある。1 回換気量と呼吸数を少なくし，呼気時間を長くするアプローチによって auto-PEEP と圧外傷のリスクを最小化に抑えられる可能性がある[8]。
3. 呼気能力が十分でない喘息患者の呼吸重積は，胸腔内圧の増加，静脈還流および冠動脈灌流圧の減少，心停止にいたる可能性がある[9-11]。これは，患者の換気の困難，人工呼吸器の高気道内圧アラーム，血圧の急低下として現れることがある。人工呼吸器を短時間外したり，バッグマスク換気を中断したり，胸郭を圧迫して呼気を補助したりすることが，過膨張を緩和する可能性がある。

このトピックは，直近で 2010 年に正式なエビデンスレビューを受けている[4]。

参考資料

1. Moorman JE, Akinbami LJ, Bailey CM, Zahran HS, King ME, Johnson CA, Liu X. National surveillance of asthma: United States, 2001–2010.Vital Health Stat 3.2012:1-58.
2. Centers for Disease Control and Prevention.AsthmaStats: asthma as the underlying cause of death.2016. https://www.cdc.gov/asthma/asthma_stats/documents/AsthmStat_Mortality_2001-2016-H.pdf.Accessed April 20, 2020.
3. Molfino NA, Nannini LJ, Martelli AN, Slutsky AS.Respiratory arrest in near-fatal asthma.N Engl J Med.1991;324:285-288. doi: 10.1056/NEJM199101313240502
4. Vanden Hoek TL, Morrison LJ, Shuster M, Donnino M, Sinz E, Lavonas EJ, Jeejeebhoy FM, Gabrielli A. Part 12: cardiac arrest in special situations: 2010 American Heart Association Guidelines for Cardiopulmonary Resuscitation and Emergency Cardiovascular Care.Circulation.2010;122 (suppl 3):S829-S861. doi: 10.1161/CIRCULATIONAHA.110.971069
5. Leigh-Smith S, Christey G. Tension pneumothorax in asthma.Resuscitation.2006;69:525-527. doi: 10.1016/j.resuscitation.2005.10.011
6. Metry AA.Acute severe asthma complicated with tension pneumothorax and hemopneumothorax.Int J Crit Illn Inj Sci.2019;9:91-95. doi: 10.4103/IJCIIS.IJCIIS_83_18
7. Karakaya Z, Demir S, Sagay SS, Karakaya O, Ozdinç S. Bilateral spontaneous pneumothorax, pneumomediastinum, and subcutaneous emphysema: rare and fatal complications of asthma.Case Rep Emerg Med.2012;2012:242579. doi: 10.1155/2012/242579
8. Leatherman J. Mechanical ventilation for severe asthma. Chest.2015;147:1671-1680. doi: 10.1378/chest.14-1733
9. Myles PS, Madder H, Morgan EB.Intraoperative cardiac arrest after unrecognized dynamic hyperinflation.Br J Anaesth.1995;74:340-342. doi: 10.1093/bja/74.3.340
10. Mercer M. Cardiac arrest after unrecognized dynamic inflation.Br J Anaesth.1995;75:252. doi: 10.1093/bja/75.2.252
11. Berlin D. Hemodynamic consequences of auto-PEEP.J Intensive Care Med.2014;29:81-86. doi: 10.1177/0885066612445712

心臓手術後の心停止

心臓手術後の心停止に関する 推奨事項

COR	LOE	推奨事項
1	B-NR	1. 緊急の胸骨再切開を直ちに行えなければ，胸骨圧迫を行う。
1	C-LD	2. 訓練されたプロバイダーが心臓手術後患者の心停止を目撃したら，VF/VT に対して直ちに除細動を行う。1 分以内に除細動が成功しなければ CPR を開始する。
1	C-EO	3. 訓練されたプロバイダー がペーシングリードを留置された心臓手術後患者の心停止を目撃したら，心静止または徐脈性心停止に対して直ちにペーシングを開始することを推奨する。1 分以内にペーシングが成功しなければ CPR を開始する。
2a	B-NR	4. 心臓手術後患者の心停止では，適切なスタッフと設備を有する ICU において早期に胸骨再切開を行うことは妥当である。
2a	C-LD	5. 開胸または開腹手術の術中または心臓胸部手術の術後早期に心停止が起きたときには，開胸 CPR を行える可能性がある。
2b	C-LD	6. 標準的な蘇生手技が困難な心臓術後患者では，体外循環式心肺蘇生により転帰が改善する可能性がある。

「概要」

心臓手術後には，1%～8%の患者で心停止が起きる[1-8]。病因としては，VTやVFなどの頻拍性不整脈，房室ブロックや心静止などの徐脈性不整脈，タンポナーデや気胸などの閉塞性の原因，置換された弁の機能障害や移植されたグラフトの閉塞や出血などの技術的な要因がある。あらゆる心停止患者と同様に，当面の目標はCPRによる灌流の再開，ACLSの開始，心停止の原因の早急な特定と修正である。他の多くの心停止とは異なり，これらの患者の心停止は，ICUのような高度の監視体制の下で，救命処置を行える高度な訓練を受けたスタッフのいる状況で発生するのが通例である。

これらのガイドラインは全てを網羅するものではない。この項目に関しては，米国胸部外科学会（Society of Thoracic Surgeons）が最近声明を発表した[9]。

「推奨事項の裏付けとなる解説」

1. 胸骨圧迫による心臓損傷の報告がわずかにあった[10-14]。しかし，他の多くの症例報告ではそのような損傷はみられず，一定の状況下では胸骨圧迫が血流を発生させる唯一の手段であることに変わりはない。胸骨圧迫による心臓損傷は血流停止による確実な死亡に較べれば遙かに軽微なリスクである。

2. VFは，心臓手術後の心停止の25%～50%の患者で見られる心リズムである。訓練されたプロバイダーによる迅速な除細動はこれらの患者に明白な利点をもたらすが，胸骨圧迫や胸骨再切開に関連する後遺症は回復に重大な影響を及ぼす恐れがある。この問題を取り上げた報告は乏しく，異なる波形と出力を用いて体外式除細動器による除細動の成功の閾値を調べた少数の報告に限られる[15-17]。これらの研究の多くで90%以上の初回ショック成功率が観察されたが，15の研究結果を蓄積すると，初回のショックで78%，2回目のショックで35%，3回目のショックで14%の成功率であった[18]。米国胸部外科学会の心臓手術後の蘇生に関するタスクフォース，および欧州心臓胸部外科学会は，CPRを開始する前に，1分以内に3回連続で除細動を行うことを推奨している。このような標準的なACLSからの逸脱は，高度な監視体制の下，胸骨圧迫と胸骨再切開が固有のリスクを有する心臓手術後においては正当化されるかもしれない。

3. ペーシングリードを留置された心臓手術後患者がICUにおいて心静止または徐脈性心停止になれば，訓練されたプロバイダーが直ちにペーシングを開始できる。血行動態監視装置と脈拍触知を組み合わせれば，ペースメーカーによる捕捉と十分な心機能を確認できる。ペーシングが迅速に確立しなければ，CPRを含む標準的なACLSを行う。このプロトコールは外科学会に支持されているが[9,18]，妥当性を裏付けるデータはない。

4. 胸骨再切開のタイミングに関するRCTはない。しかし，経験を積んだプロバイダーが適切な設備を備えたICUにおいて迅速に胸骨再切開を行うプロトコールは，良好な予後をもたらすことが観察されている[1,4,8,19-25]。中立的であったり，他の標準的な治療と比較して胸骨再切開の利点を否定する研究もある[3,6,26,27]。ICU外で実施された胸骨再切開は転帰不良である[1,3]。米国胸部外科学会は，少なくとも術後10日目までは胸骨再切開を蘇生の標準的な手段とすることを推奨している[9]。

5. 開胸CPRと通常のCPRとのRCTはない。2件の小規模試験で，心臓手術患者での通常の胸骨圧迫と比較して開胸CPRの血流動態の効果が改善することが示された[3,4]。

6. 症例集積研究では，標準的な蘇生が困難な場合にECMOや心肺バイパスを含む体外循環式心肺蘇生が有効である可能性を示したものが複数あった[24,28-34]。RCTは現在まで実施されていない。

このトピックは，直近で2010年に正式なエビデンスレビューを受けている[35]。これらの推奨事項は，米国胸部外科学会（Society of Thoracic Surgeons）によって発表された2017年のレビューによって補足された[9]。

参考資料

1. Mackay JH, Powell SJ, Osgathorp J, Rozario CJ.Six-year prospective audit of chest reopening after cardiac arrest.Eur J Cardiothorac Surg.2002;22:421–425. doi: 10.1016/s1010-7940(02)00294-4

2. Birdi I, Chaudhuri N, Lenthall K, Reddy S, Nashef SA.Emergency reinstitution of cardiopulmonary bypass following cardiac surgery: outcome justifies the cost.Eur J Cardiothorac Surg.2000;17:743–746. doi: 10.1016/s1010-7940(00)00453-x

3. Pottle A, Bullock I, Thomas J, Scott L. Survival to discharge following open chest cardiac compression (OCCC).A 4-year retrospective audit in a cardiothoracic specialist centre-Royal Brompton and Harefield NHS Trust, United Kingdom.Resuscitation.2002;52:269–272. doi: 10.1016/s0300-9572(01)00479-8

4. Anthi A, Tzelepis GE, Alivizatos P, Michalis A, Palatianos GM, Geroulanos S. Unexpected cardiac arrest after cardiac surgery: incidence, predisposing causes, and outcome of open chest cardiopulmonary resuscitation. Chest.1998;113:15–19. doi: 10.1378/chest.113.1.15

5. Charalambous CP, Zipitis CS, Keenan DJ.Chest reexploration in the intensive care unit after cardiac surgery: a safe alternative to returning to the operating theater.Ann Thorac Surg.2006;81:191–194. doi: 10.1016/j.athoracsur.2005.06.024

6. Wahba A, Götz W, Birnbaum DE.Outcome of cardiopulmonary resuscitation following open heart surgery.Scand Cardiovasc J. 1997;31:147–149. doi: 10.3109/14017439709058084

7. LaPar DJ, Ghanta RK, Kern JA, Crosby IK, Rich JB, Speir AM, Kron IL, Ailawadi G; and the Investigators for the Virginia Cardiac Surgery Quality Initiative.Hospital variation in mortality from cardiac arrest after cardiac surgery: an opportunity for improvement? Ann Thorac Surg.2014;98:534–539. doi: 10.1016/j.athoracsur.2014.03.030

8. el-Banayosy A, Brehm C, Kizner L, Hartmann D, Körtke H, Körner MM, Minami K, Reichelt W, Körfer R. Cardiopulmonary resuscitation after cardiac surgery: a two-year study. J Cardiothorac Vasc Anesth. 1998;12:390–392. doi: 10.1016/s1053-0770(98)90189-6
9. Society of Thoracic Surgeons Task Force on Resuscitation After Cardiac Surgery. The Society of Thoracic Surgeons expert consensus for the resuscitation of patients who arrest after cardiac surgery. Ann Thorac Surg. 2017;103:1005–1020. doi: 10.1016/j.athoracsur.2016.10.033
10. Böhrer H, Gust R, Böttiger BW. Cardiopulmonary resuscitation after cardiac surgery. J Cardiothorac Vasc Anesth. 1995;9:352. doi: 10.1016/s1053-0770(05)80355-6
11. Ricci M, Karamanoukian HL, D'Ancona G, Jajkowski MR, Bergsland J, Salerno TA. Avulsion of an H graft during closed-chest cardiopulmonary resuscitation after minimally invasive coronary artery bypass graft surgery. J Cardiothorac Vasc Anesth. 2000;14:586–587. doi: 10.1053/jcan.2000.9440
12. Kempen PM, Allgood R. Right ventricular rupture during closed-chest cardiopulmonary resuscitation after pneumonectomy with pericardiotomy: a case report. Crit Care Med. 1999;27:1378–1379. doi: 10.1097/00003246-199907000-00033
13. Sokolove PE, Willis-Shore J, Panacek EA. Exsanguination due to right ventricular rupture during closed-chest cardiopulmonary resuscitation. J Emerg Med. 2002;23:161–164. doi: 10.1016/s0736-4679(02)00504-8
14. Fosse E, Lindberg H. Left ventricular rupture following external chest compression. Acta Anaesthesiol Scand. 1996;40:502–504. doi: 10.1111/j.1399-6576.1996.tb04476.x
15. Szili-Torok T, Theuns D, Verblaauw T, Scholten M, Kimman GJ, Res J, Jordaens L. Transthoracic defibrillation of short-lasting ventricular fibrillation: a randomised trial for comparison of the efficacy of low-energy biphasic rectilinear and monophasic damped sine shocks. Acta Cardiol. 2002;57:329–334. doi: 10.2143/AC.57.5.2005448
16. Higgins SL, O'Grady SG, Banville I, Chapman FW, Schmitt PW, Lank P, Walker RG, Ilina M. Efficacy of lower-energy biphasic shocks for transthoracic defibrillation: a follow-up clinical study. Prehosp Emerg Care. 2004;8:262–267. doi: 10.1016/j.prehos.2004.02.002
17. Bardy GH, Marchlinski FE, Sharma AD, Worley SJ, Luceri RM, Yee R, Halperin BD, Fellows CL, Ahern TS, Chilson DA, Packer DL, Wilber DJ, Mattioni TA, Reddy R, Kronmal RA, Lazzara R. Multicenter comparison of truncated biphasic shocks and standard damped sine wave monophasic shocks for transthoracic ventricular defibrillation. Transthoracic Investigators. Circulation. 1996;94:2507–2514. doi: 10.1161/01.cir.94.10.2507
18. Dunning J, Fabbri A, Kolh PH, Levine A, Lockowandt U, Mackay J, Pavie AJ, Strang T, Versteegh MI, Nashef SA; EACTS Clinical Guidelines Committee. Guideline for resuscitation in cardiac arrest after cardiac surgery. Eur J Cardiothorac Surg. 2009;36:3–28. doi: 10.1016/j.ejcts.2009.01.033
19. Mackay JH, Powell SJ, Charman SC, Rozario C. Resuscitation after cardiac surgery: are we ageist? Eur J Anaesthesiol. 2004;21:66–71. doi: 10.1017/s0265021504001115
20. Raman J, Saldanha RF, Branch JM, Esmore DS, Spratt PM, Farnsworth AE, Harrison GA, Chang VP, Shanahan MX. Open cardiac compression in the postoperative cardiac intensive care unit. Anaesth Intensive Care. 1989;17:129–135. doi: 10.1177/0310057X8901700202
21. Karhunen JP, Sihvo EI, Suojaranta-Ylinen RT, Rämö OJ, Salminen US. Predictive factors of hemodynamic collapse after coronary artery bypass grafting: a case-control study. J Cardiothorac Vasc Anesth. 2006;20:143–148. doi: 10.1053/j.jvca.2005.11.005
22. Fairman RM, Edmunds LH Jr. Emergency thoracotomy in the surgical intensive care unit after open cardiac operation. Ann Thorac Surg. 1981;32:386–391. doi: 10.1016/s0003-4975(10)61761-4
23. Ngaage DL, Cowen ME. Survival of cardiorespiratory arrest after coronary artery bypass grafting or aortic valve surgery. Ann Thorac Surg. 2009;88:64–68. doi: 10.1016/j.athoracsur.2009.03.042
24. Rousou JA, Engelman RM, Flack JE III, Deaton DW, Owen SG. Emergency cardiopulmonary bypass in the cardiac surgical unit can be a lifesaving measure in postoperative cardiac arrest. Circulation. 1994;90(5 Pt 2):II280–II284.
25. Dimopoulou I, Anthi A, Michalis A, Tzelepis GE. Functional status and quality of life in long-term survivors of cardiac arrest after cardiac surgery. Crit Care Med. 2001;29:1408–1411. doi: 10.1097/00003246-200107000-00018
26. Feng WC, Bert AA, Browning RA, Singh AK. Open cardiac massage and periresuscitative cardiopulmonary bypass for cardiac arrest following cardiac surgery. J Cardiovasc Surg (Torino). 1995;36:319–321.
27. Kaiser GC, Naunheim KS, Fiore AC, Harris HH, McBride LR, Pennington DG, Barner HB, Willman VL. Reoperation in the intensive care unit. Ann Thorac Surg. 1990;49:903–7; discussion 908. doi: 10.1016/0003-4975(90)90863-2
28. Chen YS, Chao A, Yu HY, Ko WJ, Wu IH, Chen RJ, Huang SC, Lin FY, Wang SS. Analysis and results of prolonged resuscitation in cardiac arrest patients rescued by extracorporeal membrane oxygenation. J Am Coll Cardiol. 2003;41:197–203. doi: 10.1016/s0735-1097(02)02716-x
29. Dalton HJ, Siewers RD, Fuhrman BP, Del Nido P, Thompson AE, Shaver MG, Dowhy M. Extracorporeal membrane oxygenation for cardiac rescue in children with severe myocardial dysfunction. Crit Care Med. 1993;21:1020–1028. doi: 10.1097/00003246-199307000-00016
30. Ghez O, Feier H, Ughetto F, Fraisse A, Kreitmann B, Metras D. Postoperative extracorporeal life support in pediatric cardiac surgery: recent results. ASAIO J. 2005;51:513-516. doi: 10.1097/01.mat.0000178039.53714.57
31. Duncan BW, Ibrahim AE, Hraska V, del Nido PJ, Laussen PC, Wessel DL, Mayer JE Jr, Bower LK, Jonas RA. Use of rapid-deployment extracorporeal membrane oxygenation for the resuscitation of pediatric patients with heart disease after cardiac arrest. J Thorac Cardiovasc Surg. 1998;116:305–311. doi: 10.1016/s0022-5223(98)70131-x
32. Newsome LR, Ponganis P, Reichman R, Nakaji N, Jaski B, Hartley M. Portable percutaneous cardiopulmonary bypass: use in supported coronary angioplasty, aortic valvuloplasty, and cardiac arrest. J Cardiothorac Vasc Anesth. 1992;6:328–331. doi: 10.1016/1053-0770(92)90151-v
33. Parra DA, Totapally BR, Zahn E, Jacobs J, Aldousany A, Burke RP, Chang AC. Outcome of cardiopulmonary resuscitation in a pediatric cardiac intensive care unit. Crit Care Med. 2000;28:3296–3300. doi: 10.1097/00003246-200009000-00030
34. Overlie PA. Emergency use of cardiopulmonary bypass. J Interv Cardiol. 1995;8:239–247. doi: 10.1111/j.1540-8183.1995.tb00541.x
35. Vanden Hoek TL, Morrison LJ, Shuster M, Donnino M, Sinz E, Lavonas EJ, Jeejeebhoy FM, Gabrielli A. Part 12: cardiac arrest in special situations: 2010 American Heart Association Guidelines for Cardiopulmonary Resuscitation and Emergency Cardiovascular Care. Circulation. 2010;122(suppl 3):S829–S861. doi: 10.1161/CIRCULATIONAHA.110.971069

溺水

溺水に関する 推奨事項		
COR	LOE	推奨事項
1	C-LD	1. 水没から救助された傷病者に対しては、可及的早期に補助呼吸を含むCPRを行う。
1	C-LD	2. 補助呼吸単独を含む何らかの蘇生処置を必要とする水没傷病者は、例え現場で意識清明で有効な心肺機能を有しているようにみえても、全員病院に搬送して評価とモニタリングを行う。
2b	C-LD	3. 水中での口対口人工呼吸は、訓練を受けた救助者が安全性を損なわずに行う場合は有効である可能性がある。
3:利益なし	B-NR	4. 脊髄損傷を示唆する状況がない場合、頸椎をルーチンに固定することは推奨されない。

「概要」

毎年、溺水は全世界の死亡者のうちで死因の約 0.7 %を占めており、年間500,000 人以上が死亡している。[1,2] 米国でのデータを用いた最近の研究では、溺水による心停止から 13% が生還した[3]。溺水のリスクが高いのは、子ども、けいれん発作の

ある人，アルコールやその他の薬物の中毒患者などである。[1] 長時間の水没後の生存例は稀であるが，蘇生の成功例も報告されている[4-9]。そのため，死の徴候が明らかでない限り，現場で蘇生を開始し，傷病者を病院に搬送する必要がある。標準的なBLSとACLSは治療の基本であり，呼吸停止による心停止であることから気道確保と換気は特に重要である。これらの推奨事項に関するエビデンスが最後に全面的にレビューされたのは2010年である。

「推奨事項の裏付けとなる解説」

1. 溺水の結果として生じる低酸素症の持続時間とその程度は，転帰を決定する単一かつ最も重要な因子である[10,11]。水没から救助された傷病者に対しては，転帰を考慮して可及的早期にCPRを行う。適切な訓練を受けている場合は補助呼吸も行う。補助呼吸を迅速に開始することで，傷病者の生存率が向上する[12]。

2. 複数の観察評価により，主に小児患者において，淡水または塩水での溺水後の代償不全は水没から4～6時間後に発生する可能性があることが示されている[13,14]。したがって，可能な限り水没傷病者全員を病院に搬送し，少なくとも4～6時間監視を継続すべきである。

3. 溺水による死亡の直接の原因は低酸素血症である。救助者の受けた訓練に基づいて実施され，かつ現場における救助者の安全を維持できる場合のみ，水中で（「水中蘇生」）で換気を実施できる。こうすることで，水没から救助するまで換気が行われない場合と比較して，転帰を改善できる可能性がある[8]。

4. 報告によれば水没傷病者における頸髄損傷の発生率は小さい（0.009％）[15,16]。脊髄損傷を疑う状況でない限り，ルーチンの頸椎固定は利点がなく，必要な蘇生が遅れる原因になり得る[16,17]。

これらの推奨事項は，溺水における転帰要因を重視する2020年のILCOR CoSTRの結果を反映している[18]。それ以外ではこのトピックは，直近で2010年に正式なエビデンスレビューを受けている[19]。これらのガイドラインは，『Wilderness Medical Society Clinical Practice Guidelines for the Treatment and Prevention of Drowning:2019 Update』によって補足された[20]。

参考資料

1. Szpilman D, Bierens JJ, Handley AJ, Orlowski JP.Drowning.N Engl J Med.2012;366:2102-2110. doi: 10.1056/NEJMra1013317
2. Peden MM, McGee K. The epidemiology of drowning worldwide.Inj Control Saf Promot.2003;10:195-199. doi: 10.1076/icsp.10.4.195.16772
3. Reynolds JC, Hartley T, Michiels EA, Quan L. Long-Term Survival After Drowning-Related Cardiac Arrest.J Emerg Med.2019;57:129-139. doi: 10.1016/j.jemermed.2019.05.029
4. Southwick FS, Dalglish PH Jr. Recovery after prolonged asystolic cardiac arrest in profound hypothermia.A case report and literature review. JAMA.1980;243:1250-1253.
5. Siebke H, Rod T, Breivik H, Link B. Survival after 40 minutes; submersion without cerebral sequeae.Lancet.1975;1:1275-1277. doi: 10.1016/s0140-6736(75)92554-4
6. Bolte RG, Black PG, Bowers RS, Thorne JK, Corneli HM.The use of extracorporeal rewarming in a child submerged for 66 minutes. JAMA.1988;260:377-379.
7. Gilbert M, Busund R, Skagseth A, Nilsen PA, Solbø JP.Resuscitation from accidental hypothermia of 13.7 degrees C with circulatory arrest.Lancet.2000;355:375-376. doi: 10.1016/S0140-6736(00)01021-7
8. Szpilman D, Soares M. In-water resuscitation-is it worthwhile? Resuscitation.2004;63:25-31. doi: 10.1016/j.resuscitation.2004.03.017
9. Allman FD, Nelson WB, Pacentine GA, McComb G. Outcome following cardiopulmonary resuscitation in severe pediatric near-drowning.Am J Dis Child.1986;140:571-575. doi: 10.1001/archpedi.1986.02140200081033
10. Youn CS, Choi SP, Yim HW, Park KN.Out-of-hospital cardiac arrest due to drowning: An Utstein Style report of 10 years of experience from St. Mary's Hospital.Resuscitation.2009;80:778-783. doi: 10.1016/j.resuscitation.2009.04.007
11. Suominen P, Baillie C, Korpela R, Rautanen S, Ranta S, Olkkola KT.Impact of age, submersion time and water temperature on outcome in near-drowning.Resuscitation.2002;52:247-254. doi: 10.1016/s0300-9572(01)00478-6
12. Kyriacou DN, Arcinue EL, Peek C, Kraus JF.Effect of immediate resuscitation on children with submersion injury.Pediatrics.1994;94(2 Pt 1):137-142.
13. Causey AL, Tilelli JA, Swanson ME.Predicting discharge in uncomplicated near-drowning.Am J Emerg Med.2000;18:9-11. doi: 10.1016/s0735-6757(00)90039-1
14. Noonan L, Howrey R, Ginsburg CM.Freshwater submersion injuries in children: a retrospective review of seventy-five hospitalized patients.Pediatrics.1996;98(3 Pt 1):368-371.
15. Weinstein MD, Krieger BP.Near-drowning: epidemiology, pathophysiology, and initial treatment.J Emerg Med.1996;14:461-467. doi: 10.1016/0736-4679(96)00097-2
16. Watson RS, Cummings P, Quan L, Bratton S, Weiss NS.Cervical spine injuries among submersion victims.J Trauma.2001;51:658-662. doi: 10.1097/00005373-200110000-00006
17. Hwang V, Shofer FS, Durbin DR, Baren JM.Prevalence of traumatic injuries in drowning and near drowning in children and adolescents.Arch Pediatr Adolesc Med.2003;157:50-53. doi: 10.1001/archpedi.157.1.50
18. Olasveengen TM, Mancini ME, Perkins GD, Avis S, Brooks S, Castrén M, Chung SP, Considine J, Couper K, Escalante R, et al; on behalf of the Adult Basic Life Support Collaborators.Adult basic life support: 2020 International Consensus on Cardiopulmonary Resuscitation and Emergency Cardiovascular Care Science With Treatment Recommendations.Circulation.2020;142(suppl 1):S41-S91. doi: 10.1161/CIR.0000000000000892
19. Vanden Hoek TL, Morrison LJ, Shuster M, Donnino M, Sinz E, Lavonas EJ, Jeejeebhoy FM, Gabrielli A. Part 12: cardiac arrest in special situations: 2010 American Heart Association Guidelines for Cardiopulmonary Resuscitation and Emergency Cardiovascular Care.Circulation.2010;122(suppl 3):S829-S861. doi: 10.1161/CIRCULATIONAHA.110.971069
20. Schmidt AC, Sempsrott JR, Hawkins SC, Arastu AS, Cushing TA, Auerbach PS.Wilderness Medical Society Clinical Practice Guidelines for the Treatment and Prevention of Drowning: 2019 Update.Wilderness Environ Med.2019;30(4S):S70-S86. doi: 10.1016/j.wem.2019.06.007

電解質異常

心停止における電解質異常に関する 推奨事項

COR	LOE	推奨事項
1	C-LD	1. 高カリウム血症によることがわかっているか，その疑いがある心停止では，標準的な ACLS に加え，カルシウム製剤の静脈内投与を行う。
1	C-LD	2. 重篤な低マグネシウム血症による心毒性および心停止については，標準的な ACLS に加え，マグネシウム製剤の静脈内投与が推奨される。
2b	C-EO	3. 高マグネシウム血症によることがわかっているか，その疑いがある心停止では，標準的な ACLS に加え，経験的なカルシウム製剤の静脈内投与が妥当かもしれない。
3：有害	C-LD	4. 低カリウム血症によることが疑われる心停止において，カリウム製剤の静脈内ボーラス投与は推奨されない。

「概要」

電解質異常は，心停止を引き起こすか，心停止の一因となる可能性があり，また，蘇生努力を妨げ，心停止後の血行動態回復に影響する可能性がある。高カリウム血症と高マグネシウム血症の症例では，標準的な ACLS の他，特定の治療介入が救命につながることがある。

高カリウム血症は腎不全が原因となっていることが多く，不整脈や心停止を誘発することがある。6.5 mmol/L を超える重篤な高カリウム血症に伴う臨床的兆候として，弛緩性麻痺，知覚異常，深部腱反射減弱，息切れなどがある[1-3]。初期段階で心電図上に見られる兆候として，尖鋭な T 波の後に続く T 波の平坦化または消失，PR 間隔の延長，QRS 幅の拡大，S 波の増高，S 波と T 波の融合などがある[4,5]。高カリウム血症が進行すると，心電図上に心室固有調律が現れ，正弦波パターンが形成されて，心静止性心停止に発展することがある[4,5]。重篤な低カリウム血症は稀であるが，消化管や腎臓に損失がある状況で発生することがあり，致死的な心室不整脈の原因となることがある[6-8]。重篤な高マグネシウム血症は，産婦人科領域において，マグネシウム製剤の静脈内投与による子癇前症や子癇の治療中に起こりやすい。血中マグネシウム濃度が極めて高値になると，意識障害，徐脈，心室性不整脈，心停止が起こることがある[9,10]。低マグネシウム血症は，特に消化管疾患や栄養障害がある場合に発生することがあり，重篤になると，心房不整脈と心室不整脈双方の原因となることがある[11]。

推奨事項の裏付けとなる解説

1. 致死的な高カリウム血症の治療法としては，標準的な ACLS に加え，複数の方法が推奨されてきた[12]。それらには，カルシウム製剤や重炭酸の静脈内投与，GI 療法，アルブテロールの吸入などがある。非経口カルシウムは，心筋細胞膜を安定化する効果があることから，心停止の治療で効果が期待でき，静脈路と骨髄路から投与できる。通常，10% 塩化カルシウム製剤 5～10 mL，または 10% グルコン酸カルシウム製剤 15～30 mL を静脈路または骨髄路から 2～5 分かけて投与する[12]。ポリエチレンスルホン酸ナトリウム（ケイキサレート）の標準的な使用は，効能が不十分であること，腸管合併症のリスクがあることから，現在では推奨されていない。致死的な高カリウム血症に対しては，院内での緊急血液透析が引き続き確実な治療法である。

2. QT 延長を伴わない患者の VF/VT に対するマグネシウム製剤の静脈内投与の効果は明らかではない．一方，QT 延長を伴う患者の心停止では使用を考慮することが望ましい[13]。低マグネシウム血症は，QT 延長の発生要因または悪化要因となることがあり，複数の不整脈を伴い，心停止を誘発することもある[11]。これが血中マグネシウム濃度を正常値に戻す生理学的根拠である．一方で，標準的な ACLS が治療の基本であることに変わりはない．トルサード・ド・ポワントトに推奨される治療法については，「QRS 幅の広い頻拍」セクションで取り上げている。

3. 高カリウム血症に推奨される投与量のカルシウム製剤を静脈路や骨髄路から投与すると，重篤なマグネシウム中毒において血行動態を改善できることがある。そのため，直接的なエビデンスを欠くにもかかわらず，心停止での使用が支持されている[14]。

4. 重篤な低カリウム血症に起因する心室不整脈に対して，カリウム製剤を注意深く静脈内に投与することは有用と考えられるが，多くの症例報告ではボーラス投与ではなく分割投与である[15]。合併症を伴わないボーラス投与の報告は少なくとも 1 編あって，心臓手術の患者に高度な監視下で麻酔科医が投与しているが，心停止に対する効果が不明で，安全性への懸念も残る[16]。

このトピックは，直近で 2010 年に正式なエビデンスレビューを受けている[12]。

参考資料

1. Weiner ID, Wingo CS.Hyperkalemia: a potential silent killer.J Am Soc Nephrol.1998;9:1535-1543.
2. Weiner M, Epstein FH.Signs and symptoms of electrolyte disorders.Yale J Biol Med.1970;43:76-109.
3. Rastegar A, Soleimani M, Rastergar A. Hypokalaemia and hyperkalaemia. Postgrad Med J. 2001;77:759-764. doi: 10.1136/pmj.77.914.759
4. Mattu A, Brady WJ, Robinson DA.Electrocardiographic manifestations of hyperkalemia.Am J Emerg Med.2000;18:721-729. doi: 10.1053/ajem.2000.7344
5. Frohnert PP, Giuliani ER, Friedberg M, Johnson WJ, Tauxe WN.Statistical investigation of correlations between serum potassium levels and electrocardiographic findings in patients on intermittent hemodialysis therapy. Circulation.1970;41:667-676. doi: 10.1161/01.cir.41.4.667
6. Gennari FJ.Hypokalemia.N Engl J Med.1998;339:451-458. doi: 10.1056/NEJM199808133390707
7. Clausen TG, Brocks K, Ibsen H. Hypokalemia and ventricular arrhythmias in acute myocardial infarction.Acta Med Scand.1988;224:531-537. doi: 10.1111/j.0954-6820.1988.tb19623.x
8. Slovis C, Jenkins R. ABC of clinical electrocardiography: Conditions not primarily affecting the heart.BMJ.2002;324:1320-1323. doi: 10.1136/bmj.324.7349.1320

9. McDonnell NJ, Muchatuta NA, Paech MJ.Acute magnesium toxicity in an obstetric patient undergoing general anaesthesia for caesarean delivery.Int J Obstet Anesth.2010;19:226–231. doi: 10.1016/j.ijoa.2009.09.009
10. McDonnell NJ.Cardiopulmonary arrest in pregnancy: two case reports of successful outcomes in association with perimortem Caesarean delivery.Br J Anaesth.2009;103:406–409. doi: 10.1093/bja/aep176
11. Hansen BA, Bruserud Ø.Hypomagnesemia in critically ill patients.J Intensive Care.2018;6:21. doi: 10.1186/s40560-018-0291-y
12. Vanden Hoek TL, Morrison LJ, Shuster M, Donnino M, Sinz E, Lavonas EJ, Jeejeebhoy FM, Gabrielli A. Part 12: cardiac arrest in special situations: 2010 American Heart Association Guidelines for Cardiopulmonary Resuscitation and Emergency Cardiovascular Care.Circulation.2010;122(suppl 3):S829–S861. doi: 10.1161/CIRCULATIONAHA.110.971069
13. Panchal AR, Berg KM, Kudenchuk PJ, Del Rios M, Hirsch KG, Link MS, Kurz MC, Chan PS, Cabañas JG, Morley PT, Hazinski MF, Donnino MW.2018 American Heart Association Focused Update on Advanced Cardiovascular Life Support Use of Antiarrhythmic Drugs During and Immediately After Cardiac Arrest: An Update to the American Heart Association Guidelines for Cardiopulmonary Resuscitation and Emergency Cardiovascular Care. Circulation.2018;138:e740–e749. doi: 10.1161/CIR.0000000000000613
14. Van Hook JW.Endocrine crises.Hypermagnesemia.Crit Care Clin. 1991;7:215–223.
15. Curry P, Fitchett D, Stubbs W, Krikler D. Ventricular arrhythmias and hypokalaemia.Lancet.1976;2:231–233. doi: 10.1016/s0140-6736(76)91029-1
16. McCall BB, Mazzei WJ, Scheller MS, Thomas TC.Effects of central bolus injections of potassium chloride on arterial potassium concentration in patients undergoing cardiopulmonary bypass.J Cardiothorac Anesth.1990;4:571–576. doi: 10.1016/0888-6296(90)90406-6

オピオイドの過量摂取

「緒言」

進行中のオピオイドの蔓延によりオピオイド関連のOHCAが増加している．米国での1日の死者は約115人で，主に25歳から65歳の患者に悪影響を及ぼしている[1-3]．単一のオピオイド中毒では，最初に中枢神経系（CNS）の機能低下と呼吸抑制をきたし，次いで呼吸停止から心停止に至る．オピオイド関連死の大半は，複数薬物の摂取もしくは医学的，精神的な問題を合併している[4-7]．

この推奨事項の作成では，執筆陣はオピオイド関連の蘇生緊急事態と，他の原因による心肺停止との正確な鑑別が困難であることに配慮した．オピオイド関連の蘇生緊急事態は，原因としてオピオイドの毒性が疑われる心停止，呼吸停止，または重篤で致死的な不安定性（重度のCNS機能低下，呼吸抑制，低血圧，不整脈など）と定義される．このような状況下でのケアの中心が，緊急事態の早期認識と救急対応システムの発動であることに変わりはない（図13，14）．オピオイドの過量摂取により気道閉塞と呼吸停止による心肺停止が起こる．したがって，心停止直前の患者では気道確保と換気が最優先である．その後の，CPRとナロキソン投与を含むケアについては後述する．

オピオイド過量摂取の対応に関する教育への詳しい推奨事項は「第6章：蘇生教育科学」で取り上げている．

オピオイド過量摂取の急性期ケアについての推奨事項

COR	LOE	推奨事項
1	C-LD	1. 呼吸停止の患者では，自発呼吸再開まで補助呼吸またはバッグマスク換気を続ける．自発呼吸が再開しなければ，標準的なBLSまたはACLSを継続する．
1	C-EO	2. 心停止またはその疑いがある患者でのナロキソン投与は有効性が明らかではないため，標準的な蘇生処置がナロキソン投与よりも優先されるから，質の高いCPR（胸骨圧迫と換気）に重点を置く．
1	C-EO	3. 市民救助者や訓練された救助者は，ナロキソンや他の処置に患者が反応するのを待っている間，緊急対応システムの発動を遅らせてはならない．
2a	B-NR	4. オピオイドの過量摂取が疑われる患者では，確実な脈拍が触知されるが正常な呼吸がないか，死戦期呼吸のみ（呼吸停止）の場合，標準的なBLSまたはACLSに加えてナロキソンを投与することは妥当である．

「推奨事項の裏付けとなる解説」

1. 初期管理では，患者の気道と呼吸のサポートに重点を置く必要がある．気道を確保し補助呼吸を行う．その場合は，バッグマスクまたは感染防護具の使用が理想的である[8-10]．自発呼吸の回復が見られない場合は，ACLSを引き続き実施する必要がある．
2. 心停止ではナロキソン投与が転帰を改善することを示す研究がないので，初期治療ではCPRの実施に重点を置くべきである[3]．質の高いCPRの妨げにならなければ，標準的なACLSを実施しながらナロキソンを投与してよい．
3. オピオイドの過量摂取が疑われる患者では，救急対応システムの迅速な発動が重要である．現場での患者の状態が，オピオイド誘発の呼吸抑制のみに起因するか否かの判断は困難である．脈拍触知に確信を持てない場合の応急処置や[11,12]．ナロキソンはオピオイド以外の薬物過量や他の原因による心停止など，オピオイド過量摂取以外の病態では無効である．ナロキソン投与が奏功しても，CNS機能低下や呼吸抑制が再発することがあるため，安全に退院するまでの長期間にわたって観察を継続する必要がある[13-16]．
4. 呼吸停止でのナロキソンの使用を検討した試験が12件あり，そのうちの5件では，ナロキソンの筋注投与，静注投与，経鼻投与を比較している（2

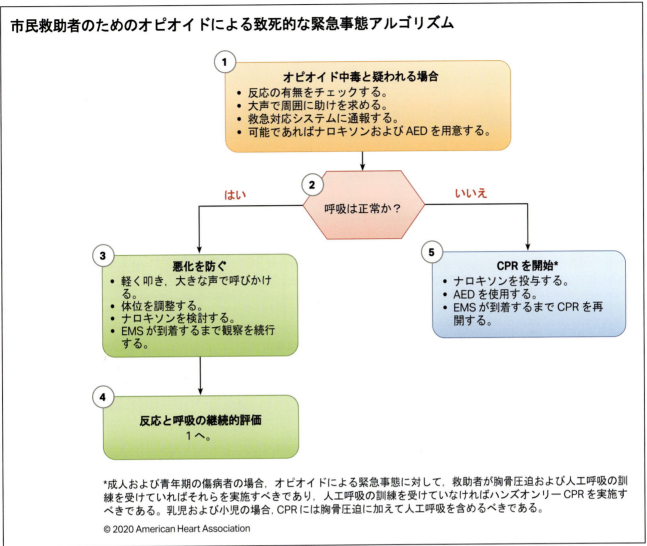

図 13. 市民救助者のためのオピオイドによる致死的な緊急事態アルゴリズム。
AED：自動体外式除細動器（automated external defibrillator），CPR：心肺蘇生（cardiopulmonary resuscitation），EMS：救急医療サービス（emergency medical services）。

件のRCT[17,18] 3件の非RCT[19-21]）。また，9件ではナロキソン使用の安全性を評価するか，またはその観察研究を実施している[22-30]。これらの試験では，ナロキソンが安全で，オピオイドによって誘発された呼吸抑制の治療に効果があること，合併症の発生はまれで，投与量に関連していることが報告されている。

オピオイド過量摂取の蘇生後ケアについての推奨事項		
COR	LOE	推奨事項
1	C-LD	1. 自発呼吸再開後も，オピオイド中毒の再発のリスクが小さくなり，意識レベルやバイタルサインが正常化するまでは医療施設で観察を続ける。
2a	C-LD	2. オピオイド中毒の再発には，ナロキソンの少量反復投与が有用なことがある。

推奨事項の裏付けとなる解説

1. ナロキソンの投与が奏功した患者では，CNSまたは呼吸抑制（あるいはその両方）が再発することがある。フェンタニル，モルヒネ，またはヘロインを過量摂取した患者の場合，短期間の観察で十分なこともあるが[28,30-34]，長時間作用型または徐放型オピオイドの致死的過量摂取の患者が安全に退院するまでには，長時間の観察が必要となることがある[13-15]。病院前搬送に携わるプロバイダーが致死的なオピオイド過量摂取の治療後の搬送を拒否する場面に遭遇したら，患者が治療拒否の判断力を有しているかどうかを決める地域のプロトコルと慣行に従うことが推奨される。
2. ナロキソンの作用時間がオピオイドの呼吸抑制作用時間よりも短い場合がある。特に長時間作用性の製剤に対しては，ナロキソンの反復投与または持続投与が必要になることがある[13-15]。

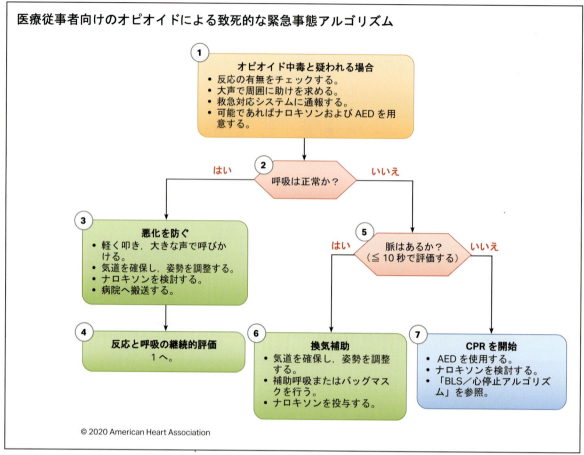

図14. 医療従事者のためのオピオイドによる致死的な緊急事態アルゴリズム。
AED：自動体外式除細動器（automated external defibrillator），BLS：一次救命処置（basic life support）。

これらの推奨事項は，オピオイドに伴う OHCA に関して 2020 年に AHA が作成した科学的ステートメントで支持されている[3]。

参考資料

1. Scholl L, Seth P, Kariisa M, Wilson N, Baldwin G. Drug and opioid-involved overdose deaths—United States, 2013-2017.MMWR Morb Mortal Wkly Rep.2018;67:1419-1427. doi: 10.15585/mmwr.mm675152e1
2. Jones CM, Einstein EB, Compton WM.Changes in synthetic opioid involvement in drug overdose deaths in the United States, 2010-2016. JAMA.2018;319:1819-1821. doi: 10.1001/jama.2018.2844
3. Dezfulian C, Orkin AM, Maron BA, Elmer J, Girota S, Gladwin MT, Merchant RM, Panchal AR, Perman SM, Starks M, et al; on behalf of the American Heart Association Council on Cardiopulmonary, Critical Care, Perioperative and Resuscitation; Council on Arteriosclerosis, Thrombosis and Vascular Biology; Council on Cardiovascular and Stroke Nursing; and Council on Clinical Cardiology.Opioid-associated out-of-hospital cardiac arrest: distinctive clinical features and implications for healthcare and public responses: a scientific statement from the American Heart Association. Circulation.In press.
4. Jones CM, Paulozzi LJ, Mack KA; Centers for Disease Control and Prevention (CDC).Alcohol involvement in opioid pain reliever and benzodiazepine drug abuse-related emergency department visits and drug-related deaths – United States, 2010.MMWR Morb Mortal Wkly Rep.2014;63:881-885.
5. Madadi P, Hildebrandt D, Lauwers AE, Koren G. Characteristics of opioid-users whose death was related to opioid-toxicity: a population-based study in Ontario, Canada.PLoS One.2013;8:e60600. doi: 10.1371/journal.pone.0060600
6. Paulozzi LJ, Logan JE, Hall AJ, McKinstry E, Kaplan JA, Crosby AE.A comparison of drug overdose deaths involving methadone and other opioid analgesics in West Virginia.Addiction.2009;104:1541-1548. doi: 10.1111/j.1360-0443.2009.02650.x
7. Webster LR, Cochella S, Dasgupta N, Fakata KL, Fine PG, Fishman SM, Grey T, Johnson EM, Lee LK, Passik SD, Peppin J, Porucznik CA, Ray A, Schnoll SH, Stieg RL, Wakeland W. An analysis of the root causes for opioid-related overdose deaths in the United States.Pain Med.2011;12 Suppl 2:S26-S35. doi: 10.1111/j.1526-4637.2011.01134.x
8. Kleinman ME, Brennan EE, Goldberger ZD, Swor RA, Terry M, Bobrow BJ, Gazmuri RJ, Travers AH, Rea T. Part 5: adult basic life support and cardiopulmonary resuscitation quality: 2015 American Heart Association Guidelines Update for Cardiopulmonary Resuscitation and Emergency Cardiovascular Care.Circulation.2015;132 (suppl 2):S414-S435. doi: 10.1161/CIR.0000000000000259
9. Guildner CW.Resuscitation—opening the airway: a comparative study of techniques for opening an airway obstructed by the tongue.JACEP.1976;5:588-590. doi: 10.1016/s0361-1124(76)80217-1
10. Wenzel V, Keller C, Idris AH, Dörges V, Lindner KH, Brimacombe JR.Effects of smaller tidal volumes during basic life support ventilation in patients with respiratory arrest: good ventilation, less risk? Resuscitation.1999;43:25-29. doi: 10.1016/s0300-9572 (99)00118-5
11. Bahr J, Klingler H, Panzer W, Rode H, Kettler D. Skills of lay people in checking the carotid pulse.Resuscitation.1997;35:23-26. doi: 10.1016/s0300-9572 (96)01092-1
12. Eberle B, Dick WF, Schneider T, Wisser G, Doetsch S, Tzanova I. Checking the carotid pulse check: diagnostic accuracy of first responders in patients with and without a pulse.Resuscitation.1996;33:107-116. doi: 10.1016/s0300-9572 (96)01016-7
13. Clarke SF, Dargan PI, Jones AL.Naloxone in opioid poisoning: walking the tightrope.Emerg Med J. 2005;22:612-616. doi: 10.1136/emj.2003.009613
14. Etherington J, Christenson J, Innes G, Grafstein E, Pennington S, Spinelli JJ, Gao M, Lahiffe B, Wanger K, Fernandes C. Is early discharge safe after naloxone reversal of presumed opioid overdose? CJEM.2000;2:156-162. doi: 10.1017/s1481803500004863

15. Zuckerman M, Weisberg SN, Boyer EW.Pitfalls of intranasal naloxone.Prehosp Emerg Care.2014;18:550–554. doi: 10.3109/10903127.2014.896961
16. Heaton JD, Bhandari B, Faryar KA, Huecker MR.Retrospective Review of Need for Delayed Naloxone or Oxygen in Emergency Department Patients Receiving Naloxone for Heroin Reversal.J Emerg Med.2019;56:642–651. doi: 10.1016/j.jemermed.2019.02.015
17. Kelly AM, Kerr D, Dietze P, Patrick I, Walker T, Koutsogiannis Z. Randomised trial of intranasal versus intramuscular naloxone in prehospital treatment for suspected opioid overdose.Med J Aust.2005;182:24–27.
18. Kerr D, Kelly AM, Dietze P, Jolley D, Barger B. Randomized controlled trial comparing the effectiveness and safety of intranasal and intramuscular naloxone for the treatment of suspected heroin overdose.Addiction.2009;104:2067–2074. doi: 10.1111/j.1360-0443.2009.02724.x
19. Wanger K, Brough L, Macmillan I, Goulding J, MacPhail I, Christenson JM.Intravenous vs subcutaneous naloxone for out-of-hospital management of presumed opioid overdose.Acad Emerg Med.1998;5:293–299. doi: 10.1111/j.1553-2712.1998.tb02707.x
20. Barton ED, Colwell CB, Wolfe T, Fosnocht D, Gravitz C, Bryan T, Dunn W, Benson J, Bailey J. Efficacy of intranasal naloxone as a needleless alternative for treatment of opioid overdose in the prehospital setting.J Emerg Med.2005;29:265–271. doi: 10.1016/j.jemermed.2005.03.007
21. Robertson TM, Hendey GW, Stroh G, Shalit M. Intranasal naloxone is a viable alternative to intravenous naloxone for prehospital narcotic overdose.Prehosp Emerg Care.2009;13:512–515. doi: 10.1080/10903120903144866
22. Cetrullo C, Di Nino GF, Melloni C, Pieri C, Zanoni A. [Naloxone antagonism toward opiate analgesic drugs.Clinical experimental study].Minerva Anestesiol.1983;49:199–204.
23. Osterwalder JJ.Naloxone-for intoxications with intravenous heroin and heroin mixtures-harmless or hazardous? A prospective clinical study.J Toxicol Clin Toxicol.1996;34:409–416. doi: 10.3109/15563659609013811
24. Sporer KA, Firestone J, Isaacs SM.Out-of-hospital treatment of opioid overdoses in an urban setting.Acad Emerg Med.1996;3:660–667. doi: 10.1111/j.1553-2712.1996.tb03487.x
25. Stokland O, Hansen TB, Nilsen JE. [Prehospital treatment of heroin intoxication in Oslo in 1996].Tidsskr Nor Laegeforen.1998;118:3144–3146.
26. Buajordet I, Naess AC, Jacobsen D, Brørs O. Adverse events after naloxone treatment of episodes of suspected acute opioid overdose.Eur J Emerg Med.2004;11:19–23. doi: 10.1097/00063110-200402000-00004
27. Cantwell K, Dietze P, Flander L. The relationship between naloxone dose and key patient variables in the treatment of non-fatal heroin overdose in the prehospital setting.Resuscitation.2005;65:315–319. doi: 10.1016/j.resuscitation.2004.12.012
28. Boyd JJ, Kuisma MJ, Alaspää AO, Vuori E, Repo JV, Randell TT.Recurrent opioid toxicity after pre-hospital care of presumed heroin overdose patients.Acta Anaesthesiol Scand.2006;50:1266–1270. doi: 10.1111/j.1399-6576.2006.01172.x
29. Nielsen K, Nielsen SL, Siersma V, Rasmussen LS.Treatment of opioid overdose in a physician-based prehospital EMS: frequency and long-term prognosis.Resuscitation.2011;82:1410–1413. doi: 10.1016/j.resuscitation.2011.05.027
30. Wampler DA, Molina DK, McManus J, Laws P, Manifold CA.No deaths associated with patient refusal of transport after naloxone-reversed opioid overdose.Prehosp Emerg Care.2011;15:320–324. doi: 10.3109/10903127.2011.569854
31. Vilke GM, Sloane C, Smith AM, Chan TC.Assessment for deaths in out-of-hospital heroin overdose patients treated with naloxone who refuse transport.Acad Emerg Med.2003;10:893–896. doi: 10.1111/j.1553-2712.2003.tb00636.x
32. Rudolph SS, Jehu G, Nielsen SL, Nielsen K, Siersma V, Rasmussen LS.Prehospital treatment of opioid overdose in Copenhagen-is it safe to discharge on-scene? Resuscitation.2011;82:1414–1418. doi: 10.1016/j.resuscitation.2011.06.027
33. Moss ST, Chan TC, Buchanan J, Dunford JV, Vilke GM.Outcome study of prehospital patients signed out against medical advice by field paramedics.Ann Emerg Med.1998;31:247–250. doi: 10.1016/s0196-0644(98)70315-4
34. Christenson J, Etherington J, Grafstein E, Innes G, Pennington S, Wanger K, Fernandes C, Spinelli JJ, Gao M. Early discharge of patients with presumed opioid overdose: development of a clinical prediction rule.Acad Emerg Med.2000;7:1110–1118. doi: 10.1111/j.1553-2712.2000.tb01260.x

妊娠中の心停止
「緒言」

米国では産入院の 12,000 件のうち約 1 件で母体に心停止が発生している[1]。このような心停止はまれではあるものの，増加傾向にある[2]。母体および胎児／新生児の生存率として報告された数字には大きな幅がある[3-8]。母体と胎児双方に最良の転機を実現するには，母体の無事な蘇生が最良の手段であることは変わりない。母体の心停止の原因として多く見られるものは，出血，心不全，羊水塞栓，敗血症，誤嚥性肺炎，静脈血栓塞栓症，子癇前症／子癇，麻酔合併症などである[1,4,6]。

最新の文献の多くは観察研究であり，いくつかの治療方針の判断は，主に妊娠の生理学および心停止がない妊娠状態からの推定に基づいている[9]。このような集団では，心停止で最も可能性のある原因を対象とした質の高い蘇生的介入と治療的介入がきわめて重要である。子宮の大きさが 20 週間以上になった時点での死戦期帝王切開（PMCD）は，蘇生によって短時間で ROSC に至らなかった母体の心停止で転機を改善できるものと考えられる。このような PMCD は蘇生的帝王切開とも呼ばれることがある（図 15）[10-14]。また，心停止から切開分娩までの時間が短いほど，母体と新生児の転帰が改善される[15]。ただし，医師とチームのトレーニングレベルや患者因子（心停止の原因，在胎期間など），およびシステムのリソースが異なるため，妊産婦の心停止に関連した PMCD の実施ならびにその実施時期の臨床的決定は複雑である。最後に，心停止した母体患者に ECMO を使用した症例と症例集積研究で，母体の生存率が良好であることが報告されている[16]。妊娠後期で発生した心停止の治療には大きな科学的ギャップが見られる。

妊娠中の心停止の計画・準備に関する 推奨事項		
COR	LOE	推奨事項
1	C-LD	1. 妊娠中の心停止に対するチームの計画は，産科，新生児科，救急科，麻酔科，集中治療科，心停止対応チームが協力して作成すべきである。
1	C-LD	2. 即時の ROSC を常に実現できるとは限らないため，妊娠後半期の女性において心停止が認識され次第，死戦期帝王切開用の地域の医療リソースを招集すべきである。
1	C-EO	3. 蘇生措置を継続しながら，死戦期帝王切開をただちに実施できる機能を備えた施設へのタイムリーな搬送を容易にするために，妊娠中の OHCA を管理するためのプロトコルを作成しておく必要がある。

「推奨事項の裏付けとなる解説」

1. 母体を確実に蘇生できるように，関与が予想されるすべての関係者は，PMCD が必要になる可能性も含め，妊娠中の心停止に備えた計画とトレーニングに参加する必要がある。同様にまれではあるが，時間が重要

な治療に基づき，計画，シミュレーションによるトレーニング，模擬救急を実施することは，施設の準備態勢を整えるうえで効果的である[17-21]。

2. 当初の母体蘇生が功を奏さないことも考えられるので，蘇生の早期段階でPMCDの準備に着手すべきである。PMCDへの移行時間が短いほど，母体と胎児の転帰が良好になるからである[8]。

3. 入院前の段階で母体が心停止に陥った場合は，PMCDと新生児蘇生が可能な施設への迅速な直接搬送によって，良好な転帰が得られる最大の可能性が開ける。このような受け入れ先施設では，成人蘇生，産科蘇生，新生児蘇生の各担当チームが早期段階で活動を開始する必要がある。

妊娠中の心停止からの蘇生に関する 推奨事項		
COR	LOE	推奨事項
1	C-LD	1. 心停止の妊産婦で優先する措置は，質の高いCPRの実施および子宮左方移動による大動静脈圧迫の解除である。
1	C-LD	2. 妊娠患者は低酸素症を発症しやすいので，妊娠中の心停止からの蘇生では，酸素投与と気道確保を優先する必要がある。
1	C-EO	3. 母体の蘇生の妨げとなる可能性があるため，妊娠中の心停止中に胎児のモニタリングを実施してはならない。
1	C-EO	4. 心停止からの蘇生後に昏睡状態である妊産婦に対し，目標体温管理が推奨される。
1	C-EO	5. 妊娠患者の目標体温管理中，潜在的な合併症としての徐脈が胎児に発生しないように持続的にモニターすることが推奨されるので，産科および新生児科に相談するべきである。

「推奨事項の裏付けとなる解説」

1. 妊娠子宮は下大静脈を圧迫し，静脈還流を妨げ，それにより1回拍出量および心拍出量を減少させうる。仰臥位では，単体妊娠の20週頃（子宮底長が臍の高さ以上になる時期）から大動静脈の圧迫が始まることがある[22]。用手的子宮左方移動を行うと，低血圧患者における大動静脈圧迫が効果的に緩和される（図16）[23,23a,23b]。

2. 妊娠中は，気道確保，換気，および酸素投与が特に重要になる。妊産婦の代謝上昇，および妊娠子宮に起因する機能的予備容量の低下のため，妊娠患者は低酸素症を発症しやすくなるからである。また，有害な影響として胎児の低酸素症があることもわかっている。どちら

の考慮事項も，早期段階で妊娠患者に高度な気道確保を実現するうえで効果的である。

3. 母体と胎児双方の生存率向上につながることから，必要に応じたPMCDの実施も含め，妊産婦の蘇生が最優先の措置である[9]。胎児をモニタリングすると，この目標を達成できず，母体の蘇生措置を阻害することもある。特に，除細動がある場合や，PMCDのために腹部を備える場合に重要である。

4. 妊娠中にTTMを使用した無作為試験は実施されていない。しかし，心停止後にTTMを使用して母体と胎児に良好な転帰が得られたことを示す症例報告はいくつか存在する[24,25]。

5. 母体を蘇生できても，出産前の胎児では，低体温症，アシドーシス，低酸素血症，低血圧症の影響を受けやすい状態が続いている。これらのどの疾患も，TTMを使用したROSC治療後に発症する可能性がある。また，胎児の状態悪化は，母体の代償不全を示す早期の警告兆候であることも考えられる。

心停止とPMCDに関する 関する推奨事項		
COR	LOE	推奨事項
1	C-LD	1. 子宮底が臍以上の高さにある心停止中の妊産婦に，通常の蘇生処置と用手的子宮左方移動を実施してもROSCにいたらなかった場合は，蘇生処置を継続しながら，子宮内容除去の準備に取りかかることが望ましい。
1	C-LD	2. 母体に生存不可能な外傷がある場合や，長時間脈拍がない場合など，母体の蘇生措置が明らかに無益である場合，死戦期帝王切開が適切な患者に対し，その実施を遅らせる理由はない。
2a	C-EO	3. 理想的には心停止から5分以内などの早期段階で出産を実現するには，当初のBLSとACLSの治療介入を継続しながら，死戦期帝王切開の準備にただちに着手することが妥当である。

「推奨事項の裏付けとなる解説」

1. 妊娠子宮の内容を除去することで，大動静脈の圧迫が緩和されるので，ROSCにいたる可能性が高くなることがある[10-14]。妊娠後期では，胎児の生育可能性にかかわらず，PMCDを母体蘇生の一手段と見なすことができる[26]。

2. 早期段階で出産することで，母体と新生児の生存率が高くなる[15]。母体の生存率が伴わない状況でも，胎児の早期段階出産により，新生児としての生存率が高くなる可能性がある[26]。

3. PMCDの最適な実施時期は，まだ十分には確立されておらず，救助者の一連の手技と利用できる資源と利用できるリソース，および患

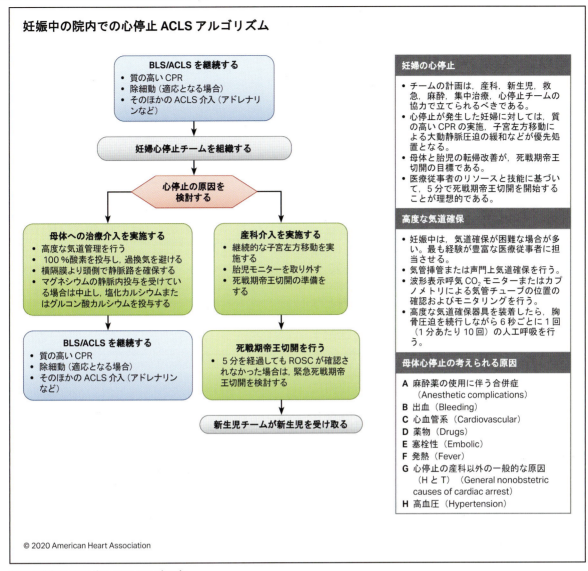

図15. 妊娠中の院内での心停止ACLSアルゴリズム。
ACLS：二次救命処置（advanced cardiovascular life support），BLS：一次救命処置（basic life support），CPR：心肺蘇生（cardiopulmonary resuscitation），ROSC：自己心拍再開（return of spontaneous circulation）。

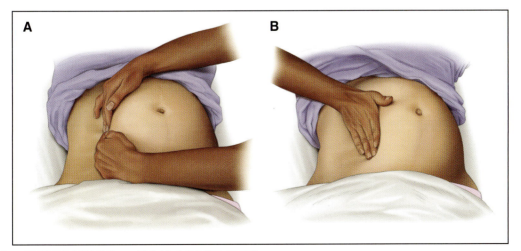

図16. A，両手での用手的子宮左側方移動。B，蘇生中における片手での手技。

者と心停止の特性に基づいて論理的に異なる。各種文献の系統的なレビューにより，妊娠中の心停止の症例報告すべてにおけるPMCDの実施時期が評価されているが，症例の多様性がきわめて幅広く，報告にも偏りがあることから，いまだに結論には至っていない[15]。母体の心停止発生から最大で39分の時点でも，母体が生存していたとの報告がある[4,10,27-29]。1980年から2010年の間に発表された文献のシステマティックレビューによると，母体の心停止から出産までの時間の中央値は，母体が生存していた場合は9分，母体が生存していなかった場合は20分となっている[15]。同じ研究によると，PMCDの実施までの時間の中央値は，母体が生存していた場合は10分，生存していなかった場合は20分である。報告された症例57件のうち4件（7%）でのみ，出産までの時間が4分以内となっている[15]。英国のコホート研究では[4]，虚脱からPMCDまでの時間の中央値は，母体が生存していた場合は3分であることに対し，生存していなかった場合は12分である。この研究によれば，母体の心停止から5分以内に実施されたPMCDでは，25件中24件で乳児が生存しているが，心停止から5分を超過して実施されたPMCDで乳児が生存しているのは10件中7件である。新生児の生存については，母体の心停止発生から最大で30分までに実施されたPMCDを対象とした報告がある[10]。心停止におけるPMCDの実施時期は，心停止から5分以内を重要な目標とすることが専門家による推奨事項となっているが，この目標が達成されることはまれである[9]。生存の具体的な閾値を4分とすることのエビデンスは存在していない[8]。

これらの各種推奨事項は，『Cardiac Arrest in Pregnancy: a Scientific Statement From the AHA』[9]および2020年のエビデンス更新で指示されている[30]。

参考資料

1. Mhyre JM, Tsen LC, Einav S, Kuklina EV, Leffert LR, Bateman BT.Cardiac arrest during hospitalization for delivery in the United States, 1998–2011.Anesthesiology.2014;120:810–818. doi: 10.1097/ALN.0000000000000159
2. Centers for Disease Control and Prevention.Pregnancy-related deaths: data from 14 U.S. maternal mortality review committees, 2008–2017.https://www.cdc.gov/reproductivehealth/maternal-mortality/erase-mm/mmr-data-brief.html.Accessed April 22, 2020.
3. Kobori S, Toshimitsu M, Nagaoka S, Yaegashi N, Murotsuki J. Utility and limitations of perimortem cesarean section: A nationwide survey in Japan.J Obstet Gynaecol Res.2019;45:325–330. doi: 10.1111/jog.13819
4. Beckett VA, Knight M, Sharpe P. The CAPS Study: incidence, management and outcomes of cardiac arrest in pregnancy in the UK: a prospective, descriptive study.BJOG.2017;124:1374–1381. doi: 10.1111/1471-0528.14521
5. Maurin O, Lemoine S, Jost D, Lanoë V, Renard A, Travers S, The Paris Fire Brigade Cardiac Arrest Work Group, Lapostolle F, Tourtier JP.Maternal out-of-hospital cardiac arrest: A retrospective observational study.Resuscitation.2019;135:205–211. doi: 10.1016/j.resuscitation.2018.11.001
6. Schaap TP, Overtoom E, van den Akker T, Zwart JJ, van Roosmalen J, Bloemenkamp KWM.Maternal cardiac arrest in the Netherlands: A nationwide surveillance study.Eur J Obstet Gynecol Reprod Biol.2019;237:145–150. doi: 10.1016/j.ejogrb.2019.04.028
7. Lipowicz AA, Cheskes S, Gray SH, Jeejeebhoy F, Lee J, Scales DC, Zhan C, Morrison LJ; Rescu Investigators.Incidence, outcomes and guideline compliance of out-of-hospital maternal cardiac arrest resuscitations: A population-based cohort study.Resuscitation.2018;132:127–132. doi: 10.1016/j.resuscitation.2018.09.003
8. Benson MD, Padovano A, Bourjeily G, Zhou Y. Maternal collapse: Challenging the four-minute rule.EBioMedicine.2016;6:253–257. doi: 10.1016/j.ebiom.2016.02.042
9. Jeejeebhoy FM, Zelop CM, Lipman S, Carvalho B, Joglar J, Mhyre JM, Katz VL, Lapinsky SE, Einav S, Warnes CA, Page RL, Griffin RE, Jain A, Dainty KN, Arafeh J, Windrim R, Koren G, Callaway CW; American Heart Association Emergency Cardiovascular Care Committee, Council on Cardiopulmonary, Critical Care, Perioperative and Resuscitation, Council on Cardiovascular Diseases in the Young, and Council on Clinical Cardiology.Cardiac Arrest in Pregnancy: A Scientific Statement From the American Heart Association.Circulation.2015;132:1747–1773. doi: 10.1161/CIR.0000000000000300
10. Dijkman A, Huisman CM, Smit M, Schutte JM, Zwart JJ, van Roosmalen JJ, Oepkes D. Cardiac arrest in pregnancy: increasing use of perimortem caesarean section due to emergency skills training? BJOG.2010;117:282–287. doi: 10.1111/j.1471-0528.2009.02461.x
11. Page-Rodriguez A, Gonzalez-Sanchez JA.Perimortem cesarean section of twin pregnancy: case report and review of the literature.Acad Emerg Med.1999;6:1072–1074. doi: 10.1111/j.1553-2712.1999.tb01199.x
12. Cardosi RJ, Porter KB.Cesarean delivery of twins during maternal cardiopulmonary arrest.Obstet Gynecol.1998;92 (4 Pt 2):695–697. doi: 10.1016/s0029-7844(98)00127-6
13. Rose CH, Faksh A, Traynor KD, Cabrera D, Arendt KW, Brost BC.Challenging the 4- to 5-minute rule: from perimortem cesarean to resuscitative hysterotomy. Am J Obstetr Gynecol.2015;213:653–656. doi: 10.1016/j.ajog.2015.07.019
14. Tambawala ZY, Cherawala M, Maqbool S, Hamza LK.Resuscitative hysterotomy for maternal collapse in a triplet pregnancy.BMJ Case Rep.2020;13:e235328. doi: 10.1136/bcr-2020-235328
15. Einav S, Kaufman N, Sela HY.Maternal cardiac arrest and perimortem caesarean delivery: evidence or expert-based? Resuscitation.2012;83:1191–1200. doi: 10.1016/j.resuscitation.2012.05.005
16. Biderman P, Carmi U, Setton E, Fainblut M, Bachar O, Einav S. Maternal Salvage With Extracorporeal Life Support: Lessons Learned in a Single Center. Anesth Analg.2017;125:1275–1280. doi: 10.1213/ANE.0000000000002262
17. Lipman SS, Daniels KI, Arafeh J, Halamek LP.The case for OBLS: a simulation-based obstetric life support program.Semin Perinatol.2011;35:74–79. doi: 10.1053/j.semperi.2011.01.006
18. Petrone P, Talving P, Browder T, Teixeira PG, Fisher O, Lozornio A, Chan LS.Abdominal injuries in pregnancy: a 155-month study at two level 1 trauma centers.Injury.2011;42:47–49. doi: 10.1016/j.injury.2010.06.026
19. Al-Foudri H, Kevelighan E, Catling S. CEMACH 2003-5 Saving Mothers' Lives: lessons for anaesthetists.Continuing Education in Anaesthesia Critical Care & Pain.2010;10:81–87. doi: 10.1093/bjaceaccp/mkq009
20. The Joint Commission.TJC Sentinel Event Alert 44: preventing maternal death. https://www.jointcommission.org/resources/patient-safety-topics/sentinel-event/sentinel-event-alert-newsletters/sentinel-event-alert-issue-44-preventing-maternal-death/.Accessed May 11, 2020.
21. The Joint Commission.Sentinel Event Alert: Preventing infant death and injury during delivery.2004. https://www.jointcommission.org/resources/patient-safety-topics/sentinel-event/sentinel-event-alert-newsletters/sentinel-event-alert-issue-30-preventing-infant-death-and-injury-during-delivery/.Accessed February 28, 2020.
22. Goodwin AP, Pearce AJ.The human wedge.A manoeuvre to relieve aortocaval compression during resuscitation in late pregnancy.Anaesthesia.1992;47:433–434. doi: 10.1111/j.1365-2044.1992.tb02228.x
23. Cyna AM, Andrew M, Emmett RS, Middleton P, Simmons SW.Techniques for preventing hypotension during spinal anaesthesia for caesarean section. Cochrane Database Syst Rev. 2006:CD002251. doi: 10.1002/14651858.CD002251.pub2
23a. Rees SG, Thurlow JA, Gardner IC, Scrutton MJ, Kinsella SM.Maternal cardiovascular consequences of positioning after spinal anaesthesia for Caesarean section: left 15 degree table tilt vs. left lateral.Anaesthesia.2002;57:15–20. doi: 10.1046/j.1365-2044.2002.02325.x
23b. Mendonca C, Griffiths J, Ateleanu B, Collis RE.Hypotension following combined spinal-epidural anaesthesia for Caesarean section.Left lateral position vs. tilted supine position.Anaesthesia.2003;58:428–431. doi: 10.1046/j.1365-2044.2003.03090.x
24. Rittenberger JC, Kelly E, Jang D, Greer K, Heffner A. Successful outcome utilizing hypothermia after cardiac arrest in pregnancy: a case report.Crit Care Med.2008;36:1354–1356. doi: 10.1097/CCM.0b013e318169ee99
25. Chauhan A, Musunuru H, Donnino M, McCurdy MT, Chauhan V, Walsh M. The use of therapeutic hypothermia after cardiac arrest in a pregnant patient.Ann Emerg Med.2012;60:786–789. doi: 10.1016/j.annemergmed.2012.06.004
26. Svinos H. Towards evidence based emergency medicine: best BETs from the Manchester Royal Infirmary.BET 1.Emergency caesarean section in cardiac

27. Kam CW.Perimortem caesarean sections (PMCS).J Accid Emerg Med.1994;11:57-58. doi: 10.1136/emj.11.1.57-b
28. Kupas DF, Harter SC, Vosk A. Out-of-hospital perimortem cesarean section.Prehosp Emerg Care.1998;2:206-208. doi: 10.1080/10903129808958874
29. Oates S, Williams GL, Rees GA.Cardiopulmonary resuscitation in late pregnancy.BMJ.1988;297:404-405. doi: 10.1136/bmj.297.6645.404
30. Berg KM, Soar J, Andersen LW, Böttiger BW, Cacciola S, Callaway CW, Couper K, Cronberg T, D'Arrigo S, Deakin CD, et al; on behalf of the Adult Advanced Life Support Collaborators.Adult advanced life support: 2020 International Consensus on Cardiopulmonary Resuscitation and Emergency Cardiovascular Care Science With Treatment Recommendations.Circulation.2020;142 (suppl 1):S92-S139. doi: 10.1161/CIR.0000000000000893

肺塞栓症

肺塞栓症に関する 推奨事項		
COR	LOE	推奨事項
2a	C-LD	1. 心停止の悪化要因として肺塞栓症（PE）が確定診断された患者の救急処置として，血栓溶解療法，外科的塞栓摘出，および機械的塞栓摘出が妥当な治療選択肢である。
2b	C-LD	2. 心停止が肺塞栓症に起因することが疑われる場合は，血栓溶解療法による治療が考えられる。

「概要」

このトピックは，ILCORによる2020年のシステマティックレビューで確認されている[1]。PEはショックおよび心停止の可逆的原因となりうる。肺動脈閉塞および血管作用物質の放出による右室圧の急激な上昇は，心原性ショックをもたらし，速やかに心血管虚脱に進行することがある。急性PEの管理方法は疾患の重症度によって決まる[2]。心停止または重度の不安定な血行動態を特徴とする劇症型PEは，ここでの推奨事項で重点的に取り上げられている広範型PEの一部と定義されている。PEが関連する心停止の心リズムのうち36～53％が無脈静電気活動であり，ショック適応が見られることは少ない[3-5]。

広範型PEおよび亜広範型PEの患者には，数週間にわたって血栓の増大を予防し，内因性の血栓溶解を促すために，迅速な全身への抗凝固療法が適用されるのが一般的である。劇症型PEの患者には，抗凝固療法のみでは治療として不十分である。劇症型PEをはじめとする広範型PEの主な治療方法として，肺動脈閉塞を迅速に取り除き，十分な肺循環と体循環を回復する薬物療法と機械療法が取り入れられるようになってきた[2,6]。現時点における高度な治療方法として，血栓溶解薬全身投与，外科的血栓摘出または経皮的機械的血栓摘出，ECPRなどがある。

「推奨事項の裏付けとなる解説」

1. ILCORによる2020年のシステマティックレビューでは，確定診断されたPEによる心停止の治療を扱った無作為試験の存在は確認されていない。PEが疑われる症例に適用した血栓溶解療法の観察研究には著しいバイアスが見られ，転帰の改善に関しては，複数の要因による結果が混在していることがみて取れる[3,7-10]。外科的血栓摘出術を施行されCPRを受けている患者の合計21人を対象とした2件の症例集積研究では，30日後の生存率がそれぞれ12.5％と71.4％であったことが報告されている[11,12]。経皮手段による機械的血栓摘出を受けた患者7人のうち，6人（86％）がROSCに達したことを報告しているPE関連心停止の症例集積研究がある[13]。副作用の可能性に関しては，血栓溶解治療とCPRを受けた患者で大出血が発生するリスクは比較的低いことが，1件の臨床試験と数件の観察研究で示されている[7-9]。心停止の死亡リスクは，血栓溶解による出血のリスクと外科的介入と機械的介入のリスクを上回るが，これらの治療の利点については不明確である。一方の手法に対する他方の手法の利点が明確でないことから，血栓溶解または外科的／機械的な血栓摘出のどちらを選択するかは，その時期と治療における専門性に左右される。

2. PEが疑われるもののそれが確定診断されていない心停止では，誤診によって患者を無益な出血のリスクにさらす可能性があることから，その対応方法が不明確である。しかし，血栓溶解を受けた心停止患者であっても，大出血のリスクが顕著に高いわけではないことを示唆するエビデンスが最近は見られる[8]。心停止中はPEの診断が困難であるが，患者がROSCに達しない場合はPEの疑いが強いので，このようなエビデンスは血栓摘出を検討する根拠となる[1]。

これらの推奨事項は，ILCORによる2020年のシステマティックレビューで支持されている[1]。

参考資料

1. Berg KM, Soar J, Andersen LW, Böttiger BW, Cacciola S, Callaway CW, Couper K, Cronberg T, D'Arrigo S, Deakin CD, et al; on behalf of the Adult Advanced Life Support Collaborators.Adult advanced life support: 2020 International Consensus on Cardiopulmonary Resuscitation and Emergency Cardiovascular Care Science With Treatment Recommendations.Circulation.2020;142 (suppl 1):S92-S139. doi: 10.1161/CIR.0000000000000893
2. Jaff MR, McMurtry MS, Archer SL, Cushman M, Goldenberg N, Goldhaber SZ, Jenkins JS, Kline JA, Michaels AD, Thistlethwaite P, Vedantham S, White RJ, Zierler BK; American Heart Association Council on Cardiopulmonary, Critical Care, Perioperative and Resuscitation; American Heart Association Council on Peripheral Vascular Disease; American Heart Association Council on Arteriosclerosis, Thrombosis and Vascular Biology.Management of massive and submassive pulmonary embolism, iliofemoral deep vein thrombosis, and chronic thromboembolic pulmonary hypertension: a scientific statement from the American Heart Association. Circulation.2011;123:1788-1830. doi: 10.1161/CIR.0b013e318214914f

3. Kürkciyan I, Meron G, Sterz F, Janata K, Domanovits H, Holzer M, Berzlanovich A, Bankl HC, Laggner AN.Pulmonary embolism as a cause of cardiac arrest: presentation and outcome.Arch Intern Med.2000;160:1529–1535. doi: 10.1001/archinte.160.10.1529
4. Courtney DM, Kline JA.Prospective use of a clinical decision rule to identify pulmonary embolism as likely cause of outpatient cardiac arrest.Resuscitation.2005;65:57–64. doi: 10.1016/j.resuscitation.2004.07.018
5. Comess KA, DeRook FA, Russell ML, Tognazzi-Evans TA, Beach KW.The incidence of pulmonary embolism in unexplained sudden cardiac arrest with pulseless electrical activity.Am J Med.2000;109:351–356. doi: 10.1016/s0002-9343(00)00511-8
6. Wood KE.Major pulmonary embolism: review of a pathophysiologic approach to the golden hour of hemodynamically significant pulmonary embolism.Chest.2002;121:877–905. doi: 10.1378/chest.121.3.877
7. Böttiger BW, Arntz HR, Chamberlain DA, Bluhmki E, Belmans A, Danays T, Carli PA, Adgey JA, Bode C, Wenzel V; TROICA Trial Investigators; European Resuscitation Council Study Group.Thrombolysis during resuscitation for out-of-hospital cardiac arrest.N Engl J Med.2008;359:2651–2662. doi: 10.1056/NEJMoa070570
8. Javaudin F, Lascarrou JB, Le Bastard Q, Bourry Q, Latour C, De Carvalho H, Le Conte P, Escutnaire J, Hubert H, Montassier E, Leclère B; Research Group of the French National Out-of-Hospital Cardiac Arrest Registry (GR-RéAC).Thrombolysis During Resuscitation for Out-of-Hospital Cardiac Arrest Caused by Pulmonary Embolism Increases 30-Day Survival: Findings From the French National Cardiac Arrest Registry.Chest.2019;156:1167–1175. doi: 10.1016/j.chest.2019.07.015
9. Yousuf T, Brinton T, Ahmed K, Iskander J, Woznicka D, Kramer J, Kopiec A, Chadaga AR, Ortiz K. Tissue Plasminogen Activator Use in Cardiac Arrest Secondary to Fulminant Pulmonary Embolism.J Clin Med Res.2016;8:190–195. doi: 10.14740/jocmr2452w
10. Janata K, Holzer M, Kürkciyan I, Losert H, Riedmüller E, Pikula B, Laggner AN, Laczika K. Major bleeding complications in cardiopulmonary resuscitation: the place of thrombolytic therapy in cardiac arrest due to massive pulmonary embolism.Resuscitation.2003;57:49–55. doi: 10.1016/s0300-9572(02)00430-6
11. Doerge HC, Schoendube FA, Loeser H, Walter M, Messmer BJ.Pulmonary embolectomy: review of a 15-year experience and role in the age of thrombolytic therapy.Eur J Cardiothorac Surg.1996;10:952–957. doi: 10.1016/s1010-7940(96)80396-4
12. Konstantinov IE, Saxena P, Koniuszko MD, Alvarez J, Newman MA.Acute massive pulmonary embolism with cardiopulmonary resuscitation: management and results.Tex Heart Inst J. 2007;34:41–5; discussion 45.
13. Fava M, Loyola S, Bertoni H, Dougnac A. Massive pulmonary embolism: percutaneous mechanical thrombectomy during cardiopulmonary resuscitation.J Vasc Interv Radiol.2005;16:119–123. doi: 10.1097/01.RVI.0000146173.85401.BA

中毒：ベンゾジアゼピン系薬物

COR	LOE	推奨事項
3：有害	B-R	1. 鑑別不能な昏睡患者へのフルマゼニルの投与は危険性を伴い，推奨されない。

「概要」

ベンゾジアゼピン系薬物の過量投与は CNS 抑制と呼吸抑制の原因となり，特にオピオイドなどの他の鎮静薬とともに投与した場合は呼吸停止と心停止を引き起こすことがある。ベンゾジアゼピン特異的拮抗薬であるフルマゼニルには，意識，気道保護反射，呼吸応答を回復する効果があるが，けいれん発作や不整脈などの顕著な副作用を伴うことがある[1]。ベンゾジアゼピン依存症の患者および環状抗うつ薬を含む複数薬物投与を受けている患者で，このようなリスクが高くなる。フルマゼニルの半減期は多くのベンゾジアゼピン系薬物よりも短いので，フルマゼニルの投与後は慎重なモニタリングを必要とする[2]。フルマゼニル投与の代替となる治療は，バッグマスク換気およびそれに続く ETI と人工呼吸による呼吸補助を，ベンゾジアゼピン系薬物が代謝されるまで継続することである。

「推奨事項の裏付けとなる解説」

1. 13 件の RCT（評価可能な 990 人の患者を対象）を基にした最新のメタアナリシスでは，無作為でフルマゼニルに割り付けた患者には，プラセボに割り付けた患者よりも有害事象と重篤な有害事象が多いことが見出されている（害必要数：すべての有害事象では 5.5 人，重篤な有害事象では 50 人）[1]。最も多く見られる有害事象として，精神面の事象（不安，興奮，攻撃行動）があり，重篤な有害事象として，頻拍，上室不整脈，心室性期外収縮，けいれん発作，低血圧などが報告されている。これらの臨床試験で死亡した患者はいないが，まれであるがフルマゼニルの投与に伴う死亡の症例の報告がある[3,4]。過量投与の診断が未確定の患者にフルマゼニルを投与すると，不必要なリスクに患者をさらすことになるので，対症療法に重点を置くことが最良の手段となる。

このトピックは，直近で 2010 年に正式なエビデンスレビューを受けている[5]。

参考資料

1. Penninga EI, Graudal N, Ladekarl MB, Jürgens G. Adverse Events Associated with Flumazenil Treatment for the Management of Suspected Benzodiazepine Intoxication-A Systematic Review with Meta-Analyses of Randomised Trials.Basic Clin Pharmacol Toxicol.2016;118:37–44. doi: 10.1111/bcpt.12434
2. Bowden CA, Krenzelok EP.Clinical applications of commonly used contemporary antidotes.A US perspective.Drug Saf.1997;16:9–47. doi: 10.2165/00002018-199716010-00002
3. Katz Y, Boulos M, Singer P, Rosenberg B. Cardiac arrest associated with flumazenil.BMJ.1992;304:1415. doi: 10.1136/bmj.304.6839.1415-b
4. Burr W, Sandham P, Judd A. Death after flumazepil.BMJ.1989;298:1713. doi: 10.1136/bmj.298.6689.1713-a
5. Vanden Hoek TL, Morrison LJ, Shuster M, Donnino M, Sinz E, Lavonas EJ, Jeejeebhoy FM, Gabrielli A. Part 12: cardiac arrest in special situations: 2010 American Heart Association Guidelines for Cardiopulmonary Resuscitation and Emergency Cardiovascular Care.Circulation.2010;122 (suppl 3):S829–S861. doi: 10.1161/CIRCULATIONAHA.110.971069

中毒：βアドレナリン遮断薬およびカルシウム拮抗薬

「緒言」

βアドレナリン受容体遮断薬（「βアドレナリン遮断薬」）および L 型カルシウムチャネル拮抗薬（「カルシウム拮抗薬」）の投与は，血圧管理と心拍数管理で一般的な薬物療法である。βアドレナリン受容体には，L 型カルシウムチャネルの活動を制御する効果があるので[1]，これらの薬物の過量投与は互いに似たような結果をもたらし，血管収縮薬の注入などの標準的な治療では対処できない致死的な低血圧や徐脈の原因となる[2,3]。治療困難で不安定な血行動態

の患者に適用する療法として，高用量インスリン，静注カルシウム，またはグルカゴンの投与がある。また，最適な療法を判断するうえで，中毒学者や地域の中毒センターによる助言が効果的なこともある。βアドレナリン遮断薬またはカルシウム拮抗薬の過量投与に起因する心停止から患者が蘇生した後は，標準的な蘇生ガイドラインに従う。

βアドレナリン遮断薬の過量投与に関する推奨事項

COR	LOE	推奨事項
2a	C-LD	1. βアドレナリン遮断薬の過量投与を受けた患者に難治性ショックが発生している場合は，高用量インスリンとグルコースの投与が妥当な治療である。
2a	C-LD	2. βアドレナリン遮断薬の過量投与を受けた患者に難治性ショックが発生している場合は，静注グルカゴンの投与が妥当な治療である。
2b	C-LD	3. βアドレナリン遮断薬の過量投与を受けた患者に難治性ショックが発生している場合は，検討すべき治療としてカルシウムの投与が考慮される。
2b	C-LD	4. βアドレナリン遮断薬の過量投与を受けた患者に，薬物療法では治療が困難なショックが発生している場合は，検討すべき治療としてECMOの使用がある。

「推奨事項の裏付けとなる解説」

1. βアドレナリン遮断薬中毒に対して高用量インスリンを投与した結果，心拍数の上昇と血行動態の改善が見られたことを報告している動物実験，症例報告，症例集積研究がある[4-6]。これらの研究で使用されたインスリンの一般的な用量は，ボーラスによる1 U/kgに続き，U/kg/時の注入を臨床効果が得られるように調節する。また，ブドウ糖とカリウムを同時に注入投与している[2,7]。このトピックに関する対照試験の存在は確認されていない。
2. 対照試験は実施されていないが，グルカゴンの投与後，徐脈と低血圧に改善が見られたことがいくつかの症例報告と小規模な症例集積研究で報告されている[8-10]。
3. 限定的な動物実験とまれな症例の報告で，βアドレナリン遮断薬中毒における心拍数と低血圧の改善において，カルシウムに有用である可能性が示唆されている[11-13]。
4. βアドレナリン遮断薬の過量投与で難治性ショックを示していた患者がECMO処置後に生存した症例が，症例報告と少なくとも1件の後ろ向き観察研究とで発表されている[14,15]。あらゆる心停止に対するECMOのエビデンスはきわめて限られているが，薬物中毒などの治癒可能な原因による難治性ショックは，ECMOによる効果が見込める状況と考えられるだろう。

徐脈と心伝導遅延を示す患者の評価と管理に関して，米国心臓学会議（American College of Cardiology, ACC），AHA，およびHeart Rhythm Society（HRS）が2018年に発表したガイドラインで，これらの推奨事項が支持されている[16]。

カルシウム拮抗薬の過量投与に関する推奨事項

COR	LOE	推奨事項
2a	C-LD	1. カルシウム拮抗薬の過量投与を受けた患者に難治性ショックが発生している場合は，カルシウムの投与が妥当な治療である。
2a	C-LD	2. カルシウム拮抗薬の過量投与を受けた患者に難治性ショックが発生している場合は，高用量インスリンとグルコースの投与が妥当な治療である。
2b	C-LD	3. カルシウム拮抗薬の過量投与を受けた患者に難治性ショックが発生している場合は，検討すべき治療として静注グルカゴンの投与が考慮される。
2b	C-LD	4. カルシウム拮抗薬の過量投与を受けた患者に，薬物療法では治療が困難なショックが発生している場合は，検討すべき治療としてECMOの使用がある。

「推奨事項の裏付けとなる解説」

1. カルシウム拮抗薬中毒に対する静注カルシウムの効果を確認した対照試験は存在しない[16]。発生率の低い副作用とともに，さまざまな効能が症例集積研究と症例報告とで報告されている。動物実験では一貫性のある利点が得られているが，人体では結果に一貫性がないことを指摘しているシステマティックレビューがある[17-21]。この治療に関するエビデンスの確実性は非常に低いと認識されているが，専門家による2017年のコンセンサスステートメントでは，カテコラミンに起因する難治性ショックの第一選択薬としてカルシウムが推奨されている[22]。
2. 2件のシステマティックレビューでは，カルシウム拮抗薬中毒に高用量インスリンを投与した後，心拍数の上昇と血行動態の改善が見られたことを報告している動物実験，症例報告，人体の観察研究があることを確認している[4,16,21,23,24]。βアドレナリン遮断薬の過量投与の場合と同様に，これらの研究で使用されたインスリンの一般的な用量は，ボーラスによる1 U/kgに続き，システマティックレビュー 1 U/kg/時の注入を臨床効果が得られるように調節する。また，ブドウ糖とカリウムを同時に注入投与している[2,4,7,21]。
3. カルシウム拮抗薬中毒でグルカゴンが示す効果については，動物実験および人体での症例報告／症例集積研究で，心拍数が上昇した報告もあれば，効果が認められなかった報告もあり，所見に一貫性が見いだせない状況が続いている[21]。
4. 薬物中毒から心停止または難治性ショックに陥った患者にECMOを使用し，転帰が改善したことを報告している後ろ向き研究が少なくとも1件ある[14]。すべての後ろ向き研究同様に，どの患者をECMOで治療するかを判断する際に考慮するべき事項が他にもあることから，この研究でもバイアスのリスクは高くなっている。薬物中毒などの治癒可能な原因による難治性ショックに対しては，最近のコンセンサスステートメントでECMOの使用が支持されている[22]。

米国心臓学会議（American College of Cardiology, ACC），AHA，および Heart Rhythm Society（HRS）が 2018 年に発表したガイドラインで，徐脈と心伝導遅延を示す患者の評価と管理に関してこれらの推奨事項が支持されている[16]。

参考資料

1. van der Heyden MA, Wijnhoven TJ, Opthof T. Molecular aspects of adrenergic modulation of cardiac L-type Ca2+ channels.Cardiovasc Res.2005;65:28-39. doi: 10.1016/j.cardiores.2004.09.028
2. Graudins A, Lee HM, Druda D. Calcium channel antagonist and beta-blocker overdose: antidotes and adjunct therapies.Br J Clin Pharmacol.2016;81:453-461. doi: 10.1111/bcp.12763
3. Levine M, Curry SC, Padilla-Jones A, Ruha AM.Critical care management of verapamil and diltiazem overdose with a focus on vasopressors: a 25-year experience at a single center.Ann Emerg Med.2013;62:252-258. doi: 10.1016/j.annemergmed.2013.03.018
4. Engebretsen KM, Kaczmarek KM, Morgan J, Holger JS.High-dose insulin therapy in beta-blocker and calcium channel-blocker poisoning.Clin Toxicol (Phila).2011;49:277-283. doi: 10.3109/15563650.2011.582471
5. Seegobin K, Maharaj S, Deosaran A, Reddy P. Severe beta blocker and calcium channel blocker overdose: Role of high dose insulin.Am J Emerg Med.2018;36:736.e5-736.e6. doi: 10.1016/j.ajem.2018.01.038
6. Doepker B, Healy W, Cortez E, Adkins EJ.High-dose insulin and intravenous lipid emulsion therapy for cardiogenic shock induced by intentional calcium-channel blocker and Beta-blocker overdose: a case series.J Emerg Med.2014;46:486-490. doi: 10.1016/j.jemermed.2013.08.135
7. Holger JS, Stellpflug SJ, Cole JB, Harris CR, Engebretsen KM.High-dose insulin: a consecutive case series in toxin-induced cardiogenic shock.Clin Toxicol (Phila).2011;49:653-658. doi: 10.3109/15563650.2011.593522
8. Love JN, Sachdeva DK, Bessman ES, Curtis LA, Howell JM.A potential role for glucagon in the treatment of drug-induced symptomatic bradycardia. Chest.1998;114:323-326. doi: 10.1378/chest.114.1.323
9. Bailey B. Glucagon in beta-blocker and calcium channel blocker overdoses: a systematic review.J Toxicol Clin Toxicol.2003;41:595-602. doi: 10.1081/clt-120023761
10. Peterson CD, Leeder JS, Sterner S. Glucagon therapy for beta-blocker overdose.Drug Intell Clin Pharm.1984;18:394-398. doi: 10.1177/106002808401800507
11. Pertoldi F, D'Orlando L, Mercante WP.Electromechanical dissociation 48 hours after atenolol overdose: usefulness of calcium chloride.Ann Emerg Med.1998;31:777-781. doi: 10.1016/s0196-0644(98)70241-0
12. Love JN, Hanfling D, Howell JM.Hemodynamic effects of calcium chloride in a canine model of acute propranolol intoxication.Ann Emerg Med.1996;28:1-6. doi: 10.1016/s0196-0644(96)70129-4
13. Teo LK, Tham DJW, Chong CP.A case of massive atenolol overdose successfully managed with intravenous calcium chloride.East J Med.2018;21:213-215.
14. Masson R, Colas V, Parienti JJ, Lehoux P, Massetti M, Charbonneau P, Saulnier F, Daubin C. A comparison of survival with and without extracorporeal life support treatment for severe poisoning due to drug intoxication.Resuscitation.2012;83:1413-1417. doi: 10.1016/j.resuscitation.2012.03.028
15. Rotella JA, Greene SL, Koutsogiannis Z, Graudins A, Hung Leang Y, Kuan K, Baxter H, Bourke E, Wong A. Treatment for beta-blocker poisoning: a systematic review.Clin Toxicol (Phila).2020:1-41. doi: 10.1080/15563650.2020.1752918
16. Kusumoto FM, Schoenfeld MH, Barrett C, Edgerton JR, Ellenbogen KA, Gold MR, Goldschlager NF, Hamilton RM, Joglar JA, Kim RJ, Lee R, Marine JE, McLeod CJ, Oken KR, Patton KK, Pellegrini CN, Selzman KA, Thompson A, Varosy PD.2018 ACC/AHA/HRS Guideline on the Evaluation and Management of Patients With Bradycardia and Cardiac Conduction Delay: A Report of the American College of Cardiology/American Heart Association Task Force on Practice Guidelines Circulation.2019;140:e382-e482. doi: 10.1161/CIR.0000000000000628
17. Howarth DM, Dawson AH, Smith AJ, Buckley N, Whyte IM.Calcium channel blocking drug overdose: an Australian series.Hum Exp Toxicol.1994;13:161-166. doi: 10.1177/096032719401300304
18. Crump BJ, Holt DW, Vale JA.Lack of response to intravenous calcium in severe verapamil poisoning.Lancet.1982;2:939-940. doi: 10.1016/s0140-6736(82)90912-6
19. Ghosh S, Sircar M. Calcium channel blocker overdose: experience with amlodipine.Indian J Crit Care Med.2008;12:190-193. doi: 10.4103/0972-5229.45080
20. Henry M, Kay MM, Viccellio P. Cardiogenic shock associated with calcium-channel and beta blockers: reversal with intravenous calcium chloride.Am J Emerg Med.1985;3:334-336. doi: 10.1016/0735-6757(85)90060-9
21. St-Onge M, Dubé PA, Gosselin S, Guimont C, Godwin J, Archambault PM, Chauny JM, Frenette AJ, Darveau M, Le Sage N, Poitras J, Provencher J, Juurlink DN, Blais R. Treatment for calcium channel blocker poisoning: a systematic review.Clin Toxicol (Phila).2014;52:926-944. doi: 10.3109/15563650.2014.965827
22. St-Onge M, Anseeuw K, Cantrell FL, Gilchrist IC, Hantson P, Bailey B, Lavergne V, Gosselin S, Kerns W II, Laliberté M, Lavonas EJ, Juurlink DN, Muscedere J, Yang CC, Sinuff T, Rieder M, Mégarbane B. Experts Consensus Recommendations for the Management of Calcium Channel Blocker Poisoning in Adults.Crit Care Med.2017;45:e306-e315. doi: 10.1097/CCM.0000000000002087
23. Greene SL, Gawarammana I, Wood DM, Jones AL, Dargan PI.Relative safety of hyperinsulinaemia/euglycaemia therapy in the management of calcium channel blocker overdose: a prospective observational study.Intensive Care Med.2007;33:2019-2024. doi: 10.1007/s00134-007-0768-y
24. Espinoza TR, Bryant SM, Aks SE.Hyperinsulin therapy for calcium channel antagonist poisoning: a seven-year retrospective study.Am J Ther.2013;20:29-31. doi: 10.1097/MJT.0b013e31824d5fbd

中毒：コカイン

COR	LOE	推奨事項
2a	B-NR	1. コカイン誘発性の高血圧，頻拍，興奮，または胸部不快感を呈する患者の場合，ベンゾジアゼピン，α遮断薬，カルシウム拮抗薬，ニトログリセリン，および／またはモルヒネが有益な場合がある。
2b	C-LD	2. 相反するエビデンスが存在するものの，コカイン中毒の影響下においてはβアドレナリン遮断薬の単独使用を避けることが妥当と考えられる。

「概要」

コカイン中毒は心血管系の有害事象（不整脈，高血圧，頻拍，冠動脈攣縮，心伝導遅延など）を引き起こすことがある。これらの事象は，急性冠症候群および脳卒中を誘発することもある。臨床試験データにより，ベンゾジアゼピン系薬物（ジアゼパム，ロラゼパム），α遮断薬（フェントラミン），カルシウム拮抗薬（ベラパミル），モルヒネ，およびニトログリセリンはすべて，コカイン中毒患者に対して安全であり，有益な可能性があると示唆されている。これらのアプローチを比較するデータは得られていない[1-5]。βアドレナリン遮断薬の使用に関しては，相反するデータが存在している[6-8]。コカイン中毒患者は，摂取量とその時期によって急速に悪化することがある。コカイン中毒の結果として心停止を起こした際，重度の心毒性または神経毒性のエビデンスがある場合は，必要に応じて心拍再開後に実施する具体的な治療戦略を含めて，標準の BLS および ALS ガイドラインからの逸脱を勧めるエビデンスはない。ROSC 後，速やかに中毒学者または地域の中毒センターに問い合わせることが推奨される。

「推奨事項の裏付けとなる解説」

1. 急性コカイン中毒患者に対するさまざまな治療戦略を評価する大規模な RCT は存在しない。文献の体系的レビューで 5 件の小規

模な前向き試験，3件の後ろ向き研究，および相反する結果を含む複数の症例報告と症例集積研究が確認されている。良好な転帰が報告されている文献もあれば，明らかな有害事象が報告されている文献もある[9]。

2. 適切に実施された臨床試験では，プロプラノロール投与でコカインへの曝露患者の冠動脈血流が減少したことが示された[8]。最近の体系的レビューで，βアドレナリン遮断薬の使用が有害ではない可能性が示唆されているが，[6,7] 安全な代替薬が入手可能である。

このトピックが正式なエビデンスレビューを最後に受けたのは2010年である[10]。

参考資料

1. Baumann BM, Perrone J, Hornig SE, Shofer FS, Hollander JE. Randomized, double-blind, placebo-controlled trial of diazepam, nitroglycerin, or both for treatment of patients with potential cocaine-associated acute coronary syndromes. Acad Emerg Med. 2000;7:878-885. doi: 10.1111/j.1553-2712.2000.tb02065.x
2. Negus BH, Willard JE, Hillis LD, Glamann DB, Landau C, Snyder RW, Lange RA. Alleviation of cocaine-induced coronary vasoconstriction with intravenous verapamil. Am J Cardiol. 1994;73:510-513. doi: 10.1016/0002-9149(94)90684-x
3. Saland KE, Hillis LD, Lange RA, Cigarroa JE. Influence of morphine sulfate on cocaine-induced coronary vasoconstriction. Am J Cardiol. 2002;90:810-811. doi: 10.1016/s0002-9149(02)02622-x
4. Hollander JE, Hoffman RS, Gennis P, Fairweather P, DiSano MJ, Schumb DA, Feldman JA, Fish SS, Dyer S, Wax P. Nitroglycerin in the treatment of cocaine associated chest pain-clinical safety and efficacy. J Toxicol Clin Toxicol. 1994;32:243-256. doi: 10.3109/15563659409017957
5. Honderick T, Williams D, Seaberg D, Wears R. A prospective, randomized, controlled trial of benzodiazepines and nitroglycerine or nitroglycerine alone in the treatment of cocaine-associated acute coronary syndromes. Am J Emerg Med. 2003;21:39-42. doi: 10.1053/ajem.2003.50010
6. Pham D, Addison D, Kayani W, Misra A, Jneid H, Resar J, Lakkis N, Alam M. Outcomes of beta blocker use in cocaine-associated chest pain: a meta-analysis. Emerg Med J. 2018;35:559-563. doi: 10.1136/emermed-2017-207065
7. Shin D, Lee ES, Bohra C, Kongpakpaisarn K. In-Hospital and Long-Term Outcomes of Beta-Blocker Treatment in Cocaine Users: A Systematic Review and Meta-analysis. Cardiol Res. 2019;10:40-47. doi: 10.14740/cr831
8. Lange RA, Cigarroa RG, Flores ED, McBride W, Kim AS, Wells PJ, Bedotto JB, Danziger RS, Hillis LD. Potentiation of cocaine-induced coronary vasoconstriction by beta-adrenergic blockade. Ann Intern Med. 1990;112:897-903. doi: 10.7326/0003-4819-112-12-897
9. Richards JR, Garber D, Laurin EG, Albertson TE, Derlet RW, Amsterdam EA, Olson KR, Ramoska EA, Lange RA. Treatment of cocaine cardiovascular toxicity: a systematic review. Clin Toxicol (Phila). 2016;54:345-364. doi: 10.3109/15563650.2016.1142090
10. Vanden Hoek TL, Morrison LJ, Shuster M, Donnino M, Sinz E, Lavonas EJ, Jeejeebhoy FM, Gabrielli A. Part 12: cardiac arrest in special situations: 2010 American Heart Association Guidelines for Cardiopulmonary Resuscitation and Emergency Cardiovascular Care. Circulation. 2010;122(suppl 3):S829-S861. doi: 10.1161/CIRCULATIONAHA.110.971069

中毒：局所麻酔薬

COR	LOE	推奨事項
2b	C-LD	1. 局所麻酔薬全身毒性（LAST）を呈した患者，とくにブピバカイン中毒による前駆的神経毒性または心停止を伴う患者に対して，標準的蘇生治療と並行して脂肪乳剤を静注投与することは妥当と考えられる。

ベンゾジアゼピン系薬物の過量投与に関する 局所麻酔薬過剰投与

「概要」

局所麻酔薬過量投与（「局所麻酔薬全身毒性」（local anesthetic systemic toxicity, LAST）とも呼ばれる）は致死的な緊急事態であり，神経毒性または劇症心血管虚脱を呈することがある[1,2]。LASTに関して最も一般的に報告されている薬剤はブピバカイン，リドカイン，およびロピバカインである[2]。

定義により，LASTとは標準的なBLSおよびALSに加えて代替アプローチを検討すべき特殊な状況である。症例報告および動物試験データでは，脂肪乳剤の静注が有益である可能性が示唆されている[2-5]。LASTは，細胞膜の電位依存性チャネル（とくにナトリウム伝達）に重度の阻害を引き起こす。静注の脂肪乳剤について起こりえる作用機序には，局所麻酔薬を能動的に心臓および脳から迅速に排出する作用，心筋収縮力増加，血管収縮，および心保護の効果が含まれる[1]。

報告されたLASTの発生数は，神経ブロック1000件につき0～2件である[2]が，毒性の認識および手技が向上した結果，減少しているとみられる[1]。

「推奨事項の裏付けとなる解説」

1. 前回これらの推奨事項が正式にレビューされた[6]後，米国区域麻酔疼痛治療学会（American Society of Regional Anesthesia and Pain Medicine, ASRA）から詳細かつ体系的なレビューが複数，また診療推奨事項書が1本発行された[1-5]。標準の蘇生治療と比較したRCTまたは研究はいまだ発行されていない。臨床試験データは，2014年までに発行された約100本の症例報告書[6]，および2014年～2016年11月の35本の文献に含まれる追加症例47件から得たが，このうち患者がCPRを受けた症例は10件のみであった[2]。対照群がないため，特定された症例の結果を脂肪乳剤の静注によるものと安易に解釈したり，脂肪乳剤の静注を原因とすることはできない。脂肪乳剤の使用により膵炎，および急性呼吸窮迫症候群の併発がみられたが，脂肪乳剤の静注投与は比較的良性と考えられている[7]。

このトピックが正式なエビデンスレビューを最後に受けたのは2015年である[6]。

参考資料

1. Neal JM, Barrington MJ, Fettiplace MR, Gitman M, Memtsoudis SG, Morwald EE, Rubin DS, Weinberg G. The Third American Society of Regional Anesthesia and Pain Medicine Practice advisory on local anesthetic systemic toxicity: executive summary 2017. Reg Anesth Pain Med. 2018;43:113-123. doi: 10.1097/AAP.0000000000000720
2. Gitman M, Barrington MJ. Local Anesthetic Systemic Toxicity: A Review of Recent Case Reports and Registries. Reg Anesth Pain Med. 2018;43:124-130. doi: 10.1097/AAP.0000000000000721
3. Cao D, Heard K, Foran M, Koyfman A. Intravenous lipid emulsion in the emergency department: a systematic review of recent literature. J Emerg Med. 2015;48:387-397. doi: 10.1016/j.jemermed.2014.10.009
4. Gosselin S, Hoegberg LC, Hoffman RS, Graudins A, Stork CM, Thomas SH, Stellpflug SJ, Hayes BD, Levine M, Morris M, Nesbitt-Miller A, Turgeon AF, Bailey B, Calello DP, Chuang R, Bania TC, Mégarbane B, Bhalla A, Lavergne V. Evidence-based recommendations on the use of intravenous lipid emulsion therapy in poisoning. Clin Toxicol (Phila). 2016;54:899-923. doi: 10.1080/15563650.2016.1214275

5. Hoegberg LC, Bania TC, Lavergne V, Bailey B, Turgeon AF, Thomas SH, Morris M, Miller-Nesbitt A, Mégarbane B, Magder S, Gosselin S; Lipid Emulsion Workgroup.Systematic review of the effect of intravenous lipid emulsion therapy for local anesthetic toxicity.Clin Toxicol (Phila).2016;54:167-193. doi: 10.3109/15563650.2015.1121270
6. Lavonas EJ, Drennan IR, Gabrielli A, Heffner AC, Hoyte CO, Orkin AM, Sawyer KN, Donnino MW.Part 10: special circumstances of resuscitation: 2015 American Heart Association Guidelines Update for Cardiopulmonary Resuscitation and Emergency Cardiovascular Care.Circulation.2015;132(suppl 2):S501-S518. doi: 10.1161/CIR.0000000000000264
7. Levine M, Skolnik AB, Ruha AM, Bosak A, Menke N, Pizon AF.Complications following antidotal use of intravenous lipid emulsion therapy.J Med Toxicol.2014;10:10-14. doi: 10.1007/s13181-013-0356-1

中毒：ナトリウムチャネル遮断薬（三環系抗うつ薬など）

COR	LOE	推奨事項
2a	C-LD	1. ナトリウムチャネル遮断薬／三環系抗うつ薬（TCA）の過量投与に起因する心停止または致死的な心伝導遅延（すなわち120 msを超えるQRS延長）に対して，炭酸水素ナトリウムの投与は有益な場合がある。
2b	C-LD	2. ナトリウムチャネル遮断薬／TCAの中毒に起因する心停止または治療抵抗性ショックに対して，ECMOの使用を検討してもよい。

カルシウム拮抗薬の過量投与に関する ナトリウムチャネル遮断薬（三環系抗うつ薬など）に起因する心停止に関する推奨事項

「概要」

TCAおよびその他の薬物（コカイン，フレカイニド，シタロプラムなど）のようなナトリウムチャネル遮断薬の過量投与によって，低血圧，不整脈，および死亡が引き起こされることがあり，これは，他の機序のうち，とりわけ心臓ナトリウムチャネルの遮断による。ECGの特徴的な所見として，頻拍および右脚パターンでのQRS延長がある[1,2]。TCA中毒により，ブルガダ1型に似たECGパターンが出現する可能性がある[3]。

ナトリウムチャネル遮断薬中毒による低血圧または心毒性の標準治療は，ナトリウムボーラス投与と血清のアルカリ化であり，通常は炭酸水素ナトリウムボーラスの投与で実現される。このアプローチは，動物実験および症例報告によって裏付けられており，最近，体系的レビューを受けている[4]。

臨床試験で，TCA誘発性の低血圧，アシドーシス，および／またはQRS延長を呈する患者に対して，炭酸水素ナトリウム投与にマグネシウム投与を加えた研究を行った[5]。マグネシウム投与群は全体的な転帰に優れていたが，死亡率において統計的に有意な効果は見られなかった。マグネシウム投与患者は研究開始時点で対照群よりも症状が大幅に軽度であり，この方法論的な問題のため，これは予備研究と見なされる。

いくつかの症例報告書では，ナトリウムチャネル遮断薬による重度の心毒性に対して，ECMOを使用し[6]，脂肪乳剤の静注治療[7-10]を行った後の良好な転帰が記載されているが，ヒトにおける対照試験は見つからず，限定的な動物データは脂肪乳剤の有効性を裏付けるものではない[11]。

TCA中毒による心停止の治療を評価するヒトの対照試験は見つからなかったが，1件の研究ではイヌのアミトリプチリン誘発性VTの消失が示された[12]。

「推奨事項の裏付けとなる解説」

1. TCAおよびその他の毒物によるナトリウムチャネル遮断の治療として，高張炭酸水素ナトリウム水溶液（8.4％，1 mEq/mL）の投与がヒトの観察研究[13,14]および動物実験により実証されている[12,15-22]。この文献は最近，体系的なレビューを受けている[4]。用量設定試験の結果は得られていないが，1～2 mEq/kg（1 mEq/mL [8.4％]）の炭酸水素ナトリウムを1～2 mL/kg初回投与し，極度の低ナトリウム血症またはアルカリ血症を予防しつつ，必要に応じて反復投与し，臨床的安定に至らせることが歴史的に推奨されており，効果的と見られている。

2. いくつかの症例報告書で，TCA中毒による治療抵抗性ショックを呈した患者へのECMOの使用が実証されている[23,24]。TCA中毒は心原性ショック／心停止の治療可能な原因であるため，ECPRによる転帰の改善については総合的なエビデンスが限られているが，他の治療法に抵抗性があり，致死的な中毒を示した患者に対するECPR/ECMOの使用は論理的である。

このトピックについて最後に正式なエビデンスレビューを受けたのは2010年である[25]。

参考資料

1. Harrigan RA, Brady WJ.ECG abnormalities in tricyclic antidepressant ingestion.Am J Emerg Med.1999;17:387-393. doi: 10.1016/s0735-6757(99)90094-3
2. Thanacoody HK, Thomas SH.Tricyclic antidepressant poisoning: cardiovascular toxicity.Toxicol Rev. 2005;24:205-214. doi: 10.2165/00139709-200524030-00013
3. Bebarta VS, Phillips S, Eberhardt A, Calihan KJ, Waksman JC, Heard K. Incidence of Brugada electrocardiographic pattern and outcomes of these patients after intentional tricyclic antidepressant ingestion.Am J Cardiol.2007;100:656-660. doi: 10.1016/j.amjcard.2007.03.077
4. Bruccoleri RE, Burns MM.A Literature Review of the Use of Sodium Bicarbonate for the Treatment of QRS Widening.J Med Toxicol.2016;12:121-129. doi: 10.1007/s13181-015-0483-y
5. Emamhadi M, Mostafazadeh B, Hassanijirdehi M. Tricyclic antidepressant poisoning treated by magnesium sulfate: a randomized, clinical trial.Drug Chem Toxicol.2012;35:300-303. doi: 10.3109/01480545.2011.614249
6. Koschny R, Lutz M, Seckinger J, Schwenger V, Stremmel W, Eisenbach C. Extracorporeal life support and plasmapheresis in a case of severe polyintoxication.J Emerg Med.2014;47:527-531. doi: 10.1016/j.jemermed.2014.04.044
7. Kiberd MB, Minor SF.Lipid therapy for the treatment of a refractory amitriptyline overdose.CJEM.2012;14:193-197. doi: 10.2310/8000.2011.110486
8. Agarwala R, Ahmed SZ, Wiegand TJ.Prolonged use of intravenous lipid emulsion in a severe tricyclic antidepressant overdose.J Med Toxicol.2014;10:210-214. doi: 10.1007/s13181-013-0353-4
9. Cao D, Heard K, Foran M, Koyfman A. Intravenous lipid emulsion in the emergency department: a systematic review of recent literature.J Emerg Med.2015;48:387-397. doi: 10.1016/j.jemermed.2014.10.009
10. Odigwe CC, Tariq M, Kotecha T, Mustafa U, Senussi N, Ikwu I, Bhattarcharya A, Ngene JI, Ojiako K, Iroegbu N. Tricyclic antidepressant overdose treated with adjunctive lipid rescue and plasmapheresis.Proc (Bayl Univ Med Cent).2016;29:284-287. doi: 10.1080/08998280.2016.11929437
11. Varney SM, Bebarta VS, Vargas TE, Boudreau S, Castaneda M. Intravenous lipid emulsion therapy does not improve hypotension compared to sodium bicarbonate for tricyclic antidepressant toxicity: a randomized, controlled pilot study in a swine model.Acad Emerg Med.2014;21:1212-1219. doi: 10.1111/acem.12513

12. Sasyniuk BI, Jhamandas V, Valois M. Experimental amitriptyline intoxication: treatment of cardiac toxicity with sodium bicarbonate.Ann Emerg Med.1986;15:1052–1059. doi: 10.1016/s0196-0644(86)80128-7
13. Köppel C, Wiegreffe A, Tenczer J. Clinical course, therapy, outcome and analytical data in amitriptyline and combined amitriptyline/chlordiazepoxide overdose.Hum Exp Toxicol.1992;11:458–465. doi: 10.1177/096032719201100604
14. Hoffman JR, Votey SR, Bayer M, Silver L. Effect of hypertonic sodium bicarbonate in the treatment of moderate-to-severe cyclic antidepressant overdose.Am J Emerg Med.1993;11:336–341. doi: 10.1016/0735-6757(93)90163-6
15. Brown TC.Tricyclic antidepressant overdosage: experimental studies on the management of circulatory complications.Clin Toxicol.1976;9:255–272. doi: 10.3109/15563657608988129
16. Nattel S, Mittleman M. Treatment of ventricular tachyarrhythmias resulting from amitriptyline toxicity in dogs.J Pharmacol Exp Ther.1984;231:430–435.
17. Pentel P, Benowitz N. Efficacy and mechanism of action of sodium bicarbonate in the treatment of desipramine toxicity in rats.J Pharmacol Exp Ther.1984;230:12–19.
18. Hedges JR, Baker PB, Tasset JJ, Otten EJ, Dalsey WC, Syverud SA.Bicarbonate therapy for the cardiovascular toxicity of amitriptyline in an animal model.J Emerg Med.1985;3:253–260. doi: 10.1016/0736-4679(85)90427-5
19. Knudsen K, Abrahamsson J. Epinephrine and sodium bicarbonate independently and additively increase survival in experimental amitriptyline poisoning.Crit Care Med.1997;25:669–674. doi: 10.1097/00003246-199704000-00019
20. Tobis JM, Aronow WS.Effect of amitriptyline antidotes on repetitive extrasystole threshold.Clin Pharmacol Ther.1980;27:602–606. doi: 10.1038/clpt.1980.85
21. McCabe JL, Cobaugh DJ, Menegazzi JJ, Fata J. Experimental tricyclic antidepressant toxicity: a randomized, controlled comparison of hypertonic saline solution, sodium bicarbonate, and hyperventilation.Ann Emerg Med.1998;32 (3 Pt 1):329–333. doi: 10.1016/s0196-0644(98)70009-5
22. Bou-Abboud E, Nattel S. Relative role of alkalosis and sodium ions in reversal of class I antiarrhythmic drug-induced sodium channel blockade by sodium bicarbonate.Circulation.1996;94:1954–1961. doi: 10.1161/01.cir.94.8.1954
23. Goodwin DA, Lally KP, Null DM Jr. Extracorporeal membrane oxygenation support for cardiac dysfunction from tricyclic antidepressant overdose.Crit Care Med.1993;21:625–627. doi: 10.1097/00003246-199304000-00025
24. de Lange DW, Sikma MA, Meulenbelt J. Extracorporeal membrane oxygenation in the treatment of poisoned patients.Clin Toxicol (Phila).2013;51:385–393. doi: 10.3109/15563650.2013.800876
25. Vanden Hoek TL, Morrison LJ, Shuster M, Donnino M, Sinz E, Lavonas EJ, Jeejeebhoy FM, Gabrielli A. Part 12: cardiac arrest in special situations: 2010 American Heart Association Guidelines for Cardiopulmonary Resuscitation and Emergency Cardiovascular Care.Circulation.2010;122(suppl 3):S829–S861. doi: 10.1161/CIRCULATIONAHA.110.971069

毒性：一酸化炭素，ジゴキシン，およびシアン化物

COR	LOE	推奨事項
1	B-R	1. 重度の強心配糖体中毒を示す患者には，抗ジゴキシン Fab 抗体を投与すべきである。
2b	B-R	2. 高圧酸素療法は，重度の中毒を示す急性一酸化炭素中毒患者の治療に役立つことがある。
2a	C-LD	3. ヒドロキソコバラミンと 100 ％の酸素（チオ硫酸ナトリウムの併用を問わない）は，シアン化物中毒に有益な場合がある。

「概要」

ジゴキシン中毒により，重度の徐脈，房室結節伝導抑制，および致死的な心室不整脈を引き起こすことがある。セイヨウキョウチクトウ，キツネノテブクロ，ジギトキシンなど，その他の強心配糖体の中毒も類似の症状を示す。強心配糖体中毒の速やかな治療には致死的不整脈の予防または治療が重要である。

一酸化炭素中毒はヘモグロビンの酸素運搬能力を低下させ，また脳細胞および心筋細胞に直接損傷を与え，死亡に至らしめるか，神経傷害および心筋傷害の長期リスクをもたらす。一酸化炭素中毒による心停止はほとんどの場合に致命的であるが，重大度のより低い一酸化炭素中毒による神経学的後遺症に関する試験が必要かもしれない。

シアン化物中毒は主に好気性細胞の代謝が停止することによる。シアン化物はミトコンドリアのチトクロム酸化酵素の鉄イオンと可逆的に結合し，細胞の呼吸とアデノシン三リン酸の生成を停止させる。シアン化物中毒の原因として，煙の吸引，産業曝露，服毒，テロリズム，またはニトロプルシドナトリウムの投与がある。症状は通常数分以内に現れ，所見に含まれる症状には不整脈，無呼吸，徐脈を伴う低血圧，けいれん発作，心血管虚脱などの症状を呈する[1]。乳酸アシドーシスは，感度と特異度の高い所見である[2,3]。迅速な解毒剤としてヒドロキソコバラミンと亜硝酸塩があるが，前者がはるかに安全性に優れている。チオ硫酸ナトリウムは，シアン化物の解毒作用を促進することにより亜硝酸塩の有効性を高めるが，ヒドロキソコバラミンを投与した患者における効果は定かではない[4]。新規の解毒剤が開発中である。

「推奨事項の裏付けとなる解説」

1. ジゴキシン過量投与に対して（とくに心停止の状況において），解毒剤の使用を評価できるデータはない。1 件の RCT[5]，および 4 件の症例収集研究[6-9]では，ジギタリスとその他の強心配糖体の過量投与により誘発された重篤な心不整脈の治療として，抗ジゴキシン Fab フラグメントが安全かつ効果的であるとされている。

2. まれな良好な転帰が記述されることがあるが，一酸化炭素中毒により心停止を起こして生存退院した患者は，ROSC 後の治療の内容に関係なく，ほとんどいない[10-12]。一酸化炭素中毒による神経傷害を防ぐための高圧酸素療法の臨床試験では，相反する結果が得られている。心停止を起こした患者はすべての試験から除外されている[13,14]。高圧酸素療法の副作用の発生率は低い。

3. シアン化物中毒が既にわかっているか，またはその疑いがあり，不安定な心血管系または心停止を呈した患者にヒドロキソコバラミン（シアン化物スカベンジャー）[2,15-19] 静注をただちに行った場合，致死的な毒性を拮抗させることが数件の試験で示された。チオ硫酸ナトリウム（シアン化物代謝の補助因子）の追加投与によりヒドロキソコバラミンの解毒効果が向上するかどうかは議論が分かれてい

る。4件の動物試験[20-23]および2件の臨床試験で[2,24]チオ硫酸ナトリウムの同時投与によりヒドロキソコバラミンの有効性向上が示されたが，他のモデルでは示されていない[4]。このトピックについて最後に正式なエビデンスレビューを受けたのは2010年である[25]。

参考資料

1. Parker-Cote JL, Rizer J, Vakkalanka JP, Rege SV, Holstege CP. Challenges in the diagnosis of acute cyanide poisoning. Clin Toxicol (Phila). 201856:609-617. doi: 10.1080/15563650.2018.1435886
2. Baud FJ, Barriot P, Toffis V, Riou B, Vicaut E, Lecarpentier Y, Bourdon R, Astier A, Bismuth C. Elevated blood cyanide concentrations in victims of smoke inhalation. N Engl J Med. 1991;325:1761-1766. doi: 10.1056/NEJM199112193252502
3. Baud FJ, Borron SW, Bavoux E, Astier A, Hoffman Jr Relation between plasma lactate and blood cyanide concentrations in acute cyanide poisoning. BMJ. 1996;312:26-27. doi: 10.1136/bmj.312.7022.26
4. Bebarta VS, Pitotti RL, Dixon P, Lairet Jr, Bush A, Tanen DA. Hydroxocobalamin versus sodium thiosulfate for the treatment of acute cyanide toxicity in a swine (Sus scrofa) model. Ann Emerg Med. 201259:532-539. doi: 10.1016/j.annemergmed.2012.01.022
5. Eddleston M, Rajapakse S, Rajakanthan, Jayalath S, Sjöström L, Santharaj W, Thenabadu PN, Sheriff MH, Warrell DA. Anti-digoxin Fab fragments in cardiotoxicity induced by ingestion of yellow oleander: a randomised controlled trial. Lancet. 2000;355:967-972. doi: 10.1016/s0140-6736(00)90014-x
6. Smith M. tw, Butler VP Jr, Haber E, Fozzard H, Marcus FI, Bremner WF, Schulman IC, Phillips A. Treatment of life-threatening digitalis intoxication with digoxin-specific Fab antibody fragments: experience in 26 cases. N Engl J Med. 1982;307:1357-1362. doi: 10.1056/NEJM198211253072201
7. Antman EM, Wenger TL, Butler VP Jr, Haber E, Smith M. tw Treatment of 150 cases of life-threatening digitalis intoxication with digoxin-specific Fab antibody fragments.Final report of a multicenter study. Circulation. 1990;81:1744-1752. doi: 10.1161/01.cir.81.6.1744
8. Wenger TL, Butler VP Jr, Haber E, Smith M. tw Treatment of 63 severely digitalis-toxic patients with digoxin-specific antibody fragments. J Am Coll Cardiol. 1985;5 (suppl A):118A-123A. doi: 10.1016/s0735-1097(85)80471-x
9. Hickey AR, Wenger TL, Carpenter VP, Tilson HH, Hlatky mA, Furberg CD, Kirkpatrick CH, Strauss HC, Smith M. tw Digoxin Immune Fab therapy in the management of digitalis intoxication: safety and efficacy results of an observational surveillance study. J Am Coll Cardiol. 1991;17:590-598. doi: 10.1016/s0735-1097 (10)80170-6
10. Hampson NB, Zmaeff JL. Outcome of patients experiencing cardiac arrest with carbon monoxide poisoning treated with hyperbaric oxygen. Ann Emerg Med. 2001;38:36-41. doi: 10.1067/mem.2001.115532
11. Sloan EP, Murphy DG, Hart R, Cooper mA, Turnbull T, Barreca RS, Ellerson B. Complications and protocol considerations in carbon monoxide-poisoned patients who require hyperbaric oxygen therapy: report from a ten-year experience. Ann Emerg Med. 1989;18:629-634. doi: 10.1016/s0196-0644 (89)80516-5
12. Mumma BE :, Shellenbarger D, Callaway CW, Katz KD, Guyette FX, Rittenberger JC. Neurologic recovery following cardiac arrest due to carbon monoxide poisoning. Resuscitation. 2009;80:835. doi: 10.1016/j.resuscitation.2009.03.027
13. Buckley NA, Juurlink DN, Isbister G, Bennett MH, Lavonas EJ. Hyperbaric oxygen for carbon monoxide poisoning. Cochrane Database Syst Rev. 2011:CD002041. doi: 10.1002/14651858.CD002041.pub3
14. American College of Emergency Physicians Clinical Policies Subcommittee on Carbon Monoxide Poisoning, Wolf SJ, Maloney GE, Shih RD, Shy BD, Brown MD. Clinical policy: critical issues in the evaluation and management of adult patients presenting to the emergency department with acute carbon monoxide poisoning. Ann Emerg Med. 201769:98.e6-107.e6. doi: 10.1016/j.annemergmed.2016.11.003
15. Borron SW, Baud FJ, Barriot P, Imbert M, Bismuth C. Prospective study of hydroxocobalamin for acute cyanide poisoning in smoke inhalation. Ann Emerg Med. 200749:794-801, 801.e1. doi: 10.1016/j.annemergmed.2007.01.026
16. Fortin JL, Giocanti JP, Ruttimann M, Kowalski JJ. Prehospital administration of hydroxocobalamin for smoke inhalation-associated cyanide poisoning: 8 years of experience in the Paris Fire Brigade. Clin Toxicol (Phila). 200644 (suppl 1):37-44. doi: 10.1080/15563650600811870
17. Borron SW, Baud FJ, Mégarbane B, Bismuth C. Hydroxocobalamin for severe acute cyanide poisoning by ingestion or inhalation. Am J Emerg Med. 200725:551-558. doi: 10.1016/j.ajem.2006.10.010
18. Houeto P, Hoffman Jr, Imbert M, Levillain P, Baud FJ. Relation of blood cyanide to plasma cyanocobalamin concentration after a fixed dose of hydroxocobalamin in cyanide poisoning. Lancet. 1995;346:605-608. doi: 10.1016/s0140-6736 (95)91437-4
19. Espinoza OB, Perez M, Ramirez MS. Bitter cassava poisoning in eight children: a case report. Vet Hum Toxicol. 1992;34:65.
20. Hall AH, Rumack BH. Hydroxycobalamin/sodium thiosulfate as a cyanide antidote. J Emerg Med. 1987;5:115-121. doi: 10.1016/0736-4679 (87)90074-6
21. Höbel M, Engeser P, Nemeth L, Pill J. The antidote effect of thiosulphate and hydroxocobalamin in formation of nitroprusside intoxication of rabbits. Arch Toxicol. 1980;46:207-213. doi: 10.1007/BF00310436
22. Mengel K, Krämer W, Isert B, Friedberg KD. Thiosulphate and hydroxocobalamin prophylaxis in progressive cyanide poisoning in guinea-pigs. Toxicology. 1989;54:335-342. doi: 10.1016/0300-483x (89)90068-1
23. Friedberg KD, Shukla UR. The efficiency of aquocobalamine as an antidote in cyanide poisoning when given alone or combined with sodium thiosulfate. Arch Toxicol. 1975;33:103-113. doi: 10.1007/BF00353235
24. Forsyth JC, Mueller TL., Becker CE, Osterloh J, Benowitz NL, Rumack BH, Hall AH. Hydroxocobalamin as a cyanide antidote: safety, efficacy and pharmacokinetics in heavily smoking normal volunteers. J Toxicol Clin Toxicol. 1993;31:277-294. doi: 10.3109/15563659309000395
25. Vanden Hoek TL, Morrison LJ, Shuster M, Donnino M, Sinz E, Lavonas EJ, Jeejeebhoy FM, Gabrielli A. Part 12: cardiac arrest in special situations: 2010 American Heart Association Guidelines for Cardiopulmonary Resuscitation and Emergency Cardiovascular Care. Circulation. 2010122 (suppl 3):S829-S861. doi: 10.1161/CIRCULATIONAHA.110.971069

今後の課題と研究の優先順位

これらのガイドラインを作成する作業全体の一部として，執筆グループは成人の心停止の管理に関する膨大な文献をレビューすることができた。このプロセスで直面すると予測された課題の1つは，心停止研究の多くの分野でデータが不足していることであった。この課題には，『ガイドライン2010』および『ガイドラインアップデート2015』の両プロセスで直面した。このとき，高グレードLOE（A）に基づくガイドラインの推奨事項はわずかな割合のみ（1％）であり，約75％の推奨事項は低グレードLOE（C）に基づいていた。[1]

同様の課題には，『ガイドライン2020』のプロセスでも直面した。このときに成人の心停止の管理に関する今後の課題が多数判明した。これらのトピックは，情報が確認されなかった分野だけでなく，進行中の研究が推奨事項に直接影響を及ぼす可能性のある分野としても特定された。推奨事項の裏付けとなる解説全体を通して，これらの疑問を解き明かす次のステップを推進するための具体的な研究の必要性が明らかとなった。

重要な今後の課題は表4にまとめている。

参考資料

1. Morrison LJ, Gent LM, Lang E, Nunnally ME, Parker MJ, Callaway CW, Nadkarni VM, Fernandez AR, Billi JE, Egan Jr, et al. Part 2: evidence evaluation and management of conflicts of interest: 2015 American Heart Association Guidelines Update for Cardiopulmonary Resuscitation and Emergency Cardiovascular Care. Circulation. 2015132 (suppl 2):S368-S382. doi: 10.1161/CIR.0000000000000253

表4. 2020 成人ガイドラインの重要な今後の課題

蘇生の手順	
蘇生開始	市民救助者の CPR 技能を向上させる最善の戦略は？
質の高い CPR の指標	最良な CPR のデューティサイクル（胸骨圧迫と圧迫解除のサイクルの合計時間に対する圧迫時間の割合）は？
質の高い CPR の指標	挿管されていない患者での $ETCO_2$ の有効性と信頼性は？
質の高い CPR の指標	動脈ラインが挿入されている患者の場合，特定の血圧目標値を設定した CPR は転帰を改善するか？
質の高い CPR の指標	個人の蘇生スキルの能力と比較して，統合されたチームの能力は蘇生の転帰に影響するか？
除細動	CPR サイクルにおける除細動器の充電の最適な時間は？
除細動	実際の臨床現場において CPR 中の ECG 心リズム解析用アーチファクトフィルタリングアルゴリズムは，胸骨圧迫の休止を減少して転帰を改善できるか？
除細動	ショック実施前の波形解析は転帰改善につながるか？
除細動	二重連続手動式電気ショック，および／または除細動器パッド装着位置の変更は，ショック適応のリズムを呈する心停止の転帰に影響するか？
血管路確保	心停止の場合に薬物の骨髄内投与は安全かつ有効であるか？また有効性は穿刺部位によって異なるか？
心停止中の血管収縮薬の投与	心停止後早期にアドレナリンを投与した場合，良好な神経学的転帰を伴って生存率が改善するか？
心停止中の非血管収縮薬の投与	心停止に対して抗不整脈薬を併用すると，ショック適応のリズムを呈する心停止の転帰が改善するか？
心停止中の非血管収縮薬の投与	除細動の成功後，ROSC 時に抗不整脈薬を予防的に投与すると，不整脈の再発が減少して転帰が改善するか？
心停止中の非血管収縮薬の投与	ROSC 後に低血圧のままである患者に対して，ステロイド薬はショックまたはその他の転帰を改善するか？
CPR の補助用具	心停止中におけるベッドサイドでの心臓の超音波検査は転帰を改善するか？
CPR の補助用具	CPR 中に特定の $ETCO_2$ の目標値を設定することは有益か？また，$ETCO_2$ 値がどの程度上昇したら ROSC を示すか？
蘇生終了	心停止中の予後予測に，他の指標と組み合わせて $ETCO_2$ を使用できるか？
蘇生終了	ベッドサイドでの心臓の超音波検査は，他の因子と組み合わせて蘇生終了の判断材料にできるか？
蘇生に使用する高度な手技および器具	
高度な気道確保器具の留置	IHCA の場合，高度な気道確保のための最適なアプローチは何か？
高度な気道確保器具の留置	気道確保のアプローチを選択する上で，とくに患者の因子と，プロバイダーの経験，訓練，ツールおよびスキルのマッチングに関してさらに研究が必要である。
高度な気道確保器具の留置	習熟度を維持するための気道確保の訓練経験の具体的な種類は何か？またその量と間隔は？
CPR の代替手法および装置	ECPR が最も有益な可能性をもつ集団は？
不整脈の具体的な管理	
心室レートの速い心房細動または心房粗動	心房細動および心房粗動の電気ショックに必要な最適エネルギーは？
徐脈	症候性徐脈の管理に最適なアプローチ，血管収縮薬，または経皮ペーシングは何か？
ROSC 後の治療	
蘇生後の治療	心拍再開後に高酸素症の回避は転帰改善につながるか？
蘇生後の治療	心停止後の転帰に対する低炭酸ガス血症や高炭酸ガス血症の影響は何か？
蘇生後の治療	心拍再開後の患者に一般的に見られる非けいれん性てんかん発作の治療は，患者の転帰を改善するか？
蘇生後の治療	心拍再開後のけいれん発作の管理に最良の薬物療法は何か？
蘇生後の治療	神経保護薬は，心停止後の神経学的転帰を良好に改善するか？
蘇生後の治療	薬物介入，カテーテル介入，または植込み型機器を含めて，心停止後の心原性ショックに最も効果のある管理アプローチは何か？
蘇生後の治療	ROSC 後に抗不整脈薬の予防的投与が果たす役割はあるか？
目標体温管理	正常体温の厳格な維持と比較して，目標体温管理は転帰を改善するか？
目標体温管理	目標体温管理の最適な体温目標値は？
目標体温管理法	復温前に目標体温管理を実施する最適な期間は？
目標体温管理	目標体温管理による処置後，心拍再開後の患者を復温する最善のアプローチは何か？
心拍再開後の PCI	VF/VT 心停止後，ROSC した患者で，非 STEMI のショックの兆候，または電気生理学的に不安定な兆候がある場合，緊急 PCI を行うと転帰が改善するか？
神経学的予後予測	瞳孔対光反射，角膜反射，ミオクローヌス／ミオクローヌス重積状態などの身体診察の所見について，評価者間の一致率は？
神経学的予後予測	心停止後の神経学的予後不良を予測可能な一定の NSE および S100B の閾値を特定できるか？
神経学的予後予測	ROSC 後 72 時間以降にチェックしたとき，NSE および S100B は役立つか？

（続く）

表 4. （続き）

神経学的予後予測		グリア線維性酸性タンパク質，血清τタンパク質，およびはニューロフィラメント軽鎖は神経学的予後予測に役立つか？
神経学的予後予測		複数の研究にわたる予後予測能の比較を可能にするには，「てんかん重積状態」，「悪性 EEG パターン」，およびその他の EEG パターンについて，より不変な定義が必要である。
神経学的予後予測		予後予測を行うために最適な頭部 CT 検査のタイミングは？
神経学的予後予測		予後予測を行うための一定の GWR または ADC の閾値はあるか？
神経学的予後予測		GWR および ADC の定量方法の標準化が有用と考えられる。
回復		
	心停止後の回復と生存	心停止からの生存に関する観点での転帰の尺度はどのようなものであるか？また，その尺度は，一般的な尺度または医師観点での尺度とどのように異なるか？
	心停止後の回復と生存	心停止後の身体機能障害の軽減または予防を可能にする院内介入は存在するか？
	心停止後の回復と生存	心停止後に感情障害を発症したり，精神が不安定になるのはどのような患者か？またそれらの症状の治療／予防／回復は可能か？
	心停止後の回復と生存	心停止からの生存者用に病院主体でプロトコール化した退院計画は，リハビリテーションサービスへのアクセス／紹介，または患者の転帰を改善するか？
特殊な蘇生の状況		
	偶発性低体温症	復温しても患者に生存の可能性がまったくないと判定可能な所見の組み合わせは何か？
	偶発性低体温症	重度の低体温症患者には，挿管および機械的換気または単なる加温加湿酸素の供給のいずれを行うべきか？
	偶発性低体温症	VF の症状を呈する重度の低体温症患者が初回の除細動の試みに失敗した場合，追加の除細動を行うべきか？
	偶発性低体温症	心停止を起こしている重度の低体温症患者には，アドレナリンまたはその他の蘇生薬物を投与すべきか？投与する場合，使用すべき投与量とスケジュールは？
	溺水	溺水傷病者の蘇生が無益なのはどのような状況か？
	溺水	軽度の溺水事故の後，どの程度の期間，遅発性呼吸困難の発生に備えて患者を観察すべきか？
	電解質異常	致死的な不整脈または心停止による高カリウム血症に対して最善の治療は何か？
	オピオイド過量投与	オピオイド過量投与による呼吸抑制にナロキシン拮抗薬を投与した後，最短の安全観察期間はどの程度か？この期間は関与したオピオイドによって異なるか？
	オピオイド過量投与	オピオイド関連の心停止を起こし，換気を伴う CPR を受けている患者にナロキシン投与は有益か？
	オピオイド過量投与	オピオイド過量投与の大部分がフェンタニルおよびフェンタニルアナログである場合，ナロキシンの最良の初回投与量は？
	オピオイド過量投与	オピオイド過量投与が疑われ，信頼性の高い脈拍確認ができない非医療従事者が対処する場合，CPR の開始は有益か？
	妊娠	心停止を起こしている妊婦に PMCD を実施する最良のタイミングは？
	肺塞栓症	心停止の原因が肺塞栓症と「疑われる」場合，蘇生中の緊急血栓溶解が有益なのはどのような患者か？
	中毒：βアドレナリン遮断薬およびカルシウム拮抗薬	βアドレナリン遮断薬またはカルシウム拮抗薬の過量投与による治療抵抗性ショックの場合，モダリティ（従来の昇圧薬，カルシウム，グルカゴン，高容量インスリン）の最良の実施順序は？
	中毒：局所麻酔薬	脂肪乳剤静注法の最良の投与量と処方は？
	中毒：一酸化炭素，ジゴキシン，およびシアン化物	シアン化物中毒で解毒療法が有益なのはどのような患者か？
	中毒：一酸化炭素，ジゴキシン，およびシアン化物	シアン化物中毒を起こし，ヒドロキソコバラミンが投与されている患者にチオ硫酸ナトリウムを投与するとさらに有益か？

ADC：見かけ上の拡散係数（apparent diffusion coefficient），CPR：心肺蘇生（cardiopulmonary resuscitation），CT：コンピュータ断層撮影（computed tomography），ECG：心電図（electrocardiogram），ECPR：体外循環式心肺蘇生法（extracorporeal cardiopulmonary resuscitation），EEG：脳波図，$ETCO_2$：呼気終末二酸化炭素（end-tidal carbon dioxide），GWR：灰白質／白質比（gray-white ratio），IHCA：院内心停止（in-hospital cardiac arrest），IO：骨髄内（intraosseous），IV：静脈内（intravascular），NSE：ニューロン特異的エノラーゼ（neuron-specific enolase），PCI：経皮的冠動脈インターベンション（percutaneous coronary intervention），PMCD：死戦期帝王切開（perimortem cesarean delivery），ROSC：自己心拍再開（return of spontaneous circulation），S100B：S100 カルシウム結合タンパク質（S100 calcium binding protein），STEMI：ST 上昇型心筋梗塞（ST-segment elevation myocardial infarction），VF：心室細動（ventricular fibrillation）。

文献情報

アメリカ心臓協会は，この文書の引用時に次の記載を含めることを要求する。Panchal AR, Bartos JA, Cabañas JG, Donnino MW, Drennan IR, Hirsch KG, Kudenchuk PJ, Kurz MC, Lavonas EJ, Morley PT, O'Neil BJ, Peberdy MA, Rittenberger JC, Rodriguez AJ, Sawyer KN, Berg KM; on behalf of the Adult Basic and Advanced Life Support Writing Group.Part 3: adult basic and advanced life support: 2020 American Heart Association Guidelines for Cardiopulmonary Resuscitation and Emergency Cardiovascular Care.循環.2020;142(suppl 2):S366-S468. doi: 10.1161/CIR.0000000000000916

謝辞

執筆グループは次の寄稿者に感謝する；Julie Arafeh, RN, MSN；Justin L. Benoit, MD, MS；Maureen Chase, MD, MPH；Antonio Fernandez；EdisonFerreiradePaiva, MD, PhD；BryanL.Fischberg, NRP；Gustavo E. Flores, MD, EMT-P；Peter Fromm, MPH, RN；Raul Gazmuri, MD, PhD；Blayke Courtney Gibson, MD；Theresa Hoadley, MD, PhD；Cindy H. Hsu, MD, PhD；Mahmoud Issa, MD；Adam Kessler, DO；Mark S. Link, MD；David J. Magid, MD, MPH；Keith Marrill, MD；Tonia Nicholson, MBBS；Joseph P. Ornato, MD；Garrett Pacheco, MD；Michael Parr, MB；Rahul Pawar, MBBS, MD；James Jaxton, MD；Sarah M. Perman, MD, MSCE；James Pribble, MD；Derek Robinett, MD；Daniel Rolston, MD；Comilla Sasson, MD, PhD；Sree Veena Satyapriya, MD；Travis Sharkey, MD, PhD；Jasmeet Soar, MA, MB, BChir；Deb Torman, MBA, MEd, AT, ATC, EMT-P；Benjamin Von Schweinitz；Anezi Uzendu, MD；Carolyn M. Zelop, MD。

また，執筆グループは，David J. Magid, MD, MPH の多大な貢献に対して感謝の意を表す。

情報開示

付録 1　執筆グループの情報開示

執筆グループメンバー	所属	研究助成金	その他の研究支援	講演／謝礼金	鑑定人	株式所有	コンサルタント／顧問	その他
Ashish R. Panchal	The Ohio State University	なし	なし	なし	なし	なし	なし	なし
Katherine M. Berg	Beth Israel Deaconess Medical Center	NHLBI Grant K23 HL128814†	なし	なし	なし	なし	なし	なし
Jason A. Bartos	University of Minnesota	なし	なし	なし	なし	なし	なし	Abbott Labs*, Biotronik Inc*, Edwards Lifesciences Corp*, Inari Medical, Inc*, Maquet Cardiovascular US Sales, LLC*, Stryker Corp*, Zoll Circulation, Inc*
José G. Cabañas	Wake County Emergency Medical Services	なし	なし	なし	なし	なし	なし	なし
Michael W. Donnino	Beth Israel Deaconess Medical Center	NIH†，General Electric*，Kaneka（研究者主導）*	なし	心停止のトピックに関する取り組みの講演*	なし	なし	なし	なし
Ian R. Drennan	Sunnybrook Health Sciences Center	なし	なし	なし	なし	なし	なし	なし
Karen G. Hirsch	Stanford University	NIH（心停止に関する研究活動への給与支援）*，AHA（心停止に関する研究への給与支援）*	なし	なし	なし	なし	なし	なし
Peter J. Kudenchuk	University of Washington	NIH（AHA での SIREN ネットワークの PI）†	なし	なし	なし	なし	なし	なし
Michael C. Kurz	University of Alabama at Birmingham	DOD（PACT 試験の DSMB メンバー）*，NIH（OHCA における肥満細胞脱顆粒試験の R21 検査の CO-I）*	なし	Zoll Medical Corp*	なし	なし	Zoll Circulation, Inc†	Zoll Circulation, Inc†
Eric J. Lavonas	Denver Health Emergency Medicine	BTG Pharmaceuticals（Denver Health（Lavonas 医師の勤務先）は研究，コールセンター，コンサルティング，指導に関する契約を BTG Pharmaceuticals と締結している。BTG はジゴキシン解毒剤 DigiFab を製造している。Lavonas 医師は，賞与またはインセンティブを受け取っておらず，前述の契約に関連する製品はない。これらのガイドラインの作成時に，Lavonas 医師はジゴキシン中毒に関する議論に参加しなかった）†。	なし	なし	なし	なし	なし	アメリカ心臓協会（American Heart Association, AHA）（上級科学編集者）†

（続く）

付録 1（続き）

執筆グループメンバー	所属	研究助成金	その他の研究支援	講演／謝礼金	鑑定人	株式所有	コンサルタント／顧問	その他
Peter T. Morley	University of Melbourne, Royal Melbourne Hospital（オーストラリア）	なし	なし	なし	なし	なし	なし	なし
Brian J. O'Neil	Wayne State University	SIREN ネットワーク（NHLBI による臨床試験ネットワーク）*	なし	Zoll circulation*, Genentech*	なし	なし	なし	なし
Mary Ann Peberdy	Virginia Commonwealth University	なし	なし	なし	なし	なし	なし	なし
Jon C. Rittenberger	Guthrie Medical Center	NIH–SIREN（ICECAP 試験）*, AHA（助成金）*	なし	なし	Bailey Glasser*	なし	Hibernaid, LLC*	なし
Amber J. Rodriguez	American Heart Association	なし	なし	なし	なし	なし	なし	なし
Kelly N. Sawyer	University of Pittsburgh – 医師	なし	なし	なし	なし	なし	なし	なし

この表は，執筆グループの全メンバーに回答および提出が求められる情報開示アンケート（Disclosure Questionnaire）の結果に基づき実在の利益相反または合理的に認定できる利益相反とみなされる可能性のある，執筆グループメンバーの関係を示している。メンバーと該当団体との関係が「顕著」であると考えられるのは，次のいずれかの状況が存在する場合である。（a）当該メンバーが団体から受領する金額が過去いずれの 12 か月間に $10,000 以上であるか，メンバーの総収入の 5 ％以上である，（b）団体の議決権株式の 5 ％以上，またはその団体の公正市場価値の $10,000 以上を保有している。この定義において「重大」に相当するレベルに満たない場合，その関係は「軽度」とみなされる。

*軽度
†重大

付録 2　レビューアーの情報開示

レビューアー	所属	研究助成金	その他の研究支援	講演／謝礼金	鑑定人	所有権	コンサルタント／顧問	その他
Clifton Callaway	University of Pittsburgh – 医師	NIH（心停止および心血管緊急状態の治療を含む救急医療の研究に対する助成）†	なし	なし	なし	なし	なし	なし
Alix Carter	Dalhousie University（カナダ）	Maritime Heart（OHCA 生存の記述因子）*	なし	なし	なし	なし	なし	なし
Henry Halperin	Johns Hopkins University	Zoll Circulation（CPR 研究）†, NIH（CPR 研究）†	なし	なし	なし	なし	なし	なし
Timothy Henry	The Christ Hospital	なし	なし	なし	なし	なし	なし	なし
Jonathan Jui	Oregon Health and Science University	NIH（HL 126938）*	なし	なし	なし	なし	なし	なし
Tommaso Pellis	Friuli Occidentale（イタリア）	なし	なし	なし	なし	なし	なし	なし
Fred Severyn	Denver Health and Hospital Authority, University of Colorado Anschutz Medical Campus, University of Arkansas for Medical Sciences	なし	なし	なし	なし	なし	なし	なし
Andrew H. Travers	Emergency Health Services, Nova Scotia（カナダ）	なし	なし	なし	なし	なし	なし	なし

この表は，執筆グループの全メンバーに回答および提出が求められる情報開示アンケート（Disclosure Questionnaire）の結果に基づき実在の利益相反または合理的に認定できる利益相反とみなされる可能性のある，執筆グループメンバーの関係を示している。メンバーと該当団体との関係が「顕著」であると考えられるのは，次のいずれかの状況が存在する場合である。（a）当該メンバーが団体から受領する金額が過去いずれの 12 か月間に $10,000 以上であるか，メンバーの総収入の 5 ％以上である，（b）団体の議決権株式の 5 ％以上，またはその団体の公正市場価値の $10,000 以上を保有している。この定義において「重大」に相当するレベルに満たない場合，その関係は「軽度」とみなされる。

*軽度
†重大

Circulation

第4章：小児一次救命処置と二次救命処置
AHA 心肺蘇生と救急心血管治療のためのガイドライン 2020

覚えておくべき重要な事項トップ 10

1. 質の高い心肺蘇生（CPR）は蘇生成功の基礎である。新規のデータから質の高い CPR の次の重要な要素が確認された。適切なテンポと深さの胸骨圧迫を行って，CPR の中断を最小限にし，胸郭が完全に元に戻ってから次の圧迫を開始し，過換気を避けること。
2. 乳児および小児に対し，（a）高度な気道確保器具を用いて CPR を実施する場合，または（b）脈拍があり補助呼吸を実施する場合の呼吸数が，20〜30 回/分となった。
3. ショック不適応リズム患者の場合，CPR 開始後，早期にアドレナリンを投与するほど，患者の生存率が高くなる。
4. カフ付き気管チューブの使用により，気管チューブ交換の必要性が低下する。
5. 輪状軟骨圧迫法のルーチン使用は，バッグマスク換気中の逆流のリスクが低下せず，挿管成功の妨げになる可能性がある。
6. 院外心停止の場合，バッグマスク換気は気管挿管などの高度な気道確保の処置と同様の蘇生転帰をもたらす。
7. 蘇生は，自己心拍再開（ROSC）で終了ではない。優れた心拍再開後の治療は，最善の患者転帰のために極めて重要である。ROSC 後に意識が回復しない小児の場合，心拍再開後の治療には，目標体温管理および継続的な脳波モニタリングが含まれる。低血圧，高酸素症または低酸素症，および高炭酸ガス血症または低炭酸ガス血症の予防および／または治療が重要である。
8. 退院後に，心停止からの生存者は身体的，認知的，および感情的な問題を抱える場合があり，進行中の治療および介入の継続を要する可能性がある。
9. ナロキソンはオピオイド過量投与に起因する呼吸停止を回復させられるが，心停止の患者にナロキソンが有効というエビデンスはない。
10. 敗血症での輸液蘇生では，患者の反応に基づく頻回の再評価が必要である。調整晶質液，不調整晶質液および膠質液はすべて敗血症の蘇生に認められる。アドレナリンまたはノルアドレナリン注入を，輸液抵抗性の敗血症性ショックに使用する。

Alexis A. Topjian, MD, MSCE, Chair
Tia T. Raymond, MD, Vice-Chair
Dianne Atkins, MD
Melissa Chan, MD
Jonathan P. Duff, MD, MEd
Benny L. Joyner Jr, MD, MPH
Javier J. Lasa, MD
Eric J. Lavonas, MD, MS
Arielle Levy, MD, MEd
Melissa Mahgoub, PhD
Garth D. Meckler, MD, MSHS
Kathryn E. Roberts, MSN, RN
Robert M. Sutton, MD, MSCE
Stephen M. Schexnayder, MD
On behalf of the Pediatric Basic and Advanced Life Support Collaborators

キーワード：AHA による科学的提言 ■ 不整脈 ■ 心肺蘇生 ■ 除細動 ■ 心停止 ■ 小児科学 ■ 心拍再開後の治療

© 2020 American Heart Association, Inc.

https://www.ahajournals.org/journal/circ

前文

米国では毎年，20,000 人を超える乳児および小児の心停止が発生している[1-4]。2015 年に，救急医療サービスで記録された院外心停止（OHCA）が，7000 人を超える乳児および小児で発生した[4]。小児 OHCA 患者の約 11.4 ％が生存して退院したが，予後は年齢により異なり，青年期で

17.1％，小児で13.2％，乳児で4.9％であった。同年の小児の院内心停止（IHCA）発生は入院中の乳児および小児1000人あたり12.66件で，全生存退院率が41.1％であった[4]。神経学的転帰を小児の年齢範囲全体で評価するのは困難な状態であり，OHCAおよびIHCAの両研究全体で指標とフォローアップ期間の報告にばらつきがある。良好な神経学的転帰が，生存退院者の最大47％で報告されている[5]。IHCAからの生存は増加しているものの，生存転帰と神経学的転帰を改善するためにさらに多くを成し遂げる必要がある[6]。

国際蘇生連絡委員会（International Liaison Committee on Resuscitation, ILCOR）の生存のための方程式（Formula for Survival）では良好な蘇生転帰を得るための3つの基本的な要素を強調している。すなわち，健全な蘇生科学に基づくガイドライン，市民および蘇生を行うプロバイダーの効果的な教育，適切に機能する救命の連鎖の実施である[7]。

これらのガイドラインは，新生児期を除く小児の一次救命処置と二次救命処置に関する推奨事項を含み，利用可能な最良の蘇生科学に基づいている。現在心停止からの回復を含む範囲までに拡張されている救命の連鎖（セクション2）では，さまざまな分野の医療専門家の連携した取り組みや，OHCAの場合，バイスタンダー，救急通信指令員，および第1救助者の連携した取り組みが必要である。さらに，蘇生を行うプロバイダーの訓練についての具体的な推奨事項を，第6章：蘇生教育科学に記載し，治療システムについての推奨事項を第7章に記載する。

概要
ガイドラインの範囲

これらのガイドラインは，市民救助者と医療従事者に対する，心停止前，心停止中および心拍再開後の各状態で乳児および小児を見極めて治療するためのリソースとなることを目的とする。これらは，地域社会，病院前，病院環境などの多数の状況で乳児および小児に適用できる。心停止前，心停止中，および心拍再開後の各トピックで，先天性心疾患患者のような特殊な状況での心停止を含め総説する。

小児の二次救命処置ガイドラインを目的とするため，小児患者は乳児，小児，および18歳までの青年とし，新生児は除外する。小児の一次救命処置（BLS）の場合，ガイドラインは以下のとおりである。

- 乳児のガイドラインは，概ね1歳未満の乳児に適用する。
- 小児のガイドラインは，概ね1歳から思春期までの小児に適用する。指導する際は，女性では乳房の発達，男性では腋毛が生えた時期を思春期と定義する。
- 思春期の徴候がある者と思春期を過ぎた者については，成人の一次救命処置ガイドラインに従う必要がある。

新生児の蘇生については，「第5章：新生児の蘇生」に記載し，通常，出生後の初回入院期間中のみの新生児に適用する。小児一次救命処置と二次救命処置ガイドラインは，退院後の新生児（生後＜30日）に適用される。

「新型コロナウイルス感染症ガイダンス」

他の専門家組織とともに，アメリカ心臓協会（AHA）は，新型コロナウイルス感染症（COVID-19）の疑い例または確定例の成人，小児および新生児における一次救命処置と二次救命処置の暫定ガイダンスを提供している。エビデンスとガイダンスがCOVID-19の状況に伴い変化し続けているため，この暫定ガイダンスを救急心血管治療（ECC）ガイドラインから切り離している。最新のガイダンスについては，AHAサイトを参照されたい[8]。

小児執筆委員会（Pediatric Writing Committee）の組織

小児執筆グループ（Pediatric Writing Group）を，集中治療専門医，心臓集中治療専門医，心臓病専門医，救急医療医，中毒学者，および看護師を含む小児科医で構成した。蘇生の専門知識を有することが認められたボランティアが，執筆グループの共同委員長により指名され，AHA ECC委員会によって選出される。AHAには，厳格な利益相反方針とガイドライン作成中のバイアスや不適切な影響のリスクを最小化するための手順がある[9]。指名に先立ち，執筆グループメンバーと査読者は，すべての商業的な関係と他の利益相反の可能性（知的財産など）を開示した。ガイドラインの変更につながる研究をしている執筆グループメンバーは，考察中にその相反を公表し，特定の推奨事項に関する投票を棄権するよう求めた。このプロセスについては，「第2章：エビデンス評価とガイドライン作成」に詳細に記載する。執筆グループメンバーの開示情報を，付録1に収載する。

方法論とエビデンスのレビュー

これらの小児ガイドラインは，ILCORとILCOR加盟団体を併せて実施した広範なエビデンス評価に基づくものである。3種類のエビデンスレビュー（システマティックレビュー，スコーピングレビュー，最新のエビデンス）をガイドライン2020プロセスに使用した[10,11]。ILCOR科学諮問

表1. 患者ケアにおける臨床上の戦略，介入，治療，または診断検査への推奨事項のクラスとエビデンスレベルの適用（2019年5月更新）*

推奨事項のクラス（強さ）
クラス1（強い）　　　　　　　　　　利益＞＞＞リスク
推奨事項文に適した表現例： • 推奨される • 適応／有用／有効／有益である • 実施／投与（など）すべきである • 比較に基づく有効性の表現例†： 　− 治療Bよりも治療／治療戦略Aが推奨される／適応である 　− 治療Bよりも治療Aを選択すべきである
クラス2a（中等度）　　　　　　　　　利益＞＞リスク
推奨事項文に適した表現例： • 妥当である • 有用／有効／有益でありうる • 比較に基づく有効性の表現例†： 　− 治療Bよりも治療／治療戦略Aがおそらく推奨される／適応である 　− 治療Bよりも治療Aを選択することが妥当である
クラス2b（弱い）　　　　　　　　　　利益≧リスク
推奨事項文に適した表現例： • 妥当としてよい／よいだろう • 考慮してもよい／よいだろう • 有用性／有効性は不明／不明確／不確実である，あるいは十分に確立されていない
クラス3：利益なし（中等度）　　　　　利益＝リスク **（一般にLOE AまたはBの使用に限る）**
推奨事項文に適した表現例： • 推奨しない • 適応／有用／有効／有益ではない • 実施／投与（など）すべきでない
クラス3：有害（強い）　　　　　　　　リスク＞利益
推奨事項文に適した表現例： • 有害な可能性がある • 有害となる • 合併症発生率／死亡率の上昇を伴う • 実施／投与（など）すべきでない

エビデンスレベル（質）‡
レベルA
• 複数のRCTから得られた質の高いエビデンス‡ • 質の高いRCTのメタアナリシス • 質の高い症例登録試験によって裏付けられた1件以上のRCT
レベルB-R　　　　　　　　　　　　　（無作為化）
• 1件以上のRCTから得られた質が中等度のエビデンス‡ • 質が中等度のRCTのメタアナリシス
レベルB-NR　　　　　　　　　　　　（非無作為化）
• 1件以上の綿密にデザインされ，適切に実施された非無作為化試験，観察研究，または症例登録試験から得られた質が中等度のエビデンス‡ • そのような試験のメタアナリシス
レベルC-LD　　　　　　　　　　　　（限定的なデータ）
• デザインまたは実施に限界がある無作為化または非無作為化観察研究または症例登録試験 • そのような試験のメタアナリシス • ヒトを対象にした生理学的試験または反応機構研究
レベルC-EO　　　　　　　　　　　　（専門家の見解）
• 臨床経験に基づく専門家の見解のコンセンサス

CORおよびLOEは個別に決定する（CORとLOEのあらゆる組み合わせが可能）。

LOE Cの推奨事項は，その推奨事項が弱いことを意味するわけではない。ガイドラインが扱っている重要な医療上の問題の多くは，臨床試験の対象となっていない。RCTが行われていなくても，特定の検査あるいは治療法の有用性／有効性について，臨床上非常に明確なコンセンサスが得られている場合がある。

* 介入の成果または結果を記述すべきである（臨床転帰の改善，または診断精度の向上，または予後情報の増加）。

† 比較に基づく有効性の推奨事項（COR 1および2a，LOE AおよびBのみ）に関しての推奨事項の裏付けとなる試験は，評価する治療または治療戦略を直接比較しているものでなければならない。

‡ 標準化され，広く用いられていて，望ましくは検証されている複数のエビデンス評価ツールを活用する，システマティックレビューについてはエビデンスレビュー委員会を設けるなど，質を評価する方法は進化している。

COR：推奨事項のクラス（Class of Recommendation），EO：専門家の見解（expert opinion），LD：限定的なデータ（limited data），LOE：エビデンスレベル（Level of Evidence），NR：非無作為化（nonrandomized），R：無作為化（randomized），RCT：無作為化比較試験（randomized controlled trial）。

委員会（Science Advisory Committee）委員長によるレビュー後，最新のエビデンスワークシートを『2020 ILCOR Consensus on CPR and ECC Science With Treatment Recommendations』の付録Cに収載した。[11a]　それぞれの結果はガイドラインの策定に使用した文献の記述として示した。このプロセスについては，「第2章：エビデンス評価とガイドライン作成」に詳細に記載する[12]。

推奨事項のクラスおよびエビデンスレベル

執筆グループは，すべての関連する現行の『AHA心肺蘇生と救急心血管治療のためのガイドライン（AHA Guidelines for Cardiopulmonary Resuscitation (CPR) and ECC）』とすべての関連する『2020 ILCOR Consensus on CPR and ECC Science With Treatment Recommendations』のエビデンスと推奨事項をレビューして，現行のガイドラインを見直す，修正する，もしくは廃止する必要があるか，または新規の推奨事項が必要かどうかを決定した。次に執筆グループは，推奨事項の原案を作成し，レビューし，承認して，推奨事項のクラス（COR，すなわち強さ）とエビデンスレベル（LOE，すなわち品質と確実性）をそれぞれに割り当てた。各CORとLOEの基準を表1に記載する。

ガイドラインの構成

ガイドライン2020は，特定のトピックや管理上の問題に関する情報を個々のモジュールにまとめている[13]。各モジュールの「ナレッジチャンク」には，AHAの標準的なCORとLOEの表記法に従っ

て推奨事項表を示す。推奨事項はCORの順序，すなわち利益の可能性が最も高い（クラス 1），次に利益の確実性が低い（クラス 2），最後に有害な可能性がある，または利益のない（クラス 3）の順に示される。CORに続き，推奨事項を，LOEを裏付ける確実性，すなわち，レベル A（高品質の無作為化比較試験）からレベル C-EO（専門家の見解）で順序付ける。この順序は，治療を提供すべき順序を反映するものではない。

簡潔な概略と短い「概要」を示し，重要な背景情報と包括的な管理概念や治療概念のある推奨事項の内容を説明する。「推奨事項の裏付けとなる解説」で，推奨事項を裏付ける根拠と重要な研究データを明らかにする。必要に応じてフローチャートまたは補助的な表を掲載した。すばやくアクセスして確認できるようにハイパーリンク付きの参考資料を提供する。

文書のレビューと承認

本ガイドラインを盲検下での査読のため，AHAが指名した対象分野の専門家5人に提出した。査読者のフィードバックを草案の形で，さらに最終的な形でガイドラインに含めた。本ガイドラインは，AHA科学諮問委員会調整委員会（AHA Science Advisory and Coordinating Committee）およびAHA実行委員会（AHA Executive Committee）による出版物の審査と承認を受けた。査読者の開示情報を，付録2に収載する。

略語

略語	意味／語句
ACLS	二次救命処置（advanced cardiovascular life support）
AED	自動体外式除細動器（automated external defibrillator）
ALS	二次救命処置（advanced life support）
AHA	アメリカ心臓協会（American Heart Association）
BLS	一次救命処置（basic life support）
COI	利益相反（conflict of interest）
COR	推奨事項のクラス（Class of Recommendation）
CPR	心肺蘇生（cardiopulmonary resuscitation）
ECC	救急心血管治療（emergency cardiovascular care）
ECLS	体外生命維持（extracorporeal life support）
ECMO	体外膜型人工肺（extracorporeal membrane oxygenation）
ECPR	体外循環補助を用いた心肺蘇生（extracorporeal cardiopulmonary resuscitation）
EO	専門家の見解（Expert Opinion）
ETI	気管挿管（endotracheal intubation）
FBAO	異物による気道閉塞（foreign body airway obstruction）
IHCA	院内心停止（in-hospital cardiac arrest）
ILCOR	国際蘇生連絡協議会（International Liaison Committee on Resuscitation）
LD	限定的なデータ（limited data）
LOE	エビデンスレベル（Level of Evidence）
MCS	機械的循環補助（mechanical circulatory support）
NR	非無作為化（nonrandomized）
OHCA	院外心停止（out-of-hospital cardiac arrest）
PALS	小児の二次救命処置（pediatric advanced life support）
PICO	集団，介入，比較，転帰（population, intervention, comparator, outcome）
無脈性VT	無脈性心室頻拍（pulseless ventricular tachycardia）
RCT	無作為化試験（randomized clinical trial）
ROSC	自己心拍再開（return of spontaneous circulation）
SGA	声門上器具（supraglottic airway）
TTM	目標体温管理（targeted temperature management）
VF	心室細動（ventricular fibrillation）

参考文献

1. Holmberg MJ, Ross CE, Fitzmaurice GM, Chan PS, Duval-Arnould J, Grossestreuer AV, Yankama T, Donnino MW, Andersen LW; American Heart Association's Get With The Guidelines-Resuscitation Investigators. Annual Incidence of Adult and Pediatric In-Hospital Cardiac Arrest in the United States. Circ Cardiovasc Qual Outcomes. 2019;12:e005580.
2. Atkins DL, Everson-Stewart S, Sears GK, Daya M, Osmond MH, Warden CR, Berg RA; Resuscitation Outcomes Consortium Investigators. Epidemiology and outcomes from out-of-hospital cardiac arrest in children: the Resuscitation Outcomes Consortium Epistry-Cardiac Arrest. Circulation. 2009;119:1484-1491. doi: 10.1161/CIRCULATIONAHA.108.802678
3. Knudson JD, Neish SR, Cabrera AG, Lowry AW, Shamszad P, Morales DL, Graves DE, Williams EA, Rossano JW. Prevalence and outcomes of pediatric in-hospital cardiopulmonary resuscitation in the United States: an analysis of the Kids' Inpatient Database*. Crit Care Med.2012;40:2940-2944. doi: 10.1097/CCM.0b013e31825feb3f
4. Virani SS, Alonso A, Benjamin EJ, Bittencourt MS, Callaway CW, Carson AP, Chamberlain AM, Chang AR, Cheng S, Delling FN, et al: on behalf of the American Heart Association Council on Epidemiology and Prevention Statistics Committee and Stroke Statistics Subcommittee. Heart disease and stroke statistics—2020 update: a report from the American Heart Association. Circulation. 2020;141:e139-e596. doi: 10.1161/CIR.0000000000000757
5. Matos RI, Watson RS, Nadkarni VM, Huang HH, Berg RA, Meaney PA, Carroll CL, Berens RJ, Praestgaard A, Weissfeld L, Spinella PC; American Heart Association's Get With The Guidelines-Resuscitation (Formerly the National Registry of Cardiopulmonary Resuscitation) Investigators. Duration of cardiopulmonary resuscitation and illness category impact survival and neurologic outcomes for in-hospital pediatric cardiac arrests. Circulation.2013;127:442-451. doi: 10.1161/CIRCULATIONAHA.112.125625
6. Girotra S, Spertus JA, Li Y, Berg RA, Nadkarni VM, Chan PS; American Heart Association Get With the Guidelines-Resuscitation Investigators. Survival trends in pediatric in-hospital cardiac arrests: an analysis from Get With the Guidelines-Resuscitation. Circ Cardiovasc Qual Outcomes.2013;6:42-49. doi: 10.1161/CIRCOUTCOMES.112.967968
7. Søreide E, Morrison L, Hillman K, Monsieurs K, Sunde K, Zideman D, Eisenberg M, Sterz F, Nadkarni VM, Soar J, Nolan JP; Utstein Formula for Survival Collaborators. The formula for survival in resuscitation. Resuscitation.2013;84:1487-1493. doi: 10.1016/j.resuscitation.2013.07.020
8. American Heart Association. CPR & ECC. https://cpr.heart.org/. Accessed June 19, 2020.
9. American Heart Association. Conflict of interest policy. https://www.heart.org/en/about-us/statements-and-policies/conflict-of-interest-policy. Accessed December 31, 2019.
10. International Liaison Committee on Resuscitation (ILCOR). Continuous evidence evaluation guidance and templates: 2020 evidence update process final. https://www.ilcor.org/documents/continuous-evidence-evaluation-guidance-and-templates. Accessed December 31, 2019.
11. Institute of Medicine (US) Committee of Standards for Systematic Reviews of Comparative Effectiveness Research. Finding What Works in Health Care: Standards for Systematic Reviews. Eden J, Levit L, Berg A, Morton S, eds. Washington, DC: The National Academies Press; 2011.
11a. Maconochie IK, Aickin R, Hazinski MF, Atkins DL, Bingham R, Couto TB, Guerguerian A-M, Nadkarni VM, Ng K-C, Nuthall GA, et al; on behalf of the Pediatric Life Support Collaborators. Pediatric life support: 2020 International Consensus on Cardiopulmonary Resuscitation and Emergency

Cardiovascular Care Science With Treatment Recommendations.Circulation. 2020;142 (suppl 1):S140-S184. doi: 10.1161/CIR.0000000000000894

12. Magid DJ, Aziz K, Cheng A, Hazinski MF, Hoover AV, Mahgoub M, Panchal AR, Sasson C, Topjian AA, Rodriguez AJ, et al. Part 2: evidence evaluation and guidelines development: 2020 American Heart Association Guidelines for Cardiopulmonary Resuscitation and Emergency Cardiovascular Care.Circulation. 2020;142 (suppl 2):S358-S365. doi: 10.1161/CIR.0000000000000898

13. Levine GN, O'Gara PT, Beckman JA, Al-Khatib SM, Birtcher KK, Cigarroa JE, de Las Fuentes L, Deswal A, Fleisher LA, Gentile F, Goldberger ZD, Hlatky MA, Joglar JA, Piano MR, Wijeysundera DN. Recent Innovations, Modifications, and Evolution of ACC/AHA Clinical Practice Guidelines: An Update for Our Constituencies: A Report of the American College of Cardiology/American Heart Association Task Force on Clinical Practice Guidelines. Circulation.2019;139:e879-e886. doi: 10.1161/CIR.0000000000000651

主要な概念

小児の心停止に関する疫学，病態生理学，および多く見られる病因は，成人および新生児の心停止とは異なっている。乳児や小児では，心停止の一次的原因が心臓そのものにないことが多い。むしろ，呼吸不全またはショックが進行した最終的な結果である。これらの患者では，心停止に先行してさまざまな悪化期間が認められ，その最終的な結果として心肺機能不全，徐脈，および心停止にいたる。先天性心疾患の小児において，心停止は心臓の原因疾患によることが多いものの，その病因は成人と異なっている。

小児 IHCA の予後はこの 20 年にわたり改善されてきた。その一部は早期の認知，質の高い CPR，心拍再開後の治療，および体外循環補助を用いた心肺蘇生（ECPR）の理由による[1,2]。大規模な多施設共同，病院内心停止登録である Get With The Guidelines Resuscitation Registry の最近の解析では，小児の退院にいたる心停止からの生存率が 2000 年に 19 %，2018 年には 38 %となった[2]。生存率は平均して 1 年に 0.67 %上昇してきたものの，その上昇は 2010 年以降に頭打ちとなっている[2]。心停止からの生存率を向上させるためには，研究と治療の新しい方向性が必要と考えられる。多くの心停止イベントが今も集中治療室（ICU）環境で生じているため，心停止リスクがある患者をより早く特定し，より高度の医療提供のレベルに移すことが推奨される[3]。

OHCA からの生存率は芳しくない状態である。多施設共同 OHCA 登録である Resuscitation Outcomes Consortium Epidemiological Registry の最近の解析では，2007～2012 年の小児 OHCA で退院にいたる年間生存率は，地域と患者の年齢に依存して 6.7～10.2 %の範囲となった[4]。これらの生存率には長期にわたる有意な変化がなく，他の国内登録（日本の登録，オーストラリアおよびニュージーランドの登録）のものとも一致した[5,6]。Resuscitation Outcomes Consortium Epidemiological Registry では，救急医療サービスによって目撃された心停止が多い地域と，バイスタンダーによる CPR 率がより高い地域で OHCA の生存率がより高く，これらの患者の早期の認知と早期の治療の重要性が強調された[4]。

小児の心停止からの生存率が上昇するにつれて，生存者の神経発達的，身体的，および感情的な予後により多くの焦点が移行している。最近の研究で，良好な予後を有する患者の 4 分の 1 に広範な認知障害があり，良好な予後を有すると報告された年長児の 85 %に特定の神経心理学的障害があることが明らかになった[7]。

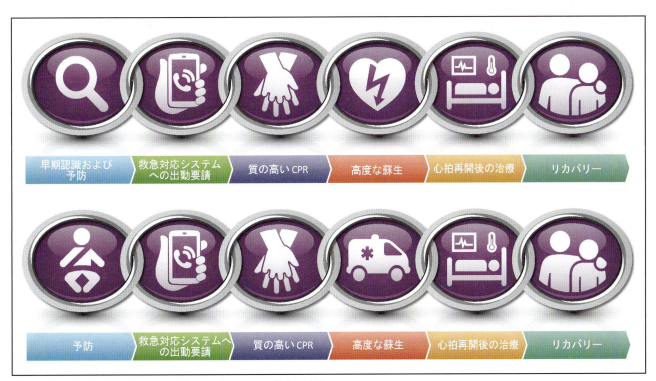

図 1. 院内（上）と院外（下）の心停止に備えた小児の救命の連鎖。
CPR = 心肺蘇生。

小児の救命の連鎖

これまで，心停止の治療では主として心停止そのものの管理に集中し，質の高いCPR，早期除細動，効果的なチームワークが強調されていた。しかし，予後の改善に極めて重要となる心停止前治療と心拍再開後治療が存在する。小児の心停止からの生存率が頭打ちになるにつれ，心停止の予防がより重要になっている。院外環境では，安全性イニシアチブ（例えば，二輪車のヘルメット着用法），乳幼児突然死の予防，市民救助者のCPR訓練，および救急医療への早期アクセスが含まれる。OHCAが発生した場合，早期のバイスタンダーによるCPRが予後の改善に極めて重要となる。院内環境での心停止の予防は，心臓の外科的治療を受けている新生児や，急性劇症型心筋炎，急性非代償性心不全，または肺高血圧を呈する患者のような心停止のリスクがある患者の早期の認識と早期の治療である。

心停止からの蘇生後に，心停止後症候群（脳機能障害，低心拍出量を伴う心機能障害，および虚血や再灌流傷害が認められることもある）の管理が，低血圧などの二次的損傷にいたる既知の要因を避けるために重要となる[8,9]。正確な神経学的予後予測は，養育者との話し合いや意思決定を進めるために重要である。最後に，心停止からの生存者における高リスクの神経発達障害を考慮すると，リハビリテーション評価および介入を目的とする早期の紹介が重要な点である。

心停止の管理におけるこれらのあらゆる面を明らかにするため，小児の救命の連鎖を更新した（図1）。個々のOHCAの救命の連鎖を作成して，OHCAとIHCAとの相違を区別している。OHCA連鎖とIHCA連鎖のいずれにも，短期および長期の治療評価に重点を置く回復の重要性を強調し，生存者とその家族を支援するため，6番目の鎖を追加した。両方の救命の連鎖では，救急対応システムへの通報後，直ちに質の高いCPRが開始される。近くに助けが得られる場合や携帯電話が利用できる場合，救急対応システムへの通報とCPRの開始がほぼ同時に起こり得る。しかし，院外環境で，携帯電話を利用できない単独の救助者は，助けを呼ぶ前に乳児と小児に対しCPR（胸骨圧迫－気道確保－人工呼吸）を開始するべきである。その理由として，呼吸停止が心停止の最も多い原因であり，近くに助けが得られない可能性が挙げられる。突然の卒倒を目撃した場合，早期除細動が救命になり得るため，救助者は利用できる自動体外式除細動器（AED）を使用する必要がある。

参考文献

1. Girotra S, Spertus JA, Li Y, Berg RA, Nadkarni VM, Chan PS; American Heart Association Get With the Guidelines-Resuscitation Investigators.Survival trends in pediatric in-hospital cardiac arrests: an analysis from Get With the Guidelines-Resuscitation.Circ Cardiovasc Qual Outcomes.2013;6:42-49. doi: 10.1161/CIRCOUTCOMES.112.967968
2. Holmberg MJ, Wiberg S, Ross CE, Kleinman M, Hoeyer-Nielsen AK, Donnino MW, Andersen LW. Trends in Survival After Pediatric In-Hospital Cardiac Arrest in the United States. Circulation.2019;140:1398-1408. doi: 10.1161/CIRCULATIONAHA.119.041667
3. Berg RA, Sutton RM, Holubkov R, Nicholson CE, Dean JM, Harrison R, Heidemann S, Meert K, Newth C, Moler F, Pollack M, Dalton H, Doctor A, Wessel D, Berger J, Shanley T, Carcillo J, Nadkarni VM; Eunice Kennedy Shriver National Institute of Child Health and Human Development Collaborative Pediatric Critical Care Research Network and for the American Heart Association's Get With the Guidelines-Resuscitation (formerly the National Registry of Cardiopulmonary Resuscitation) Investigators. Ratio of PICU versus ward cardiopulmonary resuscitation events is increasing. Crit Care Med.2013;41:2292-2297. doi: 10.1097/CCM.0b013e31828cf0c0
4. Fink EL, Prince DK, Kaltman JR, Atkins DL, Austin M, Warden C, Hutchison J, Daya M, Goldberg S, Herren H, Tijssen JA, Christenson J, Vaillancourt C, Miller R, Schmicker RH, Callaway CW; Resuscitation Outcomes Consortium. Unchanged pediatric out-of-hospital cardiac arrest incidence and survival rates with regional variation in North America. Resuscitation.2016;107:121-128. doi: 10.1016/j.resuscitation.2016.07.244
5. Kitamura T, Iwami T, Kawamura T, Nitta M, Nagao K, Nonogi H, Yonemoto N, Kimura T; Japanese Circulation Society Resuscitation Science Study Group. Nationwide improvements in survival from out-of-hospital cardiac arrest in Japan. Circulation.2012;126:2834-2843. doi: 10.1161/CIRCULATIONAHA.112.109496
6. Straney LD, Schlapbach LJ, Yong G, Bray JE, Millar J, Slater A, Alexander J, Finn J; Australian and New Zealand Intensive Care Society Paediatric Study Group. Trends in PICU Admission and Survival Rates in Children in Australia and New Zealand Following Cardiac Arrest. Pediatr Crit Care Med.2015;16:613-620. doi: 10.1097/PCC.0000000000000425
7. Slomine BS, Silverstein FS, Christensen JR, Page K, Holubkov R, Dean JM, Moler FW. Neuropsychological Outcomes of Children 1 Year After Pediatric Cardiac Arrest: Secondary Analysis of 2 Randomized Clinical Trials. JAMA Neurol. 2018;75:1502-1510. doi: 10.1001/jamaneurol.2018.2628
8. Topjian AA, de Caen A, Wainwright MS, Abella BS, Abend NS, Atkins DL, Bembea MM, Fink EL, Guerguerian AM, Haskell SE, Kilgannon JH, Lasa JJ, Hazinski MF. Pediatric Post-Cardiac Arrest Care: A Scientific Statement From the American Heart Association. Circulation.2019;140:e194-e233. doi: 10.1161/CIR.0000000000000697
9. Laverriere EK, Polansky M, French B, Nadkarni VM, Berg RA, Topjian AA. Association of Duration of Hypotension With Survival After Pediatric Cardiac Arrest. Pediatr Crit Care Med.2020;21:143-149. doi: 10.1097/PCC.0000000000002119

蘇生の順序

心停止の迅速な認識，質の高い胸骨圧迫の即時開始，および有効な換気の実施が，心停止の転帰を改善するために極めて重要である。市民救助者は，「生存の徴候」が認められない小児へのCPRの開始を遅延してはならない。CPRの開始が10秒以上遅れない限り，医療従事者は脈拍の有無の評価を検討してもよい。脈拍の有無を目的とした触診は，心停止の唯一の決定因子としても，胸骨圧迫の必要性を判断するうえも信頼できない。乳児や小児では，呼吸原性心停止が心原性心停止より多い。このため，小児の蘇生時には有効な換気が重要となる。CPRを開始する場合，順序は胸骨圧迫－気道確保－人工呼吸である。

質の高い CPR によって，重要臓器への血流が生じ，自己心拍再開（ROSC）の可能性が増大する。質の高い CPR の 5 つの主要な要素は，(1) 十分な胸骨圧迫の深さ，(2) 最適な胸骨圧迫のテンポ，(3) CPR の中断の最小化（すなわち，胸骨圧迫の割合または心停止に対し実施した胸骨圧迫時間の割合を最大にする），(4) 胸骨圧迫の合間に胸郭が十分に戻るようにする，(5) 過剰な換気の回避である。不十分な深さとテンポの圧迫，[1,2] 不完全な胸郭の戻り，[3] および多い換気回数[4,5]が小児の蘇生時によく見られる。

CPR の開始

CPR の開始に関する推奨事項

COR	LOE	推奨事項
1	C-LD	1. 市民救助者は，反応のない傷病者，正常に呼吸していない傷病者，および生存の徴候がない傷病者に対し CPR を開始すること。脈拍は確認しない[6-20]。
2a	C-LD	2. 生存の徴候がない乳児および小児には，医療従事者の場合，10 秒以内に脈拍を確認し，確実に脈拍を触知できない限り胸骨圧迫を開始するのが妥当である[21-23]。
2b	C-EO	3. 気道確保－人工呼吸－胸骨圧迫よりも，胸骨圧迫－気道確保－人工呼吸で CPR を開始するのが妥当と考えられる[24]。

「推奨事項の裏付けとなる解説」
1. 市民救助者は，脈拍の有無を確実に判定できない。[6-20]
2. 手動の脈拍チェックと「生存の徴候」とを比較した臨床試験は存在しない。しかし，成人と小児を対象とした研究では，訓練を受けた救助者による脈拍チェック時に高い誤判別率と有害な CPR の中断を認めた[21-23]。1 件の研究では，医療従事者による脈拍触診の正確さが 78 ％であり[21]，対する市民救助者による脈拍触診の正確さは 5 秒で 47 ％，10 秒で 73 ％ であった[6]。
3. 小児を対象とした 1 件の研究では，胸骨圧迫－気道確保－人工呼吸による補助呼吸の開始の遅れは，気道確保－人工呼吸－胸骨圧迫と比較してごくわずか（5.74 秒）なことを示した[24]。このエビデンスは確実性の低いものであるが，おそらく推奨の胸骨圧迫－気道確保－人工呼吸を続けることで補助呼吸の遅れが最小限となり，成人および小児での心停止の治療への一貫したアプローチが可能となる。

質の高い CPR の構成要素

質の高い CPR の構成要素に関する推奨事項

COR	LOE	推奨事項
1	B-NR	1. 心停止の乳児と小児には，補助呼吸を伴う胸骨圧迫による CPR を実施すべきである[25-29]。
1	B-NR	2. 乳児および小児に対し，バイスタンダーが補助呼吸の実施を望まない，または実施できない場合，救助者は胸骨圧迫のみを行うことを推奨する[27,28]。
1	C-EO	3. 圧迫のたびに胸郭が完全に元に戻るようにすること[2,3,30]。
2a	C-LD	4. 乳児および小児に対し，≈100～120 回/分の胸骨圧迫のテンポの使用が妥当である[31,32]。
2a	C-LD	5. 乳児および小児では，救助者が胸部を胸郭前後径の 3 分の 1 以上まで押し込む胸骨圧迫を実施するのが妥当である。胸郭前後径の 3 分の 1 は乳児で約 4 cm（1.5 インチ），小児で 5 cm（2 インチ）に相当する。小児が思春期を迎えた場合，成人用の胸骨圧迫の深さ（≧5～＜6 cm）を使用するのが妥当である[33-36]。
2a	C-EO	6. 医療従事者の場合，心リズムチェック（継続時間：＜ 10 秒，約 2 分ごと）の実施が妥当である。
2a	C-EO	7. CPR 中に，100 ％酸素で換気するのが妥当である。
2a	C-EO	8. 高度な気道確保器具を用いずに CPR を行う場合，救助者 1 人では胸骨圧迫と人工呼吸の比率 30:2 の実施が妥当であり，救助者 2 人では胸骨圧迫と人工呼吸の比率 15:2 の実施が妥当である[25]。
2b	C-LD	9. 高度な気道確保器具を挿入している乳児および小児の CPR を実施する場合は，年齢および臨床状態に応じて，2～3 秒ごとに 1 回（20～30 回/分）の呼吸数を目標とすることを妥当としてよい。これらの推奨事項を超える呼吸数は，血行動態に悪影響を及ぼす可能性がある[5]。

「推奨事項の裏付けとなる解説」
1. OHCA を経験した小児の大規模な観察研究では，胸骨圧迫－換気 CPR による最善の予後が示されているものの，OHCA を経験した乳児は蘇生法に関係なく予後不良になることが多い[25-29]。
2. OHCA を経験した小児の大規模な観察研究では，胸骨圧迫のみの CPR のほうがバイスタンダーによる CPR を受けていない場合より優れていることが示されているものの，OHCA を経験した乳児は予後不良になることが多い[27,28]。
3. 胸郭を完全に再拡張することで，CPR 時に心臓に戻る血流が改善し，それによって身体への血流が向上する。CPR 中の胸部への

寄りかかりの影響を評価する小児を対象とした研究はないものの，小児 CPR 時の寄りかかりは多く見られる[2,3]。小児を麻酔下で侵襲的にモニターした 1 件の観察研究では，寄りかかりによって心充満圧が上昇し，結果として洞調律中の冠動脈灌流圧が低下した[30]。

4. 小規模の観察研究では，小児 IHCA に対する CPR 時に，100 回/分以上の圧迫のテンポが収縮期および拡張期血圧の改善と関係していることを認めた[31]。1 件の小児 IHCA の多施設共同観察研究では，100〜120 回/分の胸骨圧迫のテンポでの収縮期血圧が 120 回/分を超えるテンポでの収縮期血圧よりも上昇したことを示した[32]。100 回/分未満のテンポでは，100〜120 回/分のテンポと比較して生存率が向上した。しかし，このより遅いカテゴリーのテンポ中央値は，約 95 回/分（すなわち，100 回/分に非常に近い値）であった[32]。

5. 3 件の身体計測学的研究では，胸腔内の臓器に損傷がない場合，小児の胸郭は胸郭前後径の 3 分の 1 まで圧迫し得ることを示している[33-35]。1 件の観察研究では，CPR 30 秒間値の 60 ％以上が小児 IHCA で 5 cm を超える平均胸骨圧迫深さに達する場合に，ROSC 率と 24 時間生存率の改善を認めた[36]。

6. 現行の推奨事項には，モニターまたは AED を利用できる場合に 2 分ごとの短い心リズムチェックが含まれている。

7. CPR 中のさまざまな吸入酸素濃度が乳児および小児の予後に及ぼす影響について記載したヒト試験はない。

8. 最適な胸骨圧迫と人工呼吸の比率は不明である。OHCA を経験した小児の大規模な観察研究では，胸骨圧迫のみの CPR と比較して，15:2 または 30:2 の比による胸骨圧迫-換気 CPR でより良好な転帰を示した[25]。

9. 挿管した小児患者を対象とした 1 件の小規模の多施設共同観察研究では，換気回数（1 歳未満の小児で 30 回/分以上，より年上の小児で 25 回/分以上）が ROSC 率と生存率の向上に関連することを認めた[5]。しかし，小児では換気回数の増加に伴い収縮期血圧が低下する。高度な気道確保器具を装着した小児での連続胸骨圧迫中の最適な換気回数は，限定的なデータに基づくものであるため，さらなる研究が必要である。

推奨事項 1 および 2 は，『2017 American Heart Association Focused Update on Pediatric Basic Life Support and Cardiopulmonary Resuscitation Quality: An Update to the American Heart Association Guidelines for Cardiopulmonary Resuscitation and Emergency Cardiovascular Care』で概説された[37]。

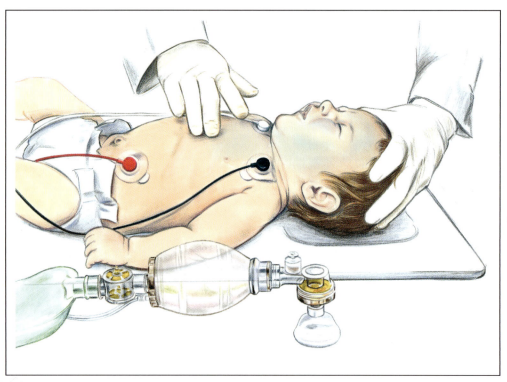

図 2. 2 本指圧迫法

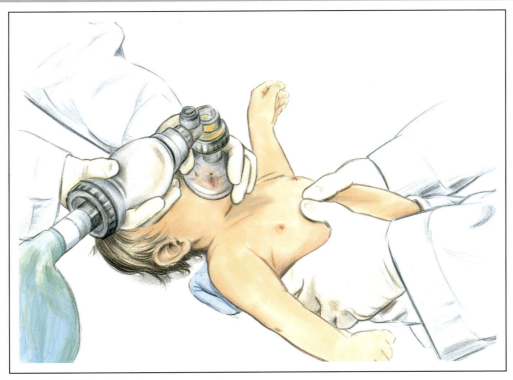

図 3. 胸郭包み込み両母指圧迫法 encircling hands compressions.

CPR 手技

COR	LOE	推奨事項
1	C-LD	1. 乳児に対し，救助者 1 人の場合（市民救助者，医療従事者のいずれでも），指 2 本で胸骨を圧迫する（図 2），または両手の親指 2 本を乳頭間線の真下に当てて胸骨を圧迫すること[38-41]。
1	C-LD	2. 乳児に対し，救助者 2 人が CPR を実施する場合，胸郭包み込み両母指圧迫法（図 3）が推奨される。救助者が傷病者の胸部に指を回すことができない場合は，胸骨を指 2 本で圧迫する[42-46]。
2b	C-LD	3. 小児では，片手圧迫法または両手圧迫法のいずれかを使用して胸骨圧迫するのが妥当と考えられる[47-49]。
2b	C-EO	4. 乳児で，救助者がガイドライン推奨事項の圧迫の深さ（胸郭前後径の 3 分の 1 以上）を達成できない場合，片手の手のひらの付け根を使用するのが妥当と考えられる。

「推奨事項の裏付けとなる解説」

1. 身体計測学的研究 1 件[38] と 放射線学的研究 3 件[39-41] では，指を乳頭間線の真下に当てる場合に，最適な心臓圧迫が生じることを認めた。小児を対象とした 1 件の観察研究で，胸骨中央部と比較して胸骨下部 3 分の 1 の範囲で胸骨圧迫を実施する場合に，血圧がより高くなることが明らかになった[41]。2 本指圧迫法については図 2 を参照。
2. システマティックレビューでは，2 本指圧迫法と比較する場合，胸郭包み込み両母指圧迫法は CPR の質を，特に圧迫深さに対して改善できることを示唆している[42,43]。しかし，最近のマネキンによる研究では，特に救助者が 1 人で実施する場合に，胸郭包み込み両母指圧迫法が胸骨圧迫の割合（胸骨圧迫を実施した心停止時間の割合）の低下[44]や，不完全な胸郭の戻り[45,46] に関連する可能性を示唆した。胸郭包み込み両母指圧迫法については，図 3 を参照。
3. 片手圧迫法または両手圧迫法が CPR を受けている小児に良好な予後をもたらすかどうかを判断するための小児用の臨床データは存在しない。マネキンによる研究では，両手による圧迫法が圧迫の深さの向上[47]，圧迫力の向上[48]，および救助者の疲労軽減[49] と関連した。
4. 乳児での片手圧迫法と胸郭包み込み両母指圧迫法を比較したヒト研究は存在しなかった。

CPR に適した支持面

COR	LOE	推奨事項
1	C-LD	1. IHCA 時に，可能な場合，ベッドの「CPR モード」を有効にしてマットレスの硬さを強める[50-53]。
2a	C-LD	2. 硬い表面上で胸骨圧迫を行うのが妥当である[53-59]。
2a	C-LD	3. IHCA 時にバックボードを使用して胸骨圧迫の深さを向上させるのが妥当である[53,55,56,60-63]。

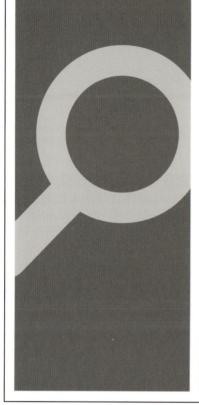
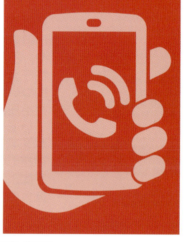
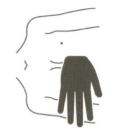

図 4. 市民救助者向けの小児の BLS。
AED：自動体外式除細動器，BLS：一次救命処置，CPR：心肺蘇生，EMS：救急医療サービス

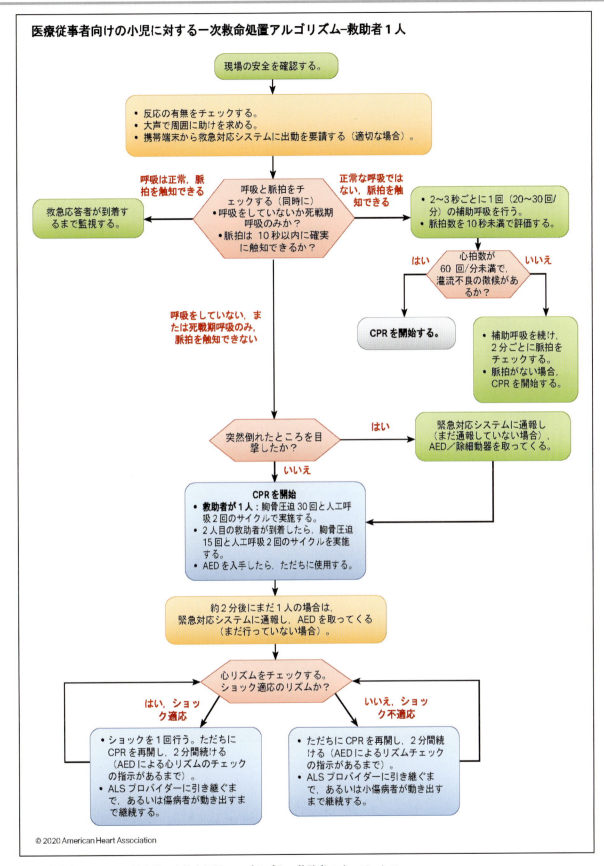

図 5. 医療従事者向けの小児に対する一次救命処置アルゴリズム—救助者 1 人。 Single Rescuer.
AED：自動体外式除細動器，ALS：二次救命処置，CPR：心肺蘇生，HR：心拍数

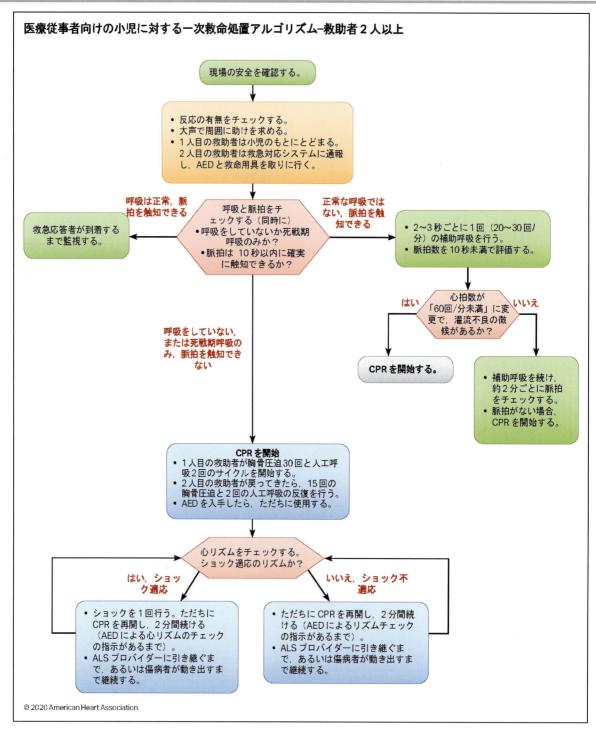

図6. 医療従事者向けの小児に対する一次救命処置アルゴリズム―救助者2人以上。2 or More Rescuers.
AED：自動体外式除細動器，ALS：二次救命処置，CPR：心肺蘇生，HR：心拍数

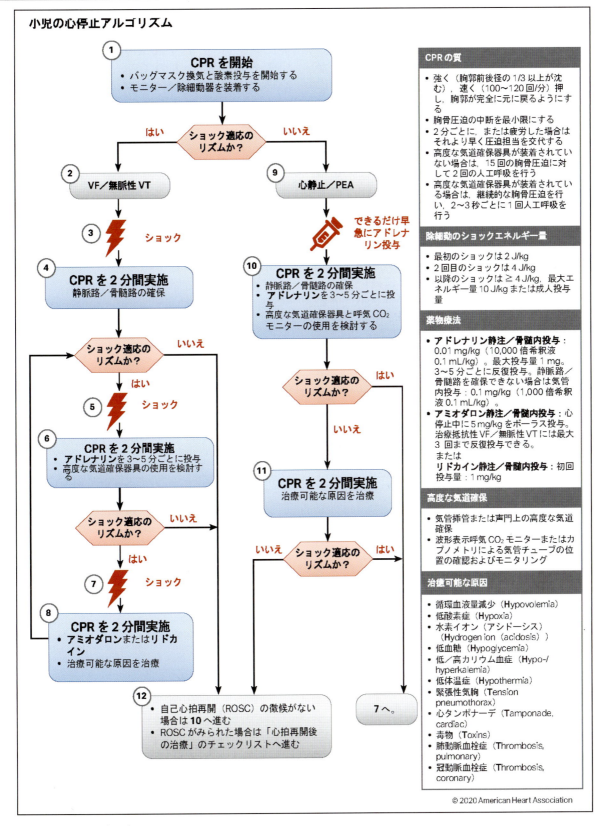

図7. 小児の心停止アルゴリズム。
ASAP：できるだけ早急に，CPR：心肺蘇生，HR：心拍数，PEA：無脈性電気活動，VF／無脈性VT：心室細動／無脈性心室頻拍

「推奨事項の裏付けとなる解説」

1. 「CPR モード」は一部の病院用ベッドで利用でき，CPR 時にマットレスを硬くする。マネキンモデルでは，マットレスの圧縮が全ての胸骨圧迫の深さの 12〜57 %範囲に及び，柔らかいマットレスで最大の圧縮になることを示した[50-53]。これは，胸骨変位の低下と有効な胸骨圧迫の深さの減少をもたらすことがある。
2. マネキンによる研究と 1 件の小児の症例集積研究では，CPR プロバイダーが総合的な胸骨圧迫の深さを増してマットレスの圧縮を補う場合，有効な胸骨圧迫の深さが柔らかい表面でも達成できることを示している[53-59]。
3. 6 件の研究報告[53,56,60-63]のメタアナリシスでは，マットレスまたはベッドの上に置いたマネキンで CPR を実施した場合，バックボードを使用することで胸骨圧迫の深さが 3 mm（95 % CI：1〜4 mm）向上することを示した。

気道確保

気道確保に関する推奨事項

COR	LOE	推奨事項
1	C-LD	1. 頸椎損傷が疑われない限り，頭部後屈―あご先挙上法を使用して気道を確保する[64]。
1	C-EO	2. 頸椎損傷が疑われる外傷患者には，頭部後屈をせずに下顎挙上法を使用して気道を確保する。
1	C-EO	3. 頸椎損傷が疑われる外傷患者で，下顎挙上法では気道確保ができない場合，頭部後屈―あご先挙上法を使用する。

「推奨事項の裏付けとなる解説」

1. 気道確保や気道開存を維持する理想的な方法を直接検討したデータはない。1 件の後向きコホート研究では，診断 MRI を受ける新生児と幼若乳児でさまざまな頭部後屈角度を評価し，回帰分析を基に気道開存の最大の割合が 144〜150 度の頭部後屈角度であることを見出した[64]。
2. 気道確保を目的に下顎挙上法と頭部後屈―あご先挙上法を比較評価する小児を対象とした研究は存在しないものの，下顎挙上法は気道を確保する有効な方法として広く認められている。この手技は頭部後屈―あご先挙上法と比較して頸部の動作を理論的に制限する。
3. 頸椎損傷が疑われる外傷患者において頭部後屈―あご先挙上法の気道確保に対する影響を評価している小児を対象とした研究は存在しない。しかし，プロバイダーが気道を確保できず，下顎挙上法を用いて有効な換気を実施する場合，気道開存の重要性を考慮すると，頭部後屈―あご先挙上法の使用が推奨される。

図 4，5，6，および 7 に，市民救助者向けの小児 BLS の解説画像，現行の医療従事者向けの小児に対する BLS アルゴリズム，救助者 1 人の CPR と救助者 2 人の CPR，および現行の小児の心停止に対するアルゴリズムを示す。

参考文献

1. Niles DE, Duval-Arnould J, Skellett S, Knight L, Su F, Raymond TT, Sweberg T, Sen AI, Atkins DL, Friess SH, de Caen AR, Kurosawa H, Sutton RM, Wolfe H, Berg RA, Silver A, Hunt EA, Nadkarni VM; pediatric Resuscitation Quality (pediRES-Q) Collaborative Investigators. Characterization of Pediatric In-Hospital Cardiopulmonary Resuscitation Quality Metrics Across an International Resuscitation Collaborative. Pediatr Crit Care Med.2018;19:421-432. doi: 10.1097/PCC.0000000000001520
2. Sutton RM, Niles D, Nysaether J, Abella BS, Arbogast KB, Nishisaki A, Maltese MR, Donoghue A, Bishnoi R, Helfaer MA, Myklebust H, Nadkarni V. Quantitative analysis of CPR quality during in-hospital resuscitation of older children and adolescents. Pediatrics.2009;124:494-499. doi: 10.1542/peds.2008-1930
3. Niles D, Nysaether J, Sutton R, Nishisaki A, Abella BS, Arbogast K, Maltese MR, Berg RA, Helfaer M, Nadkarni V. Leaning is common during in-hospital pediatric CPR, and decreased with automated corrective feedback. Resuscitation.2009;80:553-557. doi: 10.1016/j.resuscitation.2009.02.012
4. McInnes AD, Sutton RM, Orioles A, Nishisaki A, Niles D, Abella BS, Maltese MR, Berg RA, Nadkarni V. The first quantitative report of ventilation rate during in-hospital resuscitation of older children and adolescents. Resuscitation.2011;82:1025-1029. doi: 10.1016/j.resuscitation.2011.03.020
5. Sutton RM, Reeder RW, Landis WP, Meert KL, Yates AR, Morgan RW, Berger JT, Newth CJ, Carcillo JA, McQuillen PS, Harrison RE, Moler FW, Pollack MM, Carpenter TC, Notterman DA, Holubkov R, Dean JM, Nadkarni VM, Berg RA; Eunice Kennedy Shriver National Institute of Child Health and Human Development Collaborative Pediatric Critical Care Research Network (CPCCRN). Ventilation Rates and Pediatric In-Hospital Cardiac Arrest Survival Outcomes. Crit Care Med.2019;47:1627-1636. doi: 10.1097/CCM.0000000000003898
6. Bahr J, Klingler H, Panzer W, Rode H, Kettler D. Skills of lay people in checking the carotid pulse. Resuscitation.1997;35:23-26. doi: 10.1016/s0300-9572(96)01092-1
7. Brearley S, Shearman CP, Simms MH. Peripheral pulse palpation: an unreliable physical sign. Ann R Coll Surg Engl. 1992;74:169-171.
8. Cavallaro DL, Melker RJ. Comparison of two techniques for detecting cardiac activity in infants. Crit Care Med.1983;11:189-190. doi: 10.1097/00003246-198303000-00009
9. Inagawa G, Morimura N, Miwa T, Okuda K, Hirata M, Hiroki K. A comparison of five techniques for detecting cardiac activity in infants. Paediatr Anaesth. 2003;13:141-146. doi: 10.1046/j.1460-9592.2003.00970.x
10. Kamlin CO, O'Donnell CP, Everest NJ, Davis PG, Morley CJ. Accuracy of clinical assessment of infant heart rate in the delivery room. Resuscitation.2006;71:319-321. doi: 10.1016/j.resuscitation.2006.04.015
11. Lee CJ, Bullock LJ. Determining the pulse for infant CPR: time for a change? Mil Med. 1991;156:190-193.
12. Mather C, O'Kelly S. The palpation of pulses. Anaesthesia.1996;51:189-191. doi: 10.1111/j.1365-2044.1996.tb07713.x
13. Ochoa FJ, Ramalle-Gómara E, Carpintero JM, García A, Saralegui I. Competence of health professionals to check the carotid pulse. Resuscitation.1998;37:173-175. doi: 10.1016/s0300-9572(98)00055-0
14. Owen CJ, Wyllie JP. Determination of heart rate in the baby at birth. Resuscitation.2004;60:213-217. doi: 10.1016/j.resuscitation.2003.10.002
15. Sarti A, Savron F, Casotto V, Cuttini M. Heartbeat assessment in infants: a comparison of four clinical methods. Pediatr Crit Care Med.2005;6:212-215. doi: 10.1097/01.PCC.0000154952.59176.E0
16. Sarti A, Savron F, Ronfani L, Pelizzo G, Barbi E. Comparison of three sites to check the pulse and count heart rate in hypotensive infants. Paediatr Anaesth.2006;16:394-398. doi: 10.1111/j.1460-9592.2005.01803.x
17. Tanner M, Nagy S, Peat JK. Detection of infant's heart beat/pulse by caregivers: a comparison of 4 methods. J Pediatr.2000;137:429-430. doi: 10.1067/mpd.2000.107188
18. Whitelaw CC, Goldsmith LJ. Comparison of two techniques for determining the presence of a pulse in an infant. Acad Emerg Med.1997;4:153-154. doi: 10.1111/j.1553-2712.1997.tb03725.x

19. Dick WF, Eberle B, Wisser G, Schneider T. The carotid pulse check revisited: what if there is no pulse? Crit Care Med. 2000;28 (suppl):N183-N185. doi: 10.1097/00003246-200011001-00002
20. Eberle B, Dick WF, Schneider T, Wisser G, Doetsch S, Tzanova I. Checking the carotid pulse check: diagnostic accuracy of first responders in patients with and without a pulse. Resuscitation.1996;33:107-116. doi: 10.1016/s0300-9572(96)01016-7
21. Tibballs J, Russell P. Reliability of pulse palpation by healthcare personnel to diagnose paediatric cardiac arrest. Resuscitation.2009;80:61-64. doi: 10.1016/j.resuscitation.2008.10.002
22. Tibballs J, Weeranatna C. The influence of time on the accuracy of healthcare personnel to diagnose paediatric cardiac arrest by pulse palpation. Resuscitation.2010;81:671-675. doi: 10.1016/j.resuscitation.2010.01.030
23. O'Connell KJ, Keane RR, Cochrane NH, Sandler AB, Donoghue AJ, Kerrey BT, Myers SR, Vazifedan T, Mullan PC. Pauses in compressions during pediatric CPR: Opportunities for improving CPR quality. Resuscitation.2019;145:158-165. doi: 10.1016/j.resuscitation.2019.08.015
24. Lubrano R, Cecchetti C, Bellelli E, Gentile I, Loayza Levano H, Orsini F, Bertazzoni G, Messi G, Rugolotto S, Pirozzi N, Elli M. Comparison of times of intervention during pediatric CPR maneuvers using ABC and CAB sequences: a randomized trial. Resuscitation.2012;83:1473-1477. doi: 10.1016/j.resuscitation.2012.04.011
25. Kitamura T, Iwami T, Kawamura T, Nagao K, Tanaka H, Nadkarni VM, Berg RA, Hiraide A; implementation working group for All-Japan Utstein Registry of the Fire and Disaster Management Agency. Conventional and chest-compression-only cardiopulmonary resuscitation by bystanders for children who have out-of-hospital cardiac arrests: a prospective, nationwide, population-based cohort study. Lancet.2010;375:1347-1354. doi: 10.1016/S0140-6736(10)60064-5
26. Goto Y, Maeda T, Goto Y. Impact of dispatcher-assisted bystander cardiopulmonary resuscitation on neurological outcomes in children with out-of-hospital cardiac arrests: a prospective, nationwide, population-based cohort study. J Am Heart Assoc. 2014;3:e000499. doi: 10.1161/JAHA.113.000499
27. Naim MY, Burke RV, McNally BF, Song L, Griffis HM, Berg RA, Vellano K, Markenson D, Bradley RN, Rossano JW. Association of Bystander Cardiopulmonary Resuscitation With Overall and Neurologically Favorable Survival After Pediatric Out-of-Hospital Cardiac Arrest in the United States: A Report From the Cardiac Arrest Registry to Enhance Survival Surveillance Registry. JAMA Pediatr. 2017;171:133-141. doi: 10.1001/jamapediatrics.2016.3643
28. Fukuda T, Ohashi-Fukuda N, Kobayashi H, Gunshin M, Sera T, Kondo Y, Yahagi N. Conventional Versus Compression-Only Versus No-Bystander Cardiopulmonary Resuscitation for Pediatric Out-of-Hospital Cardiac Arrest. Circulation.2016;134:2060-2070. doi: 10.1161/CIRCULATIONAHA.116.023831
29. Ashoor HM, Lillie E, Zarin W, Pham B, Khan PA, Nincic V, Yazdi F, Ghassemi M, Ivory J, Cardoso R, Perkins GD, de Caen AR, Tricco AC; ILCOR Basic Life Support Task Force. Effectiveness of different compression-to-ventilation methods for cardiopulmonary resuscitation: A systematic review. Resuscitation.2017;118:112-125. doi: 10.1016/j.resuscitation.2017.05.032
30. Glatz AC, Nishisaki A, Niles DE, Hanna BD, Eilevstjonn J, Diaz LK, Gillespie MJ, Rome JJ, Sutton RM, Berg RA, Nadkarni VM. Sternal wall pressure comparable to leaning during CPR impacts intrathoracic pressure and haemodynamics in anaesthetized children during cardiac catheterization. Resuscitation.2013;84:1674-1679. doi: 10.1016/j.resuscitation.2013.07.010
31. Sutton RM, French B, Nishisaki A, Niles DE, Maltese MR, Boyle L, Stavland M, Eilevstjønn J, Arbogast KB, Berg RA, et al. American Heart Association cardiopulmonary resuscitation quality targets are associated with improved arterial blood pressure during pediatric cardiac arrest. Resuscitation.2013;84:168-172. doi: 10.1016/j.resuscitation.2012.08.335
32. Sutton RM, Reeder RW, Landis W, Meert KL, Yates AR, Berger JT, Newth CJ, Carcillo JA, McQuillen PS, Harrison RE, Moler FW, Pollack MM, Carpenter TC, Notterman DA, Holubkov R, Dean JM, Nadkarni VM, Berg RA; Eunice Kennedy Shriver National Institute of Child Health and Human Development Collaborative Pediatric Critical Care Research Network (CPCCRN) Investigators. Chest compression rates and pediatric in-hospital cardiac arrest survival outcomes. Resuscitation.2018;130:159-166. doi: 10.1016/j.resuscitation.2018.07.015
33. Kao PC, Chiang WC, Yang CW, Chen SJ, Liu YP, Lee CC, Hsidh MJ, Ko PC, Chen SC, Ma MH. What is the correct depth of chest compression for infants and children? A radiological study. Pediatrics.2009;124:49-55. doi: 10.1542/peds.2008-2536
34. Sutton RM, Niles D, Nysaether J, Arbogast KB, Nishisaki A, Maltese MR, Bishnoi R, Helfaer MA, Nadkarni V, Donoghue A. Pediatric CPR quality monitoring: analysis of thoracic anthropometric data. Resuscitation.2009;80:1137-1141. doi: 10.1016/j.resuscitation.2009.06.031
35. Braga MS, Dominguez TE, Pollock AN, Niles D, Meyer A, Myklebust H, Nysaether J, Nadkarni V. Estimation of optimal CPR chest compression depth in children by using computer tomography. Pediatrics.2009;124:e69-e74. doi: 10.1542/peds.2009-0153
36. Sutton RM, French B, Niles DE, Donoghue A, Topjian AA, Nishisaki A, Leffelman J, Wolfe H, Berg RA, Nadkarni VM, et al. 2010 American Heart Association recommended compression depths during pediatric in-hospital resuscitations are associated with survival. Resuscitation. 2014;85:1179-1184. doi: 10.1016/j.resuscitation.2014.05.007
37. Atkins DL, de Caen AR, Berger S, Samson RA, Schexnayder SM, Joyner BL Jr, Bigham BL, Niles DE, Duff JP, Hunt EA, Meaney PA. 2017 American Heart Association Focused Update on Pediatric Basic Life Support and Cardiopulmonary Resuscitation Quality: An Update to the American Heart Association Guidelines for Cardiopulmonary Resuscitation and Emergency Cardiovascular Care. Circulation.2018;137:e1-e6. doi: 10.1161/CIR.0000000000000540
38. Clements F, McGowan J. Finger position for chest compressions in cardiac arrest in infants. Resuscitation.2000;44:43-46. doi: 10.1016/s0300-9572(99)00165-3
39. Finholt DA, Kettrick RG, Wagner HR, Swedlow DB. The heart is under the lower third of the sternum. Implications for external cardiac massage. Am J Dis Child. 1986;140:646-649. doi: 10.1001/archpedi.1986.02140210044022
40. Phillips GW, Zideman DA. Relation of infant heart to sternum: its significance in cardiopulmonary resuscitation. Lancet.1986;1:1024-1025. doi: 10.1016/s0140-6736(86)91284-5
41. Orlowski JP. Optimum position for external cardiac compression in infants and young children. Ann Emerg Med.1986;15:667-673. doi: 10.1016/s0196-0644(86)80423-1
42. Douvanas A, Koulouglioti C, Kalafati M. A comparison between the two methods of chest compression in infant and neonatal resuscitation: a review according to 2010 CPR guidelines. J Matern Fetal Neonatal Med. 2018;31:805-816. doi: 10.1080/14767058.2017.1295953
43. Lee JE, Lee J, Oh J, Park CH, Kang H, Lim TH, Yoo KH. Comparison of two-thumb encircling and two-finger technique during infant cardiopulmonary resuscitation with single rescuer in simulation studies: a systematic review and meta-analysis. Medicine (Baltimore). 2019;98:e17853. doi: 10.1097/MD.0000000000017853
44. Lee SY, Hong JY, Oh JH, Son SH. The superiority of the two-thumb over the two-finger technique for single-rescuer infant cardiopulmonary resuscitation. Eur J Emerg Med.2018;25:372-376. doi: 10.1097/MEJ.0000000000000461
45. Tsou JY, Kao CL, Chang CJ, Tu YF, Su FC, Chi CH. Biomechanics of two-thumb versus two-finger chest compression for cardiopulmonary resuscitation in an infant manikin model. Eur J Emerg Med.2020;27:132-136. doi: 10.1097/MEJ.0000000000000631
46. Pellegrino JL, Bogumil D, Epstein JL, Burke RV. Two-thumb-encircling advantageous for lay responder infant CPR: a randomised manikin study. Arch Dis Child. 2019;104:530-534. doi: 10.1136/archdischild-2018-314893
47. Kim MJ, Lee HS, Kim S, Park YS. Optimal chest compression technique for paediatric cardiac arrest victims. Scand J Trauma Resusc Emerg Med. 2015;23:36. doi: 10.1186/s13049-015-0118-y
48. Stevenson AG, McGowan J, Evans AL, Graham CA. CPR for children: one hand or two? Resuscitation.2005;64:205-208. doi: 10.1016/j.resuscitation.2004.07.012
49. Peska E, Kelly AM, Kerr D, Green D. One-handed versus two-handed chest compressions in paediatric cardio-pulmonary resuscitation. Resuscitation.2006;71:65-69. doi: 10.1016/j.resuscitation.2006.02.007
50. Lin Y, Wan B, Belanger C, Hecker K, Gilfoyle E, Davidson J, Cheng A. Reducing the impact of intensive care unit mattress compressibility during CPR: a simulation-based study. Adv Simul (Lond). 2017;2:22. doi: 10.1186/s41077-017-0057-y
51. Noordergraaf GJ, Paulussen IW, Venema A, van Berkom PF, Woerlee PH, Scheffer GJ, Noordergraaf A. The impact of compliant surfaces on in-hospital chest compressions: effects of common mattresses and a backboard. Resuscitation.2009;80:546-552. doi: 10.1016/j.resuscitation.2009.03.023
52. Oh J, Chee Y, Song Y, Lim T, Kang H, Cho Y. A novel method to decrease mattress compression during CPR using a mattress compression cover and a vacuum pump. Resuscitation.2013;84:987-991. doi: 10.1016/j.resuscitation.2012.12.027

53. Song Y, Oh J, Lim T, Chee Y. A new method to increase the quality of cardiopulmonary resuscitation in hospital. Conf Proc IEEE Eng Med Biol Soc. 2013;2013:469-472. doi: 10.1109/EMBC.2013.6609538
54. Beesems SG, Koster RW. Accurate feedback of chest compression depth on a manikin on a soft surface with correction for total body displacement. Resuscitation.2014;85:1439-1443. doi: 10.1016/j.resuscitation.2014.08.005
55. Nishisaki A, Maltese MR, Niles DE, Sutton RM, Urbano J, Berg RA, Nadkarni VM. Backboards are important when chest compressions are provided on a soft mattress. Resuscitation.2012;83:1013-1020. doi: 10.1016/j.resuscitation.2012.01.016
56. Sato H, Komasawa N, Ueki R, Yamamoto N, Fujii A, Nishi S, Kaminoh Y. Backboard insertion in the operating table increases chest compression depth: a manikin study. J Anesth.2011;25:770-772. doi: 10.1007/s00540-011-1196-2
57. Lee S, Oh J, Kang H, Lim T, Kim W, Chee Y, Song Y, Ahn C, Cho JH. Proper target depth of an accelerometer-based feedback device during CPR performed on a hospital bed: a randomized simulation study. Am J Emerg Med. 2015;33:1425-1429. doi: 10.1016/j.ajem.2015.07.010
58. Oh J, Song Y, Kang B, Kang H, Lim T, Suh Y, Chee Y. The use of dual accelerometers improves measurement of chest compression depth. Resuscitation.2012;83:500-504. doi: 10.1016/j.resuscitation.2011.09.028
59. Ruiz de Gauna S, González-Otero DM, Ruiz J, Gutiérrez JJ, Russell JK. A feasibility study for measuring accurate chest compression depth and rate on soft surfaces using two accelerometers and spectral analysis. Biomed Res Int. 2016;2016:6596040. doi: 10.1155/2016/6596040
60. Andersen LØ, Isbye DL, Rasmussen LS. Increasing compression depth during manikin CPR using a simple backboard. Acta Anaesthesiol Scand. 2007;51:747-750. doi: 10.1111/j.1399-6576.2007.01304.x
61. Fischer EJ, Mayrand K, Ten Eyck RP. Effect of a backboard on compression depth during cardiac arrest in the ED: a simulation study. Am J Emerg Med.2016;34:274-277. doi: 10.1016/j.ajem.2015.10.035
62. Perkins GD, Smith CM, Augre C, Allan M, Rogers H, Stephenson B, Thickett DR. Effects of a backboard, bed height, and operator position on compression depth during simulated resuscitation. Intensive Care Med.2006;32:1632-1635. doi: 10.1007/s00134-006-0273-8
63. Sanri E, Karacabey S. The Impact of Backboard Placement on Chest Compression Quality: A Mannequin Study. Prehosp Disaster Med. 2019;34:182-187. doi: 10.1017/S1049023X19000153
64. Bhalala US, Hemani M, Shah M, Kim B, Gu B, Cruz A, Arunachalam P, Tian E, Yu C, Punnoose J, Chen S, Petrillo C, Brown A, Munoz K, Kitchen G, Lam T, Bosemani T, Huisman TA, Allen RH, Acharya S. Defining Optimal Head-Tilt Position of Resuscitation in Neonates and Young Infants Using Magnetic Resonance Imaging Data. PLoS One.2016;11:e0151789. doi: 10.1371/journal.pone.0151789

CPR時の高度な気道確保

ほとんどの小児の心停止は，呼吸の悪化によって引き起こされる。気道確保と有効な換気が小児の蘇生に不可欠である。大多数の患者はバッグマスク換気による換気に成功するものの，この方法には胸骨圧迫の中断が必要であり，誤嚥および圧外傷のリスクを伴う。

声門上器具（SGA）の留置や気管挿管（ETI）などの高度な気道確保器具は，換気を改善し，誤嚥リスクを低減する可能性があり，継続的な胸骨圧迫の実施が可能である。しかし，気道確保器具の留置は胸骨圧迫を中断する可能性や，装置の位置ずれを生じる可能性がある。高度な気道確保器具の留置には専門の器材や熟練したプロバイダーが必要であり，小児への挿管を日常的に行っていない専門家にとって困難な場合がある。

CPR時の高度な気道確保に関する推奨事項

COR	LOE	推奨事項
2a	C-LD	1. 院外で心停止を起こした小児の管理において，バッグマスク換気の使用は，高度な気道確保（SGAとETI）と比較して妥当である[1-4]。

「推奨事項の裏付けとなる解説」

1. 臨床試験1件と傾向マッチ法による2件の後ろ向き研究では，ETIとバッグマスク換気がOHCAの小児患者において良好な神経機能の生存率と生存退院は，同程度であることを示した[1-3]。傾向マッチ法による後ろ向き研究でも，OHCAが全ての小児でSGAとバッグマスク換気とを比較する場合，良好な神経機能と生存退院を伴う同程度の生存率を示した[2,3]。SGAの転帰とETIの転帰との間に差を認めなかった[2,3]。IHCAの管理で，バッグマスク換気の転帰とETIの転帰を比較するためのデータは限定的であり[4]，SGAに関する病院ベースの研究は存在しない。IHCAでの高度な気道確保器具の使用に関する推奨事項を裏付けるデータは不十分である。早期の高度な気道確保が有益となる具体的な状況や集団が存在する可能性がある。

この推奨事項は，『2019 American Heart Association Focused Update on Pediatric Advanced Life Support: An Update to the American Heart Association Guidelines for Cardiopulmonary Resuscitation and Emergency Cardiovascular Care』で概説された[5]。

参考文献

1. Gausche M, Lewis RJ, Stratton SJ, Haynes BE, Gunter CS, Goodrich SM, Poore PD, McCollough MD, Henderson DP, Pratt FD, et al. Effect of out-of-hospital pediatric endotracheal intubation on survival and neurological outcome: a controlled clinical trial. JAMA.2000;283:783-790.
2. Hansen ML, Lin A, Eriksson C, Daya M, McNally B, Fu R, Yanez D, Zive D, Newgard C; CARES surveillance group. A comparison of pediatric airway management techniques during out-of-hospital cardiac arrest using the CARES database. Resuscitation.2017;120:51-56. doi: 10.1016/j.resuscitation.2017.08.015
3. Ohashi-Fukuda N, Fukuda T, Doi K, Morimura N. Effect of prehospital advanced airway management for pediatric out-of-hospital cardiac arrest. Resuscitation.2017;114:66-72. doi: 10.1016/j.resuscitation.2017.03.002
4. Andersen LW, Raymond TT, Berg RA, Nadkarni VM, Grossestreuer AV, Kurth T, Donnino MW; American Heart Association's Get With The Guidelines-Resuscitation Investigators. Association Between Tracheal Intubation During Pediatric In-Hospital Cardiac Arrest and Survival. JAMA.2016;316:1786-1797. doi: 10.1001/jama.2016.14486
5. Duff JP, Topjian AA, Berg MD, Chan M, Haskell SE, Joyner BL Jr, Lasa JJ, Ley SJ, Raymond TT, Sutton RM, Hazinski MF, Atkins DL. 2019 American Heart Association Focused Update on Pediatric Advanced Life Support: An Update to the American Heart Association Guidelines for Cardiopulmonary Resuscitation and Emergency Cardiovascular Care.Circulation.2019;140:e904-e914. doi: 10.1161/CIR.0000000000000731

CPR中の薬物投与

アドレナリンなどの血管作用薬を心停止中に使用して冠動脈灌流を最適化し、脳灌流を維持することで自己心拍を再開できるが、投与の有益性と最適なタイミングは不明である[1,2]。抗不整脈薬は、除細動後の心室細動（VF）の再発と無脈性心室頻拍（無脈性VT）のリスクを低減し、除細動の成功を向上する可能性がある。炭酸水素ナトリウムとカルシウムのルーチン使用を裏付ける現行のデータはない[3-7]。しかし、電解質不均衡やある種の薬物中毒など、これらの投与が必要な特定の状況が存在する。

小児に対する薬物投与は体重に基づくため、緊急時に体重を得るのが困難なことが多い。実体重を得られない場合に、体重を推定する方法が多数存在する[8]。

心停止中の薬物投与

心停止中の薬物投与に関する推奨事項

COR	LOE	推奨事項
2a	C-LD	1. 小児患者の場合、どのような状況でも、アドレナリンを投与するのが妥当である。IV/IOが気管チューブ（ETT）による投与よりも望ましい[2,9-11]。
2a	C-LD	2. 小児患者の場合、どのような状況でも、胸骨圧迫の開始から5分以内に初回投与量のアドレナリンを投与することが妥当である[12-16]。
2a	C-LD	3. 小児患者の場合、どのような状況でも、ROSCに達するまでアドレナリンを3～5分ごとに投与することが妥当である[17,18]。
2b	C-LD	4. ショック治療抵抗性VF／無脈性VTに対しては、アミオダロンまたはリドカインを用いてもよい[19,20]。
3: 有害	B-NR	5. 炭酸水素ナトリウムのルーチン投与は、高カリウム血症またはナトリウムチャネル遮断薬（例えば、三環系抗うつ薬）中毒がない場合の小児の心停止に対し推奨されない[5-7,21-25]。
3: 有害	B-NR	6. カルシウムのルーチン投与は、低カルシウム血症、カルシウムチャネル遮断薬の過量投与、高マグネシウム血症、高カリウム血症が判明していない小児の心肺停止で、推奨されない[3,4,23]。

「推奨事項の裏付けとなる解説」

1. 任意の状況でアドレナリン投与とアドレナリンの不投与を比較した小児のデータは限定的である。小児65名を対象としたOHCA研究で、患者12名は投与経路がないためアドレナリン投与を受けずに、1児のみがROSCに至った[2]。スポーツまたは運動中に心停止した9児を対象とするOHCA研究では、生存率が67%で、内83%がアドレナリン投与を受けなかった。すべての生存者は、早期の胸骨圧迫（5分以内）と早期の除細動（10分以内）を施された。初期心停止リズムがショック適応のリズムであった[9]。可能であれば、アドレナリンの静脈内／骨髄内（IV/IO）投与のほうがETT投与よりも望ましい[10,11]。

2. 初期のショック非適応リズムに対してアドレナリンの投与を受けたIHCAの小児の後ろ向き観察研究1件で、アドレナリンの投与が1分間遅れるたびに、ROSC、24時間生存率、生存退院率、良好な神経学的転帰を伴う生存率が有意に低下することが明らかになった[12]。CPRから5分以内にアドレナリンが投与された患者は、CPR開始から5分を超えてからアドレナリンが投与された患者よりも生存退院率が高い傾向が強かった[12]。4件の小児OHCAの観察研究では、アドレナリン投与が早期であるほどROSC率[13,14]、ICU入室生存率[14]、生存退院率[14,16]、および30日生存率[15]が上昇することを明らかにした。

3. 1件の観察研究では、5分未満の間隔でアドレナリン投与を受けた群における1年時点の生存率の上昇を示した[17]。1件の小児IHCAの観察研究では、平均アドレナリン投与間隔5～8分と8～10分が、投与間隔1～5分と比較した場合、生存確率の上昇に関連することを明らかにした[18]。両方の研究[17,18]で、さまざまな期間の蘇生全体としての投与間隔における変化の可能性を考慮せずに、総心停止時間にわたる全投与量を平均することでアドレナリン投与の平均間隔を算出した。アドレナリンの投与頻度に関する小児のOHCA研究を確認できなかった。

4. 2件の研究では、乳児および小児のVF／無脈性VTの薬物療法について検討した[19,20]。Valdes et alの研究では、アミオダロンではなくリドカインの投与が、高値のROSC率と高値の生存入院率に関連していた[19]。リドカインもアミオダロンも、退院生存の確率に有意な影響を及ぼさなかった。神経学的転帰は未評価であった。IHCA登録の傾向マッチ研究では、リドカイン投与を受けた患者の転帰をアミオダロン投与と比較し、差を認めなかった[20]。

5. 最近のエビデンスレビューで，心停止中の炭酸水素ナトリウム投与に関する 8 件の観察研究を確認した[5-7,21-25]。炭酸水素塩の投与は，IHCA と OHCA の両方で生存転帰の悪化に関連した。高カリウム血症や，三環系抗うつ薬によるものも含むナトリウムチャネル遮断薬中毒などの，炭酸水素塩を使用する特殊な状況が存在する。
6. 心停止中のカルシウム投与を検討した 2 件の観察研究では，カルシウム投与による生存率および ROSC 率の悪化を示した[4,23]。低カルシウム血症，カルシウムチャネル遮断薬の過量投与，高マグネシウム血症，高カリウム血症などの，カルシウム投与を使用する特殊な状況が存在する[3]。

推奨事項 4 は，『2018 American Heart Association Focused Update on Pediatric Advanced Life Support: An Update to the American Heart Association Guidelines for Cardiopulmonary Resuscitation and Emergency Cardiovascular Care』で概説された[26]。

蘇生薬の体重に基づく投与量

蘇生薬の体重に基づく投与量に関する推奨事項

COR	LOE	推奨事項
1	C-EO	1. 蘇生薬を投与する場合，小児の体重を用いて蘇生薬の投与量を算出し，さらに成人の推奨投与量を超えないようにすることが推奨される[27-31]。
2b	B-NR	2. 可能な場合，体型や体組成を含めることで，身長を基に推定した体重の正確さを改善できる[8]。
2b	C-LD	3. 小児の体重が不明な場合，蘇生薬の用法と用量を求めるために体重推定用の身長テープや他の認知支援ツールを検討してもよい[29,32,33]。

「推奨事項の裏付けとなる解説」

1. 実体重の使用について（特に体重過多や肥満の患者で）理論上の懸案が多数存在する[27-29]。しかし，肥満患者の薬物投与量を調整することの安全性と有効性に関するデータはない。そのような調整によって，不正確な薬物投与量となる可能性もある[30,31]。
2. 複数の研究では，体型や体組成を含めることで，身長測定値を用いる体重推定値がさらに絞り込まれ，改善されることを示唆している[8]。しかし，これらの方法には大きなばらつきがあるため，これらの測定値の使用に必要な訓練はあらゆる意味で実用的とはいえない。
3. 認知支援ツールは，体重の正確な概算値を求める際に役立つことがある（測定した全体重の 10～20 ％以内といわれる）。最近の複数の研究では，体重推定値の大きなばらつきを示し，全体重を少なく見積り，しかも理想的な体重に近づけようとする傾向を明らかにした[29,32,33]。

参考文献

1. Campbell ME, Byrne PJ. Cardiopulmonary resuscitation and epinephrine infusion in extremely low birth weight infants in the neonatal intensive care unit. J Perinatol. 2004;24:691-695. doi: 10.1038/sj.jp.7211174
2. Dieckmann RA, Vardis R. High-dose epinephrine in pediatric out-of-hospital cardiopulmonary arrest. Pediatrics.1995;95:901-913.
3. Kette F, Ghuman J, Parr M. Calcium administration during cardiac arrest: a systematic review. Eur J Emerg Med.2013;20:72-78. doi: 10.1097/MEJ.0b013e328358e336
4. Lasa JJ, Alali A, Minard CG, Parekh D, Kutty S, Gaies M, Raymond TT, Guerguerian AM, Atkins D, Foglia E, et al; on behalf of the American Heart Association's Get With the Guidelines-Resuscitation Investigators. Cardiopulmonary resuscitation in the pediatric cardiac catheterization laboratory: A report from the American Heart Association's Get With the Guidelines-Resuscitation Registry. Pediatr Crit Care Med.2019;20:1040-1047. doi: 10.1097/PCC.0000000000002038
5. Matamoros M, Rodriguez R, Callejas A, Carranza D, Zeron H, Sánchez C, Del Castillo J, López-Herce J; Iberoamerican Pediatric Cardiac Arrest Study Network (RIBEPCI). In-hospital pediatric cardiac arrest in Honduras. Pediatr Emerg Care.2015;31:31-35. doi: 10.1097/PEC.0000000000000323
6. Nehme Z, Namachivayam S, Forrest A, Butt W, Bernard S, Smith K. Trends in the incidence and outcome of paediatric out-of-hospital cardiac arrest: A 17-year observational study. Resuscitation.2018;128:43-50. doi: 10.1016/j.resuscitation.2018.04.030
7. Raymond TT, Stromberg D, Stigall W, Burton G, Zaritsky A; American Heart Association's Get With The Guidelines-Resuscitation Investigators. Sodium bicarbonate use during in-hospital pediatric pulseless cardiac arrest – a report from the American Heart Association Get With The Guidelines®-Resuscitation. Resuscitation.2015;89:106-113. doi: 10.1016/j.resuscitation.2015.01.007
8. Young KD, Korotzer NC. Weight Estimation Methods in Children: A Systematic Review. Ann Emerg Med. 2016;68:441-451.e10. doi: 10.1016/j.annemergmed.2016.02.043
9. Enright K, Turner C, Roberts P, Cheng N, Browne G. Primary cardiac arrest following sport or exertion in children presenting to an emergency department: chest compressions and early defibrillation can save lives, but is intravenous epinephrine always appropriate? Pediatr Emerg Care.2012;28:336-339. doi: 10.1097/PEC.0b013e31824d8c78
10. Niemann JT, Stratton SJ, Cruz B, Lewis RJ. Endotracheal drug administration during out-of-hospital resuscitation: where are the survivors? Resuscitation.2002;53:153-157. doi: 10.1016/s0300-9572 (02)00004-7
11. Niemann JT, Stratton SJ. Endotracheal versus intravenous epinephrine and atropine in out-of-hospital "primary" and postcountershock asystole. Crit Care Med.2000;28:1815-1819. doi: 10.1097/00003246-200006000-00022
12. Andersen LW, Berg KM, Saindon BZ, Massaro JM, Raymond TT, Berg RA, Nadkarni VM, Donnino MW; American Heart Association Get With the Guidelines-Resuscitation Investigators. Time to Epinephrine and Survival After Pediatric In-Hospital Cardiac Arrest. JAMA.2015;314:802-810. doi: 10.1001/jama.2015.9678
13. Lin YR, Wu MH, Chen TY, Syue YJ, Yang MC, Lee TH, Lin CM, Chou CC, Chang CF, Li CJ. Time to epinephrine treatment is associated with the risk of mortality in children who achieve sustained ROSC after traumatic out-of-hospital cardiac arrest. Crit Care. 2019;23:101. doi: 10.1186/s13054-019-2391-z
14. Lin YR, Li CJ, Huang CC, Lee TH, Chen TY, Yang MC, Chou CC, Chang CF, Huang HW, Hsu HY, Chen WL. Early Epinephrine Improves the Stabilization of Initial Post-resuscitation Hemodynamics in Children With Non-shockable Out-of-Hospital Cardiac Arrest. Front Pediatr. 2019;7:220. doi: 10.3389/fped.2019.00220
15. Fukuda T, Kondo Y, Hayashida K, Sekiguchi H, Kukita I. Time to epinephrine and survival after paediatric out-of-hospital cardiac arrest. Eur Heart J Cardiovasc Pharmacother. 2018;4:144-151. doi: 10.1093/ehjcvp/pvx023
16. Hansen M, Schmicker RH, Newgard CD, Grunau B, Scheuermeyer F, Cheskes S, Vithalani V, Alnaji F, Rea T, Idris AH, Herren H, Hutchison J, Austin M, Egan D, Daya M; Resuscitation Outcomes Consortium Investigators. Time to Epinephrine Administration and Survival From Nonshockable Out-of-Hospital Cardiac Arrest Among Children and Adults. Circulation.2018;137:2032-2040. doi: 10.1161/CIRCULATIONAHA.117.033067

17. Meert K, Telford R, Holubkov R, Slomine BS, Christensen JR, Berger J, Ofori-Amanfo G, Newth CJL, Dean JM, Moler FW. Paediatric in-hospital cardiac arrest: factors associated with survival and neurobehavioural outcome one year later. Resuscitation.2018;124:96-105. doi: 10.1016/j.resuscitation.2018.01.013
18. Hoyme DB, Patel SS, Samson RA, Raymond TT, Nadkarni VM, Gaies MG, Atkins DL; American Heart Association Get With The Guidelines-Resuscitation Investigators. Epinephrine dosing interval and survival outcomes during pediatric in-hospital cardiac arrest. Resuscitation.2017;117:18-23. doi: 10.1016/j.resuscitation.2017.05.023
19. Valdes SO, Donoghue AJ, Hoyme DB, Hammond R, Berg MD, Berg RA, Samson RA; American Heart Association Get With The Guidelines-Resuscitation Investigators. Outcomes associated with amiodarone and lidocaine in the treatment of in-hospital pediatric cardiac arrest with pulseless ventricular tachycardia or ventricular fibrillation. Resuscitation.2014;85:381-386. doi: 10.1016/j.resuscitation.2013.12.008
20. Holmberg MJ, Ross CE, Atkins DL, Valdes SO, Donnino MW, Andersen LW; on behalf of the American Heart Association's Get With The Guidelines-Resuscitation Pediatric Research Task Force. Lidocaine versus amiodarone for pediatric in-hospital cardiac arrest: an observational study. Resuscitation. 2020:Epub ahead of print. doi: 10.1016/j.resuscitation.2019.12.033
21. López-Herce J, del Castillo J, Cañadas S, Rodríguez-Núñez A, Carrillo A; Spanish Study Group of Cardiopulmonary Arrest in Children. In-hospital pediatric cardiac arrest in Spain. Rev Esp Cardiol (Engl Ed). 2014;67:189-195. doi: 10.1016/j.rec.2013.07.017
22. Wolfe HA, Sutton RM, Reeder RW, Meert KL, Pollack MM, Yates AR, Berger JT, Newth CJ, Carcillo JA, McQuillen PS, Harrison RE, Moler FW, Carpenter TC, Notterman DA, Holubkov R, Dean JM, Nadkarni VM, Berg RA; Eunice Kennedy Shriver National Institute of Child Health; Human Development Collaborative Pediatric Critical Care Research Network; Pediatric Intensive Care Quality of Cardiopulmonary Resuscitation Investigators. Functional outcomes among survivors of pediatric in-hospital cardiac arrest are associated with baseline neurologic and functional status, but not with diastolic blood pressure during CPR. Resuscitation.2019;143:57-65. doi: 10.1016/j.resuscitation.2019.08.006
23. Mok YH, Loke AP, Loh TF, Lee JH. Characteristics and Risk Factors for Mortality in Paediatric In-Hospital Cardiac Events in Singapore: Retrospective Single Centre Experience. Ann Acad Med Singapore. 2016;45:534-541.
24. Del Castillo J, López-Herce J, Cañadas S, Matamoros M, Rodríguez-Núñez A, Rodríguez-Calvo A, Carrillo A; Iberoamerican Pediatric Cardiac Arrest Study Network RIBEPCI. Cardiac arrest and resuscitation in the pediatric intensive care unit: a prospective multicenter multinational study. Resuscitation.2014;85:1380-1386. doi: 10.1016/j.resuscitation.2014.06.024
25. Wu ET, Li MJ, Huang SC, Wang CC, Liu YP, Lu FL, Ko WJ, Wang MJ, Wang JK, Wu MH. Survey of outcome of CPR in pediatric in-hospital cardiac arrest in a medical center in Taiwan. Resuscitation.2009;80:443-448. doi: 10.1016/j.resuscitation.2009.01.006
26. Duff JP, Topjian A, Berg MD, Chan M, Haskell SE, Joyner BL Jr, Lasa JJ, Ley SJ, Raymond TT, Sutton RM, Hazinski MF, Atkins DL. 2018 American Heart Association Focused Update on Pediatric Advanced Life Support: An Update to the American Heart Association Guidelines for Cardiopulmonary Resuscitation and Emergency Cardiovascular Care.Circulation.2018;138:e731-e739. doi: 10.1161/CIR.0000000000000612
27. Wells M, Goldstein LN, Bentley A. It is time to abandon age-based emergency weight estimation in children! A failed validation of 20 different age-based formulas. Resuscitation.2017;116:73-83. doi: 10.1016/j.resuscitation.2017.05.018
28. Tanner D, Negaard A, Huang R, Evans N, Hennes H. A Prospective Evaluation of the Accuracy of Weight Estimation Using the Broselow Tape in Overweight and Obese Pediatric Patients in the Emergency Department. Pediatr Emerg Care.2017;33:675-678. doi: 10.1097/PEC.0000000000000894
29. Waseem M, Chen J, Leber M, Giambrone AE, Gerber LM. A reexamination of the accuracy of the Broselow tape as an instrument for weight estimation. Pediatr Emerg Care.2019;35:112-116. doi: 10.1097/PEC.0000000000000982
30. van Rongen A, Brill MJE, Vaughns JD, Välitalo PAJ, van Dongen EPA, van Ramshorst B, Barrett JS, van den Anker JN, Knibbe CAJ. Higher midazolam clearance in obese adolescents compared with morbidly obese adults. Clin Pharmacokinet. 2018;57:601-611. doi: 10.1007/s40262-017-0579-4
31. Vaughns JD, Ziesenitz VC, Williams EF, Mushtaq A, Bachmann R, Skopp G, Weiss J, Mikus G, van den Anker JN. Use of fentanyl in adolescents with clinically severe obesity undergoing bariatric surgery: a pilot study. Paediatr Drugs. 2017;19:251-257. doi: 10.1007/s40272-017-0216-6
32. Shrestha K, Subedi P, Pandey O, Shakya L, Chhetri K, House DR. Estimating the weight of children in Nepal by Broselow, PAWPER XL and Mercy method. World J Emerg Med. 2018;9:276-281. doi: 10.5847/wjem.j.1920-8642.2018.04.007
33. Wells M, Goldstein LN, Bentley A. The accuracy of paediatric weight estimation during simulated emergencies: the effects of patient position, patient cooperation, and human errors. Afr J Emerg Med. 2018;8:43-50. doi: 10.1016/j.afjem.2017.12.003

VF／無脈性VTの管理

VF／無脈性 VT のリスクは，青少年層全体で着実に上昇しているものの，その頻度は成人よりも低い状態である。VF／無脈性 VT の初期リズムによる心停止は，ショック非適応の初期リズムによる心停止よりも，良好な神経機能を維持したまま，生存退院できる割合が高い。ショック適応のリズムは心停止の初期リズム（一次性 VF／無脈性 VT）である場合も，蘇生中に発生する場合もある（二次性 VF／無脈性 VT）。除細動が VF／無脈性 VT の根治治療である。VF／無脈性 VT の持続時間が短いほど，ショックによって循環を生み出すリズムがもたらされる可能性が高い。手動式除細動器と AED はともに，小児の VF／無脈性 VT を治療するためのものである。医療従事者がショック適応のリズムを確認した場合は，手動式除細動器が望ましい。患者の体重に合わせてエネルギー量を調整できるためである。AED には，小児のショック適応のリズムを認識するうえでの高い特異性がある。VF／無脈性 VT の停止に要するエネルギーが少なく，副作用も少ないため，単相性ではなく二相性の除細動器を推奨する。多くの AED は，8 歳より低年齢の乳児および小児に適用できるようにエネルギー量を減衰（低下）する性能を備えている。

エネルギー量

エネルギー量に関する推奨事項

COR	LOE	推奨事項
2a	C-LD	1. 除細動を目的とした単相性または二相性波形の初回エネルギー量として 2〜4 J/kg を使用するのが妥当であるが，教えやすさという点で，2 J/kg を初回エネルギー量としてもかまわない[1-7]。
2b	C-LD	2. 治療抵抗性 VF の場合は，除細動エネルギー量を 4 J/kg まで上げることが妥当と考える[1-7]。
2b	C-LD	3. 以降のエネルギーレベルとして，エネルギー量 4 J/kg が妥当と考える。より高いエネルギーレベルを考慮してもかまわないが，10 J/kg または成人の最大エネルギー量を超えてはならない[1-7]。

「推奨事項の裏付けとなる解説」

1. 1，2，および 3。システマティックレビュー[1]により，エネルギー量といかなる転帰との間にも関連性がないことが明らかになった。無作為化比較試験はなく，大部分の研究は初回ショックを評価するだけであった。患者 27 例のショック 71 件を対象とした IHCA 症例集積では，2J/kg で VF が停止すると結論付けたが，

以降のリズムも蘇生転帰についても報告がない[2]。長期 OHCA に関する小規模の症例集積では、2～4 J/kg のショックにより患者 11 例で 14 回の VF が停止したが、心静止または無脈性電気活動の発生を認め、生存退院者はいなかった[3]。1 件の IHCA の観察研究[4]において、3～5 J/kg より高い初回エネルギー用量では、1～3 J/kg の場合よりも ROSC に達する効果が低くなった。3 件の小児の IHCA[3,5] および OHCA[6] の小規模な観察研究では、除細動の成功に関わる特定の初回エネルギー量を見い出せなかった。1 件の研究では、特に二次性 VF の場合、2 J/kg が効果のないエネルギー量であることを示唆した[7]。

ショックと CPR の連携

「ショックと CPR の連携に関する推奨事項」		
COR	LOE	推奨事項
1	C-EO	1. 装置でショックを実行する準備ができるまで CPR を実施する[8-12]。
1	C-EO	2. 1 回のショック後に、直ちに胸骨圧迫を行うことを VF／無脈性 VT の小児に対し推奨する[13,14]。
1	C-EO	3. 胸骨圧迫の中断は最小限に抑える[13,15]。

「推奨事項の裏付けとなる解説」
1. 除細動より前の CPR の最適なタイミングに関して入手できる小児データはない。成人を対象とした研究では、初回除細動より前の長時間の CPR は無益なことを明らかにしている[8-12]。
2. ショックと CPR の連携に関する最善の順序を示す小児データは現在存在しない。VF の治療にショックを 1 回のみ行うプロトコールと 3 回連続して行うプロトコールを比較する成人を対象とした研究では、ショックを 1 回のみ行うプロトコールの有意な生存効果を示唆した[13,14]。
3. 胸骨圧迫の長期にわたる中断は、脳や心臓などの重要臓器への血流と酸素輸送を低下させ、生存率の低下を招く[13,15]。

除細動器のパドルサイズ、種類、および位置

「除細動器のパドルサイズ、種類、および位置に関する推奨事項」		
COR	LOE	推奨事項
1	C-EO	1. パッド間／パドル間の距離を適切に離して小児の胸部に適合する最大のパドルまたは粘着性の電極を使用する[16-18]。
2b	C-LD	2. 粘着性のパッドを取り付ける場合、前外側方向の貼り付け、または前後方向の貼り付けが妥当であろう[7,19]。
2b	C-LD	3. パドルと粘着性のパッドには、同等の電流放出効果があるとみなしてもよい[20]。

「推奨事項の裏付けとなる解説」
1. パッドサイズやパドルサイズが大きいほど、電流放出の主な決定要因となる経胸壁インピーダンスが低下する[16-18]。
2. 1 件のヒト試験と 1 件のブタ試験では、前外側方向の位置と前後方向の位置を比較した場合、ショックの成功や ROSC に有意差を認めなかった[7,19]。
3. 1 件の研究では、ショックまでに要する時間の中央値は、パドルと粘着性パッドによる比較で有意差はなかった[20]。

除細動器の種類

「除細動器の種類に関する推奨事項」		
COR	LOE	推奨事項
1	C-LD	1. 乳児と小児（＜8 歳）で AED を使用する場合、小児用減衰システムの使用を推奨する[21-32]。
1	C-EO	2. 訓練を受けた医療従事者がケアする乳児では、ショック適応のリズムを認める場合、手動式除細動器を推奨する[33,34]。
2b	C-EO	3. 手動式除細動器も小児用減衰システムを備えた AED もない場合、エネルギー減衰システムを備えていない AED を使用してもよい[26-28,30,35]。

「推奨事項の裏付けとなる解説」
1. ショック適応のリズムは乳児でまれである[21,22]。リズム判定アルゴリズムの研究では、乳児および小児におけるショック適応のリズムの高い特異性を明らかにした[23-25]。小児用減衰システムを備えた AED と減衰システムのない AED によるショックを直接比較した報告はないが、複数の症例報告と症例集積は小児用減衰システムを使用した場合に、生存を伴うショックの成功を記載している[26-32]。
2. 乳児または小児で手動式除細動器と AED を比較している具体的な研究はない。患者の体重に合わせてエネルギー量を調整できるため、院内で使用する場合は手動式除細動器が望ましい。成人では、院内での AED 使用で、生存率は向上せず[33]、リズム解析に要するショック前後の休止期が長くなった[34]。
3. 小児用に調整できない AED は 120～360 J のエネルギーを放出するため、体重 25 kg 未満の小児では推奨エネルギー量を超える。しかし、乳児および若齢幼児でエネルギー量が 2～4 J/kg を超えた場合の安全かつ有効な AED 使用の報告がある[26-28,30,35]。除細動は VF に対する唯一の有効な治療法であるため、エネルギー減衰システムのない AED が救命につながる可能性がある。

参考文献

1. Mercier E, Laroche E, Beck B, Le Sage N, Cameron PA, Émond M, Berthelot S, Mitra B, Ouellet-Pelletier J. Defibrillation energy dose during pediatric cardiac arrest: Systematic review of human and animal model studies. Resuscitation.2019;139:241-252. doi: 10.1016/j.resuscitation.2019.04.028
2. Gutgesell HP, Tacker WA, Geddes LA, Davis S, Lie JT, McNamara DG. Energy dose for ventricular defibrillation of children. Pediatrics. 1976;58:898-901.
3. Berg MD, Samson RA, Meyer RJ, Clark LL, Valenzuela TD, Berg RA. Pediatric defibrillation doses often fail to terminate prolonged out-of-hospital ventricular fibrillation in children. Resuscitation.2005;67:63-67. doi: 10.1016/j.resuscitation.2005.04.018
4. Meaney PA, Nadkarni VM, Atkins DL, Berg MD, Samson RA, Hazinski MF, Berg RA; American Heart Association National Registry of Cardiopulmonary Resuscitation Investigators. Effect of defibrillation energy dose during in-hospital pediatric cardiac arrest. Pediatrics.2011;127:e16-e23. doi: 10.1542/peds.2010-1617
5. Rodríguez-Núñez A, López-Herce J, del Castillo J, Bellón JM; and the Iberian-American Paediatric Cardiac Arrest Study Network RIBEPCI. Shockable rhythms and defibrillation during in-hospital pediatric cardiac arrest. Resuscitation.2014;85:387-391. doi: 10.1016/j.resuscitation.2013.11.015
6. Rossano JW, Quan L, Kenney MA, Rea TD, Atkins DL. Energy doses for treatment of out-of-hospital pediatric ventricular fibrillation. Resuscitation.2006;70:80-89. doi: 10.1016/j.resuscitation.2005.10.031
7. Tibballs J, Carter B, Kiraly NJ, Ragg P, Clifford M. External and internal biphasic direct current shock doses for pediatric ventricular fibrillation and pulseless ventricular tachycardia. Pediatr Crit Care Med.2011;12:14-20. doi: 10.1097/PCC.0b013e3181dbb4fc
8. Baker PW, Conway J, Cotton C, Ashby DT, Smyth J, Woodman RJ, Grantham H; Clinical Investigators. Defibrillation or cardiopulmonary resuscitation first for patients with out-of-hospital cardiac arrests found by paramedics to be in ventricular fibrillation? A randomised control trial. Resuscitation.2008;79:424-431. doi: 10.1016/j.resuscitation.2008.07.017
9. Jacobs IG, Finn JC, Oxer HF, Jelinek GA. CPR before defibrillation in out-of-hospital cardiac arrest: a randomized trial. Emerg Med Australas. 2005;17:39-45. doi: 10.1111/j.1742-6723.2005.00694.x
10. Ma MH, Chiang WC, Ko PC, Yang CW, Wang HC, Chen SY, Chang WT, Huang CH, Chou HC, Lai MS, Chien KL, Lee BC, Hwang CH, Wang YC, Hsiung GH, Hsiao YW, Chang AM, Chen WJ, Chen SC. A randomized trial of compression first or analyze first strategies in patients with out-of-hospital cardiac arrest: results from an Asian community. Resuscitation.2012;83:806-812. doi: 10.1016/j.resuscitation.2012.01.009
11. Stiell IG, Nichol G, Leroux BG, Rea TD, Ornato JP, Powell J, Christenson J, Callaway CW, Kudenchuk PJ, Aufderheide TP, Idris AH, Daya MR, Wang HE, Morrison LJ, Davis D, Andrusiek D, Stephens S, Cheskes S, Schmicker RH, Fowler R, Vaillancourt C, Hostler D, Zive D, Pirrallo RG, Vilke GM, Sopko G, Weisfeldt M; ROC Investigators. Early versus later rhythm analysis in patients with out-of-hospital cardiac arrest. N Engl J Med.2011;365:787-797. doi: 10.1056/NEJMoa1010076
12. Wik L, Hansen TB, Fylling F, Steen T, Vaagenes P, Auestad BH, Steen PA. Delaying defibrillation to give basic cardiopulmonary resuscitation to patients with out-of-hospital ventricular fibrillation: a randomized trial. JAMA.2003;289:1389-1395. doi: 10.1001/jama.289.11.1389
13. Bobrow BJ, Clark LL, Ewy GA, Chikani V, Sanders AB, Berg RA, Richman PB, Kern KB. Minimally interrupted cardiac resuscitation by emergency medical services for out-of-hospital cardiac arrest. JAMA.2008;299:1158-1165. doi: 10.1001/jama.299.10.1158
14. Rea TD, Helbock M, Perry S, Garcia M, Cloyd D, Becker L, Eisenberg M. Increasing use of cardiopulmonary resuscitation during out-of-hospital ventricular fibrillation arrest: survival implications of guideline changes. Circulation.2006;114:2760-2765. doi: 10.1161/CIRCULATIONAHA.106.654715
15. Sutton RM, Case E, Brown SP, Atkins DL, Nadkarni VM, Kaltman J, Callaway C, Idris A, Nichol G, Hutchison J, Drennan IR, Austin M, Daya M, Cheskes S, Nuttall J, Herren H, Christenson J, Andrusiek D, Vaillancourt C, Menegazzi JJ, Rea TD, Berg RA; ROC Investigators. A quantitative analysis of out-of-hospital pediatric and adolescent resuscitation quality-A report from the ROC epistry-cardiac arrest. Resuscitation.2015;93:150-157. doi: 10.1016/j.resuscitation.2015.04.010
16. Atkins DL, Kerber RE. Pediatric defibrillation: current flow is improved by using "adult" electrode paddles. Pediatrics.1994;94:90-93.
17. Samson RA, Atkins DL, Kerber RE. Optimal size of self-adhesive preapplied electrode pads in pediatric defibrillation. Am J Cardiol. 1995;75:544-545. doi: 10.1016/s0002-9149(99)80606-7
18. Atkins DL, Sirna S, Kieso R, Charbonnier F, Kerber RE. Pediatric defibrillation: importance of paddle size in determining transthoracic impedance. Pediatrics.1988;82:914-918.
19. Ristagno G, Yu T, Quan W, Freeman G, Li Y. Comparison of defibrillation efficacy between two pads placements in a pediatric porcine model of cardiac arrest. Resuscitation.2012;83:755-759. doi: 10.1016/j.resuscitation.2011.12.010
20. Bhalala US, Balakumar N, Zamora M, Appachi E. Hands-On Defibrillation Skills of Pediatric Acute Care Providers During a Simulated Ventricular Fibrillation Cardiac Arrest Scenario. Front Pediatr.2018;6:107. doi: 10.3389/fped.2018.00107
21. Atkins DL, Everson-Stewart S, Sears GK, Daya M, Osmond MH, Warden CR, Berg RA; Resuscitation Outcomes Consortium Investigators. Epidemiology and outcomes from out-of-hospital cardiac arrest in children: the Resuscitation Outcomes Consortium Epistry-Cardiac Arrest.Circulation.2009;119:1484-1491. doi: 10.1161/CIRCULATIONAHA.108.802678
22. Samson RA, Nadkarni VM, Meaney PA, Carey SM, Berg MD, Berg RA; American Heart Association National Registry of CPR Investigators. Outcomes of in-hospital ventricular fibrillation in children. N Engl J Med.2006;354:2328-2339. doi: 10.1056/NEJMoa052917
23. Cecchin F, Jorgenson DB, Berul CI, Perry JC, Zimmerman AA, Duncan BW, Lupinetti FM, Snyder D, Lyster TD, Rosenthal GL, Cross B, Atkins DL. Is arrhythmia detection by automatic external defibrillator accurate for children?: sensitivity and specificity of an automatic external defibrillator algorithm in 696 pediatric arrhythmias. Circulation.2001;103:2483-2488. doi: 10.1161/01.cir.103.20.2483
24. Atkinson E, Mikysa B, Conway JA, Parker M, Christian K, Deshpande J, Knilans TK, Smith J, Walker C, Stickney RE, Hampton DR, Hazinski MF. Specificity and sensitivity of automated external defibrillator rhythm analysis in infants and children. Ann Emerg Med.2003;42:185-196. doi: 10.1067/mem.2003.287
25. Atkins DL, Scott WA, Blaufox AD, Law IH, Dick M II, Geheb F, Sobh J, Brewer JE. Sensitivity and specificity of an automated external defibrillator algorithm designed for pediatric patients. Resuscitation.2008;76:168-174. doi: 10.1016/j.resuscitation.2007.06.032
26. Atkins DL, Jorgenson DB. Attenuated pediatric electrode pads for automated external defibrillator use in children. Resuscitation.2005;66:31-37. doi: 10.1016/j.resuscitation.2004.12.025
27. Bar-Cohen Y, Walsh EP, Love BA, Cecchin F. First appropriate use of automated external defibrillator in an infant. Resuscitation.2005;67:135-137. doi: 10.1016/j.resuscitation.2005.05.003
28. Divekar A, Soni R. Successful parental use of an automated external defibrillator for an infant with long-QT syndrome. Pediatrics.2006;118:e526-e529. doi: 10.1542/peds.2006-0129
29. Hoyt WJ Jr, Fish FA, Kannankeril PJ. Automated external defibrillator use in a previously healthy 31-day-old infant with out-of-hospital cardiac arrest due to ventricular fibrillation. J Cardiovasc Electrophysiol. 2019;30:2599-2602. doi: 10.1111/jce.14125
30. Gurnett CA, Atkins DL. Successful use of a biphasic waveform automated external defibrillator in a high-risk child. Am J Cardiol.2000;86:1051-1053. doi: 10.1016/s0002-9149(00)01151-6
31. Mitani Y, Ohta K, Yodoya N, Otsuki S, Ohashi H, Sawada H, Nagashima M, Sumitomo N, Komada Y. Public access defibrillation improved the outcome after out-of-hospital cardiac arrest in school-age children: a nationwide, population-based, Utstein registry study in Japan. Europace. 2013;15:1259-1266. doi: 10.1093/europace/eut053
32. Pundi KN, Bos JM, Cannon BC, Ackerman MJ. Automated external defibrillator rescues among children with diagnosed and treated long QT syndrome. Heart Rhythm. 2015;12:776-781. doi: 10.1016/j.hrthm.2015.01.002
33. Chan PS, Krumholz HM, Spertus JA, Jones PG, Cram P, Berg RA, Peberdy MA, Nadkarni V, Mancini ME, Nallamothu BK. Automated external defibrillators and survival after in-hospital cardiac arrest. JAMA.2010;304:2129-2136. doi: 10.1001/jama.2010.1576
34. Cheskes S, Schmicker RH, Christenson J, Salcido DD, Rea T, Powell J, Edelson DP, Sell R, May S, Menegazzi JJ, Van Ottingham L, Olsufka M, Pennington S, Simonini J, Berg RA, Stiell I, Idris A, Bigham B, Morrison L; Resuscitation Outcomes Consortium (ROC) Investigators. Perishock pause: an independent predictor of survival from out-of-hospital shockable cardiac arrest. Circulation.2011;124:58-66. doi: 10.1161/CIRCULATIONAHA.110.010736
35. König B, Benger J, Goldsworthy L. Automatic external defibrillation in a 6 year old. Arch Dis Child.2005;90:310-311. doi: 10.1136/adc.2004.054981

蘇生の質の評価

質の高いCPRを開始して維持することで、ROSC率と生存率が向上し、良好な神経学的転帰につながるのの、測定したCPRの質はしばしば最適とは言えない[1-3]。CPRの質を評価し指針にするために非侵襲的および侵襲的モニタリング法を使用できる。CPR中の観血的動脈圧モニタリングにより、圧迫および薬物によって発生する血圧を洞察することが可能である[4]。呼気終末CO_2（$ETCO_2$）は、生成される心拍出量と換気効果の両方を反映するため、CPRの質に関するフィードバックを得られる場合がある[5]。$ETCO_2$の急激な上昇は、ROSCの初期徴候となり得る[6]。CPRフィードバック装置（すなわち、指導、聴覚、および視聴覚装置）により、質の高いCPRを目的とする訓練や品質保証の範囲内で、胸骨圧迫のテンポ、深さ、および圧迫解除が改善する可能性がある。CPR時のベッドサイド超音波検査、特に心エコー法が、心停止の治療可能な原因を特定するために重んじられる。蘇生の質を評価するための技術として、CPR中の近赤外分光法を使用した非侵襲的な脳酸素化の測定などの方法が評価されつつある。

蘇生の質の評価に関する推奨事項

COR	LOE	推奨事項
2a	C-LD	1. 心停止時に連続的に観血的動脈圧モニタリングを行っていた患者について、プロバイダーが拡張期血圧を使用してCPRの質を評価することは妥当である[4]。
2b	C-LD	2. $ETCO_2$モニタリングを胸骨圧迫の質を評価するために検討してもよいが、小児では治療につながる特性値を確立できていない[7,8]。
2b	C-EO	3. 継続的な蘇生の質向上システムの一環として十分な胸骨圧迫のテンポおよび深さを最適化するために、救助者がCPRフィードバック装置を使用するのが妥当な場合もある[9,10]。
2b	C-EO	4. 適切な訓練を受けた要員がいる場合、心停止の潜在的に治療可能な原因（心タンポナーデや不十分な心室充満など）を特定するために心エコー法を検討してもよいが、胸骨圧迫を中断するという既知の有害な転帰と対比して潜在的利益を吟味する必要がある[11-13]。

「推奨事項の裏付けとなる解説」

1. CPRの最初の10分間に観血的動脈圧モニタリングを行った小児患者の前向き観察研究では、拡張期血圧が乳児で≧25 mm Hg、小児で≧30 mm Hgである場合、良好な神経学的転帰となる割合が高いことを示した[4]。なお、拡張期血圧トレース図のカットポイントを、事後の波形解析により分析したため、前向き評価を必要とした。

2. 乳児を対象とした院内CPRの単一施設後向き研究では、$ETCO_2$値17〜18 mm HgでROSCの陽性的中率が0.885になることを示した[7]。IHCAの前向き多施設共同観察研究では、平均$ETCO_2$値と予後との間に関連性を認めなかった[8]。

3. 小児科医療従事者のシミュレーション試験では、（フィードバックを受けていない場合と比較して）視覚フィードバックを受けた場合に、胸骨圧迫の深さおよびテンポの適合性が有意に改善したが、全体的な胸骨圧迫の質は不十分な状態であることを明らかにした[9]。IHCAの小児8例を対象とした1件の小規模の観察研究では、視聴覚フィードバックの有無と生存退院率との間に関連性を見出せなかったが、フィードバックにより過剰な胸骨圧迫のテンポが低下した[10]。

4. 複数の症例集積で、肺塞栓症を含む心停止の治療可能な原因を特定するためのベッドサイド心エコー法の使用を評価している[11,12]。ICU入院児（心停止なし）を対象とした1件の前向き観察研究では、救急医がベッドサイドで使用する限定的心エコー法と心臓病専門医が実施するを正式な心エコー法との間で短縮率および下大静脈容積の推定値が良好に一致することを報告した[13]。

参考文献

1. Niles DE, Duval-Arnould J, Skellett S, Knight L, Su F, Raymond TT, Sweberg T, Sen AI, Atkins DL, Friess SH, de Caen AR, Kurosawa H, Sutton RM, Wolfe H, Berg RA, Silver A, Hunt EA, Nadkarni VM; pediatric Resuscitation Quality (pediRES-Q) Collaborative Investigators.Characterization of Pediatric In-Hospital Cardiopulmonary Resuscitation Quality Metrics Across an International Resuscitation Collaborative.Pediatr Crit Care Med.2018;19:421-432. doi: 10.1097/PCC.0000000000001520

2. Sutton RM, Case E, Brown SP, Atkins DL, Nadkarni VM, Kaltman J, Callaway C, Idris A, Nichol G, Hutchison J, Drennan IR, Austin M, Daya M, Cheskes S, Nuttall J, Herren H, Christenson J, Andrusiek D, Vaillancourt C, Menegazzi JJ, Rea TD, Berg RA; ROC Investigators.A quantitative analysis of out-of-hospital pediatric and adolescent resuscitation quality-A report from the ROC epistry–cardiac arrest.Resuscitation.2015;93:150-157. doi: 10.1016/j.resuscitation.2015.04.010

3. Wolfe H, Zebuhr C, Topjian AA, Nishisaki A, Niles DE, Meaney PA, Boyle L, Giordano RT, Davis D, Priestley M, Apkon M, Berg RA, Nadkarni VM, Sutton RM. Interdisciplinary ICU cardiac arrest debriefing improves survival outcomes*. Crit Care Med. 2014;42:1688-1695. doi: 10.1097/CCM.0000000000000327

4. Berg RA, Sutton RM, Reeder RW, Berger JT, Newth CJ, Carcillo JA, McQuillen PS, Meert KL, Yates AR, Harrison RE, Moler FW, Pollack MM, Carpenter TC, Wessel DL, Jenkins TL, Notterman DA, Holubkov R, Tamburro RF, Dean JM, Nadkarni VM; Eunice Kennedy Shriver National Institute of Child Health and Human Development Collaborative Pediatric Critical Care Research Network (CPCCRN) PICqCPR (Pediatric Intensive Care Quality of Cardio-Pulmonary Resuscitation) Investigators. Association Between Diastolic Blood Pressure During Pediatric In-Hospital Cardiopulmonary Resuscitation and Survival. Circulation.2018;137:1784-1795. doi: 10.1161/CIRCULATIONAHA.117.032270

5. Hamrick JL, Hamrick JT, Lee JK, Lee BH, Koehler RC, Shaffner DH. Efficacy of chest compressions directed by end-tidal CO2 feedback in a pediatric resuscitation model of basic life support. J Am Heart Assoc.2014;3:e000450. doi: 10.1161/JAHA.113.000450

6. Hartmann SM, Farris RW, Di Gennaro JL, Roberts JS. Systematic Review and Meta-Analysis of End-Tidal Carbon Dioxide Values Associated With Return of Spontaneous Circulation During Cardiopulmonary Resuscitation. J Intensive Care Med. 2015;30:426-435. doi: 10.1177/0885066614530839
7. Stine CN, Koch J, Brown LS, Chalak L, Kapadia V, Wyckoff MH. Quantitative end-tidal CO_2 can predict increase in heart rate during infant cardiopulmonary resuscitation. Heliyon. 2019;5:e01871. doi: 10.1016/j.heliyon.2019.e01871
8. Berg RA, Reeder RW, Meert KL, Yates AR, Berger JT, Newth CJ, Carcillo JA, McQuillen PS, Harrison RE, Moler FW, Pollack MM, Carpenter TC, Notterman DA, Holubkov R, Dean JM, Nadkarni VM, Sutton RM; Eunice Kennedy Shriver National Institute of Child Health and Human Development Collaborative Pediatric Critical Care Research Network (CPCCRN) Pediatric Intensive Care Quality of Cardio-Pulmonary Resuscitation (PICqCPR) investigators. End-tidal carbon dioxide during pediatric in-hospital cardiopulmonary resuscitation. Resuscitation. 2018;133:173-179. doi: 10.1016/j.resuscitation.2018.08.013
9. Cheng A, Brown LL, Duff JP, Davidson J, Overly F, Tofil NM, Peterson DT, White ML, Bhanji F, Bank I, et al; on behalf of the International Network for Simulation-Based Pediatric Innovation, Research, & Education (INSPIRE) CPR Investigators. Improving cardiopulmonary resuscitation with a CPR feedback device and refresher simulations (CPR CARES Study): a randomized clinical trial. JAMA Pediatr. 2015;169:137-144. doi: 10.1001/jamapediatrics.2014.2616
10. Sutton RM, Niles D, French B, Maltese MR, Leffelman J, Eilevstjonn J, Wolfe H, Nishisaki A, Meaney PA, Berg RA, et al. First quantitative analysis of cardiopulmonary resuscitation quality during in-hospital cardiac arrests of young children. Resuscitation. 2014;85:70-74. doi: 10.1016/j.resuscitation.2013.08.014
11. Steffen K, Thompson WR, Pustavoitau A, Su E. Return of Viable Cardiac Function After Sonographic Cardiac Standstill in Pediatric Cardiac Arrest. Pediatr Emerg Care. 2017;33:58-59. doi: 10.1097/PEC.0000000000001002
12. Morgan RW, Stinson HR, Wolfe H, Lindell RB, Topjian AA, Nadkarni VM, Sutton RM, Berg RA, Kilbaugh TJ. Pediatric In-Hospital Cardiac Arrest Secondary to Acute Pulmonary Embolism. Crit Care Med. 2018;46:e229-e234. doi: 10.1097/CCM.0000000000002921
13. Pershad J, Myers S, Plouman C, Rosson C, Elam K, Wan J, Chin T. Bedside limited echocardiography by the emergency physician is accurate during evaluation of the critically ill patient. Pediatrics. 2004;114:e667-e671. doi: 10.1542/peds.2004-0881

体外循環補助を用いた心肺蘇生

体外循環補助を用いた心肺蘇生（ECPR）を、ROSCを維持できない患者に対する静動脈体外式膜型人工肺（ECMO）の迅速な装着と定義する。従来、この方法は、心疾患小児の管理に関する専門知識を有するプロバイダーが存在する大規模な小児科医療センターに限られた、リソース集約型の複雑な多岐専門分野にわたる治療である。特定の患者集団に対し、専用の高い実施経験のある環境内でECPRを賢明に使用することで、特に治療可能な原因を有するIHCAの場合に、蘇生に成功している[1]。ECPRの使用率は上昇しており、成人および小児を対象とした単一施設報告では、より幅広い患者集団にこの治療法を適用することで心停止後の生存を改善する可能性があることを示唆している[2-4]。

小児OHCA後の予後の改善を示すECPRの研究は存在しない。

体外循環補助を用いた心肺蘇生の使用に関する推奨事項

COR	LOE	推奨事項
2b	C-LD	1. 適切なプロトコールと経験を有し、器材が使用可能な場合は、IHCAを呈した心疾患診断を有する小児に対しECPRの使用を考慮してもよい[5,6]。

「推奨事項の裏付けとなる解説」

1. 1件の心臓手術後の小児IHCAに対するECPR観察登録研究では、従来のCPRよりもECPRが高い生存退院率を伴うことを明らかにした[5]。同一の登録を用いて従来のCPRと比較したECPRの傾向マッチ解析では、あらゆる病因のIHCA患者でECPRが良好な神経学的転帰と関連することを認めた[6]。OHCAを発症した小児患者、または従来のCPRに抵抗性のIHCAを発症した非心疾患の小児患者に対してECPRを使用することを推奨または反対するには、エビデンスが不十分である。

この推奨事項は、『2019 American Heart Association Focused Update on Pediatric Advanced Life Support: An Update to the American Heart Association Guidelines for Cardiopulmonary Resuscitation and Emergency Cardiovascular Care』で概説された[7]。

参考文献

1. Brunetti MA, Gaynor JW, Retzloff LB, Lehrich JL, Banerjee M, Amula V, Bailly D, Klugman D, Koch J, Lasa J, Pasquali SK, Gaies M. Characteristics, Risk Factors, and Outcomes of Extracorporeal Membrane Oxygenation Use in Pediatric Cardiac ICUs: A Report From the Pediatric Cardiac Critical Care Consortium Registry. Pediatr Crit Care Med. 2018;19:544-552. doi: 10.1097/PCC.0000000000001571
2. Sakamoto T, Morimura N, Nagao K, Asai Y, Yokota H, Nara S, Hase M, Tahara Y, Atsumi T; SAVE-J Study Group. Extracorporeal cardiopulmonary resuscitation versus conventional cardiopulmonary resuscitation in adults with out-of-hospital cardiac arrest: a prospective observational study. Resuscitation. 2014;85:762-768. doi: 10.1016/j.resuscitation.2014.01.031
3. Stub D, Bernard S, Pellegrino V, Smith K, Walker T, Sheldrake J, Hockings L, Shaw J, Duffy SJ, Burrell A, Cameron P, Smit de V, Kaye DM. Refractory cardiac arrest treated with mechanical CPR, hypothermia, ECMO and early reperfusion (the CHEER trial). Resuscitation. 2015;86:88-94. doi: 10.1016/j.resuscitation.2014.09.010
4. Conrad SJ, Bridges BC, Kalra Y, Pietsch JB, Smith AH. Extracorporeal Cardiopulmonary Resuscitation Among Patients with Structurally Normal Hearts. ASAIO J. 2017;63:781-786. doi: 10.1097/MAT.0000000000000568
5. Ortmann L, Prodhan P, Gossett J, Schexnayder S, Berg R, Nadkarni V, Bhutta A; American Heart Association's Get With the Guidelines-Resuscitation Investigators. Outcomes after in-hospital cardiac arrest in children with cardiac disease: a report from Get With the Guidelines-Resuscitation. Circulation. 2011;124:2329-2337. doi: 10.1161/CIRCULATIONAHA.110.013466
6. Lasa JJ, Rogers RS, Localio R, Shults J, Raymond T, Gaies M, Thiagarajan R, Laussen PC, Kilbaugh T, Berg RA, Nadkarni V, Topjian A. Extracorporeal Cardiopulmonary Resuscitation (E-CPR) During Pediatric In-Hospital Cardiopulmonary Arrest Is Associated With Improved Survival to Discharge: A Report from the American Heart Association's Get With The Guidelines-Resuscitation (GWTG-R) Registry. Circulation. 2016;133:165-176. doi: 10.1161/CIRCULATIONAHA.115.016082
7. Duff JP, Topjian AA, Berg MD, Chan M, Haskell SE, Joyner BL Jr, Lasa JJ, Ley SJ, Raymond TT, Sutton RM, Hazinski MF, Atkins DL. 2019 American Heart Association Focused Update on Pediatric Advanced Life Support: An Update to the American Heart Association Guidelines for Cardiopulmonary Resuscitation and Emergency Cardiovascular Care. Circulation. 2019;140:e904-e914. doi: 10.1161/CIR.0000000000000731

心拍再開後のケア治療およびモニタリング

心停止からの蘇生に成功すると，ROSC 後の数日間に発生する可能性がある心停止後症候群が生じる。心停止後症候群の要素は，(1) 脳損傷，(2) 心筋機能障害，(3) 全身性虚血および再灌流反応，(4) 持続的な病態生理の亢進である[1,2]。心拍再開後の脳損傷は，未だに成人と小児における合併症および死亡の主な原因である。脳では虚血，充血または浮腫の耐性が抑制されているためである。小児の心拍再開後のケアは，生存および神経学的転帰を改善するためにこの複雑な生理学を予測し，識別し，治療することに重点を置く。

目標体温管理（TTM）は，患者の体温を狭い規定範囲内で継続的に維持し，同時に体温を継続的にモニタリングすることを指す。すべての形の TTM では発熱を回避し，低体温 TTM では代謝需要を減少させ，フリーラジカルの産生を減らし，アポトーシスを減らすことによって血流再灌流症候群の治療を試みる[2]。

低血圧，発熱，けいれん発作，急性腎障害，および酸素化，換気，電解質の異常のような障害の特定と治療は，予後に影響を及ぼす可能性があるため，重要である。

心拍再開後の目標体温管理

心拍再開後の目標体温管理に関する推奨事項

COR	LOE	推奨事項
1	A	1. TTM 中の深部体温の連続測定を推奨する。[3,4]
2a	B-R	2. OHCA または IHCA 後に昏睡状態が続く生後 24 時間～18 歳の乳児と小児に対し，32°C～34°C の TTM 続いて 36°C～37.5°C の TTM，または 36°C～37.5°C のみの TTM の使用が妥当である[3,4]。

「推奨事項の裏付けとなる解説」

1 および 2. ROSC 後に昏睡の小児を対象とした IHCA または OHCA 後の TTM（32°C～34°C で 48 時間，続いて 36°C～37.5°C の TTM を 3 日間と，36°C～37.5°C で合計 5 日間の TTM と比較）に関する 2 件の小児無作為化試験では，良好な神経学的転帰を伴う 1 年生存率に差を認めなかった[3,4]。TTM により高体温を効果的に予防した。両方の試験で 5 日間の TTM に対し連続深部体温モニタリングを使用した。

推奨事項 1 と 2 は，『2019 American Heart Association Focused Update on Pediatric Advanced Life Support: An Update to the American Heart Association Guidelines for Cardiopulmonary Resuscitation and Emergency Cardiovascular Care』で概説された[5]。

心拍再開後の血圧管理

心拍再開後の血圧管理に関する推奨事項

COR	LOE	推奨事項
1	C-LD	1. ROSC 後，輸液静注および／または血管作動薬を投与して，収縮期血圧を各年齢層の 5 パーセンタイルより高い値に維持することが推奨される[6-9]。
1	C-EO	2. 適切な器材が使用可能な場合は，動脈圧の連続モニタリングを行い，低血圧を同定・治療することが推奨される[6-9]。

「推奨事項の裏付けとなる解説」

1 および 2. 2 件の観察研究は，心停止後約 6～12 時間の収縮期低血圧（年齢および性別の 5 パーセンタイル未満）が生存退院率の低下に関わることを示した[6,7]。別の観察研究では，ICU 心拍再開後治療の最初の 72 時間以内に長時間の血圧低下を呈した患者で生存退院率が低下したことを認めた[8]。心停止直後と心停止中に動脈モニタリングした患者の観察研究において，ROSC 後最初の 20 分間の拡張期高血圧（90 パーセンタイル超）は，生存退院率の高い可能性と関連した[9]。心拍再開後に血圧は不安定になりがちなため，連続動脈圧モニタリングを推奨する。

心拍再開後の酸素化および換気の管理

心拍再開後の酸素化および換気の管理に関する推奨事項

COR	LOE	推奨事項
2b	C-LD	1. 救助者が特定の患者の原因疾患に適する ROSC 後の酸素正常状態を目標とするのは，妥当であろう[10-13]。
2b	C-LD	2. 救助者が 94～99 %の酸素飽和度を目標とするために酸素投与を中止するのが妥当であろう[10-12,14]。
2b	C-LD	3. 医師が ROSC 後の二酸化炭素分圧（$Paco_2$）を特定の患者の原因疾患に適する目標にし，重度の高炭酸ガス血症や低炭酸ガス血症曝露を抑制するのが妥当であろう[10,11,14]。

「推奨事項の裏付けとなる解説」

1 および 2. 100 %の動脈血酸素飽和度は約 80～500 mm Hg までの任意の Pao_2 に相当する可能性があるため，94～99 %の酸素飽和度を目標にするのは妥当である。3 件の小児の IHCA および OHCA の小規模な観察研究では，高酸素血症と予後との間に関連性を認めなかった[10,11,13]。小児 IHCA および OHCA 患者を対象とした大規模な観察研究で，ROSC 後の酸素正常状態は高酸素血症と比較した場合，ICU 生存退院率の改善と関連した[12]。

3. 1件の観察研究では、ROSC後の高炭酸ガス血症と低炭酸ガス血症がともに死亡の増加に関連することを明らかにした[11]。1件の小規模な観察研究では、高炭酸ガス血症（$Paco_2$ 50 mm Hg 超）または低炭酸ガス血症（$Paco_2$ 30 mm Hg 未満）と予後との間に関連性を示さなかった[10]。別の小児IHCAの観察研究では、高炭酸ガス血症（$Paco_2$ 50 mm Hg 以上）が生存退院率の低下と関連することを認めた[14]。高炭酸ガス血症と低炭酸ガス血症は脳血流に影響を及ぼすため、慢性高炭酸ガス血症を呈する患者を把握しながら、ROSC後の炭酸ガス正常状態を目標にすることが望ましい。

心拍再開後のEEGモニタリングおよびけいれん発作治療

心拍再開後のEEGモニタリングおよびけいれん発作治療に関する推奨事項

COR	LOE	推奨事項
1	C-LD	1. リソースを利用できる場合は、持続的脳症の患者における心停止後のけいれん発作の検出のため継続的な脳波（EEG）モニタリングが推奨される[15-18]。
1	C-LD	2. 心停止後の臨床的けいれん発作を治療することが推奨される[19,20]。
2a	C-EO	3. 専門医と相談のうえ、心停止後の非けいれん性てんかん発作重積状態を治療することは妥当である[19,20]。

「推奨事項の裏付けとなる解説」

1. 非けいれん性てんかん発作と非けいれん性てんかん発作重積状態は、小児の心停止後に多く見られる[15-18]。米国臨床神経生理学会（Clinical Neurophysiology Society）では、小児の心停止後の脳症患者に対し連続EEGモニタリングを推奨している[15]。非けいれん性発作と非けいれん性てんかん発作重積状態はEEGモニタリングを用いない限り検出できない[15]。

2 および 3. けいれん性または非けいれん性発作の治療が小児の心停止後の神経学的転帰および／または機能的転帰を改善するかどうかを判定するには、エビデンスが不十分である。けいれん性および非けいれん性発作重積状態はともに予後不良に関連する[17]。神経救急学会（Neurocritical Care Society）は、けいれんおよび脳波計上のけいれん発作活動の停止を目標にするてんかん重積状態の治療を推奨している[19]。

図8に、心拍再開後の治療に関するチェックリストを示す。

参考文献

1. Neumar RW, Nolan JP, Adrie C, Aibiki M, Berg RA, Böttiger BW, Callaway C, Clark RS, Geocadin RG, Jauch EC, Kern KB, Laurent I, Longstreth WT Jr, Merchant RM, Morley P, Morrison LJ, Nadkarni V, Peberdy MA, Rivers EP, Rodriguez-Nunez A, Sellke FW, Spaulding C, Sunde K, Vanden Hoek T. Post-cardiac arrest syndrome: epidemiology, pathophysiology, treatment, and prognostication. A consensus statement from the International Liaison Committee on Resuscitation (American Heart Association, Australian and New Zealand Council on Resuscitation, European Resuscitation Council, Heart and Stroke Foundation of Canada, InterAmerican Heart Foundation, Resuscitation Council of Asia, and the Resuscitation Council of Southern Africa); the American Heart Association Emergency Cardiovascular Care Committee; the Council on Cardiovascular Surgery and Anesthesia; the Council on Cardiopulmonary, Perioperative, and Critical Care; the Council on Clinical Cardiology; and the Stroke Council. Circulation.2008;118:2452-2483. doi: 10.1161/CIRCULATIONAHA.108.190652

2. Topjian AA, de Caen A, Wainwright MS, Abella BS, Abend NS, Atkins DL, Bembea MM, Fink EL, Guerguerian AM, Haskell SE, Kilgannon JH, Lasa JJ, Hazinski MF. Pediatric post-cardiac arrest care: a scientific statement from the American Heart Association. Circulation. 2019;140:e194-e233. doi: 10.1161/CIR.0000000000000697

3. Moler FW, Silverstein FS, Holubkov R, Slomine BS, Christensen JR, Nadkarni VM, Meert KL, Browning B, Pemberton VL, Page K, et al; on behalf of the THAPCA Trial Investigators. Therapeutic hypothermia after in-hospital cardiac arrest in children. N Engl J Med.2017;376:318-329. doi: 10.1056/NEJMoa1610493

4. Moler FW, Silverstein FS, Holubkov R, Slomine BS, Christensen JR, Nadkarni VM, Meert KL, Clark AE, Browning B, Pemberton VL, Page K, Shankaran S, Hutchison JS, Newth CJ, Bennett KS, Berger JT, Topjian A, Pineda JA, Koch JD, Schleien CL, Dalton HJ, Ofori-Amanfo G, Goodman DM, Fink EL, McQuillen P, Zimmerman JJ, Thomas NJ, van der Jagt EW, Porter MB, Meyer MT, Harrison R, Pham N, Schwarz AJ, Nowak JE, Alten J, Wheeler DS, Bhalala US, Lidsky K, Lloyd E, Mathur M, Shah S, Wu T, Theodorou AA, Sanders RC Jr, Dean JM; THAPCA Trial Investigators. Therapeutic hypothermia after out-of-hospital cardiac arrest in children. N Engl J Med.2015;372:1898-1908. doi: 10.1056/NEJMoa1411480

5. Duff JP, Topjian AA, Berg MD, Chan M, Haskell SE, Joyner BL Jr, Lasa JJ, Ley SJ, Raymond TT, Sutton RM, Hazinski MF, Atkins DL. 2019 American Heart Association focused update on pediatric advanced life support: an update to the American Heart Association Guidelines for Cardiopulmonary Resuscitation and Emergency Cardiovascular Care. Circulation.2019;140:e904-e914. doi: 10.1161/CIR.0000000000000731

6. Topjian AA, Telford R, Holubkov R, Nadkarni VM, Berg RA, Dean JM, Moler FW; on behalf of the Therapeutic Hypothermia after Pediatric Cardiac Arrest (THAPCA) Trial Investigators. The association of early post-resuscitation hypotension with discharge survival following targeted temperature management for pediatric in-hospital cardiac arrest. Resuscitation.2019;141:24-34. doi: 10.1016/j.resuscitation.2019.05.032

7. Topjian AA, Telford R, Holubkov R, Nadkarni VM, Berg RA, Dean JM, Moler FW; Therapeutic Hypothermia After Pediatric Cardiac Arrest (THAPCA) Trial Investigators. Association of Early Postresuscitation Hypotension With Survival to Discharge After Targeted Temperature Management for Pediatric Out-of-Hospital Cardiac Arrest: Secondary Analysis of a Randomized Clinical Trial. JAMA Pediatr.2018;172:143-153. doi: 10.1001/jamapediatrics.2017.4043

8. Laverriere EK, Polansky M, French B, Nadkarni VM, Berg RA, Topjian AA.Association of Duration of Hypotension With Survival After Pediatric Cardiac Arrest.Pediatr Crit Care Med.2020;21:143-149. doi: 10.1097/PCC.0000000000002119

9. Topjian AA, Sutton RM, Reeder RW, Telford R, Meert KL, Yates AR, Morgan RW, Berger JT, Newth CJ, Carcillo JA, McQuillen PS, Harrison RE, Moler FW, Pollack MM, Carpenter TC, Notterman DA, Holubkov R, Dean JM, Nadkarni VM, Berg RA, Zuppa AF, Graham K, Twelves C, Diliberto MA, Landis WP, Tomanio E, Kwok J, Bell MJ, Abraham A, Sapru A, Alkhouli MF, Heidemann S, Pawluszka A, Hall MW, Steele L, Shanley TP, Weber M, Dalton HJ, Bell A, Mourani PM, Malone K, Locandro C, Coleman W, Peterson A, Thelen J, Doctor A; Eunice Kennedy Shriver National Institute of Child Health and Human Development Collaborative Pediatric Critical Care Research Network (CPCCRN) Investigators. The association of immediate post cardiac arrest diastolic hypertension and survival following pediatric cardiac arrest. Resuscitation.2019;141:88-95. doi: 10.1016/j.resuscitation.2019.05.033

10. Bennett KS, Clark AE, Meert KL, Topjian AA, Schleien CL, Shaffner DH, Dean JM, Moler FW; Pediatric Emergency Care Medicine Applied Research Network. Early oxygenation and ventilation measurements

心拍再開後の治療の要素	確認
酸素投与と換気	
酸素化を測定する。正常範囲の94％〜99％（または小児の正常／十分な酸素飽和度）を目標とする。	☐
$PaCO_2$を測定する。患者の基礎疾患に対して適切な濃度を目標とし，極端な高炭酸ガス血症や低炭酸ガス血症を避ける。	☐
血行動態モニタリング	
心拍再開後の治療中における特定の血行動態の目標を設定し，毎日確認する。	☐
心電図モニターでモニタリングする。	☐
動脈内血圧をモニタリングする。	☐
血清乳酸値，尿量，および中心静脈血酸素飽和度をモニタリングして治療の指針に役立てる。	☐
変力作用薬または血管収縮薬の使用の有無にかかわらず非経口の輸液ボーラス投与で，収縮期血圧が年齢および性別の5パーセンタイル値を上回るように維持する。	☐
目標体温管理（TTM）	
深部体温を測定して継続的にモニタリングする。	☐
心停止直後および復温中の発熱を回避し，治療する。	☐
患者が昏睡状態の場合，TTM（32℃〜34℃）とそれに続けて36℃〜37.5℃を適用するか，またはTTM（36℃〜37.5℃）のみ適用する。	☐
震えを防止する。	☐
復温中は血圧をモニタリングし，低血圧を治療する。	☐
神経機能モニタリング	
患者に脳症があり，リソースを利用できる場合は，継続的な脳波（EEG）モニタリングを実施する。	☐
けいれんを治療する。	☐
心停止の治療可能な原因を診断するため，早期の脳画像検査を検討する。	☐
電解質と血糖	
血糖を測定して低血糖を防ぐ。	☐
致死的不整脈になる可能性を回避するため，電解質を正常範囲内に維持する。	☐
鎮静薬の投与	
鎮静薬および抗不安薬による治療を行う。	☐
予後	
単一の予測因子に対して，常に複数の方法（臨床およびそのほか）を検討する。	☐
評価はTTMまたは低体温療法により変更される場合があることに留意する。	☐
心停止発症後から7日以内に，脳波とほかの因子を組み合せて考慮する。	☐
最初の7日間にMRI検査などの神経画像検査を検討する。	☐

図8. 心拍再開後の治療チェックリスト。

after pediatric cardiac arrest: lack of association with outcome. Crit Care Med.2013;41:1534-1542. doi: 10.1097/CCM.0b013e318287f54c
11. López-Herce J, del Castillo J, Matamoros M, Canadas S, Rodriguez-Calvo A, Cecchetti C, Rodríguez-Núñez A, Carrillo Á; Iberoamerican Pediatric Cardiac Arrest Study Network RIBEPCI. Post return of spontaneous circulation factors associated with mortality in pediatric in-hospital cardiac arrest: a prospective multicenter multinational observational study. Crit Care. 2014;18:607. doi: 10.1186/s13054-014-0607-9
12. Ferguson LP, Durward A, Tibby SM. Relationship between arterial partial oxygen pressure after resuscitation from cardiac arrest and mortality in children. Circulation.2012;126:335-342. doi: 10.1161/CIRCULATIONAHA.111.085100
13. van Zellem L, de Jonge R, van Rosmalen J, Reiss I, Tibboel D, Buysse C. High cumulative oxygen levels are associated with improved survival of children treated with mild therapeutic hypothermia after cardiac arrest. Resuscitation.2015;90:150-157. doi: 10.1016/j.resuscitation.2014.12.013
14. Del Castillo J, López-Herce J, Matamoros M, Cañadas S, Rodriguez-Calvo A, Cechetti C, Rodriguez-Núñez A, Alvarez AC; Iberoamerican Pediatric Cardiac Arrest Study Network RIBEPCI. Hyperoxia, hypocapnia and hypercapnia as outcome factors after cardiac arrest in children. Resuscitation.2012;83:1456-1461. doi: 10.1016/j.resuscitation.2012.07.019
15. Herman ST, Abend NS, Bleck TP, Chapman KE, Drislane FW, Emerson RG, Gerard EE, Hahn CD, Husain AM, Kaplan PW, et al. Consensus statement on continuous EEG in critically ill adults and children, part I: indications. J Clin Neurophysiol. 2015;32:87-95. doi: 10.1097/wnp.0000000000000166
16. Abend NS, Topjian A, Ichord R, Herman ST, Helfaer M, Donnelly M, Nadkarni V, Dlugos DJ, Clancy RR. Electroencephalographic monitoring during hypothermia after pediatric cardiac arrest. Neurology. 2009;72:1931-1940. doi: 10.1212/WNL.0b013e3181a82687
17. Topjian AA, Gutierrez-Colina AM, Sanchez SM, Berg RA, Friess SH, Dlugos DJ, Abend NS. Electrographic status epilepticus is associated with mortality and worse short-term outcome in critically ill children. Crit Care Med.2013;41:215-223. doi: 10.1097/CCM.0b013e3182668035
18. Ostendorf AP, Hartman ME, Friess SH. Early Electroencephalographic Findings Correlate With Neurologic Outcome in Children Following Cardiac Arrest. Pediatr Crit Care Med.2016;17:667-676. doi: 10.1097/PCC.0000000000000791
19. Brophy GM, Bell R, Claassen J, Alldredge B, Bleck TP, Glauser T, Laroche SM, Riviello JJ Jr, Shutter L, Sperling MR, Treiman DM, Vespa PM; Neurocritical Care Society Status Epilepticus Guideline Writing Committee. Guidelines for the evaluation and management of status epilepticus. Neurocrit Care. 2012;17:3-23. doi: 10.1007/s12028-012-9695-z
20. Topjian AA, Sánchez SM, Shults J, Berg RA, Dlugos DJ, Abend NS. Early Electroencephalographic Background Features Predict Outcomes in Children Resuscitated From Cardiac Arrest. Pediatr Crit Care Med.2016;17:547-557. doi: 10.1097/PCC.0000000000000740

心停止後の予後予測

心停止からの小児生存者における神経学的転帰の早期，かつ信頼できる予後予測は，治療を進め，効率的に計画をたて，家族を支援するために不可欠である。臨床医は，予後予測の指針とするために患者および心停止の特性，心拍再開後の神経学的検査，臨床検査結果，神経学的画像検査（例えば，脳コンピュータ断層撮影，MRI），およびEEGを使用する。現時点で，ROSCの24～48時間以内に良好な予後または予後不良を確実に予測するための単独因子や有効な決定ルールは定められていない。単独で使用する場合，EEG，神経画像検査，および血清バイオマーカーでは，中等度の正確さでしか予後を予測できないため，これらの検査を個々の患者に適用する前により多くのデータが必要となる。

心停止後の予後予測に関する推奨事項

COR	LOE	推奨事項
2a	B-NR	1. 心拍再開後1週間以内のEEGは，予後予測の1つの因子として有効であり，他の情報によって増強できる[1-8]。
2a	B-NR	2. 心停止から蘇生した乳児および小児で予後を予測する場合，プロバイダーは複数の因子を考慮するのが妥当である[1,7,9-21]。
2a	B-NR	3. 非致死的な溺水後に心停止から蘇生した（生存入院）乳児および小児で予後を予測する場合，プロバイダーは複数の因子を考慮するのが妥当である[22-39]。

「推奨事項の裏付けとなる解説」

1. 8件の後ろ向き観察研究で，EEGバックグラウンドパターンが退院時の神経学的転帰に関連することが明らかになった[1-8]。睡眠紡錘波[3,4,8]，正常なバックグラウンド[2]，および反応性[7,8]の存在が良好な予後と関連する。バーストサプレッションと平坦なパターン，または減衰したEEGパターンは，神経学的転帰不良に関係する[1,2,5,8]。しかし，これらの関連性は，EEGを神経学的予後予測の単独の検査法として用いるために必要な高感度と高特異度に達していない。

2. 複数の研究で，病歴，患者特性，身体所見，画像検査およびバイオマーカーのデータと心停止後の神経学的転帰との関連性が明らかになった[1,7,9-19]。今のところ，十分な正確さの予後予測結果を示す単独因子はない。心停止後24時間以内に測定された高い血清乳酸値，pH値，または塩基欠乏量が予後不良に関連している[9,11,12,16-18,20,21]。しかし，具体的なカットオフ値は不明である。

3. 溺水時間が短いほど，小児の非致命的な溺水後の転帰は良好となる[22-25]。患者の年齢[23,26-31,38]，水の種類[30,32,33]，水温[23,25,34,35]，緊急医療サービスの応答時間[35,36]，または目撃状況[36-39]と非致命的な溺水後の神経学的転帰との明確な関連性はない。いかなる単独因子も，非致命的な溺水後の予後を正確に予測しない。

参考文献

1. Brooks GA, Park JT. Clinical and Electroencephalographic Correlates in Pediatric Cardiac Arrest: Experience at a Tertiary Care Center. Neuropediatrics. 2018;49:324-329. doi: 10.1055/s-0038-1657757
2. Topjian AA, Sánchez SM, Shults J, Berg RA, Dlugos DJ, Abend NS. Early Electroencephalographic Background Features Predict Outcomes in Children Resuscitated From Cardiac Arrest.Pediatr Crit Care Med.2016;17:547-557. doi: 10.1097/PCC.0000000000000740
3. Ostendorf AP, Hartman ME, Friess SH.Early Electroencephalographic Findings Correlate With Neurologic Outcome in Children Following Cardiac Arrest.Pediatr Crit Care Med.2016;17:667-676. doi: 10.1097/PCC.0000000000000791

4. Ducharme-Crevier L, Press CA, Kurz JE, Mills MG, Goldstein JL, Wainwright MS. Early Presence of Sleep Spindles on Electroencephalography Is Associated With Good Outcome After Pediatric Cardiac Arrest. Pediatr Crit Care Med.2017;18:452-460. doi: 10.1097/PCC.0000000000001137
5. Bourgoin P, Barrault V, Joram N, Leclair Visonneau L, Toulgoat F, Anthoine E, Loron G, Chenouard A. The Prognostic Value of Early Amplitude-Integrated Electroencephalography Monitoring After Pediatric Cardiac Arrest. Pediatr Crit Care Med.2020;21:248-255. doi: 10.1097/PCC.0000000000002171
6. Lee S, Zhao X, Davis KA, Topjian AA, Litt B, Abend NS. Quantitative EEG predicts outcomes in children after cardiac arrest. Neurology.2019;92:e2329-e2338. doi: 10.1212/WNL.0000000000007504
7. Yang D, Ryoo E, Kim HJ. Combination of Early EEG, Brain CT, and Ammonia Level Is Useful to Predict Neurologic Outcome in Children Resuscitated From Cardiac Arrest. Front Pediatr.2019;7:223. doi: 10.3389/fped.2019.00223
8. Fung FW, Topjian AA, Xiao R, Abend NS. Early EEG Features for Outcome Prediction After Cardiac Arrest in Children. J Clin Neurophysiol.2019;36:349-357. doi: 10.1097/WNP.0000000000000591
9. Meert K, Telford R, Holubkov R, Slomine BS, Christensen JR, Berger J, Ofori-Amanfo G, Newth CJL, Dean JM, Moler FW. Paediatric in-hospital cardiac arrest: Factors associated with survival and neurobehavioural outcome one year later. Resuscitation.2018;124:96-105. doi: 10.1016/j.resuscitation.2018.01.013
10. Ichord R, Silverstein FS, Slomine BS, Telford R, Christensen J, Holubkov R, Dean JM, Moler FW; THAPCA Trial Group. Neurologic outcomes in pediatric cardiac arrest survivors enrolled in the THAPCA trials. Neurology.2018;91:e123-e131. doi: 10.1212/WNL.0000000000005773
11. Meert KL, Telford R, Holubkov R, Slomine BS, Christensen JR, Dean JM, Moler FW; Therapeutic Hypothermia after Pediatric Cardiac Arrest (THAPCA) Trial Investigators. Pediatric Out-of-Hospital Cardiac Arrest Characteristics and Their Association With Survival and Neurobehavioral Outcome. Pediatr Crit Care Med.2016;17:e543-e550. doi: 10.1097/PCC.0000000000000969
12. Del Castillo J, López-Herce J, Matamoros M, Cañadas S, Rodríguez-Calvo A, Cecchetti C, Rodriguez-Núñez A, Álvarez AC; Iberoamerican Pediatric Cardiac Arrest Study Network RIBEPCI. Long-term evolution after in-hospital cardiac arrest in children: Prospective multicenter multinational study. Resuscitation.2015;96:126-134. doi: 10.1016/j.resuscitation.2015.07.037
13. Topjian AA, Telford R, Holubkov R, Nadkarni VM, Berg RA, Dean JM, Moler FW; Therapeutic Hypothermia After Pediatric Cardiac Arrest (THAPCA) Trial Investigators.Association of Early Postresuscitation Hypotension With Survival to Discharge After Targeted Temperature Management for Pediatric Out-of-Hospital Cardiac Arrest: Secondary Analysis of a Randomized Clinical Trial. JAMA Pediatr.2018;172:143-153. doi: 10.1001/jamapediatrics.2017.4043
14. Conlon TW, Falkensammer CB, Hammond RS, Nadkarni VM, Berg RA, Topjian AA. Association of left ventricular systolic function and vasopressor support with survival following pediatric out-of-hospital cardiac arrest. Pediatr Crit Care Med. 2015;16:146-154. doi: 10.1097/pcc.0000000000000305
15. Starling RM, Shekdar K, Licht D, Nadkarni VM, Berg RA, Topjian AA. Early Head CT Findings Are Associated With Outcomes After Pediatric Out-of-Hospital Cardiac Arrest. Pediatr Crit Care Med.2015;16:542-548. doi: 10.1097/PCC.0000000000000404
16. Alsoufi B, Awan A, Manlhiot C, Guechef A, Al-Halees Z, Al-Ahmadi M, McCrindle BW, Kalloghlian A. Results of rapid-response extracorporeal cardiopulmonary resuscitation in children with refractory cardiac arrest following cardiac surgery. Eur J Cardiothorac Surg. 2014;45:268-275. doi: 10.1093/ejcts/ezt319
17. Polimenakos AC, Rizzo V, El-Zein CF, Ilbawi MN. Post-cardiotomy Rescue Extracorporeal Cardiopulmonary Resuscitation in Neonates with Single Ventricle After Intractable Cardiac Arrest: Attrition After Hospital Discharge and Predictors of Outcome. Pediatr Cardiol. 2017;38:314-323. doi: 10.1007/s00246-016-1515-3
18. Scholefield BR, Gao F, Duncan HP, Tasker RC, Parslow RC, Draper ES, McShane P, Davies P, Morris KP. Observational study of children admitted to United Kingdom and Republic of Ireland Paediatric Intensive Care Units after out-of-hospital cardiac arrest. Resuscitation.2015;97:122-128. doi: 10.1016/j.resuscitation.2015.07.011
19. Kramer P, Miera O, Berger F, Schmitt K. Prognostic value of serum biomarkers of cerebral injury in classifying neurological outcome after paediatric resuscitation. Resuscitation.2018;122:113-120. doi: 10.1016/j.resuscitation.2017.09.012
20. López-Herce J, del Castillo J, Matamoros M, Canadas S, Rodriguez-Calvo A, Cecchetti C, Rodríguez-Núñez A, Carrillo Á; Iberoamerican Pediatric Cardiac Arrest Study Network RIBEPCI. Post return of spontaneous circulation factors associated with mortality in pediatric in-hospital cardiac arrest: a prospective multicenter multinational observational study.Crit Care.2014;18:607. doi: 10.1186/s13054-014-0607-9
21. Topjian AA, Clark AE, Casper TC, Berger JT, Schleien CL, Dean JM, Moler FW; Pediatric Emergency Care Applied Research Network. Early lactate elevations following resuscitation from pediatric cardiac arrest are associated with increased mortality*. Pediatr Crit Care Med.2013;14:e380-e387. doi: 10.1097/PCC.0b013e3182976402
22. Kyriacou DN, Arcinue EL, Peek C, Kraus JF. Effect of immediate resuscitation on children with submersion injury. Pediatrics. 1994;94 (2 Pt 1):137-142.
23. Suominen P, Baillie C, Korpela R, Rautanen S, Ranta S, Olkkola KT. Impact of age, submersion time and water temperature on outcome in near-drowning. Resuscitation.2002;52:247-254. doi: 10.1016/s0300-9572 (01)00478-6
24. Panzino F, Quintillá JM, Luaces C, Pou J. [Unintentional drowning by immersion. Epidemiological profile of victims attended in 21 Spanish emergency departments]. An Pediatr (Barc). 2013;78:178-184. doi: 10.1016/j.anpedi.2012.06.014
25. Quan L, Mack CD, Schiff MA. Association of water temperature and submersion duration and drowning outcome. Resuscitation.2014;85:790-794. doi: 10.1016/j.resuscitation.2014.02.024
26. Frates RC Jr. Analysis of predictive factors in the assessment of warm-water near-drowning in children. Am J Dis Child.1981;135:1006-1008. doi: 10.1001/archpedi.1981.02130350010004
27. Nagel FO, Kibel SM, Beatty DW. Childhood near-drowning-factors associated with poor outcome. S Afr Med J. 1990;78:422-425.
28. Quan L, Wentz KR, Gore EJ, Copass MK. Outcome and predictors of outcome in pediatric submersion victims receiving prehospital care in King County, Washington. Pediatrics.1990;86:586-593.
29. Niu YW, Cherng WS, Lin MT, Tsao LY. An analysis of prognostic factors for submersion accidents in children. Zhonghua Min Guo Xiao Er Ke Yi Xue Hui Za Zhi. 1992;33:81-88.
30. Mizuta R, Fujita H, Osamura T, Kidowaki T, Kiyosawa N. Childhood drownings and near-drownings in Japan. Acta Paediatr Jpn. 1993;35:186-192. doi: 10.1111/j.1442-200x.1993.tb03036.x
31. Al-Mofadda SM, Nassar A, Al-Turki A, Al-Sallounm AA. Pediatric near drowning: the experience of King Khalid University Hospital. Ann Saudi Med. 2001;21:300-303. doi: 10.5144/0256-4947.2001.300
32. Forler J, Carsin A, Arlaud K, Bosdure E, Viard L, Paut O, Camboulives J, Dubus JC. [Respiratory complications of accidental drownings in children]. Arch Pediatr. 2010;17:14-18. doi: 10.1016/j.arcped.2009.09.021
33. Al-Qurashi FO, Yousef AA, Aljoudi A, Alzahrani SM, Al-Jawder NY, Al-Ahmar AK, Al-Majed MS, Abouollo HM. A Review of Nonfatal Drowning in the Pediatric-Age Group: A 10-Year Experience at a University Hospital in Saudi Arabia. Pediatr Emerg Care.2019;35:782-786. doi: 10.1097/PEC.0000000000001232
34. Kieboom JK, Verkade HJ, Burgerhof JG, Bierens JJ, Rheenen PF, Kneyber MC, Albers MJ. Outcome after resuscitation beyond 30 minutes in drowned children with cardiac arrest and hypothermia: Dutch nationwide retrospective cohort study. BMJ. 2015;350:h418. doi: 10.1136/bmj.h418
35. Claesson A, Lindqvist J, Ortenwall P, Herlitz J. Characteristics of lifesaving from drowning as reported by the Swedish Fire and Rescue Services 1996-2010. Resuscitation.2012;83:1072-1077. doi: 10.1016/j.resuscitation.2012.05.025
36. Claesson A, Svensson L, Silfverstolpe J, Herlitz J. Characteristics and outcome among patients suffering out-of-hospital cardiac arrest due to drowning. Resuscitation.2008;76:381-387. doi: 10.1016/j.resuscitation.2007.09.003
37. Dyson K, Morgans A, Bray J, Matthews B, Smith K. Drowning related out-of-hospital cardiac arrests: characteristics and outcomes. Resuscitation.2013;84:1114-1118. doi: 10.1016/j.resuscitation.2013.01.020
38. Nitta M, Kitamura T, Iwami T, Nadkarni VM, Berg RA, Topjian AA, Okamoto Y, Nishiyama C, Nishiuchi T, Hayashi Y, Nishimoto Y, Takasu A. Out-of-hospital cardiac arrest due to drowning among children and adults from the Utstein Osaka Project. Resuscitation.2013;84:1568-1573. doi: 10.1016/j.resuscitation.2013.06.017
39. Claesson A, Lindqvist J, Herlitz J. Cardiac arrest due to drowning-changes over time and factors of importance for survival. Resuscitation.2014;85:644-648. doi: 10.1016/j.resuscitation.2014.02.006

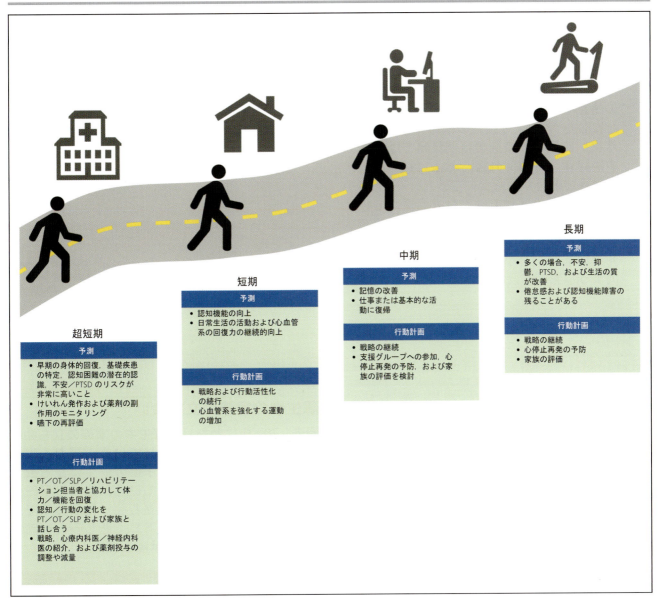

図9. 回復までの行程表。[3]

心拍再開後の回復

生存者は，短期および長期の身体的，神経学的，認知的，感情的，および社会的な病的状態の重大なリスクを有する[3]。肉眼的に「良好な予後」を有する心停止から蘇生した多くの小児には，より微小で持続的な神経心理学的障害がある[4]。脳損傷が小児の発達に及ぼす最大の影響は，心停止後数カ月〜数年が経過するまで完全に認知されない可能性がある。さらに，小児は養育者に育てられるため，心停止後の病的状態の影響は小児だけでなく家族にも及ぶ。

心停止からの生存者がその心停止後数カ月〜数年にわたり一体化した医学的支援，リハビリテーション支援，養育者支援，および地域支援の継続を必要とし得ることを発信するために，救命の連鎖内の6番目の鎖として回復を導入した（図9を参照[3]。AHAとILCORによる最近の科学的提言では，長期の神経学的転帰と健康に関連した生活の質の予後について研究する重要性を強調している[5,6]。

COR	LOE	推奨事項
1	C-LD	1. 小児の心停止からの生存者はリハビリテーションのため評価することが推奨される[4,7-11]。
2a	C-LD	2. 小児の心停止からの生存者は，少なくとも心停止から1年間は継続的な神経学的評価を受けるよう紹介することが妥当である[3,5,10-15]。

「推奨事項の裏付けとなる解説」

1. IHCAまたはOHCA後に昏睡となり1年時点で神経行動学的転帰の主要評価項目を有する小児を対象とした2件のTTMの無作為化比較試験[7,8]では，新規の病的状態が多く見られることを示した[9-11]。バインランドⅡ適応行動尺度（Vineland Adaptive Behavior Scales-II, VABS-II）で良好な神経行動学的転

帰を有する 1 年生存した多くの小児に，広範な認知機能障害と神経心理学的障害を認めた[4]。
2. 小児の心停止に対する 2 件の TTM の無作為化比較試験では，心停止後 1 年以内に一部の生存者で神経機能が改善することを明らかにした[10,11]。より長期の転帰（心停止後 1 年超）に関する複数の症例集積では，認知機能障害，身体的障害，および神経心理学的障害の進行が明らかになった[12-14]。AHA による最近の提言では，患者回復が心停止後 1 年間は継続するため，退院後の追跡調査の重要性を強調している[3,5,6,15]。小児期の発達の進行が，小児の心停止後の回復にどのような影響を及ぼすかは不明である。

参考文献

1. Deleted in proof.
2. Deleted in proof.
3. Sawyer KN, Camp-Rogers TR, Kotini-Shah P, Del Rios M, Gossip MR, Moitra VK, Haywood KL, Dougherty CM, Lubitz SA, Rabinstein AA, Rittenberger JC, Callaway CW, Abella BS, Geocadin RG, Kurz MC; American Heart Association Emergency Cardiovascular Care Committee; Council on Cardiovascular and Stroke Nursing; Council on Genomic and Precision Medicine; Council on Quality of Care and Outcomes Research; and Stroke Council. Sudden Cardiac Arrest Survivorship: A Scientific Statement From the American Heart Association.Circulation.2020;141:e654-e685. doi: 10.1161/CIR.0000000000000747
4. Slomine BS, Silverstein FS, Christensen JR, Page K, Holubkov R, Dean JM, Moler FW.Neuropsychological Outcomes of Children 1 Year After Pediatric Cardiac Arrest: Secondary Analysis of 2 Randomized Clinical Trials.JAMA Neurol.2018;75:1502-1510. doi: 10.1001/jamaneurol.2018.2628
5. Geocadin RG, Callaway CW, Fink EL, Golan E, Greer DM, Ko NU, Lang E, Licht DJ, Marino BS, McNair ND, Peberdy MA, Perman SM, Sims DB, Soar J, Sandroni C; American Heart Association Emergency Cardiovascular Care Committee. Standards for Studies of Neurological Prognostication in Comatose Survivors of Cardiac Arrest: A Scientific Statement From the American Heart Association.Circulation.2019;140:e517-e542. doi: 10.1161/CIR.0000000000000702
6. Topjian AA, Scholefield BR, Pinto NP, Fink EL, Buysse CMP, Haywood K, Maconochie I, Nadkarni VM, de Caen A, Escalante-Kanashiro R, Ng K-C, Nuthall G, Reis AG, Van de Voorde P, Suskauer SJ, Schexnayder SM, Hazinski MF, Slomine BS. P-COSCA (Pediatric Core Outcome Set for Cardiac Arrest) in children: an advisory statement from the International Liaison Committee on Resuscitation. Circulation.2020;142:e000-e000. doi: 10.1161/CIR.0000000000000911
7. Moler FW, Silverstein FS, Holubkov R, Slomine BS, Christensen JR, Nadkarni VM, Meert KL, Clark AE, Browning B, Pemberton VL, Page K, Shankaran S, Hutchison JS, Newth CJ, Bennett KS, Berger JT, Topjian A, Pineda JA, Koch JD, Schleien CL, Dalton HJ, Ofori-Amanfo G, Goodman DM, Fink EL, McQuillen P, Zimmerman JJ, Thomas NJ, van der Jagt EW, Porter MB, Meyer MT, Harrison R, Pham N, Schwarz AJ, Nowak JE, Alten J, Wheeler DS, Bhalala US, Lidsky K, Lloyd E, Mathur M, Shah S, Wu T, Theodorou AA, Sanders RC Jr, Dean JM; THAPCA Trial Investigators.Therapeutic hypothermia after out-of-hospital cardiac arrest in children.N Engl J Med.2015;372.1898-1908. doi: 10.1056/NEJMoa1411480
8. Moler FW, Silverstein FS, Holubkov R, Slomine BS, Christensen JR, Nadkarni VM, Meert KL, Browning B, Pemberton VL, Page K, et al; on behalf of the THAPCA Trial Investigators.Therapeutic hypothermia after in-hospital cardiac arrest in children.N Engl J Med.2017;376:318-329. doi: 10.1056/NEJMoa1610493
9. Slomine BS, Silverstein FS, Page K, Holubkov R, Christensen JR, Dean JM, Moler FW; Therapeutic Hypothermia after Pediatric Cardiac Arrest (THAPCA) Trial Investigators. Relationships between three and twelve month outcomes in children enrolled in the therapeutic hypothermia after pediatric cardiac arrest trials. Resuscitation.2019;139:329-336. doi: 10.1016/j.resuscitation.2019.03.020
10. Slomine BS, Silverstein FS, Christensen JR, Holubkov R, Telford R, Dean JM, Moler FW; Therapeutic Hypothermia after Paediatric Cardiac Arrest (THAPCA) Trial Investigators. Neurobehavioural outcomes in children after In-Hospital cardiac arrest. Resuscitation.2018;124:80-89. doi: 10.1016/j.resuscitation.2018.01.002
11. Slomine BS, Silverstein FS, Christensen JR, Holubkov R, Page K, Dean JM, Moler FW; on behalf of the THAPCA Trial Group. Neurobehavioral outcomes in children after out-of-hospital cardiac arrest. Pediatrics.2016;137:e20153412. doi: 10.1542/peds.2015-3412
12. van Zellem L, Buysse C, Madderom M, Legerstee JS, Aarsen F, Tibboel D, Utens EM. Long-term neuropsychological outcomes in children and adolescents after cardiac arrest. Intensive Care Med.2015;41:1057-1066. doi: 10.1007/s00134-015-3789-y
13. van Zellem L, Utens EM, Legerstee JS, Cransberg K, Hulst JM, Tibboel D, Buysse C. Cardiac Arrest in Children: Long-Term Health Status and Health-Related Quality of Life. Pediatr Crit Care Med.2015;16:693-702. doi: 10.1097/PCC.0000000000000452
14. van Zellem L, Utens EM, Madderom M, Legerstee JS, Aarsen F, Tibboel D, Buysse C. Cardiac arrest in infants, children, and adolescents: long-term emotional and behavioral functioning. Eur J Pediatr.2016;175:977-986. doi: 10.1007/s00431-016-2728-4
15. Topjian AA, de Caen A, Wainwright MS, Abella BS, Abend NS, Atkins DL, Bembea MM, Fink EL, Guerguerian AM, Haskell SE, Kilgannon JH, Lasa JJ, Hazinski MF. Pediatric Post-Cardiac Arrest Care: A Scientific Statement From the American Heart Association.Circulation.2019;140:e194-e233. doi: 10.1161/CIR.0000000000000697

蘇生中の家族の立ち会い

過去 20 年にわたり，蘇生中の家族の立ち会いを認める実施基準が増加している。調査を受けた大部分の親は，自分の子供の蘇生に立ち会うことを希望すると表明している。過去のデータは，自分の子供の死亡に立ち会った親の間で，不安やうつの発生率が低下し，悲しみの行動がより建設的になることを示唆している[1]。

蘇生中の家族の立ち会いに関する推奨事項

COR	LOE	推奨事項
1	B-NR	1. 乳児や小児の蘇生においてはできる限り，家族に蘇生に立ち会う機会を提供する[2-10]。
1	B-NR	2. 家族が蘇生に立ち会う場合，特定のチームメンバーが慰めを与え，質問に回答し，家族を支援することが有益である[11,12]。
1	C-LD	3. 家族の立ち会いが蘇生に悪影響を与えるとみなす場合は，丁寧な方法で家族に立ち会いを中止してもらうことが望ましい[13,14]。

「推奨事項の裏付けとなる解説」

1. 定性的な研究では，自分の子供の蘇生に立ち会う許可を与える場合，家族にも有益となることを示している。親が近くにいることで子供に安心感を与えられると感じ，その事実が子供の喪失に適応する助けになると親たちは述べた[2]。他の親への調査では，何が起きているのかを理解するために，できることすべてが尽くされたことを知るために，自分の子供と物理的な接触を保つために親が立ち会いを希望すると報告した[3,4]。しかし，自分の子供の蘇生に立ち会った親がすべて，再度立ち会う

ことを選択するわけではない[5]。蘇生中の家族の立ち会いについて，家族の精神的外傷，手技への干渉，技術的能力への影響，教育および臨床的判断に対する懸念などのいくつかの懸案が生じているが，これらの懸案は入手できるエビデンスで裏付けられてはいない[6-8]。経験豊かなプロバイダーのほうが，研修者よりも家族の立ち会いを支持する傾向がある[9,10]。

2. 家族を支援するファシリテーターの立ち会いが有用である[11,12]。蘇生中に精神的外傷となる出来事の処理を助ける専用のチームメンバーを家族にあてがうことが重要となるが，これは必ずしも可能ではない。ファシリテーターの不在を理由に，家族の蘇生への立ち会いを拒んではならない。

3. 大部分の調査で，家族の立ち会いにより蘇生時に混乱を来すことはないが，一部のプロバイダーがストレスの増加を感じることが示されている[13]。家族の立ち会いを多く経験したプロバイダーは，時折好ましくない経験があることを認めている[14]。

参考文献

1. Robinson SM, Mackenzie-Ross S, Campbell Hewson GL, Egleston CV, Prevost AT. Psychological effect of witnessed resuscitation on bereaved relatives. Lancet.1998;352:614-617. doi: 10.1016/s0140-6736(97)12179-1
2. Tinsley C, Hill JB, Shah J, Zimmerman G, Wilson M, Freier K, Abd-Allah S. Experience of families during cardiopulmonary resuscitation in a pediatric intensive care unit. Pediatrics.2008;122:e799-e804. doi: 10.1542/peds.2007-3650
3. Maxton FJ. Parental presence during resuscitation in the PICU: the parents' experience. Sharing and surviving the resuscitation: a phenomenological study. J Clin Nurs. 2008;17:3168-3176. doi: 10.1111/j.1365-2702.2008.02525.x
4. Stewart SA. Parents' Experience During a Child's Resuscitation: Getting Through It. J Pediatr Nurs. 2019;47:58-67. doi: 10.1016/j.pedn.2019.04.019
5. Curley MA, Meyer EC, Scoppettuolo LA, McGann EA, Trainor BP, Rachwal CM, Hickey PA. Parent presence during invasive procedures and resuscitation: evaluating a clinical practice change. Am J Respir Crit Care Med. 2012;186:1133-1139. doi: 10.1164/rccm.201205-0915OC
6. McClenathan BM, Torrington KG, Uyehara CF. Family member presence during cardiopulmonary resuscitation: a survey of US and international critical care professionals. Chest. 2002;122:2204-2211. doi: 10.1378/chest.122.6.2204
7. Vavarouta A, Xanthos T, Papadimitriou L, Kouskouni E, Iacovidou N. Family presence during resuscitation and invasive procedures: physicians' and nurses' attitudes working in pediatric departments in Greece. Resuscitation.2011;82:713-716. doi: 10.1016/j.resuscitation.2011.02.011
8. Pasek TA, Licata J. Parent Advocacy Group for Events of Resuscitation. Crit Care Nurse. 2016;36:58-64. doi: 10.4037/ccn2016759
9. Fein JA, Ganesh J, Alpern ER. Medical staff attitudes toward family presence during pediatric procedures. Pediatr Emerg Care.2004;20:224-227. doi: 10.1097/01.pec.0000121241.99242.3b
10. Bradford KK, Kost S, Selbst SM, Renwick AE, Pratt A. Family member presence for procedures: the resident's perspective. Ambul Pediatr. 2005;5:294-297. doi: 10.1367/A04-024R1.1
11. Jarvis AS. Parental presence during resuscitation: attitudes of staff on a paediatric intensive care unit. Intensive Crit Care Nurs. 1998;14:3-7. doi: 10.1016/s0964-3397(98)80029-3
12. Zavotsky KE, McCoy J, Bell G, Haussman K, Joiner J, Marcoux KK, Magarelli K, Mahoney K, Maldonado L, Mastro KA, Milloria A, Tamburri LM, Tortajada D. Resuscitation team perceptions of family presence during CPR. Adv Emerg Nurs J. 2014;36:325-334. doi: 10.1097/TME.0000000000000027
13. Kuzin JK, Yborra JG, Taylor MD, Chang AC, Altman CA, Whitney GM, Mott AR. Family-member presence during interventions in the intensive care unit: perceptions of pediatric cardiac intensive care providers. Pediatrics.2007;120:e895-e901. doi: 10.1542/peds.2006-2943
14. Fulbrook P, Latour JM, Albarran JW. Paediatric critical care nurses' attitudes and experiences of parental presence during cardiopulmonary resuscitation: a European survey. Int J Nurs Stud. 2007;44:1238-1249. doi: 10.1016/j.ijnurstu.2006.05.006

原因不明の突然の心停止の評価

肥大型心筋症，冠動脈異常，および不整脈が，乳児および小児における原因不明の突然の心停止に多い原因である。原因不明の突然の心停止から蘇生しなかった若齢患者の最大3分の1で，肉眼および顕微鏡による剖検での異常を認めなかった[1-4]。原因不明の突然の心停止の病因をさぐるために，死亡後の遺伝子評価（「分子的剖検」）の使用が急速に増えている[5]。心停止の原因を解明するだけでなく，遺伝子診断により，チャネル病や心筋症などの遺伝性の心疾患を検出できるため，親族のスクリーニングや予防措置が可能となる。

原因不明の突然の心停止の評価に関する推奨事項

COR	LOE	推奨事項
1	C-EO	1. 原因不明の突然の心停止を経験した乳児，小児，若年成人はすべて，リソースが使用可能な場合，できれば心血管病理の訓練と経験を積んだ病理医が，無制限に完全剖検を行うべきである。遺伝性心疾患の有無を判定するため，遺伝子分析を目的とした生体物質の適切な保存を検討する[6-21]。
1	C-EO	2. 剖検で死因がみつからなかった患者の家族を，医療従事者または遺伝性の心疾患および心臓の遺伝カウンセリングを専門とする医療センターに紹介する[6-12,17,18,20-25]。
1	C-EO	3. 原因不明の突然の心停止から蘇生した乳児，小児，および若年成人の場合，完全な病歴および家族歴（失神発作，けいれん発作，原因不明の事故もしくは溺水，または50歳前の突然死の既往を含む）を入手し，以前の心電図を見直し，心臓病専門医に紹介する[16,17,19-21]。

「推奨事項の裏付けとなる解説」

1. 7件のコホート研究で，チャネル病の原因となる突然変異が乳児突然死症候群の乳児の2～10％で検出された[6-12]。原因不明の突然の心停止に至り剖検が正常であった青少年を対象とした9件のコホート研究では，チャネル病または心筋症に関わる遺伝子変異の同定を報告している[13-21]。

2. 7件の臨床検査（心電計，分子遺伝学的スクリーニング）によるスクリーニングのコホート研究[17,18,20,22-25]と1件の集団研究[21]では，原因不明の突然の心停止患者に関わる一親

等および二親等の近親者の 14〜53 %に不整脈原性の障害を認めた。7 件のコホート研究で，チャネル病の原因となる突然変異が乳児突然死症候群の乳児の 2〜10 %で検出された[6-12]。

3. 複数のコホート研究では，原因不明の突然の心停止後に完全な病歴と家族歴を得ること，さらに従前の心電図を見直すことの有用性を報告している。小規模の症例集積では，病歴から親族に特有の遺伝子スクリーニングが導き出されることを示唆した[20]。3 件の小規模のコホート研究と 1 件の集団研究は，原因不明の突然の心停止患者とその親族間で，けいれん発作，失神，動悸，胸痛，左腕痛，息切れなどの関連する臨床症状や合併症を報告した[16,17,19,21]。

参考文献

1. Doolan A, Langlois N, Semsarian C. Causes of sudden cardiac death in young Australians. Med J Aust.2004;180:110-112.
2. Eckart RE, Scoville SL, Campbell CL, Shry EA, Stajduhar KC, Potter RN, Pearse LA, Virmani R. Sudden death in young adults: a 25-year review of autopsies in military recruits. Ann Intern Med.2004;141:829-834. doi: 10.7326/0003-4819-141-11-200412070-00005
3. Ong ME, Stiell I, Osmond MH, Nesbitt L, Gerein R, Campbell S, McLellan B; OPALS Study Group. Etiology of pediatric out-of-hospital cardiac arrest by coroner's diagnosis. Resuscitation.2006;68:335-342. doi: 10.1016/j.resuscitation.2005.05.026
4. Puranik R, Chow CK, Duflou JA, Kilborn MJ, McGuire MA. Sudden death in the young.Heart Rhythm.2005;2:1277-1282. doi: 10.1016/j.hrthm.2005.09.008
5. Torkamani A, Muse ED, Spencer EG, Rueda M, Wagner GN, Lucas JR, Topol EJ. Molecular Autopsy for Sudden Unexpected Death. JAMA. 2016; 316:1492-1494. doi: 10.1001/jama.2016.11445
6. Ackerman MJ, Siu BL, Sturner WQ, Tester DJ, Valdivia CR, Makielski JC, Towbin JA. Postmortem molecular analysis of SCN5A defects in sudden infant death syndrome. JAMA. 2001;286:2264-2269. doi: 10.1001/jama.286.18.2264
7. Arnestad M, Crotti L, Rognum TO, Insolia R, Pedrazzini M, Ferrandi C, Vege A, Wang DW, Rhodes TE, George AL Jr, Schwartz PJ. Prevalence of long-QT syndrome gene variants in sudden infant death syndrome. Circulation.2007;115:361-367. doi: 10.1161/CIRCULATIONAHA.106.658021
8. Cronk LB, Ye B, Kaku T, Tester DJ, Vatta M, Makielski JC, Ackerman MJ. Novel mechanism for sudden infant death syndrome: persistent late sodium current secondary to mutations in caveolin-3. Heart Rhythm.2007;4:161-166. doi: 10.1016/j.hrthm.2006.11.030
9. Millat G, Kugener B, Chevalier P, Chahine M, Huang H, Malicier D, Rodriguez-Lafrasse C, Rousson R. Contribution of long-QT syndrome genetic variants in sudden infant death syndrome. Pediatr Cardiol.2009;30:502-509. doi: 10.1007/s00246-009-9417-2
10. Otagiri T, Kijima K, Osawa M, Ishii K, Makita N, Matoba R, Umetsu K, Hayasaka K. Cardiac ion channel gene mutations in sudden infant death syndrome. Pediatr Res. 2008;64:482-487. doi: 10.1203/PDR.0b013e3181841eca
11. Plant LD, Bowers PN, Liu Q, Morgan T, Zhang T, State MW, Chen W, Kittles RA, Goldstein SA. A common cardiac sodium channel variant associated with sudden infant death in African Americans, SCN5A S1103Y. J Clin Invest. 2006;116:430-435. doi: 10.1172/JCI25618
12. Tester DJ, Dura M, Carturan E, Reiken S, Wronska A, Marks AR, Ackerman MJ. A mechanism for sudden infant death syndrome (SIDS): stress-induced leak via ryanodine receptors. Heart Rhythm.2007;4:733-739. doi: 10.1016/j.hrthm.2007.02.026
13. Albert CM, Nam EG, Rimm EB, Jin HW, Hajjar RJ, Hunter DJ, MacRae CA, Ellinor PT. Cardiac sodium channel gene variants and sudden cardiac death in women. Circulation.2008;117:16-23. doi: 10.1161/CIRCULATIONAHA.107.736330
14. Chugh SS, Senashova O, Watts A, Tran PT, Zhou Z, Gong Q, Titus JL, Hayflick SJ. Postmortem molecular screening in unexplained sudden death. J Am Coll Cardiol.2004;43:1625-1629. doi: 10.1016/j.jacc.2003.11.052
15. Tester DJ, Spoon DB, Valdivia HH, Makielski JC, Ackerman MJ. Targeted mutational analysis of the RyR2-encoded cardiac ryanodine receptor in sudden unexplained death: a molecular autopsy of 49 medical examiner/coroner's cases. Mayo Clin Proc. 2004;79:1380-1384. doi: 10.4065/79.11.1380
16. Scheiper S, Ramos-Luis E, Blanco-Verea A, Niess C, Beckmann BM, Schmidt U, Kettner M, Geisen C, Verhoff MA, Brion M, Kauferstein S. Sudden unexpected death in the young – Value of massive parallel sequencing in postmortem genetic analyses. Forensic Sci Int. 2018;293:70-76. doi: 10.1016/j.forsciint.2018.09.034
17. Hellenthal N, Gaertner-Rommel A, Klauke B, Paluszkiewicz L, Stuhr M, Kerner T, Farr M, Püschel K, Milting H. Molecular autopsy of sudden unexplained deaths reveals genetic predispositions for cardiac diseases among young forensic cases. Europace.2017;19:1881-1890. doi: 10.1093/europace/euw247
18. Jiménez-Jáimez J, Alcalde Martínez V, Jiménez Fernández M, Bermúdez Jiménez F, Rodríguez Vázquez Del Rey MDM, Perin F, Oyonarte Ramírez JM, López Fernández S, de la Torre I, García Orta R, González Molina M, Cabrerizo EM, Álvarez Abril B, Álvarez M, Macías Ruiz R, Correa C, Tercedor L. Clinical and Genetic Diagnosis of Nonischemic Sudden Cardiac Death. Rev Esp Cardiol (Engl Ed).2017;70:808-816. doi: 10.1016/j.rec.2017.04.024
19. Lahrouchi N, Raju H, Lodder EM, Papatheodorou E, Ware JS, Papadakis M, Tadros R, Cole D, Skinner JR, Crawford J, Love DR, Pua CJ, Soh BY, Bhalshankar JD, Govind R, Tfelt-Hansen J, Winkel BG, van der Werf C, Wijeyeratne YD, Mellor G, Till J, Cohen MC, Tome-Esteban M, Sharma S, Wilde AAM, Cook SA, Bezzina CR, Sheppard MN, Behr ER. Utility of Post-Mortem Genetic Testing in Cases of Sudden Arrhythmic Death Syndrome. J Am Coll Cardiol.2017;69:2134-2145. doi: 10.1016/j.jacc.2017.02.046
20. Anastasakis A, Papatheodorou E, Ritsatos K, Protonotarios N, Rentoumi V, Gatzoulis K, Antoniades L, Agapitos E, Koutsaftis P, Spiliopoulou C, Tousoulis D. Sudden unexplained death in the young: epidemiology, aetiology and value of the clinically guided genetic screening. Europace.2018;20:472-480. doi: 10.1093/europace/euw362
21. Hendrix A, Borleffs CJ, Vink A, Doevendans PA, Wilde AA, van Langen IM, van der Smagt JJ, Bots ML, Mosterd A. Cardiogenetic screening of first-degree relatives after sudden cardiac death in the young: a population-based approach. Europace.2011;13:716-722. doi: 10.1093/europace/euq460
22. Behr E, Wood DA, Wright M, Syrris P, Sheppard MN, Casey A, Davies MJ, McKenna W; Sudden Arrhythmic Death Syndrome Steering Group. Cardiological assessment of first-degree relatives in sudden arrhythmic death syndrome. Lancet.2003;362:1457-1459. doi: 10.1016/s0140-6736(03)14692-2
23. Behr ER, Dalageorgou C, Christiansen M, Syrris P, Hughes S, Tome Esteban MT, Rowland E, Jeffery S, McKenna WJ. Sudden arrhythmic death syndrome: familial evaluation identifies inheritable heart disease in the majority of families. Eur Heart J. 2008;29:1670-1680. doi: 10.1093/eurheartj/ehn219
24. Hofman N, Tan HL, Clur SA, Alders M, van Langen IM, Wilde AA. Contribution of inherited heart disease to sudden cardiac death in childhood. Pediatrics.2007;120:e967-e973. doi: 10.1542/peds.2006-3751
25. Tan HL, Hofman N, van Langen IM, van der Wal AC, Wilde AA. Sudden unexplained death: heritability and diagnostic yield of cardiological and genetic examination in surviving relatives. Circulation.2005;112:207-213. doi: 10.1161/CIRCULATIONAHA.104.522581

ショックにおける患者の蘇生

ショックは，組織の代謝需要を満たす酸素輸送の停止で，致死的な場合がある。小児に起こるショックのうち最も多いのは，出血に起因するショックを含む，循環血液量減少性ショックである。血流分布不均等性ショック，心原性ショック，閉塞性ショックが起こることは少ない。しばしば複数種のショックが同時に起こる

ため、プロバイダーは絶えず警戒する必要がある。早期の段階で心原性ショックを診断するのは困難なことがあるため、常に疑いを持つことが必要である。

ショックは、重症度に応じて代償性から非代償性（低血圧）ショックまで連続的に進行する。心拍出量と終末臓器への灌流をそれぞれ維持するために、代償機構が働いて頻拍と体血管抵抗の上昇（血管収縮）が起こる。代償機構が停止すると、意識障害、尿量減少、乳酸アシドーシス、中枢脈拍の減衰などの低血圧および終末臓器への灌流不足の徴候が発現する。

敗血症性ショックを治療する静注輸液の早期投与は、限定的なエビデンスに基づくが広く受け入れられている。小児の敗血症による死亡率は、近年、抗生物質および輸液の早期投与の役割を強調するガイドラインが導入されると同時に低下した[1]。敗血症性ショックの管理に関する論争として、敗血症に関連した心停止における輸液投与量と患者の反応の評価方法、昇圧薬の選択とタイミング、コルチコステロイドの使用、および患者に対する治療アルゴリズムの変更がある。以前のAHAガイドライン[2]は、マラリア、鎌状赤血球貧血、およびデングショック症候群の患者の大規模な研究を考慮していた。しかし、これらの研究結果を一般化することで問題が増える点を、これらの患者では特に考慮する必要がある。

蘇生の早期に血液製剤を使用する蘇生プロトコールが晶質液の次に血液製剤投与（crystalloid-then-blood）の概念を否定したように、出血ショックの小児に対する蘇生ガイダンスは進歩している。しかし、特定の種類の損傷に対する理想的な蘇生戦略は、不明なことが多い。

ショックにおける輸液蘇生

ショックにおける輸液蘇生に関する推奨事項

COR	LOE	推奨事項
1	C-LD	1. 各輸液ボーラス投与後に、プロバイダーは、輸液への反応があるか、体液過剰の徴候があるか、患者を再評価する必要がある[3-5]。
2a	B-R	2. 蘇生に最初に用いる輸液としては、等張晶質液または膠質液のいずれも有効でありうる[6]。
2a	B-NR	3. 蘇生に用いる輸液としては、調整溶液または不調整溶液のいずれも有効でありうる[7-9]。
2a	C-LD	4. 敗血症性ショックの患者において、10 mL/kgまたは20 mL/kgの単位で輸液を投与しながら頻回の再評価をすることが妥当である[4]。

「推奨事項の裏付けとなる解説」

1. ショック状態の乳児および小児に対する初期治療の中心は輸液であることに変わりはないが、特に循環血液量減少および敗血症性ショックにおいて、体液過剰が後遺症の増加につながる可能性がある[3]。2件の敗血症性ショック患者の無作為化試験において、大量の輸液投与[4]や急速な輸液蘇生[5]を受けた患者ほど、人工呼吸を要する割合の増加と酸素化の悪化を特徴とする臨床的に重大な体液過剰が起こる傾向が高くなった。
2. システマティックレビューで、12件の関連する研究を確認したが、11件はサハラ以南のアフリカにおけるマラリア患者、デングショック症候群患者、または「発熱性疾患」患者での膠質液または晶質液による輸液蘇生を評価したものであった[6]。確認された研究のいずれでも、第一選択の輸液療法としての明確な有益性が、晶質液にも膠質液にも認められなかった。
3. 初期蘇生輸液として調整晶質液（乳酸リンゲル液）と不調整晶質液（0.9％生理食塩水）の使用を比較した1件の実用的な無作為化比較試験では、関連する臨床転帰に差を認めなかった[7]。敗血症性ショックの小児患者を対象としたマッチ法による1件の後向きコホート研究では、予後に差を認めなかったものの[8]、傾向マッチ法による1件のデータベース研究では不調整晶質液による輸液蘇生に、72時間死亡率の上昇および血管作動薬注入日の増加との関連性を認めた[9]。
4. 小規模の無作為対照化試験において、最初に用いる輸液のボーラス量に20 mL/kgを使用した場合（10 mL/kgと比較）、予後に有意差を認めなかった。しかし、この研究は少数の被験者によるため限定的である[4]。

敗血症性ショックにおける患者の蘇生

敗血症性ショックにおける患者の蘇生に関する推奨事項

COR	LOE	推奨事項
2a	C-LD	1. 輸液抵抗性の敗血症性ショックの乳児および小児において、アドレナリンまたはノルアドレナリンを初回血管作動薬注入として使用することは妥当である[1,10-14]。
2a	C-EO	2. 心停止および敗血症の乳児および小児では、敗血症に関連した心停止に対する固有のアプローチよりも、標準の小児の二次救命処置アルゴリズムを適用するのが妥当である[15]。
2b	B-NR	3. 輸液に反応せず血管作動薬によるサポートを必要とする敗血症性ショックの乳児および小児において、ストレス用量の副腎皮質ステロイド薬を検討することを妥当としてよい[12,16-19]。
2b	C-LD	4. 輸液抵抗性の敗血症性ショックの乳児および小児において、アドレナリンまたはノルアドレナリンを使用できない場合は、ドパミンを検討してよい[10-12]。

「推奨事項の裏付けとなる解説」

1. ドパミンまたはアドレナリンの漸増投与を比較する2件の無作為化比較試験では、ドパミンよりもアドレナリンの使用により、ショックからの回復のタイミング[10]、およ

び28日死亡率[11]が改善することを明らかにした。両方の研究はリソースの限られた状況で行われ，使用した陽性変力作用薬の投与量を直接比較できないため，研究から得た結論は限定的である。ノルアドレナリンなどの体血管抵抗を増強する薬剤は，敗血症性ショック患者の妥当な最初の昇圧薬による治療となり得る[1,12-14]。最近の国際的な敗血症ガイドラインでは，患者の生理機能と臨床医の選択に従って薬剤を選択するよう推奨している[1]。

2. 敗血症に関連した心停止患者の予後を改善するために，標準の救命処置アルゴリズムからの逸脱を支持する研究は存在しない。敗血症に関連した心停止は，心停止の他の原因よりも予後不良に関連する[15]。

3. メタアナリシス[20]では，小児の血症性ショックにコルチコステロイドを使用しても生存率が変わらないことを示したが，より最近の無作為化比較試験はステロイドの使用によりショックが好転する時間が短縮することを示唆した[17]。2件の観察研究では[18,19]，ゲノム情報に基づく個々の部分集団に，ステロイド投与が有益となる集団や有害となる集団があり得ることを示唆したが，これらの部分集団を臨床的に識別するのは困難である。副腎不全のリスク患者（例えば，長期のステロイド投与患者，電撃性紫斑病患者）は，ステロイド療法が有効な可能性が高い[12]。

4. アドレナリンやノルアドレナリンを利用できない状況では，ドパミンを代替として血管作動薬注入するのが妥当である[10,11]。血管拡張性ショック患者では，高用量のドパミンを要する可能性がある[12]。

心原性ショックにおける患者の蘇生

心原性ショックにおける患者の蘇生に関する推奨事項		
COR	LOE	推奨事項
1	C-EO	1. 心原性ショックの乳児および小児の場合，早期に専門医に相談することが推奨される。
2b	C-EO	2. 心原性ショックの乳児および小児には，陽性変力作用薬注入としてアドレナリン，ドパミン，ドブタミン，ミルリノンの使用が妥当であろう。

「推奨事項の裏付けとなる解説」

1 および 2. 乳児および小児の心原性ショックはまれであり，高い死亡率を伴う。さまざまな血管作動薬投与の転帰を比較した研究は認められなかった。低血圧患者には，初期の陽性変力作用薬の投与としてアドレナリンのような薬剤がより適切となり得る。これらの症状はまれで複雑なため，心原性ショックの乳児および小児を管理する際に，専門医に相談することが推奨される。

外傷性出血性ショックにおける患者の蘇生

外傷性出血性ショックにおける患者の蘇生に関する推奨事項		
COR	LOE	推奨事項
2a	C-EO	1. 外傷による低血圧性出血性ショックの乳児および小児において，継続的な輸液蘇生には晶質液ではなく血液製剤が利用できる場合はこれを投与することが妥当である[21-27]。

「推奨事項の裏付けとなる解説」

1. 外傷性出血性ショックに対する初期の血液製剤投与と初期の晶質液投与を比較した前向きの小児データはない。スコーピングレビューでは，出血性ショックの小児間で24～48時間以内に投与を受けた晶質液蘇生の総量と患者転帰とを比較した最近の後ろ向き研究6件を特定した[21-25,28]。4件の研究では，24時間生存率，30日時点の良好な神経学的転帰を伴う生存，生存退院率に差を認めない報告をした[21,24,25,28]。研究6件中5件で，大量の輸液蘇生入院／ICU滞在期間の延長と関連していた[22-25,28]。1件の研究では，低用量群と比較して60 mL/kg以上の晶質液投与を受けた小児間での，生存退院率の低下を報告した[22]。小児のデータが限定的であるにもかかわらず，最近の東部外傷外科学会（Eastern Association for the Surgery of Trauma）[26]，米国外科学会（American College of Surgeons），および英国国立医療技術評価機構（National Institute for Health and Care Excellence）[27]による成人用ガイドラインでは，外傷に関連した出血性ショックに対し濃厚赤血球，新鮮凍結血漿，および血小板をバランスのよい比率で早期使用することを推奨している[29]。

参考文献

1. Weiss SL, Peters MJ, Alhazzani W, Agus MSD, Flori HR, Inwald DP, Nadel S, Schlapbach LJ, Tasker RC, Argent AC, Brierley J, Carcillo J, Carrol ED, Carroll CL, Cheifetz IM, Choong K, Cies JJ, Cruz AT, De Luca D, Deep A, Faust SN, De Oliveira CF, Hall MW, Ishimine P, Javouhey E, Joosten KFM, Joshi P, Karam O, Kneyber MCJ, Lemson J, MacLaren G, Mehta NM, Møller MH, Newth CJL, Nguyen TC, Nishisaki A, Nunnally ME, Parker MM, Paul RM, Randolph AG, Ranjit S, Romer LH, Scott HF, Tume LN, Verger JT, Williams EA, Wolf J, Wong HR, Zimmerman JJ, Kissoon N, Tissieres P. Surviving Sepsis Campaign International Guidelines for the Management of Septic Shock and Sepsis-Associated Organ Dysfunction in Children. Pediatr Crit Care Med.2020;21:e52-e106. doi: 10.1097/PCC.0000000000002198

2. de Caen AR, Berg MD, Chameides L, Gooden CK, Hickey RW, Scott HF, Sutton RM, Tijssen JA, Topjian A, van der Jagt EW, et al. Part 12: pediatric advanced life support: 2015 American Heart Association Guidelines Update for Cardiopulmonary Resuscitation and Emergency Cardiovascular Care.Circulation. 2015;132 (suppl 2):S526-S542. doi: 10.1161/CIR.0000000000000266

3. van Paridon BM, Sheppard C, Garcia Guerra G, Joffe AR; on behalf of the Alberta Sepsis Network. Timing of antibiotics, volume, and vasoactive infusions in children with sepsis admitted to intensive care. Crit Care.2015;19:293. doi: 10.1186/s13054-015-1010-x

4. Inwald DP, Canter R, Woolfall K, Mouncey P, Zenasni Z, O'Hara C, Carter A, Jones N, Lyttle MD, Nadel S, et al; on behalf of PERUKI (Paediatric Emergency Research in the UK and Ireland) and PICS SG (Paediatric Intensive Care Society Study Group). Restricted fluid bolus volume in early septic shock: results of the Fluids in Shock pilot trial. Arch Dis Child.2019;104:426-431. doi: 10.1136/archdischild-2018-314924

5. Sankar J, Ismail J, Sankar MJ, C P S, Meena RS. Fluid Bolus Over 15–20 Versus 5–10 Minutes Each in the First Hour of Resuscitation in Children With Septic Shock: A Randomized Controlled Trial. Pediatr Crit Care Med. 2017;18:e435-e445. doi: 10.1097/PCC.0000000000001269
6. Medeiros DN, Ferranti JF, Delgado AF, de Carvalho WB. Colloids for the Initial Management of Severe Sepsis and Septic Shock in Pediatric Patients: A Systematic Review. Pediatr Emerg Care. 2015;31:e11-e16. doi: 10.1097/PEC.0000000000000601
7. Balamuth F, Kittick M, McBride P, Woodford AL, Vestal N, Casper TC, Metheney M, Smith K, Atkin NJ, Baren JM, Dean JM, Kuppermann N, Weiss SL. Pragmatic Pediatric Trial of Balanced Versus Normal Saline Fluid in Sepsis: The PRoMPT BOLUS Randomized Controlled Trial Pilot Feasibility Study. Acad Emerg Med. 2019;26:1346-1356. doi: 10.1111/acem.13815
8. Weiss SL, Keele L, Balamuth F, Vendetti N, Ross R, Fitzgerald JC, Gerber JS. Crystalloid Fluid Choice and Clinical Outcomes in Pediatric Sepsis: A Matched Retrospective Cohort Study. J Pediatr. 2017;182:304-310.e10. doi: 10.1016/j.jpeds.2016.11.075
9. Emrath ET, Fortenberry JD, Travers C, McCracken CE, Hebbar KB. Resuscitation With Balanced Fluids Is Associated With Improved Survival in Pediatric Severe Sepsis. Crit Care Med. 2017;45:1177-1183. doi: 10.1097/CCM.0000000000002365
10. Ventura AM, Shieh HH, Bousso A, Góes PF, de Cássia F O Fernandes I, de Souza DC, Paulo RL, Chagas F, Gilio AE. Double-Blind Prospective Randomized Controlled Trial of Dopamine Versus Epinephrine as First-Line Vasoactive Drugs in Pediatric Septic Shock. Crit Care Med. 2015;43:2292-2302. doi: 10.1097/CCM.0000000000001260
11. Ramaswamy KN, Singhi S, Jayashree M, Bansal A, Nallasamy K. Double-Blind Randomized Clinical Trial Comparing Dopamine and Epinephrine in Pediatric Fluid-Refractory Hypotensive Septic Shock. Pediatr Crit Care Med. 2016;17:e502-e512. doi: 10.1097/PCC.0000000000000954
12. Davis AL, Carcillo JA, Aneja RK, Deymann AJ, Lin JC, Nguyen TC, Okhuysen-Cawley RS, Relvas MS, Rozenfeld RA, Skippen PW, Stojadinovic BJ, Williams EA, Yeh TS, Balamuth F, Brierley J, de Caen AR, Cheifetz IM, Choong K, Conway E Jr, Cornell T, Doctor A, Dugas MA, Feldman JD, Fitzgerald JC, Flori HR, Fortenberry JD, Graciano AL, Greenwald BM, Hall MW, Han YY, Hernan LJ, Irazuzta JE, Iselin E, van der Jagt EW, Jeffries HE, Kache S, Katyal C, Kissoon N, Kon AA, Kutko MC, MacLaren G, Maul T, Mehta R, Odetola F, Parbuoni K, Paul R, Peters MJ, Ranjit S, Reuter-Rice KE, Schnitzler EJ, Scott HF, Torres A Jr, Weingarten-Arams J, Weiss SL, Zimmerman JJ, Zuckerberg AL. American College of Critical Care Medicine Clinical Practice Parameters for Hemodynamic Support of Pediatric and Neonatal Septic Shock. Crit Care Med. 2017;45:1061-1093. doi: 10.1097/CCM.0000000000002425
13. Lampin ME, Rousseaux J, Botte A, Sadik A, Cremer R, Leclerc F. Noradrenaline use for septic shock in children: doses, routes of administration and complications. Acta Paediatr. 2012;101:e426-e430. doi: 10.1111/j.1651-2227.2012.02725.x
14. Deep A, Goonasekera CD, Wang Y, Brierley J. Evolution of haemodynamics and outcome of fluid-refractory septic shock in children. Intensive Care Med. 2013;39:1602-1609. doi: 10.1007/s00134-013-3003-z
15. Del Castillo J, López-Herce J, Cañadas S, Matamoros M, Rodríguez-Núnez A, Rodríguez-Calvo A, Carrillo A; Iberoamerican Pediatric Cardiac Arrest Study Network RIBEPCI. Cardiac arrest and resuscitation in the pediatric intensive care unit: a prospective multicenter multinational study. Resuscitation. 2014;85:1380-1386. doi: 10.1016/j.resuscitation.2014.06.024
16. Menon K, Ward RE, Lawson ML, Gaboury I, Hutchison JS, Hébert PC; Canadian Critical Care Trials Group. A prospective multicenter study of adrenal function in critically ill children. Am J Respir Crit Care Med. 2010;182:246-251. doi: 10.1164/rccm.200911-1738OC
17. El-Nawawy A, Khater D, Omar H, Wali Y. Evaluation of Early Corticosteroid Therapy in Management of Pediatric Septic Shock in Pediatric Intensive Care Patients: A Randomized Clinical Study. Pediatr Infect Dis J. 2017;36:155-159. doi: 10.1097/INF.0000000000001380
18. Wong HR, Atkinson SJ, Cvijanovich NZ, Anas N, Allen GL, Thomas NJ, Bigham MT, Weiss SL, Fitzgerald JC, Checchia PA, et al. Combining prognostic and predictive enrichment strategies to identify children with septic shock responsive to corticosteroids. Crit Care Med. 2016;44:e1000-e1003. doi: 10.1097/CCM.0000000000001833
19. Wong HR, Cvijanovich NZ, Anas N, Allen GL, Thomas NJ, Bigham MT, Weiss SL, Fitzgerald JC, Checchia PA, Meyer K, et al. Endotype transitions during the acute phase of pediatric septic shock reflect changing risk and treatment response. Crit Care Med. 2018;46:e242-e249. doi: 10.1097/CCM.0000000000002932
20. Menon K, McNally D, Choong K, Sampson M. A systematic review and meta-analysis on the effect of steroids in pediatric shock. Pediatr Crit Care Med. 2013;14:474-480. doi: 10.1097/PCC.0b013e31828a8125
21. Hussmann B, Lefering R, Kauther MD, Ruchholtz S, Moldzio P, Lendemans S; and the TraumaRegister DGU. Influence of prehospital volume replacement on outcome in polytraumatized children. Crit Care. 2012;16:R201. doi: 10.1186/cc11809
22. Acker SN, Ross JT, Partrick DA, DeWitt P, Bensard DD. Injured children are resistant to the adverse effects of early high volume crystalloid resuscitation. J Pediatr Surg. 2014;49:1852-1855. doi: 10.1016/j.jpedsurg.2014.09.034
23. Edwards MJ, Lustik MB, Clark ME, Creamer KM, Tuggle D. The effects of balanced blood component resuscitation and crystalloid administration in pediatric trauma patients requiring transfusion in Afghanistan and Iraq 2002 to 2012. J Trauma Acute Care Surg. 2015;78:330-335. doi: 10.1097/TA.0000000000000469
24. Coons BE, Tam S, Rubsam J, Stylianos S, Duron V. High volume crystalloid resuscitation adversely affects pediatric trauma patients. J Pediatr Surg. 2018;53:2202-2208. doi: 10.1016/j.jpedsurg.2018.07.009
25. Elkbuli A, Zajd S, Ehrhardt JD Jr, McKenney M, Boneva D. Aggressive crystalloid resuscitation outcomes in low-severity pediatric trauma. J Surg Res. 2020;247:350-355. doi: 10.1016/j.jss.2019.10.009
26. Cannon JW, Khan MA, Raja AS, Cohen MJ, Como JJ, Cotton BA, Dubose JJ, Fox EE, Inaba K, Rodriguez CJ, Holcomb JB, Duchesne JC. Damage control resuscitation in patients with severe traumatic hemorrhage: A practice management guideline from the Eastern Association for the Surgery of Trauma. J Trauma Acute Care Surg. 2017;82:605-617. doi: 10.1097/TA.0000000000001333
27. Kanani AN, Hartshorn S. NICE clinical guideline NG39: Major trauma: assessment and initial management. Arch Dis Child Educ Pract Ed. 2017;102:20-23. doi: 10.1136/archdischild-2016-310869
28. Zhu H, Chen B, Guo C. Aggressive crystalloid adversely affects outcomes in a pediatric trauma population. Eur J Trauma Emerg Surg. 2019:Epub ahead of print. doi: 10.1007/s00068-019-01134-0
29. Henry S. ATLS Advanced Trauma Life Support. 10th Edition Student Course Manual. Chicago, IL: American College of Surgeons; 2018.

呼吸不全の治療

患者の呼吸が不十分になり、酸素化と換気が不足する場合に、呼吸不全が発生する。これは、呼吸調節障害、上気道閉塞、下気道閉塞、呼吸筋疲労、または肺実質性疾患が原因で起こることがある。呼吸がない、または不十分な場合に補助換気を行うこと、異物による気道閉塞（FBAO）を解除すること、オピオイド過量投与にナロキソンを投与することで、救命が可能となる。

　窒息（例えば、FBAO）と中毒が、乳児および小児の主な原因である。風船、食品（例えば、ホットドッグ、ナッツ類、ブドウ）、および小さな家庭用品が、小児の FBAO の最も多い原因であり[1-3]、乳児では液体が最も多い原因となる[4]。軽度の FBAO（患者は咳をし、発声する）と重度の FBAO（患者は発声できない）を区別することが重要である。軽度の FBAO 患者は咳によって閉塞の解除を試みることができるが、重重度の閉塞には介入が必要である。

　米国では 2017 年にオピオイド過量投与が原因で 15 歳未満の小児が 79 人、15〜24 歳で 4094 人が死亡した[5]。ナロキソンは、麻薬の過量投与による呼吸抑制を緩解するため[6]、2014 年にアメリカ食品医薬品局（US Food and Drug Administration）は、市民救助者と医療従事者によるナロキソン自己注射器の使用を認可した。ナロキソン鼻腔内投与器も有効である。

脈拍がある不十分な呼吸の治療

COR	LOE	推奨事項
1	C-EO	1. 脈拍はあるが呼吸努力がないか不十分な乳児および小児に対し，補助呼吸を行う[7]。
2a	C-EO	2. 脈拍はあるが呼吸努力がないか不十分な乳児および小児に対して，2～3秒ごとに人工呼吸を1回（20～30回/分）行うことが妥当である[7]。

「推奨事項の裏付けとなる解説」

1および2. 脈拍があり呼吸が不十分な場合の予後に対し，さまざまな換気回数が及ぼす影響を評価した小児専用の臨床試験は存在しない。1件の多施設共同観察研究では，心停止に対し高度な気道確保器具の装着を伴うCPR中に換気回数が多いと（1歳未満の小児で30回/分以上，1歳以上の小児で25回/分以上），ROSCおよび生存率が改善することを認めた[7]。訓練が容易なため，脈拍があり呼吸が不十分な患者に対する推奨呼吸回数を，高度な気道確保器具を装着した患者の換気に関する新規CPRガイドラインの推奨事項に即して，3～5秒ごとに1回から2～3秒ごとに1回に増やした。

異物による気道閉塞

COR	LOE	推奨事項
1	C-LD	1. 小児が軽度のFBAOの場合，傷病者が咳をして気道から異物を出すまで待ち，その間重度のFBAOの徴候が出現しないか見守る[4,8,9]。
1	C-LD	2. 小児が重度のFBAOの場合，異物が排出されるか，傷病者が反応しなくなるまで，腹部突き上げ法を行う[4,8,9]。
1	C-LD	3. 重度のFBAOの乳児に対しては，異物を排出するか反応がなくなるまで，背部叩打法（手のひらで叩く）と胸骨圧迫を5回ずつ行うサイクルを繰り返す[4,9-12]。
1	C-LD	4. 重度のFBAOの乳児または小児が反応しなくなる場合，CPRを胸骨圧迫から開始する（脈拍チェックはしない）。2分間CPRを行った後，救急対応システムに出動を要請する（まだ誰も行っていない場合）[11]。
1	C-LD	5. CPRを受けているFBAOの乳児または小児で，人工呼吸を行うために気道を確保する際に，目に見える異物を取り除く[13-15]。
3: 有害	C-LD	6. ただし，見えないのに無闇に手探りで掻き出そうとしてはならない[13-15]。

「推奨事項の裏付けとなる解説」

1および2. 小児のFBAOに関する推奨事項を裏付ける高品質のデータは存在しない。多くのFBAOは，患者が咳をすることによって解除されるか，重度の場合は腹部突き上げ法を用いてバイスタンダーが治療する[4,8,9]。

3. 主に症例集積による観察研究データは，乳児に対する背部叩打法[4,9,10]または胸骨圧迫[11]の使用を支持している。腹部突き上げ法は，腹部の臓器障害を引き起こす可能性がある場合，乳児に対し推奨できない[12]。

4. 傷病者が意識消失した場合，患者の脈拍の有無を問わず，直ちに胸骨圧迫を実施することを観察研究データが裏付けている[11]。

5および6. 観察研究データでは，FBAOの管理において盲目的に指で異物を掻き出すリスクがあらゆる潜在的利益を上回ることを示唆している[13-15]。

オピオイドによる心肺停止

COR	LOE	推奨事項
1	C-LD	1. 呼吸停止の患者においては，自発呼吸が再開するまで補助呼吸またはバッグマスク換気を維持する必要があり，自発呼吸が再開しない場合は標準的な小児一次救命処置または二次救命処置を継続する必要がある[17,18]。
1	C-EO	2. 心停止が確認されている，あるいは疑われる患者については，ナロキソンの使用が有益であると証明されていないため，標準的な蘇生処置をナロキソン投与よりも優先し，質の高いCPR（胸骨圧迫および換気）を重視すべきである[19,20]。
1	C-EO	3. 市民救助者と訓練を受けた対応者は，ナロキソンまたは他の介入に対する患者の反応を待ちながら，救急対応システムに出動を要請するのを遅延してはならない[21,22]。
2a	B-NR	4. オピオイド過量投与が疑われ，はっきりとした脈拍を触知できるが普段どおりの呼吸をしていないか，死戦期呼吸のみ（呼吸停止）の患者については，救助者は標準的な小児一次救命処置または二次救命処置に加え，ナロキソンの筋注または経鼻投与することが妥当である[23-36]。

「推奨事項の裏付けとなる解説」

1. 初期管理は，患者の気道確保と呼吸の補助に集中する必要がある。気道確保から始め，次に補助呼吸を行う。理想を言えばバッグマスクまたは感染防護具を用いる[17,18]。自発呼吸の再開が起こらない場合，救命処置を続ける必要がある。

2. 心停止中のナロキソン投与による患者転帰の改善を示す研究は存在しないため，CPRの提供を初期治療の目的とする必要がある[20]。質の高いCPRの要素を遅延しない場合，標準の二次救命処置とともにナロキソンを投与できる。

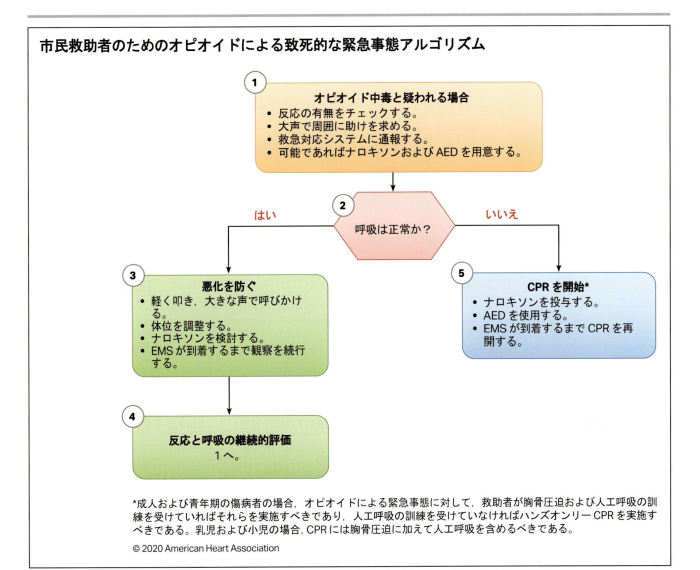

図 10. 市民救助者のためのオピオイドによる致死的な緊急事態アルゴリズム。
AED：自動体外式除細動器，CPR：心肺蘇生，EMS：救急医療サービス

3. 救急対応システムへの早期の通報は，オピオイド過量投与が疑われる患者に極めて重要である。傷病者の臨床症状がオピオイドによる呼吸抑制のみに起因することを救助者は確信できない。脈拍ありの判定が信頼できない場合，応急処置と BLS にこれが特に当てはまる[21,22]。ナロキソンは，非オピオイド薬の過量投与やあらゆる原因の心停止などの他の病状に効果はない。ナロキソン投与に反応する患者は，中枢神経系副作用および／または呼吸抑制を再発する可能性があり，安全に退院するために長期間の観察を要する場合がある[37-40]。

4. 12 件の研究が呼吸停止へのナロキソンの使用を検討し，内 5 件は，ナロキソン投与の筋肉内，静脈内および／または鼻腔内の経路を比較し（RCT 2 件[23,24]と非 RCT 3 件[25-27]），9 件はナロキソン使用の安全性を評価する研究，またはナロキソン使用の観察研究であった[28-36]。これらの研究では，オピオイドによる呼吸抑制の治療においてナロキソンが安全で効果的であること，合併症はまれで，用量依存的であることを報告した。

これらの推奨事項は，「第 3 章：成人一次救命処置と二次救命処置」[41]からの抜粋であり，2020 年 ILCOR の最新のエビデンスによりさらに裏付けられた[42]。これらの推奨事項を裏付ける小児のデータはなかった。しかし，オピオイド危機が緊急であるため，成人向け推奨事項を小児に適用する必要がある。

図 10 と 11 は，市民救助者と医療従事者向けのオピオイドによる緊急事態のアルゴリズムである。

参考文献

1. Morley RE, Ludemann JP, Moxham JP, Kozak FK, Riding KH. Foreign body aspiration in infants and toddlers: recent trends in British Columbia. J Otolaryngol. 2004;33:37-41. doi: 10.2310/7070.2004.00310

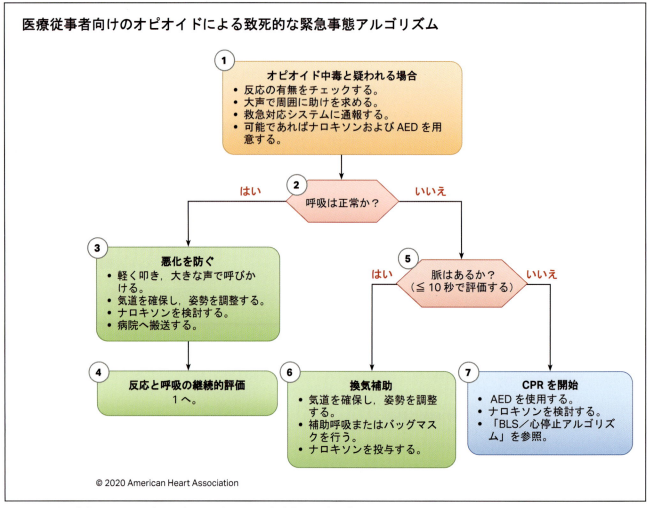

図11. 医療従事者のためのオピオイドによる致死的な緊急事態アルゴリズム。
AED：自動体外式除細動器，BLS：一次救命処置，CPR：心肺蘇生

2. Harris CS, Baker SP, Smith GA, Harris RM. Childhood asphyxiation by food. A national analysis and overview. JAMA.1984;251:2231-2235.
3. Rimell FL, Thome A Jr, Stool S, Reilly JS, Rider G, Stool D, Wilson CL. Characteristics of objects that cause choking in children. JAMA.1995;274:1763-1766.
4. Vilke GM, Smith AM, Ray LU, Steen PJ, Murrin PA, Chan TC. Airway obstruction in children aged less than 5 years: the prehospital experience. Prehosp Emerg Care.2004;8:196-199. doi: 10.1016/j.prehos.2003.12.014
5. Scholl L, Seth P, Kariisa M, Wilson N, Baldwin G. Drug and opioid-involved overdose deaths—United States, 2013-2017. MMWR Morb Mortal Wkly Rep. 2018;67:1419-1427. doi: 10.15585/mmwr.mm675152e1
6. Fischer CG, Cook DR. The respiratory and narcotic antagonistic effects of naloxone in infants. Anesth Analg.1974;53:849-852. doi: 10.1213/00000539-197453060-00007
7. Sutton RM, Reeder RW, Landis WP, Meert KL, Yates AR, Morgan RW, Berger JT, Newth CJ, Carcillo JA, McQuillen PS, Harrison RE, Moler FW, Pollack MM, Carpenter TC, Notterman DA, Holubkov R, Dean JM, Nadkarni VM, Berg RA; Eunice Kennedy Shriver National Institute of Child Health and Human Development Collaborative Pediatric Critical Care Research Network（CPCCRN).Ventilation Rates and Pediatric In-Hospital Cardiac Arrest Survival Outcomes.Crit Care Med.2019;47:1627-1636. doi: 10.1097/CCM.0000000000003898
8. Heimlich HJ. A life-saving maneuver to prevent food-choking. JAMA.1975;234:398-401.
9. Sternbach G, Kiskaddon RT. Henry Heimlich: a life-saving maneuver for food choking. J Emerg Med.1985;3:143-148. doi: 10.1016/0736-4679(85)90047-2
10. Redding JS. The choking controversy: critique of evidence on the Heimlich maneuver. Crit Care Med.1979;7:475-479.
11. Kinoshita K, Azuhata T, Kawano D, Kawahara Y. Relationships between pre-hospital characteristics and outcome in victims of foreign body airway obstruction during meals. Resuscitation.2015;88:63-67. doi: 10.1016/j.resuscitation.2014.12.018
12. Lee SL, Kim SS, Shekherdimian S, Ledbetter DJ. Complications as a result of the Heimlich maneuver. J Trauma. 2009;66:E34-E35. doi: 10.1097/01.ta.0000219291.27245.90
13. Abder-Rahman HA. Infants choking following blind finger sweep. J Pediatr（Rio J). 2009;85:273-275. doi: 10.2223/JPED.1892
14. Hartrey R, Bingham RM. Pharyngeal trauma as a result of blind finger sweeps in the choking child. J Accid Emerg Med. 1995;12:52-54. doi: 10.1136/emj.12.1.52
15. Kabbani M, Goodwin SR. Traumatic epiglottis following blind finger sweep to remove a pharyngeal foreign body. Clin Pediatr（Phila). 1995;34:495-497. doi: 10.1177/000992289503400908
16. Deleted in proof.
17. Guildner CW. Resuscitation—opening the airway: a comparative study of techniques for opening an airway obstructed by the tongue. JACEP. 1976;5:588-590. doi: 10.1016/s0361-1124(76)80217-1
18. Wenzel V, Keller C, Idris AH, Dörges V, Lindner KH, Brimacombe JR. Effects of smaller tidal volumes during basic life support ventilation in patients with respiratory arrest: good ventilation, less risk? Resuscitation.1999;43:25-29. doi: 10.1016/s0300-9572 (99)00118-5
19. Saybolt MD, Alter SM, Dos Santos F, Calello DP, Rynn KO, Nelson DA, Merlin MA. Naloxone in cardiac arrest with suspected opioid overdoses. Resuscitation.2010;81:42-46. doi: 10.1016/j.resuscitation.2009.09.016
20. Dezfulian C, Orkin AM, Maron BA, Elmer J, Girota S, Gladwin MT, Merchant RM, Panchal AR, Perman SM, Starks M, et al; on behalf of the American Heart Association Council on Cardiopulmonary, Critical Care, Perioperative and Resuscitation; Council on Arteriosclerosis, Thrombosis and Vascular Biology; Council on Cardiovascular and Stroke Nursing; and Council on Clinical Cardiology. Opioid-associated out-of-hospital cardiac arrest: distinctive clinical features and implications for healthcare and public responses:

a scientific statement from the American Heart Association.Circulation. In press.
21. Bahr J, Klingler H, Panzer W, Rode H, Kettler D. Skills of lay people in checking the carotid pulse.Resuscitation.1997;35:23-26. doi: 10.1016/s0300-9572 (96)01092-1
22. Eberle B, Dick WF, Schneider T, Wisser G, Doetsch S, Tzanova I. Checking the carotid pulse check: diagnostic accuracy of first responders in patients with and without a pulse.Resuscitation.1996;33:107-116. doi: 10.1016/s0300-9572 (96)01016-7
23. Kelly AM, Kerr D, Dietze P, Patrick I, Walker T, Koutsogiannis Z. Randomised trial of intranasal versus intramuscular naloxone in prehospital treatment for suspected opioid overdose. Med J Aust.2005;182:24-27.
24. Kerr D, Kelly AM, Dietze P, Jolley D, Barger B. Randomized controlled trial comparing the effectiveness and safety of intranasal and intramuscular naloxone for the treatment of suspected heroin overdose. Addiction.2009;104:2067-2074. doi: 10.1111/j.1360-0443.2009.02724.x
25. Wanger K, Brough L, Macmillan I, Goulding J, MacPhail I, Christenson JM. Intravenous vs subcutaneous naloxone for out-of-hospital management of presumed opioid overdose.Acad Emerg Med.1998;5:293-299. doi: 10.1111/j.1553-2712.1998.tb02707.x
26. Barton ED, Colwell CB, Wolfe T, Fosnocht D, Gravitz C, Bryan T, Dunn W, Benson J, Bailey J. Efficacy of intranasal naloxone as a needleless alternative for treatment of opioid overdose in the prehospital setting. J Emerg Med.2005;29:265-271. doi: 10.1016/j.jemermed.2005.03.007
27. Robertson TM, Hendey GW, Stroh G, Shalit M. Intranasal naloxone is a viable alternative to intravenous naloxone for prehospital narcotic overdose. Prehosp Emerg Care.2009;13:512-515. doi: 10.1080/10903120903144866
28. Cetrullo C, Di Nino GF, Melloni C, Pieri C, Zanoni A. [Naloxone antagonism toward opiate analgesic drugs. Clinical experimental study]. Minerva Anestesiol. 1983;49:199-204.
29. Osterwalder JJ. Naloxone-for intoxications with intravenous heroin and heroin mixtures-harmless or hazardous? A prospective clinical study. J Toxicol Clin Toxicol. 1996;34:409-416. doi: 10.3109/15563659609013811
30. Sporer KA, Firestone J, Isaacs SM. Out-of-hospital treatment of opioid overdoses in an urban setting.Acad Emerg Med.1996;3:660-667. doi: 10.1111/j.1553-2712.1996.tb03487.x
31. Stokland O, Hansen TB, Nilsen JE. [Prehospital treatment of heroin intoxication in Oslo in 1996]. Tidsskr Nor Laegeforen. 1998;118:3144-3146.
32. Buajordet I, Naess AC, Jacobsen D, Brørs O. Adverse events after naloxone treatment of episodes of suspected acute opioid overdose. Eur J Emerg Med.2004;11:19-23. doi: 10.1097/00063110-200402000-00004
33. Cantwell K, Dietze P, Flander L. The relationship between naloxone dose and key patient variables in the treatment of non-fatal heroin overdose in the prehospital setting. Resuscitation.2005;65:315-319. doi: 10.1016/j.resuscitation.2004.12.012
34. Boyd JJ, Kuisma MJ, Alaspää AO, Vuori E, Repo JV, Randell TT. Recurrent opioid toxicity after pre-hospital care of presumed heroin overdose patients. Acta Anaesthesiol Scand.2006;50:1266-1270. doi: 10.1111/j.1399-6576.2006.01172.x
35. Nielsen K, Nielsen SL, Siersma V, Rasmussen LS. Treatment of opioid overdose in a physician-based prehospital EMS: frequency and long-term prognosis. Resuscitation.2011;82:1410-1413. doi: 10.1016/j.resuscitation.2011.05.027
36. Wampler DA, Molina DK, McManus J, Laws P, Manifold CA. No deaths associated with patient refusal of transport after naloxone-reversed opioid overdose. Prehosp Emerg Care.2011;15:320-324. doi: 10.3109/10903127.2011.569854
37. Clarke SF, Dargan PI, Jones AL. Naloxone in opioid poisoning: walking the tightrope. Emerg Med J. 2005;22:612-616. doi: 10.1136/emj.2003.009613
38. Etherington J, Christenson J, Innes G, Grafstein E, Pennington S, Spinelli JJ, Gao M, Lahiffe B, Wanger K, Fernandes C. Is early discharge safe after naloxone reversal of presumed opioid overdose? CJEM. 2000;2:156-162. doi: 10.1017/s1481803500004863
39. Zuckerman M, Weisberg SN, Boyer EW. Pitfalls of intranasal naloxone. Prehosp Emerg Care. 2014;18:550-554. doi: 10.3109/10903127.2014.896961
40. Heaton JD, Bhandari B, Faryar KA, Huecker MR. Retrospective Review of Need for Delayed Naloxone or Oxygen in Emergency Department Patients Receiving Naloxone for Heroin Reversal. J Emerg Med.2019;56:642-651. doi: 10.1016/j.jemermed.2019.02.015
41. Panchal AR, Bartos JA, Cabañas JG, Donnino MW, Drennan IR, Hirsch KG, Kudenchuk PJ, Kurz MC, Lavonas EJ, Morley PT, et al; on behalf of the Adult Basic and Advanced Life Support Writing Group. Part 3: adult basic and advanced life support: 2020 American Heart Association Guidelines for Cardiopulmonary Resuscitation and Emergency Cardiovascular Care.Circulation. 2020;142 (suppl 2):S366-S468 doi: 10.1161/CIR.0000000000000916
42. Olasveengen TM, Mancini ME, Perkins GD, Avis S, Brooks S, Castrén M, Chung SP, Considine J, Couper K, Escalante R, et al; on behalf of the Adult Basic Life Support Collaborators. Adult basic life support: 2020 International Consensus on Cardiopulmonary Resuscitation and Emergency Cardiovascular Care Science With Treatment Recommendations.Circulation.2020;142 (suppl 1):S41-S91. doi: 10.1161/CIR.0000000000000892

挿管

小児の挿管に適した器材および薬剤を選択することが重要である。小児の正常な気道は声帯の下で狭くなり、チューブの先端側周辺で解剖学的に閉鎖されるため、これまでカフなしのETTが幼児には好ましいとされた。急性期の状況で、肺コンプライアンスが低い場合、カフなしのETTをカフ付ETTに変更する必要があり得る。カフ付のチューブは、カプノグラフィの正確さを向上し、（高リスクの再挿管や圧迫の遅れをもたらす）ETTを入れ替える必要性を減らし、圧力と1回換気量の流入を向上する。しかし、カフが高圧になると、気道の粘膜損傷を生じる場合がある。複数の研究で、カフ付チューブを使用すると、チューブの交換が少なくなるため実際に気道の外傷を減らす可能性があることを明らかにしたものの、正しいチューブサイズとカフの膨張圧を選択するよう注意しなければならない[1]。ETTのカフ圧は、高地での輸送時[2]と気道浮腫の悪化により変動する。

挿管はリスクの高い手技である。患者の血行動態、換気力学、および気道の状態によって、挿管中の心停止リスクが高まる場合がある。そのため、挿管前に適切な蘇生を実施することが重要である。

気道内に胃内容物が流入するリスクを最小化するため、バッグマスク換気および挿管時の輪状軟骨圧迫をこれまで使用してきたが、気管を圧迫して、効果的なバッグマスク換気と挿管の成功を妨げる可能性があるという懸案もある。

循環を生み出すリズムがある患者へのETT留置は、呼吸音の聴診、チューブ内の曇り、または胸の上がりでは確実には確認できない。比色計またはカプノグラフィ（$ETCO_2$）のいずれかを使用して最初のETT留置を評価できる。低心拍出量または心停止により肺血流量が低下した患者では、$ETCO_2$が信頼できない場合がある。

カフ付き気管チューブの挿管への使用

カフ付き気管チューブの挿管への使用に関する推奨事項		
COR	LOE	推奨事項
1	C-EO	1. カフ付きETTを使用する場合は、ETTのサイズ、位置、カフの膨張圧（通常はく20～25 cm H_2O）に注意を払う必要がある[3]。
2a	C-LD	2. 乳児および小児への挿管において、カフなしのETTよりもカフ付きETTを選択するほうが妥当である[4-15]。

「推奨事項の裏付けとなる解説」

1. 小児 2953 名を対象とした後向き研究では、気道に 25 cm H_2O の圧力をかけ ETT 周辺に軽微な漏れがある場合、臨床的に重大な声門下狭窄例はなく、再挿管を要する喘鳴の発生率は 1％未満であったことを報告した[3]。
2. システマティックレビュー 3 件、無作為化比較試験 2 件、および後向きレビュー 2 件が、カフ付ETTの安全性とETT交換の必要性の低減を裏付けている[4-10]。これらの研究は、ほぼすべて周術期の患者集団で行われ、熟練したプロバイダーにより挿管が実施されたものである。そのため、ETT の使用期間が重篤な患者でより短い可能性がある。カフ付 ETT の使用は、低い再挿管率、換気の高い成功率、およびカプノグラフィの正確さの向上と関連し、合併症リスクは上昇しない[7,9-13]。カフ付き ETT により、誤嚥のリスクを低減することができる[14,15]。

挿管時の輪状軟骨圧迫法の使用

挿管時の輪状軟骨圧迫法の使用に関する推奨事項		
COR	LOE	推奨事項
2b	C-LD	1. バッグマスク換気中の輪状軟骨圧迫には、胃膨満を軽減していると考えても良い[16,17]。
3: 利益なし	C-LD	2. 小児患者の気管挿管時に、輪状軟骨圧迫法のルーチン使用は推奨されない[16,17]。
3: 有害	C-LD	3. 輪状軟骨圧迫法を使用する場合、換気、スピード、または挿管のしやすさを妨げることがあれば輪状軟骨圧迫を中止すること[16,17]。

「推奨事項の裏付けとなる解説」

1、2、および3. 大規模な小児 ICU 挿管登録に由来する後ろ向き傾向スコアマッチ法による研究では、気管挿管前の導入およびバッグマスク換気中の輪状軟骨圧迫は逆流率の低下に関連しないことを示した[17]。同一の小児 ICU データベースに由来する研究では、外的喉頭操作（external laryngeal manipulation）が最初の気管挿管の低い成功率と関連することを報告した[16]。

挿管へのアトロピンの使用

挿管へのアトロピンの使用に関する推奨事項		
COR	LOE	推奨事項
2b	C-LD	1. 徐脈のリスクが高い場合（例えば、サクシニルコリンの投与時）、緊急挿管時の徐脈を予防する前投薬としてアトロピンを使用するのが妥当な場合がある[18,19]。
2b	C-LD	2. 緊急挿管時の前投薬としてアトロピンを使用する場合、アトロピン投与量 0.02 mg/kg（最小投与量なし）を考慮してもよい[20]。

「推奨事項の裏付けとなる解説」

1. 『2019 French Society of Anesthesia and Intensive Care Medicine』ガイドラインでは、敗血症性ショック、循環血液量減少、またはサクシニルコリンを投与した生後 28 日～8 歳の小児の挿管前投与薬としてアトロピンを使用しても「おそらくよい」と記載している[18,19]。
2. 1 件の非無作為化単一施設介入研究では、0.1 mg 未満のアトロピン投与量と徐脈または不整脈との関連性を認めなかった[20]。

高度な気道確保器具を装着した患者の呼気 CO_2 のモニタリング

高度な気道確保器具を装着した患者の呼気 CO_2 のモニタリングに関する推奨事項		
COR	LOE	推奨事項
1	C-LD	1. すべての状況で、循環を生み出すリズムを呈する乳児および小児に対し、ETT の留置を確認するために呼気 CO_2 検出（比色計またはカプノグラフィ）を使用する[21-27]。
2a	C-LD	2. 循環を生み出すリズムを呈する乳児および小児で、院外および院内／病院間の搬送時に呼気 CO_2 をモニター（比色計またはカプノグラフィ）するのが有益である[21,22,28-30]。

「推奨事項の裏付けとなる解説」

1. $ETCO_2$ の使用と臨床転帰とを関連付けた無作為化比較試験は存在しないものの、王立麻酔科学会と difficult airway 学会による第 4 回国内監査プロジェクト（Fourth National Audit Project of the Royal College of Anesthetists and Difficult Airway Society）では、カプノグラフィの使用やカプノグラフィの適切な解釈ができないことが ICU 関連死などの有害事象の原因になると結論付けた（成人と小児の混合データ）[21,22]。1 件の小規模の無作為化試験は、分娩室で挿管した早産新生児においてカプノグラフィが臨床的評価よりも迅速なことを示した[23]。定性的検出器（比色法）と定量的（カプノグラフィまたは数値表示）$ETCO_2$ 検出器との間で患者転帰に差異を認めなかった[24-27]。
2. 成人を対象とした文献は、挿管患者におけるカプノグラフィのモニタリングと正しい解釈により有害事象を防止できることを示唆している[21,22,28]。この点は、小児シナリオ

シミュレーションで実証され，カプノグラフィによって ETT が外れた可能性を認識するプロバイダーが多くなった[29,30]。

参考文献

1. Tobias JD. Pediatric airway anatomy may not be what we thought: implications for clinical practice and the use of cuffed endotracheal tubes. Paediatr Anaesth.2015;25:9-19. doi: 10.1111/pan.12528
2. Orsborn J, Graham J, Moss M, Melguizo M, Nick T, Stroud M. Pediatric Endotracheal Tube Cuff Pressures During Aeromedical Transport. Pediatr Emerg Care.2016;32:20-22. doi: 10.1097/PEC.0000000000000365
3. Black AE, Hatch DJ, Nauth-Misir N. Complications of nasotracheal intubation in neonates, infants and children: a review of 4 years' experience in a children's hospital. Br J Anaesth. 1990;65:461-467. doi: 10.1093/bja/65.4.461
4. Chen L, Zhang J, Pan G, Li X, Shi T, He W. Cuffed versus uncuffed endotracheal tubes in pediatrics: a meta-analysis. Open Med (Wars). 2018;13:366-373. doi: 10.1515/med-2018-0055
5. Shi F, Xiao Y, Xiong W, Zhou Q, Huang X. Cuffed versus uncuffed endotracheal tubes in children: a meta-analysis. J Anesth.2016;30:3-11. doi: 10.1007/s00540-015-2062-4
6. De Orange FA, Andrade RG, Lemos A, Borges PS, Figueiroa JN, Kovatsis PG. Cuffed versus uncuffed endotracheal tubes for general anaesthesia in children aged eight years and under. Cochrane Database Syst Rev. 2017;11:CD011954. doi: 10.1002/14651858.CD011954.pub2
7. Chambers NA, Ramgolam A, Sommerfield D, Zhang G, Ledowski T, Thurm M, Lethbridge M, Hegarty M, von Ungern-Sternberg BS. Cuffed vs. uncuffed tracheal tubes in children: a randomised controlled trial comparing leak, tidal volume and complications. Anaesthesia.2018;73:160-168. doi: 10.1111/anae.14113
8. de Wit M, Peelen LM, van Wolfswinkel L, de Graaff JC. The incidence of postoperative respiratory complications: A retrospective analysis of cuffed vs uncuffed tracheal tubes in children 0-7 years of age. Paediatr Anaesth.2018;28:210-217. doi: 10.1111/pan.13340
9. Schweiger C, Marostica PJ, Smith MM, Manica D, Carvalho PR, Kuhl G. Incidence of post-intubation subglottic stenosis in children: prospective study. J Laryngol Otol. 2013;127:399-403. doi: 10.1017/S002221511300025X
10. Dorsey DP, Bowman SM, Klein MB, Archer D, Sharar SR. Perioperative use of cuffed endotracheal tubes is advantageous in young pediatric burn patients. Burns. 2010;36:856-860. doi: 10.1016/j.burns.2009.11.011
11. Khine HH, Corddry DH, Kettrick RG, Martin TM, McCloskey JJ, Rose JB, Theroux MC, Zagnoev M. Comparison of cuffed and uncuffed endotracheal tubes in young children during general anesthesia. Anesthesiology. 1997;86:627-31; discussion 27A. doi: 10.1097/00000542-199703000-00015
12. Weiss M, Dullenkopf A, Fischer JE, Keller C, Gerber AC; European Paediatric Endotracheal Intubation Study Group. Prospective randomized controlled multi-centre trial of cuffed or uncuffed endotracheal tubes in small children. Br J Anaesth.2009;103:867-873. doi: 10.1093/bja/aep290
13. James I. Cuffed tubes in children. Paediatr Anaesth.2001;11:259-263. doi: 10.1046/j.1460-9592.2001.00675.x
14. Gopalareddy V, He Z, Soundar S, Bolling L, Shah M, Penfil S, McCloskey JJ, Mehta DI. Assessment of the prevalence of microaspiration by gastric pepsin in the airway of ventilated children. Acta Paediatr.2008;97:55-60. doi: 10.1111/j.1651-2227.2007.00578.x
15. Browning DH, Graves SA. Incidence of aspiration with endotracheal tubes in children. J Pediatr.1983;102:582-584. doi: 10.1016/s0022-3476(83)80191-7
16. Kojima T, Laverriere EK, Owen EB, Harwayne-Gidansky I, Shenoi AN, Napolitano N, Rehder KJ, Adu-Darko MA, Nett ST, Spear D, et al; and the National Emergency Airway Registry for Children (NEAR4KIDS) Collaborators and Pediatric Acute Lung Injury and Sepsis Investigators (PALISI). Clinical impact of external laryngeal manipulation during laryngoscopy on tracheal intubation success in critically ill children. Pediatr Crit Care Med.2018;19:106-114. doi: 10.1097/PCC.0000000000001373
17. Kojima T, Harwayne-Gidansky I, Shenoi AN, Owen EB, Napolitano N, Rehder KJ, Adu-Darko MA, Nett ST, Spear D, Meyer K, Giuliano JS Jr, Tarquinio KM, Sanders RC Jr, Lee JH, Simon DW, Vanderford PA, Lee AY, Brown CA III, Skippen PW, Breuer RK, Toedt-Pingel I, Parsons SJ, Gradidge EA, Glater LB, Culver K, Nadkarni VM, Nishisaki A; National Emergency Airway Registry for Children (NEAR4KIDS) and Pediatric Acute Lung Injury and Sepsis Investigators (PALISI). Cricoid Pressure During Induction for Tracheal Intubation in Critically Ill Children: A Report From National Emergency Airway Registry for Children. Pediatr Crit Care Med.2018;19:528-537. doi: 10.1097/PCC.0000000000001531
18. Quintard H, l'Her E, Pottecher J, Adnet F, Constantin JM, De Jong A, Diemunsch P, Fesseau R, Freynet A, Girault C, Guitton C, Hamonic Y, Maury E, Mekontso-Dessap A, Michel F, Nolent P, Perbet S, Prat G, Roquilly A, Tazarourte K, Terzi N, Thille AW, Alves M, Gayat E, Donetti L. Experts' guidelines of intubation and extubation of the ICU patient of French Society of Anaesthesia and Intensive Care Medicine (SFAR) and French-speaking Intensive Care Society (SRLF): In collaboration with the pediatric Association of French-speaking Anaesthetists and Intensivists (ADARPEF), French-speaking Group of Intensive Care and Paediatric emergencies (GFRUP) and Intensive Care physiotherapy society (SKR). Ann Intensive Care. 2019;9:13. doi: 10.1186/s13613-019-0483-1
19. Jones P, Ovenden N, Dauger S, Peters MJ. Estimating 'lost heart beats' rather than reductions in heart rate during the intubation of critically-ill children. PLoS One.2014;9:e86766. doi: 10.1371/journal.pone.0086766
20. Eisa L, Passi Y, Lerman J, Raczka M, Heard C. Do small doses of atropine (<0.1 mg) cause bradycardia in young children? Arch Dis Child.2015;100:684-688. doi: 10.1136/archdischild-2014-307868
21. Cook TM, Woodall N, Harper J, Benger J; on behalf of the Fourth National Audit Project. Major complications of airway management in the UK: results of the Fourth National Audit Project of the Royal College of Anaesthetists and the Difficult Airway Society, part 2: intensive care and emergency departments. Br J Anaesth.2011;106:632-642. doi: 10.1093/bja/aer059
22. Cook TM. Strategies for the prevention of airway complications – a narrative review. Anaesthesia.2018;73:93-111. doi: 10.1111/anae.14123
23. Hosono S, Inami I, Fujita H, Minato M, Takahashi S, Mugishima H. A role of end-tidal CO(2) monitoring for assessment of tracheal intubations in very low birth weight infants during neonatal resuscitation at birth. J Perinat Med. 2009;37:79-84. doi: 10.1515/JPM.2009.017
24. Hawkes GA, Finn D, Kenosi M, Livingstone V, O'Toole JM, Boylan GB, O'Halloran KD, Ryan AC, Dempsey EM. A Randomized Controlled Trial of End-Tidal Carbon Dioxide Detection of Preterm Infants in the Delivery Room. J Pediatr.2017;182:74-78.e2. doi: 10.1016/j.jpeds.2016.11.006
25. Hunt KA, Yamada Y, Murthy V, Srihari Bhat P, Campbell M, Fox GF, Milner AD, Greenough A. Detection of exhaled carbon dioxide following intubation during resuscitation at delivery. Arch Dis Child Fetal Neonatal Ed. 2019;104:F187-F191. doi: 10.1136/archdischild-2017-313982
26. Langhan ML, Emerson BL, Nett S, Pinto M, Harwayne-Gidansky I, Rehder KJ, Krawiec C, Meyer K, Giuliano JS Jr, Owen EB, Tarquinio KM, Sanders RC Jr, Shepherd M, Bysani GK, Shenoi AN, Napolitano N, Gangadharan S, Parsons SJ, Simon DW, Nadkarni VM, Nishisaki A; for Pediatric Acute Lung Injury and Sepsis Investigators (PALISI) and National Emergency Airway Registry for Children (NEAR4KIDS) Investigators. End-Tidal Carbon Dioxide Use for Tracheal Intubation: Analysis From the National Emergency Airway Registry for Children (NEAR4KIDS) Registry. Pediatr Crit Care Med.2018;19:98-105. doi: 10.1097/PCC.0000000000001372
27. Hawkes GA, Kenosi M, Ryan CA, Dempsey EM. Quantitative or qualitative carbon dioxide monitoring for manual ventilation: a mannequin study. Acta Paediatr.2015;104:e148-e151. doi: 10.1111/apa.12868
28. Fanara B, Manzon C, Barbot O, Desmettre T, Capellier G. Recommendations for the intra-hospital transport of critically ill patients. Crit Care.2010;14:R87. doi: 10.1186/cc9018
29. Langhan ML, Ching K, Northrup V, Alletag M, Kadia P, Santucci K, Chen L. A randomized controlled trial of capnography in the correction of simulated endotracheal tube dislodgement. Acad Emerg Med.2011;18:590-596. doi: 10.1111/j.1553-2712.2011.01090.x
30. Langhan ML, Auerbach M, Smith AN, Chen L. Improving detection by pediatric residents of endotracheal tube dislodgement with capnography: a randomized controlled trial. J Pediatr.2012;160:1009-14.e1. doi: 10.1016/j.jpeds.2011.12.012

徐脈の管理

血行動態障害を伴う徐脈は，触知可能な脈拍があっても，心停止の先駆けとなる場合がある。そのため，60 回/分の心拍数を下回る徐脈には，心肺機能障害の緊急評価が必要である。心肺機能障害が存在する場合，小児患者の初期管理として，病因の評価と気道確保，換気および酸素化による治療を同時に行う必要がある。有効な酸素化と換気にもかかわらず心肺機能障害を伴

う徐脈を認める場合，直ちに CPR を開始する必要がある。無脈性心停止に進行する前に徐脈に対する CPR を受けた小児では，予後がより良好である[1]。徐脈の原因となる治療可能な因子（すなわち，低酸素，低血圧，低血糖，低体温，アシドーシス，中毒性物質の摂取）を特定し，直ちに治療する必要がある。

徐脈の管理に関する推奨事項		
COR	LOE	推奨事項
1	C-LD	1. 徐脈の原因が迷走神経緊張亢進または一次性房室伝導ブロックである場合（すなわち，低体温などの要因に続発するものではない）は，アトロピンを投与する[2,4,6,7]。
1	C-LD	2. 酸素による有効な換気にもかかわらず心拍数が< 60 回/分で心肺機能障害を伴う場合，CPR を開始する[1,10]。
1	C-EO	3. 他の因子（例えば，低酸素症）を改善した後も徐脈が持続する場合や一時的にだけ反応する場合，アドレナリンの IV/IO 投与を行う。静脈路／骨髄路の確保ができない場合，あれば気管内投与する[1,11]。
2b	C-LD	4. 特に先天性または後天性の心疾患を呈する小児で，徐脈が換気，酸素化，胸骨圧迫および薬剤投与に反応しない完全房室ブロックや洞房結節の機能障害に起因する場合，緊急経皮ペーシングを考慮してもよい[12-16]。

「推奨事項の裏付けとなる解説」

1. 成人を対象とした 2 件の研究[2,4]と小児を対象とした 2 件の研究[6,7]では，迷走神経刺激，房室ブロック，および中毒に起因する徐脈を治療するためにアトロピンが有効なことを示した。他の原因による徐脈にアトロピンを使用するのがよいというエビデンスはない。
2. 同一のデータベースに由来する 2 件の後ろ向き分析は，徐脈および灌流不良のため CPR を受けた小児が，無脈性の心停止となり CPR を受けた小児よりも良好な予後となったことを示した[1,10]。徐脈による CPR の開始から脈拍喪失までの時間が長いほど，生存の可能性が低くなった。
3. 徐脈の治療に関する小児のデータは限定的である。脈拍がある徐脈の小児患者を対象とした最近の後ろ向き傾向スコアマッチ法による研究では，アドレナリンの投与を受けた患者が，投与を受けなかった患者よりも予後不良となることを明らかにした[11]。しかし，この研究は限定的であるため，徐脈および脈拍がある患者に対するアドレナリンの影響については，さらなる研究が必要である。
4. 小児の難治性徐脈に対する経皮ペーシングについてのデータは限定的である[12-16]。完全房室ブロックまたは洞房結節の機能障害患者では，特に先天性または後天性心疾患が原因で起こる場合，緊急経皮ペーシングを検討してもよい。ペーシングは，心拍再開後の低酸素症または虚血性心筋障害または呼吸不全による心静止や徐脈に有益でない。

図 12 に，小児の脈拍のある徐脈に関するアルゴリズムを示す。

参考文献

1. Khera R, Tang Y, Girotra S, Nadkarni VM, Link MS, Raymond TT, Guerguerian AM, Berg RA, Chan PS; on behalf of the American Heart Association's Get With the Guidelines–Resuscitation Investigators. Pulselessness after initiation of cardiopulmonary resuscitation for bradycardia in hospitalized children. Circulation.2019;140:370-378. doi: 10.1161/CIRCULATIONAHA.118.039048
2. Smith I, Monk TG, White PF. Comparison of transesophageal atrial pacing with anticholinergic drugs for the treatment of intraoperative bradycardia. Anesth Analg.1994;78:245-252. doi: 10.1213/00000539-199402000-00009
3. Deleted in proof.
4. Brady WJ, Swart G, DeBehnke DJ, Ma OJ, Aufderheide TP. The efficacy of atropine in the treatment of hemodynamically unstable bradycardia and atrioventricular block: prehospital and emergency department considerations. Resuscitation.1999;41:47-55. doi: 10.1016/s0300-9572(99)00032-5
5. Deleted in proof.
6. Zimmerman G, Steward DJ. Bradycardia delays the onset of action of intravenous atropine in infants. Anesthesiology. 1986;65:320-322.
7. Fullerton DA, St Cyr JA, Clarke DR, Campbell DN, Toews WH, See WM. Bezold-Jarisch reflex in postoperative pediatric cardiac surgical patients. Ann Thorac Surg. 1991;52:534-536. doi: 10.1016/0003-4975(91)90919-h
8. Deleted in proof.
9. Deleted in proof.
10. Donoghue A, Berg RA, Hazinski MF, Praestgaard AH, Roberts K, Nadkarni VM; American Heart Association National Registry of CPR Investigators. Cardiopulmonary resuscitation for bradycardia with poor perfusion versus pulseless cardiac arrest. Pediatrics.2009;124:1541-1548. doi: 10.1542/peds.2009-0727
11. Holmberg MJ, Ross CE, Yankama T, Roberts JS, Andersen LW; on behalf of the American Heart Association's Get With The Guidelines–Resuscitation Investigators. Epinephrine in children receiving cardiopulmonary resuscitation for bradycardia with poor perfusion. Resuscitation.2020;180-190. doi: 10.1016/j.resuscitation.2019.12.032
12. Pirasath S, Arulnithy K. Yellow oleander poisoning in eastern province: an analysis of admission and outcome. Indian J Med Sci. 2013;67:178-183. doi: 10.4103/0019-5359.125879
13. Singh HR, Batra AS, Balaji S. Pacing in children. Ann Pediatr Cardiol. 2013;6:46-51. doi: 10.4103/0974-2069.107234
14. Kugler JD, Danford DA. Pacemakers in children: an update. Am Heart J. 1989;117:665-679. doi: 10.1016/0002-8703(89)90743-6
15. Bolourchi M, Silver ES, Liberman L. Advanced heart block in children with Lyme disease. Pediatr Cardiol.2019;40:513-517. doi: 10.1007/s00246-018-2003-8
16. Nazif TM, Vazquez J, Honig LS, Dizon JM. Anti-N-methyl-D-aspartate receptor encephalitis: an emerging cause of centrally mediated sinus node dysfunction. Europace. 2012;14:1188-1194. doi: 10.1093/europace/eus014

頻脈性不整脈

規則的な，狭い QRS 幅の頻脈性不整脈（QRS 幅：0.09 秒以下）はリエントリー回路が原因で最も多く起こるが，他の機構（例えば，異所性心房頻拍，心房細動）が原因で起こる場合もある。規則的な，広い QRS 幅の頻脈性不整脈（QRS 幅：0.09 秒超）には，心室頻拍と変行伝導を伴う上室性頻拍（SVT）など複数の機序がある。

小児患者での SVT が血行動態に及ぼす影響はさまざまで，少数の患者では心血管障害（すなわち，意識障害，ショックの徴候，低血圧）が起こることもある。血行動態が安定した患者では，リエントリー性 SVT が，迷走神経刺激に

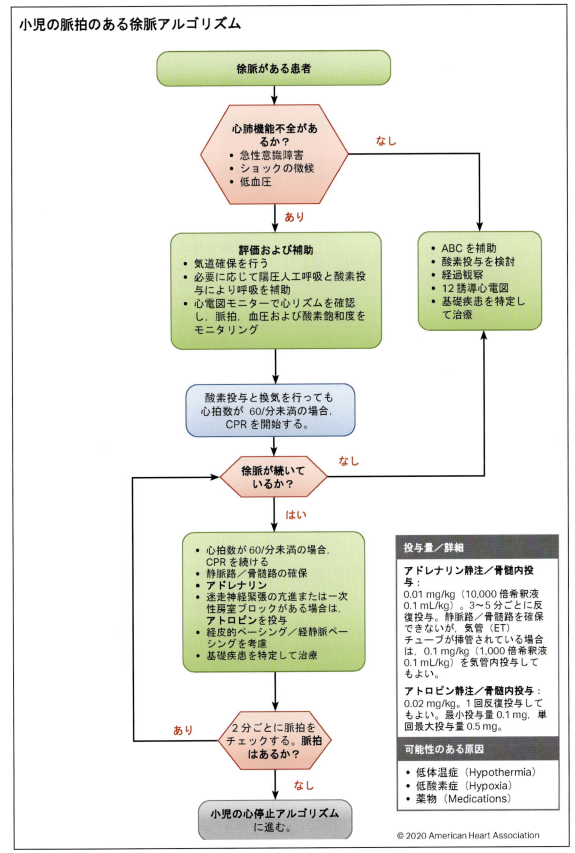

図12. 小児の脈拍のある徐脈アルゴリズム。
ABC：気道，呼吸，循環を補助，AV：房室，BP：血圧，CPR：心肺蘇生，ECG：心電図，HR：心拍数

よって停止することが多い[1,2]。アデノシンは，触知可能な脈拍があり迷走神経刺激に反応しない乳児および小児の SVT を治療するための推奨薬であり続けている。血行動態が安定した広い QRS 幅の頻拍患者で，初期治療に成功した後 SVT が繰り返し起こる場合，病因を診断し，治療法を個別に調整するために専門家の診察が重要となる。

SVT または広い QRS 幅の頻拍を呈する患者で血行動態が不安定な場合，同期電気ショックを検討することが望ましい。

脈拍がある上室性頻拍の治療

脈拍がある上室性頻拍の治療に関する推奨事項

COR	LOE	推奨事項
1	C-LD	1. 静脈路／骨髄路の確保が容易にできる場合，SVT の治療にアデノシンを推奨する[3-9]。
1	C-EO	2. 血行動態が安定した患者で，SVT が迷走神経刺激および／またはアデノシンIV 投与に反応しない場合，専門家の診察を推奨する[5-15,17]。
2a	C-LD	3. 最初に迷走神経刺激を試みるのが妥当である。ただし，患者の血行動態が不安定の場合，または化学的もしくは電気的同期電気ショックが遅延する場合を除く[1,2,4]。
2a	C-LD	4. SVT 患者の血行動態が不安定で心血管障害（すなわち，意識障害，ショックの徴候，低血圧）のエビデンスがある場合，0.5〜1 J/kg のエネルギー量で開始する電気的な同期電気ショックを実施するのが妥当である。成功しない場合は，エネルギー量を 2 J/kg に増大する[5,8,15]。
2b	C-LD	5. 不安定な SVT を有し，迷走神経刺激，アデノシンIV 投与，電気的な同期電気ショックに反応しない患者で，専門家の診察が得られていない場合，プロカインアミドまたはアミオダロンの投与を検討するのが妥当であろう[12,15]。

「推奨事項の裏付けとなる解説」

1. 静脈内アデノシン投与は，だいたい最初の 2 回以内でリエントリー性 SVT を停止する効果がある[3-6]。頻脈性不整脈の管理に関する 5 件の後ろ向き観察研究（単一施設 4 件，多施設共同 1 件）中，アデノシンと他の薬剤とを直接比較した研究はない[6-9,17]。

2. 血行動態が安定した SVT 患者で，迷走神経刺激やアデノシンに不応な場合は，複数の抗不整脈薬投与による催不整脈作用および致死的な循環虚脱の可能性を考慮して，専門家の診察に従って第二選択薬を検討する必要がある。静脈内ベラパミル，β 遮断薬，アミオダロン，プロカインアミド，ソタロール投与などの複数の薬剤が，アデノシン難治性 SVT の管理を目的とした第二選択薬として用いられている[5-15,17]。比較試験はほとんど存在しない。

3. 迷走神経刺激法は非侵襲的であり，ほとんど副作用がなく，多くの例で効果的に SVT を停止できる。各種の刺激法（すなわち，顔への氷水の適用，体位変換）の正確な成功率は不明である[4]。成人では修正バルサルバ法により成功率の向上が報告されているが[1]，バルサルバ法を適用した小児例の報告は極めて限定的である。頭部を下にする体位は，小児での効果的な迷走神経刺激の体位になり得る[2]。

4. 直流同期電気ショックは，血行動態が不安定な SVT（すなわち，意識障害，ショックの徴候，低血圧を特徴とする心血管障害）患者と標準的な治療法に反応しない SVT 患者に対する治療選択肢であり続ける。しかし，これらの症例はまれであり，SVT への電気ショックの転帰を報告するデータはわずかである[5,8,15]。リソースを利用でき，根治療法が遅延しない場合，同期電気ショックの前に鎮静剤の投与を検討する。

5. プロカインアミドおよびアミオダロン投与は，アデノシン耐性 SVT に対する中等度に効果的な治療である[12]。プロカインアミドのほうを選好する有効上のメリットは少ない可能性がある。副作用の頻度は，どちらでも頻回である。静脈内ソタロール投与は，2009 年にアメリカ食品医薬品局（US Food and Drug Administration）から SVT の治療に関する承認を得た。急性または亜急性の上室頻脈性不整脈でのソタロール使用を記載する報告は 3 件のみで，SVT と心房頻脈性不整脈の停止率は 60〜100 ％であった[9,13,14]。上述した研究では，ソタロールを，集中治療室または小児循環器病棟において小児循環器医（小児電気生理学者）の指導に従って IV 投与した。催不整脈性の可能性があるため，他の環境でソタロール IV 投与を安全にできるかどうかは不明である。現在のところ，難治性 SVT へのソタロール IV 投与に賛成または反対するためのエビデンスが不十分である。

脈拍がある広い QRS 幅の頻拍の治療

脈拍がある広い QRS 幅の頻拍の治療に関する推奨事項

COR	LOE	推奨事項
1	C-LD	1. 広い QRS 幅の頻拍患者で血行動態が安定している場合，抗不整脈薬を投与する前に専門家の診察を受けることを推奨する[18]。
2a	C-EO	2. 広い QRS 幅の頻拍患者の血行動態が不安定で心血管障害（すなわち，意識障害，ショックの徴候，低血圧）のエビデンスがある場合，0.5〜1 J/kg のエネルギー量で開始する電気的な同期電気ショックを実施するのが妥当である。成功しない場合は，エネルギー量を 2 J/kg に増量する。

「推奨事項の裏付けとなる解説」

1. 脈拍がある広い QRS 幅の頻拍（QRS 幅：0.09秒超）の発生は，小児ではまれであり，心室（心室頻拍）または心房（変行伝導を伴う SVT）に由来する可能性がある[18]。小児と成人を対象とした研究の両方で，抗不整脈治療による催不整脈作用合併症のリスクが高い潜在集団が特定され，心筋症，QT 延長症候群，ブルガダ症候群，Wolff-Parkinson-White 症候群の患者が該当した[19-23]。

2. 電気的な直流同期電気ショックは，心房または心室源の広い QRS 幅の頻拍を呈し，脈拍がある血行動態が不安定な小児の治療に対し緊急として提供することが望ましい。心血管障害は，最初の薬物療法の代わりに電気的な治療の使用を判定する際の主要な要因である。脈拍があり血行動態が安定している広い QRS 幅の頻拍の発生率について記載したエビデンスは不十分であり，脈拍がある広い QRS 幅の頻拍を呈する小児の管理に特定の抗不整脈薬を使用することへの賛成または反対はない。

図 13 に，小児の脈拍のある徐頻拍に関するアルゴリズムを示す。

参考文献

1. Appelboam A, Reuben A, Mann C, Gagg J, Ewings P, Barton A, Lobban T, Dayer M, Vickery J, Benger J; REVERT trial collaborators. Postural modification to the standard Valsalva manoeuvre for emergency treatment of supraventricular tachycardias (REVERT): a randomised controlled trial. Lancet.2015;386:1747-1753. doi: 10.1016/S0140-6736(15)61485-4
2. Bronzetti G, Brighenti M, Mariucci E, Fabi M, Lanari M, Bonvicini M, Gargiulo G, Pession A. Upside-down position for the out of hospital management of children with supraventricular tachycardia. Int J Cardiol. 2018;252:106-109. doi: 10.1016/j.ijcard.2017.10.120
3. Losek JD, Endom E, Dietrich A, Stewart G, Zempsky W, Smith K. Adenosine and pediatric supraventricular tachycardia in the emergency department: multicenter study and review. Ann Emerg Med.1999;33:185-191. doi: 10.1016/s0196-0644(99)70392-6
4. Campbell M, Buitrago SR. BET 2: Ice water immersion, other vagal manoeuvres or adenosine for SVT in children. Emerg Med J. 2017;34:58-60. doi: 10.1136/emermed-2016-206487.2
5. Clausen H, Theophilos T, Jackno K, Babl FE. Paediatric arrhythmias in the emergency department. Emerg Med J. 2012;29:732-737. doi: 10.1136/emermed-2011-200242
6. Díaz-Parra S, Sánchez-Yañez P, Zabala-Argüelles I, Picazo-Angelin B, Conejo-Muñoz L, Cuenca-Peiró V, Durán-Hidalgo I, García-Soler P. Use of adenosine in the treatment of supraventricular tachycardia in a pediatric emergency department. Pediatr Emerg Care.2014;30:388-393. doi: 10.1097/PEC.0000000000000144
7. Chu PY, Hill KD, Clark RH, Smith PB, Hornik CP. Treatment of supraventricular tachycardia in infants: Analysis of a large multicenter database. Early Hum Dev. 2015;91:345-350. doi: 10.1016/j.earlhumdev.2015.04.001
8. Lewis J, Arora G, Tudorascu DL, Hickey RW, Saladino RA, Manole MD. Acute management of refractory and unstable pediatric supraventricular tachycardia. J Pediatr. 2017;181:177.e2-182.e2. doi: 10.1016/j.jpeds.2016.10.051
9. Borquez AA, Aljohani OA, Williams MR, Perry JC. Intravenous sotalol in the young. J Am Coll Cardiol EP. 2020;6:425-432. doi: 10.1016/j.jacep.2019.11.019
10. Lim SH, Anantharaman V, Teo WS, Chan YH. Slow infusion of calcium channel blockers compared with intravenous adenosine in the emergency treatment of supraventricular tachycardia. Resuscitation.2009;80:523-528. doi: 10.1016/j.resuscitation.2009.01.017
11. Lapage MJ, Bradley DJ, Dick M II. Verapamil in infants: an exaggerated fear? Pediatr Cardiol.2013;34:1532-1534. doi: 10.1007/s00246-013-0739-8
12. Chang PM, Silka MJ, Moromisato DY, Bar-Cohen Y. Amiodarone versus procainamide for the acute treatment of recurrent supraventricular tachycardia in pediatric patients. Circ Arrhythm Electrophysiol. 2010;3:134-140. doi: 10.1161/CIRCEP.109.901629
13. Li X, Zhang Y, Liu H, Jiang H, Ge H, Zhang Y. Efficacy of intravenous sotalol for treatment of incessant tachyarrhythmias in children. Am J Cardiol.2017;119:1366-1370. doi: 10.1016/j.amjcard.2017.01.034
14. Valdés SO, Landstrom AP, Schneider AE, Miyake CY, de la Uz CM, Kim JJ. Intravenous sotalol for the management of postoperative junctional ectopic tachycardia. HeartRhythm Case Rep. 2018;4:375-377. doi: 10.1016/j.hrcr.2018.05.007
15. Sacchetti A, Moyer V, Baricella R, Cameron J, Moakes ME. Primary cardiac arrhythmias in children. Pediatr Emerg Care.1999;15:95-98. doi: 10.1097/00006565-199904000-00004
16. Deleted in proof.
17. Chandler SF, Chu E, Whitehill RD, Bevilacqua LM, Bezzerides VJ, DeWitt ES, Alexander ME, Abrams DJ, Triedman JK, Walsh EP, et al. Adverse event rate during inpatient sotalol initiation for the management of supraventricular and ventricular tachycardia in the pediatric and young adult population. Heart Rhythm. 2020;17:984-990. doi: 10.1016/j.hrthm.2020.01.022
18. Brady WJ, Mattu A, Tabas J, Ferguson JD. The differential diagnosis of wide QRS complex tachycardia. Am J Emerg Med.2017;35:1525-1529. doi: 10.1016/j.ajem.2017.07.056
19. Ramusovic S, Läer S, Meibohm B, Lagler FB, Paul T. Pharmacokinetics of intravenous amiodarone in children. Arch Dis Child.2013;98:989-993. doi: 10.1136/archdischild-2013-304483
20. Sarganas G, Garbe E, Klimpel A, Hering RC, Bronder E, Haverkamp W. Epidemiology of symptomatic drug-induced long QT syndrome and Torsade de Pointes in Germany. Europace.2014;16:101-108. doi: 10.1093/europace/eut214
21. Chen S, Motonaga KS, Hollander SA, Almond CS, Rosenthal DN, Kaufman BD, May LJ, Avasarala K, Dao DT, Dubin AM, Ceresnak SR. Electrocardiographic repolarization abnormalities and increased risk of life-threatening arrhythmias in children with dilated cardiomyopathy. Heart Rhythm.2016;13:1289-1296. doi: 10.1016/j.hrthm.2016.02.014
22. Coughtrie AL, Behr ER, Layton D, Marshall V, Camm AJ, Shakir SAW. Drugs and life-threatening ventricular arrhythmia risk: results from the DARE study cohort. BMJ Open. 2017;7:e016627. doi: 10.1136/bmjopen-2017-016627
23. Ortiz M, Martín A, Arribas F, Coll-Vinent B, Del Arco C, Peinado R, Almendral J; PROCAMIO Study Investigators. Randomized comparison of intravenous procainamide vs. intravenous amiodarone for the acute treatment of tolerated wide QRS tachycardia: the PROCAMIO study. Eur Heart J. 2017;38:1329-1335. doi: 10.1093/eurheartj/ehw230

心筋炎および心筋症の治療

劇症型心筋炎は，終末臓器の障害，完全房室ブロックなどの伝導系疾患，持続性の上室性不整脈や心室不整脈を伴う心拍出量低下を引き起こす場合があり，最終的に心停止に至ることがある[1]。患者が，腹痛，下痢，嘔吐，疲労感などの非特異的な症状を呈することがあるため，心筋炎は，他のより多く認められる疾患の症状と混同されることがある。転帰は，ICU でのモニタリングおよび治療などの早期診断と迅速な介入によって最適なものとなる。劇症型心筋炎患者での心ブロックおよび多病巣性の異所性心室興奮の突発的な発現は，心停止直前の状態とみなす必要がある。体外もしくは心内ペーシング，または抗不整脈薬による治療は成功しない可能性があるため，一時的または植え込み型の心室補助装置などの体外生命維持（ECLS）または機械的循環補助（MCS）を提供できる施設への早期の転院を推奨する[2,3]。

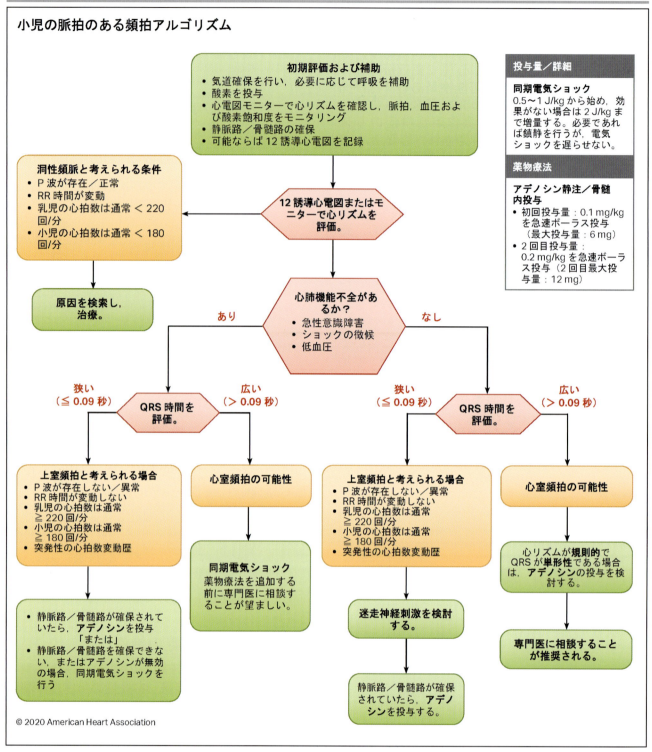

図 13. 小児の脈拍のある頻拍アルゴリズム。
CPR：心肺蘇生，ECG：心電図

感染以外を原因とする小児の心筋症には，拡張型心筋症，肥大型心筋症，収縮性心筋症，および不整脈原性右室異形成，ミトコンドリア心筋症，左室心筋緻密化障害を含むその他の（まれな）心筋症がある。機械的換気および血管作動薬の投与に不応の急性非代償性心不全を呈する心筋症患者は，心停止の前または心停止中にECMO，短期の経皮的心室補助装置または長期の植え込み型心室補助装置の形で予防的MCSを受けている[4,5]。

臨床状態が悪化している，または頻回の心室不整脈を呈する患者では，心停止の前に開始する場合，ECLSで救命できる。ECLSは，陽性変力作用を停止し，心筋の回復を支援し，必要に応じて心臓移植への橋渡しとして機能するような機会も提供する。ECLSとMCSの使用により急性心筋炎の予後が改善し，心筋機能を部分的に，または完全に回復する可能性が高くなる[2,6]。

心筋炎および心筋症の治療に関する推奨事項

COR	LOE	推奨事項
1	C-LD	1. 不整脈，房室ブロック，ST波の変化，および／または低心拍出量を示す急性心筋炎の小児は心停止を起こす危険性が高いため，ICUでのモニタリングおよび治療を受けられるように搬送を早期に検討することが推奨される[1,7,8]。
2a	B-NR	2. 心筋炎または心筋症および抵抗性低心拍出量の小児については，心停止前のECLSまたはMCSの使用が終末臓器のサポートを提供し心停止を防ぐうえで有益でありうる[9,10]。
2a	B-NR	3. 心筋炎および心筋症の小児の蘇生の成功に対するさまざまな課題を考慮し，心停止が発生した場合はECPRの早期検討が有益でありうる[9]。

「推奨事項の裏付けとなる解説」

1. 3件の後ろ向き研究では，劇症型心筋炎の予後不良の予測因子を評価し，この高リスク集団で心停止の発生率およびECLSの必要性の増加を示した[1,7,8]。1件の研究では，ほぼ半数近くの劇症型心筋炎患者がCPRを必要とし，ほぼ3分の1近くの患者がMCSを受けた[7]。左室駆出率の軽度の低下も，侵襲的な循環補助の必要性と関連している[8]。
2. ECLSまたはMCSを受けた劇症型心筋炎患者の予後は良好な場合がある。1件の研究では，MCSを要する小児28名中13名（46％）が移植なしで生存した[9]。1件の研究によると，心筋炎の診断を受けてカニューレ挿入したECPR患者の転帰のほうが，ECPRにいたる他の心停止および疾患カテゴリー（すなわち，先天性心疾患のない患者）より優れ，心筋炎を生存の向上に関わる事前のカニューレ挿入因子として示した[10]。心停止前の心筋症患者では，より新しい形状の一時的な循環補助装置により，移植への橋渡しを要する非代償性心不全に対し代替の改善され得る補助が得られている。これらの装置は，ECMOよりも延命効果を有する可能性がある[4,5]。
3. 1件の研究では，心停止後にECLSを留置した（n＝15），またはMCSを留置した（n＝1）心筋炎患児の95％が6カ月後に生存した[9]。

参考文献

1. Miyake CY, Teele SA, Chen L, Motonaga KS, Dubin AM, Balasubramanian S, Balise RR, Rosenthal DN, Alexander ME, Walsh EP, Mah DY. In-hospital arrhythmia development and outcomes in pediatric patients with acute myocarditis. Am J Cardiol.2014;113:535-540. doi: 10.1016/j.amjcard.2013.10.021
2. Wilmot I, Morales DL, Price JF, Rossano JW, Kim JJ, Decker JA, McGarry MC, Denfield SW, Dreyer WJ, Towbin JA, Jefferies JL. Effectiveness of mechanical circulatory support in children with acute fulminant and persistent myocarditis. J Card Fail. 2011;17:487-494. doi: 10.1016/j.cardfail.2011.02.008
3. Teele SA, Allan CK, Laussen PC, Newburger JW, Gauvreau K, Thiagarajan RR. Management and outcomes in pediatric patients presenting with acute fulminant myocarditis. J Pediatr.2011;158:638-643.e1. doi: 10.1016/j.jpeds.2010.10.015
4. Lorts A, Eghtesady P, Mehegan M, Adachi I, Villa C, Davies R, Gossett JG, Kanter K, Alejos J, Koehl D, Cantor RS, Morales DLS. Outcomes of children supported with devices labeled as "temporary" or short term: A report from the Pediatric Interagency Registry for Mechanical Circulatory Support. J Heart Lung Transplant. 2018;37:54-60. doi: 10.1016/j.healun.2017.10.023
5. Yarlagadda VV, Maeda K, Zhang Y, Chen S, Dykes JC, Gowen MA, Shuttleworth P, Murray JM, Shin AY, Reinhartz O, Rosenthal DN, McElhinney DB, Almond CS. Temporary Circulatory Support in U.S. Children Awaiting Heart Transplantation. J Am Coll Cardiol. 2017;70:2250-2260. doi: 10.1016/j.jacc.2017.08.072
6. Rajagopal SK, Almond CS, Laussen PC, Rycus PT, Wypij D, Thiagarajan RR. Extracorporeal membrane oxygenation for the support of infants, children, and young adults with acute myocarditis: a review of the Extracorporeal Life Support Organization registry. Crit Care Med.2010;38:382-387. doi: 10.1097/CCM.0b013e3181bc8293
7. Casadonte JR, Mazwi ML, Gambetta KE, Palac HL, McBride ME, Eltayeb OM, Monge MC, Backer CL, Costello JM. Risk Factors for Cardiac Arrest or Mechanical Circulatory Support in Children with Fulminant Myocarditis. Pediatr Cardiol.2017;38:128-134. doi: 10.1007/s00246-016-1493-5
8. Wu HP, Lin MJ, Yang WC, Wu KH, Chen CY. Predictors of Extracorporeal Membrane Oxygenation Support for Children with Acute Myocarditis. Biomed Res Int. 2017;2017:2510695. doi: 10.1155/2017/2510695
9. Schubert S, Opgen-Rhein B, Boehne M, Weigelt A, Wagner R, Müller G, Rentzsch A, Zu Knyphausen E, Fischer M, Papakostas K, Wiegand G, Ruf B, Hannes T, Reineker K, Kiski D, Khalil M, Steinmetz M, Fischer G, Pickardt T, Klingel K, Messroghli DR, Degener F; MYKKE consortium. Severe heart failure and the need for mechanical circulatory support and heart transplantation in pediatric patients with myocarditis: Results from the prospective multicenter registry "MYKKE". Pediatr Transplant. 2019;23:e13548. doi: 10.1111/petr.13548
10. Conrad SJ, Bridges BC, Kalra Y, Pietsch JB, Smith AH.Extracorporeal Cardiopulmonary Resuscitation Among Patients with Structurally Normal Hearts. ASAIO J. 2017;63:781-786. doi: 10.1097/MAT.0000000000000568

単心室患者の蘇生

小児の先天性心疾患の複雑さと多様さによって、蘇生時に固有の問題が生じる。単心室心疾患の小児には、通常、一連の段階的な姑息手術を実施する。通常、新生児期に実施する初回の姑息的手術の目的は、(1) 妨害されない体血流を構築すること、(2) 心房での混合ができるように有効な心房交通を構築すること、および (3) 過剰循環を防ぎ体心室の容量負荷を減らすために肺血流を調節することである（図 14）。第二期姑息手術時に、上大静脈肺動脈吻合術または両方向性 Glenn／hemi Fontan 手術を実施して、肺循環に直接戻る体静脈還流の再分配を補助する吻合を構築する（図 15）。Fontan 手術は最後の姑息術で、下大静脈の血流が人工血管を通じ直接肺循環に入るので、体心室である単心室への前負荷は肺血管床を介した受動的な血流に依存する。（図 16）。

単心室の生理特性を有する新生児および乳児では、(1) 体液過剰により心筋の働きが増大した結果、(2) 相対的な体血流（Qs）と肺血流（Qp）の平衡異常の結果、および (3) シャント閉塞の可能性により心停止のリスクが上昇する[1,2]。修復術の段階によって、蘇生には肺血管抵抗、酸素化、体血管抵抗、または ECLS の制御を要する可能性がある。

第一期姑息手術（Norwood/Blalock-Taussig シャント、Sano シャント）の術前および術後

第一期姑息手術（Norwood/Blalock-Taussig シャント、Sano シャント）の術前および術後に関する推奨事項		
COR	LOE	推奨事項
2a	B-NR	1. 直接（上大静脈カテーテル）および／または間接（近赤外分光法）酸素飽和度モニタリングは、第一期 Norwood 法姑息手術またはシャント留置後の重篤な新生児の傾向を把握し処置を指揮するうえで有益でありうる[3]。
2a	C-LD	2. 適切な制限的シャント術を受けた患者では、肺血管抵抗の操作はほとんど効果がない可能性があるが、全身血管拡張薬（α-アドレナリン拮抗薬および／またはホスホジエステラーゼ III 型阻害薬）を使用した体血管抵抗の低下が、酸素の使用の有無にかかわらず、全身酸素供給（DO_2）の増加に有用でありうる[4,5]。
2a	C-LD	3. 第一期手術前の高肺血流および症候性低体心拍出量および酸素輸送（DO_2）の新生児については、$Paco_2$ の目標値を 50～60 mm Hg とすることが妥当である。これは人工呼吸中に分時換気量を減らすか、神経筋遮断を伴うあるいは伴わない鎮痛／鎮静薬の投与によって達成できる[6,7]。
2a	C-LD	4. 第一期 Norwood 法姑息手術後の ECLS は低全身 DO_2 の治療に有用でありうる[8,9]。
2a	C-EO	5. シャント閉塞が確認されているまたは疑われる状況において、カテーテルまたは外科的治療の準備をする間に酸素、シャント灌流圧上昇のための血管作動薬、およびヘパリン（50～100 U/kg ボーラス）の投与が妥当である[2]。

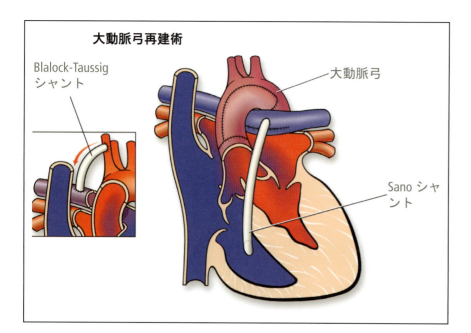

図 14. Norwood 修復術、および右鎖骨下動脈から右肺動脈までの Blalock-Taussig シャントまたは右心室から肺動脈までの Sano シャントによる単心室の第一期姑息手術。

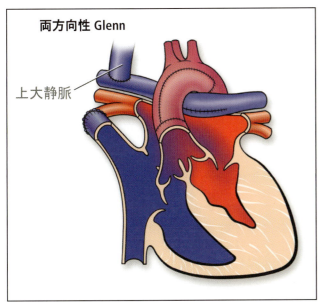

図15. 上大静脈と右肺動脈をつなぐ両方向性 Glenn シャントによる単心室の第二期姑息手術。

「推奨事項の裏付けとなる解説」

1. 術後の早期に，近赤外分光法で非侵襲的に測定した局所脳酸素飽和度と全身酸素飽和度により，第一期 Norwood 姑息手術後の早期死亡および ECLS 使用の予後を予測できる。術後近赤外分光法の測定値が目的志向型介入の目標値になり得ることを示す後ろ向きデータが存在する[3]。
2. 血管拡張薬（ニトロプルシドナトリウムまたはフェントラミン）を用いて後負荷を低減すると，ホスホジエステラーゼ III 型阻害薬（例えば，ミルリノン）投与の有無にかかわらず，シャントを要する単心室患者の術後期で体血管抵抗，血清乳酸値，動静脈血酸素較差，および ECPR の必要性が低下した[4,5]。
3. 単心室姑息手術前の期間に，制御下の低換気を慎重に使用すると，肺血管抵抗が増大しすることにより，Qp:Qs を低下させ，動静脈血酸素較差が縮小され，脳への酸素輸送が増加する。単純な低換気でも肺血管抵抗を増大できるが，望ましくない無気肺や呼吸性アシドーシスを伴うことがある[6,7]。
4. 第一期姑息修復術前後の心停止の場合，ECPR を使用すると生存率が向上する。2件の観察研究では，ECPR を要した新生児の 32〜54 %が生存し，1件の研究では，ECPR で管理された心停止患者で生存確率が向上した[8,9]。
5. 急性シャント閉塞の治療は，酸素の投与，シャントの灌流圧を最大にするための血管作用薬投与（例えば，フェニレフリン，ノルアドレナリン，アドレナリン），ヘパリンによる抗凝固療法（50〜100 U/kg ボーラス投与），カテーテル法または手術によるシャント介入，ECLS などで可能である[2]。

第二期（両方向性 Glenn／hemi Fontan）および第三期（Fontan）姑息手術後

第二期（両方向性 Glenn／半 Fontan）および第三期（Fontan）姑息手術後の治療に関する推奨事項

COR	LOE	推奨事項
2a	B-NR	1. 不十分な Qp による上大静脈肺動脈吻合生理機能および重度の低酸素血症のある心停止前の状態の患者については，脳および全身動脈血の酸素化を上昇させるため，無気肺のない軽度の呼吸性アシドーシスおよび最小限の平均気道内圧を目標とする換気法が有用でありうる[10]。
2b	B-NR	2. 上大静脈肺動脈吻合または Fontan 灌流のある患者において，治療可能な原因による低 DO_2 を治療するため，あるいは心補助装置または再置換術への橋渡しとして ECLS を検討してもよい[11]。

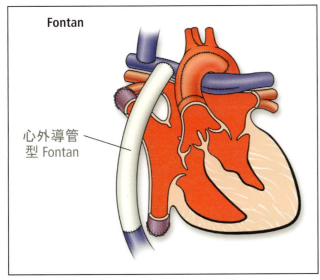

図16. 下大静脈と右肺動脈をつなぐ心外導管法による第三期 Fontan 単心室姑息手術。

「推奨事項の裏付けとなる解説」

1. 両方向性 Glenn 手術による留置直後の患者において，より高い $Paco_2$ による換気戦略で酸素化が向上した[10]。
2. 1件のExtracorporeal Life Support Organization データベースの後向き分析で，両方向性 Glenn 手術を実施した乳児と ECLS を必要とする乳児の間では，ECLS 前に心停止した患者（16/39 例，41 %）と心停止しなかった患者（26/64 例，41 %）での生存率が類似していた[11]。

これらのテーマについては，以前に『Cardiopulmonary Resuscitation in Infants and Children With Cardiac Disease: A Scientific Statement From the American Heart Association.』で概説された[12]。

参考文献

1. Feinstein JA, Benson DW, Dubin AM, Cohen MS, Maxey DM, Mahle WT, Pahl E, Villafañe J, Bhatt AB, Peng LF, et al. Hypoplastic left heart syndrome: current considerations and expectations. J Am Coll Cardiol. 2012;59 (suppl 1):S1-S42. doi: 10.1016/j.jacc.2011.09.022
2. Marino BS, Tibby SM, Hoffman GM. Resuscitation of the patient with the functionally univentricular heart. Curr Pediatr Rev. 2013;9:148-157. doi: 10.2174/1573396311309020008
3. Hoffman GM, Ghanayem NS, Scott JP, Tweddell JS, Mitchell ME, Mussatto KA. Postoperative Cerebral and Somatic Near-Infrared Spectroscopy Saturations and Outcome in Hypoplastic Left Heart Syndrome. Ann Thorac Surg.2017;103:1527-1535. doi: 10.1016/j.athoracsur.2016.09.100
4. Mills KI, Kaza AK, Walsh BK, Bond HC, Ford M, Wypij D, Thiagarajan RR, Almodovar MC, Quinonez LG, Baird CW, et al. Phosphodiesterase inhibitor-based vasodilation improves oxygen delivery and clinical outcomes following stage 1 palliation. J Am Heart Assoc. 2016;5 doi: 10.1161/JAHA.116.003554
5. Hansen JH, Schlangen J, Voges I, Jung O, Wegmann A, Scheewe J, Kramer HH. Impact of afterload reduction strategies on regional tissue oxygenation after the Norwood procedure for hypoplastic left heart syndrome. Eur J Cardiothorac Surg.2014;45:e13-e19. doi: 10.1093/ejcts/ezt538
6. Ramamoorthy C, Tabbutt S, Kurth CD, Steven JM, Montenegro LM, Durning S, Wernovsky G, Gaynor JW, Spray TL, Nicolson SC. Effects of inspired hypoxic and hypercapnic gas mixtures on cerebral oxygen saturation in neonates with univentricular heart defects. Anesthesiology.2002;96:283-288. doi: 10.1097/00000542-200202000-00010
7. Tabbutt S, Ramamoorthy C, Montenegro LM, Durning SM, Kurth CD, Steven JM, Godinez RI, Spray TL, Wernovsky G, Nicolson SC. Impact of inspired gas mixtures on preoperative infants with hypoplastic left heart syndrome during controlled ventilation. Circulation.2001;104 (suppl 1):I159-I164. doi: 10.1161/hc37t1.094818
8. Alsoufi B, Awan A, Manlhiot C, Guechef A, Al-Halees Z, Al-Ahmadi M, McCrindle BW, Kalloghlian A. Results of rapid-response extracorporeal cardiopulmonary resuscitation in children with refractory cardiac arrest following cardiac surgery.Eur J Cardiothorac Surg.2014;45:268-275. doi: 10.1093/ejcts/ezt319
9. Alsoufi B, Awan A, Manlhiot C, Al-Halees Z, Al-Ahmadi M, McCrindle BW, Alwadai A. Does single ventricle physiology affect survival of children requiring extracorporeal membrane oxygenation support following cardiac surgery? World J Pediatr Congenit Heart Surg. 2014;5:7-15. doi: 10.1177/2150135113507292
10. Zhu L, Xu Z, Gong X, Zheng J, Sun Y, Liu L, Han L, Zhang H, Xu Z, Liu J, et al. Mechanical ventilation after bidirectional superior cavopulmonary anastomosis for single-ventricle physiology: a comparison of pressure support ventilation and neurally adjusted ventilatory assist. Pediatr Cardiol.2016;37:1064-1071. doi: 10.1007/s00246-016-1392-9
11. Jolley M, Thiagarajan RR, Barrett CS, Salvin JW, Cooper DS, Rycus PT, Teele SA. Extracorporeal membrane oxygenation in patients undergoing superior cavopulmonary anastomosis. J Thorac Cardiovasc Surg. 2014;148:1512-1518. doi: 10.1016/j.jtcvs.2014.04.028
12. Marino BS, Tabbutt S, MacLaren G, Hazinski MF, Adatia I, Atkins DL, Checchia PA, DeCaen A, Fink EL, Hoffman GM, Jefferies JL, Kleinman M, Krawczeski CD, Licht DJ, Macrae D, Ravishankar C, Samson RA, Thiagarajan RR, Toms R, Tweddell J, Laussen PC; American Heart Association Congenital Cardiac Defects Committee of the Council on Cardiovascular Disease in the Young; Council on Clinical Cardiology; Council on Cardiovascular and Stroke Nursing; Council on Cardiovascular Surgery and Anesthesia; and Emergency Cardiovascular Care Committee. Cardiopulmonary Resuscitation in Infants and Children With Cardiac Disease: A Scientific Statement From the American Heart Association.Circulation.2018;137:e691-e782. doi: 10.1161/CIR.0000000000000524

肺高血圧症小児の治療に関する推奨事項

乳児および小児においてはまれな疾患である肺高血圧症は後遺症および死亡に有意に関連する。大多数の小児患者では，肺高血圧症は特発性であるか，または慢性肺疾患，先天性心疾患，まれであるが，結合組織病や血栓塞栓障害などの他の疾患に関連する[1]。肺高血圧症は先天性心疾患手術後の患者の 2～20 %で生じ，合併症および死亡率は依然として高い[2]。肺高血圧症は，心臓手術後に小児患者の 2～5 %で生じ[3]，さらに全心血管手術患者の 0.7～5 %は，術後肺高血圧クリーゼを経験する[4]。肺高血圧クリーゼは肺動脈圧の急激な上昇に伴う右（または単心室）心不全である。肺高血圧クリーゼ時には，右心室は機能せず，右心室で上昇した後負荷が心筋の酸素需要の増加を生じ，同時に冠動脈灌流圧と冠状動脈の血流が低下する。上昇した左心室圧と右心室圧が肺血流量と左室充満の低下を引き起こし，結果として心拍出量が減少する。陽性変力作用薬を投与すると右心室機能を改善でき，昇圧薬を投与すると体低血圧を治療し，冠状動脈灌流圧を改善できる。心停止が起きた時点で，肺血流がなくても左心室前負荷を維持できる解剖学的右ー左シャントが存在する場合，予後を改善できる[2]。これらのクリーゼは致死的であり，体低血圧，心筋虚血，心停止および心停止につながる場合がある。アシドーシスと低酸素血症はともに強力な肺血管収縮因子になるため，これらの状態の慎重なモニタリングと管理が肺高血圧症の管理に極めて重要である。治療には，適切な鎮痛薬，鎮静薬，および筋弛緩薬の投与も含める必要がある。吸入一酸化窒素，吸入プロスタサイクリン，吸入および静脈内プロスタサイクリンアナログ，静脈内および経口ホスホジエステラーゼⅤ型阻害薬（例えば，シルデナフィル）などの肺血管拡張薬を使用して，肺高血圧クリーゼを予防し治療する[5-8]。

肺高血圧症小児の治療に関する推奨事項

COR	LOE	推奨事項
1	B-R	1. 吸入一酸化窒素またはプロスタサイクリンは，肺血管抵抗の上昇に続発する肺高血圧緊急症または急性右心不全の初期治療として使用する必要がある[7,9-12]。
1	B-NR	2. 肺高血圧症の小児の術後治療において低酸素症およびアシドーシスを防ぐため，慎重な呼吸管理とモニタリングを提供する[13-15]。
1	C-EO	3. 肺高血圧緊急症のリスクが高い小児患者に対して，適切な鎮痛薬，鎮静薬，および神経筋遮断薬を投与する[2,11,16,17]。
2a	C-LD	4. 肺高血圧緊急症の初期治療について，肺専用の血管拡張薬の投与中に酸素投与および過換気によるアルカローシスの導入，またはアルカリ投与は有用となりうる[13-15]。
2b	C-LD	5. 最適な治療にもかかわらず低心拍出量または重度の呼吸不全の徴候を含む抵抗性肺高血圧症を発症した小児について，ECLS を検討してよい[11,18-23]。

「推奨事項の裏付けとなる解説」

1. 吸入一酸化窒素による治療で，肺高血圧クリーゼの頻度が低減し，抜管までの時間を短縮できる[9]。房室中隔欠損の修復および重度の術後肺高血圧症患者において，吸入一酸化窒素の投与は，死亡率の低下に関連する[7,10]。吸入プロスタサイクリンでは一時的に肺血管拡張が生じ，酸素化が改善するものの，本薬はアルカリ性が強いため気道を刺激することがあり，また噴霧回路内で薬物が損失するため正確な投与が難しい場合がある。[11,12]。

2. 生理学的レビュー 2 件と無作為化試験 1 件では，高炭酸ガス血症，低酸素血症，アシドーシス，無気肺，および換気血流の不均衡がすべて肺血管抵抗の上昇，すなわち術後期直後の肺動脈圧の上昇につながる場合があることを明らかにした[13-15]。

3. 特定の高リスク術後心疾患患者を調べた 2 件の観察研究では，術後期にフェンタニルの投与を受けた患者でのストレス反応の減弱を認めた[2,11,16,17]。

4. 生理学的レビュー 2 件と無作為化試験 1 件では，高炭酸ガス血症，低酸素血症，アシドーシス，無気肺，および換気血流の不均衡がすべて肺血管抵抗の上昇，すなわち術後期直後の肺動脈圧の上昇につながる場合があることを明らかにした[13-15]。

5. 肺血管疾患を呈する小児では，心肺虚脱後または心拍出量の低下後に ECLS を使用している[18,19]。特定の集団では予後不良が継続するものの[20]，体外循環補助装置の技術的進歩により，MCS または移植への橋渡しが可能となるであろう[21]。ECLS を要する肺高血圧症患者では死亡率が高いものの，ECLS の導入により救命が可能である[11,22,23]。

これらのテーマについては，以前に『Cardiopulmonary Resuscitation in Infants and Children With Cardiac Disease: A Scientific Statement From the American Heart Association』[2]，および『Pediatric Pulmonary Hypertension: Guidelines From the American Heart Association and American Thoracic Society』で概説された[11]。

参考文献

1. Ivy DD, Abman SH, Barst RJ, Berger RM, Bonnet D, Fleming TR, Haworth SG, Raj JU, Rosenzweig EB, Schulze Neick I, et al. Pediatric pulmonary hypertension. J Am Coll Cardiol.2013;62 (suppl):D117-D126. doi: 10.1016/j.jacc.2013.10.028

2. Marino BS, Tabbutt S, MacLaren G, Hazinski MF, Adatia I, Atkins DL, Checchia PA, DeCaen A, Fink EL, Hoffman GM, Jefferies JL, Kleinman M, Krawczeski CD, Licht DJ, Macrae D, Ravishankar C, Samson RA, Thiagarajan RR, Toms R, Tweddell J, Laussen PC; American Heart Association Congenital Cardiac Defects Committee of the Council on Cardiovascular Disease in the Young; Council on Clinical Cardiology; Council on Cardiovascular and Stroke Nursing; Council on Cardiovascular Surgery and Anesthesia; and Emergency Cardiovascular Care Committee.Cardiopulmonary Resuscitation in Infants and Children With Cardiac Disease: A Scientific Statement From the American Heart Association.Circulation.2018;137:e691-e782. doi: 10.1161/CIR.0000000000000524

3. Bando K, Turrentine MW, Sharp TG, Sekine Y, Aufiero TX, Sun K, Sekine E, Brown JW. Pulmonary hypertension after operations for congenital heart disease: analysis of risk factors and management. J Thorac Cardiovasc Surg. 1996;112:1600-7; discussion 1607. doi: 10.1016/S0022-5223(96)70019-3

4. Lindberg L, Olsson AK, Jögi P, Jonmarker C. How common is severe pulmonary hypertension after pediatric cardiac surgery? J Thorac Cardiovasc Surg.2002;123:1155-1163. doi: 10.1067/mtc.2002.121497

5. Avila-Alvarez A, Del Cerro Marin MJ, Bautista-Hernandez V. Pulmonary Vasodilators in the Management of Low Cardiac Output Syndrome After Pediatric Cardiac Surgery. Curr Vasc Pharmacol. 2016;14:37-47. doi: 10.2174/1570161113666151014124912

6. Sabri MR, Bigdelian H, Hosseinzadeh M, Ahmadi A, Ghaderian M, Shoja M. Comparison of the therapeutic effects and side effects of tadalafil and sildenafil after surgery in young infants with pulmonary arterial hypertension due to systemic-to-pulmonary shunts. Cardiol Young. 2017;27:1686-1693. doi: 10.1017/S1047951117000981

7. Bizzarro M, Gross I, Barbosa FT. Inhaled nitric oxide for the postoperative management of pulmonary hypertension in infants and children with congenital heart disease. Cochrane Database Syst Rev. 2014:CD005055. doi: 10.1002/14651858.CD005055.pub3

8. Unegbu C, Noje C, Coulson JD, Segal JB, Romer L. Pulmonary hypertension therapy and a systematic review of efficacy and safety of PDE-5 inhibitors. Pediatrics.2017;139:e20161450. doi: 10.1542/peds.2016-1450

9. Miller OI, Tang SF, Keech A, Pigott NB, Beller E, Celermajer DS. Inhaled nitric oxide and prevention of pulmonary hypertension after congenital heart surgery: a randomised double-blind study. Lancet.2000;356:1464-1469. doi: 10.1016/S0140-6736(00)02869-5

10. Journois D, Baufreton C, Mauriat P, Pouard P, Vouhé P, Safran D. Effects of inhaled nitric oxide administration on early postoperative mortality in patients operated for correction of atrioventricular canal defects. Chest.2005;128:3537-3544. doi: 10.1378/chest.128.5.3537

11. Abman SH, Hansmann G, Archer SL, Ivy DD, Adatia I, Chung WK, Hanna BD, Rosenzweig EB, Raj JU, Cornfield D, Stenmark KR, Steinhorn R, Thébaud B, Fineman JR, Kuehne T, Feinstein JA, Friedberg MK, Earing M, Barst RJ, Keller RL, Kinsella JP, Mullen M, Deterding R, Kulik T, Mallory G, Humpl T, Wessel DL; American Heart Association Council on Cardiopulmonary, Critical Care, Perioperative and Resuscitation; Council on Clinical Cardiology; Council on

Cardiovascular Disease in the Young; Council on Cardiovascular Radiology and Intervention; Council on Cardiovascular Surgery and Anesthesia; and the American Thoracic Society. Pediatric Pulmonary Hypertension: Guidelines From the American Heart Association and American Thoracic Society. Circulation.2015;132:2037-2099. doi: 10.1161/CIR.0000000000000329

12. Kelly LK, Porta NF, Goodman DM, Carroll CL, Steinhorn RH. Inhaled prostacyclin for term infants with persistent pulmonary hypertension refractory to inhaled nitric oxide. J Pediatr.2002;141:830-832. doi: 10.1067/mpd.2002.129849

13. Morris K, Beghetti M, Petros A, Adatia I, Bohn D. Comparison of hyperventilation and inhaled nitric oxide for pulmonary hypertension after repair of congenital heart disease. Crit Care Med.2000;28:2974-2978. doi: 10.1097/00003246-200008000-00048

14. Nair J, Lakshminrusimha S. Update on PPHN: mechanisms and treatment. Semin Perinatol. 2014;38:78-91. doi: 10.1053/j.semperi.2013.11.004

15. Moudgil R, Michelakis ED, Archer SL. Hypoxic pulmonary vasoconstriction. J Appl Physiol (1985). 2005;98:390-403. doi: 10.1152/japplphysiol.00733.2004

16. Hopkins RA, Bull C, Haworth SG, de Leval MR, Stark J. Pulmonary hypertensive crises following surgery for congenital heart defects in young children. Eur J Cardiothorac Surg.1991;5:628-634. doi: 10.1016/1010-7940(91)90118-4

17. Anand KJ, Hansen DD, Hickey PR. Hormonal-metabolic stress responses in neonates undergoing cardiac surgery. Anesthesiology.1990;73:661-670. doi: 10.1097/00000542-199010000-00012

18. Kolovos NS, Bratton SL, Moler FW, Bove EL, Ohye RG, Bartlett RH, Kulik TJ. Outcome of pediatric patients treated with extracorporeal life support after cardiac surgery. Ann Thorac Surg.2003;76:1435-41; discussion 1441. doi: 10.1016/s0003-4975(03)00898-1

19. Dhillon R, Pearson GA, Firmin RK, Chan KC, Leanage R. Extracorporeal membrane oxygenation and the treatment of critical pulmonary hypertension in congenital heart disease. Eur J Cardiothorac Surg.1995;9:553-556. doi: 10.1016/s1010-7940(05)80004-1

20. Puri V, Epstein D, Raithel SC, Gandhi SK, Sweet SC, Faro A, Huddleston CB. Extracorporeal membrane oxygenation in pediatric lung transplantation. J Thorac Cardiovasc Surg.2010;140:427-432. doi: 10.1016/j.jtcvs.2010.04.012

21. Ricci M, Gaughan CB, Rossi M, Andreopoulos FM, Novello C, Salerno TA, Rosenkranz ER, Panos AL. Initial experience with the TandemHeart circulatory support system in children. ASAIO J. 2008;54:542-545. doi: 10.1097/MAT.0b013e31818312f1

22. Morrell NW, Aldred MA, Chung WK, Elliott CG, Nichols WC, Soubrier F, Trembath RC, Loyd JE. Genetics and genomics of pulmonary arterial hypertension. Eur Respir J. 2019;53:Epub ahead of print. doi: 10.1183/13993003.01899-2018

23. Frank DB, Crystal MA, Morales DL, Gerald K, Hanna BD, Mallory GB Jr, Rossano JW. Trends in pediatric pulmonary hypertension-related hospitalizations in the United States from 2000-2009. Pulm Circ. 2015;5:339-348. doi: 10.1086/681226

外傷性心停止の管理

意図しない傷害は，青少年の間で最も頻度が高い死因である[1]。多くの組織が外傷治療のガイドラインを定めているものの[2-4]，外傷性心停止の管理は不正確になりがちである。小児の重大な鈍的損傷または穿通性損傷による心停止は，非常に高い死亡率となる[5-8]。緊張性気胸，血胸，肺挫傷，または心タンポナーデが血行動態，酸素化，および換気を損なう可能性があるため，すべての胸腹部の外傷で胸部損傷を疑う必要がある。

外傷性心停止の管理に関する推奨事項		
COR	LOE	推奨事項
1	C-EO	1. 小児の外傷性心停止では，出血，緊張性気胸，心タンポナーデなどの治療可能な潜在的原因を評価し治療する[9,10]。
2b	C-LD	2. 穿通性損傷による小児の心停止で輸送時間が短い場合，蘇生的開胸術の実施が妥当であろう[11-18]。

「推奨事項の裏付けとなる解説」

1. 外傷専用の介入の実施で遅延を減らして治療可能な原因を早期に修正することで，穿通性の外傷性心停止後の生存率を向上できる[9,10]。外傷による心停止に関するガイドラインでは，出血の制御，循環血液量の回復，気道確保，および緊張性気胸の緩和を推奨している。これらの措置を，従来の蘇生と同時に実施する必要がある。

2. 最近のシステマティックレビュー[11-14]，多施設共同後ろ向き研究[15,16]および単一施設後ろ向き研究[17]では，穿通性の胸部損傷後に脈拍の触れない小児患者に対し緊急開胸術を推奨した。生存の徴候がない鈍的損傷の乳児および小児に対する緊急開胸術を裏付けるエビデンスはない[12,18]。

参考文献

1. Heron M. Deaths: leading causes for 2010. Natl Vital Stat Rep. 2013;62:1-96.

2. Western Trauma Association. Western Trauma Association algorithms. 2011. https://www.westerntrauma.org/algorithms/algorithms.html. Accessed March 6, 2020.

3. Eastern Association for the Surgery of Trauma. EAST practice management guidelines. https://www.east.org/education/practice-management-guidelines. Accessed February 3, 2020.

4. Pediatric Trauma Society. Pediatric trauma society clinical practice guidelines. https://pediatrictraumasociety.org/resources/clinical-resources.cgi. Accessed February 3, 2020.

5. Calkins CM, Bensard DD, Partrick DA, Karrer FM. A critical analysis of outcome for children sustaining cardiac arrest after blunt trauma. J Pediatr Surg.2002;37:180-184. doi: 10.1053/jpsu.2002.30251

6. Crewdson K, Lockey D, Davies G. Outcome from paediatric cardiac arrest associated with trauma. Resuscitation.2007;75:29-34. doi: 10.1016/j.resuscitation.2007.02.018

7. Perron AD, Sing RF, Branas CC, Huynh T. Predicting survival in pediatric trauma patients receiving cardiopulmonary resuscitation in the prehospital setting. Prehosp Emerg Care.2001;5:6-9. doi: 10.1080/10903120190940245

8. Lopez-Herce Cid J, Dominguez Sampedro P, Rodriguez Nunez A, Garcia Sanz C, Carrillo Alvarez A, Calvo Macias C, Bellon Cano JM. [Cardiorespiratory arrest in children with trauma]. An Pediatr (Barc).2006;65:439-447. doi: 10.1157/13094250

9. Shibahashi K, Sugiyama K, Hamabe Y. Pediatric Out-of-Hospital Traumatic Cardiopulmonary Arrest After Traffic Accidents and Termination of Resuscitation. Ann Emerg Med.2020;75:57-65. doi: 10.1016/j.annemergmed.2019.05.036

10. Alqudah Z, Nehme Z, Williams B, Oteir A, Bernard S, Smith K. A descriptive analysis of the epidemiology and management of paediatric traumatic out-of-hospital cardiac arrest. Resuscitation.2019;140:127-134. doi: 10.1016/j.resuscitation.2019.05.020

11. Nevins EJ, Bird NTE, Malik HZ, Mercer SJ, Shahzad K, Lunevicius R, Taylor JV, Misra N. A systematic review of 3251 emergency department

- thoracotomies: is it time for a national database? Eur J Trauma Emerg Surg. 2019;45:231-243. doi: 10.1007/s00068-018-0982-z
12. Moskowitz EE, Burlew CC, Kulungowski AM, Bensard DD. Survival after emergency department thoracotomy in the pediatric trauma population: a review of published data. Pediatr Surg Int. 2018;34:857-860. doi: 10.1007/s00383-018-4290-9
13. Seamon MJ, Haut ER, Van Arendonk K, Barbosa RR, Chiu WC, Dente CJ, Fox N, Jawa RS, Khwaja K, Lee JK, Magnotti LJ, Mayglothling JA, McDonald AA, Rowell S, To KB, Falck-Ytter Y, Rhee P. An evidence-based approach to patient selection for emergency department thoracotomy: A practice management guideline from the Eastern Association for the Surgery of Trauma. J Trauma Acute Care Surg. 2015;79:159-173. doi: 10.1097/TA.0000000000000648
14. Moore HB, Moore EE, Bensard DD. Pediatric emergency department thoracotomy: A 40-year review. J Pediatr Surg. 2016;51:315-318. doi: 10.1016/j.jpedsurg.2015.10.040
15. Flynn-O'Brien KT, Stewart BT, Fallat ME, Maier RV, Arbabi S, Rivara FP, McIntyre LK. Mortality after emergency department thoracotomy for pediatric blunt trauma: analysis of the National Trauma Data Bank 2007-2012. J Pediatr Surg. 2016;51:163-167. doi: 10.1016/j.jpedsurg.2015.10.034
16. Nicolson NG, Schwulst S, Esposito TA, Crandall ML. Resuscitative thoracotomy for pediatric trauma in Illinois, 1999 to 2009. Am J Surg. 2015;210:720-723. doi: 10.1016/j.amjsurg.2015.05.007
17. Easter JS, Vinton DT, Haukoos JS. Emergent pediatric thoracotomy following traumatic arrest. Resuscitation. 2012;83:1521-1524. doi: 10.1016/j.resuscitation.2012.05.024
18. Duron V, Burke RV, Bliss D, Ford HR, Upperman JS. Survival of pediatric blunt trauma patients presenting with no signs of life in the field. J Trauma Acute Care Surg. 2014;77:422-426. doi: 10.1097/TA.0000000000000394

重要な今後の課題および進行中の研究

文献レビューの過程で，小児一次救命処置と二次救命処置に関連したいくつかの重要な課題を見出した。これらの項目は，現在進行中の研究の分野であるか，またはエビデンスに基づく推奨事項を裏付ける重要な小児エビデンスが欠如しているものである。さらに，ILCORの一次救命処置作業部会（Basic Life Support Task Force）または小児救命処置作業部会（Pediatric Life Support Task Force）によるシステマティックレビューとスコーピングレビューが進行中である項目を確認し，これらのレビューが得られるまで時期尚早の推奨事項をしないことを決定した。

小児科医療でよくあるように，多くの推奨事項は成人データから推定したものである。小児蘇生のBLS要素には特にこれが当てはまる。小児の心停止の原因は，成人の心停止とはまったく異なるため，小児を対象とした研究が特に必要である。さらに，乳児，小児，および青年は，異なる患者集団である。米国で心停止を経験する乳児，小児，および青年が毎年20 000人を上回ることを考慮すると，小児専用の蘇生の研究は最優先である。

重要な今後の課題を表2にまとめた。

表2. 不十分な小児データを原因とする極めて重要な今後の課題

CPR時の最適な薬剤投与方法は何か？ IOまたはIV？
薬剤投与に備えて体重を判定するための最適な方法は何か？
脈拍の触れない心停止時のどのような期間内に，初回投与量のアドレナリンを投与すべきか？
どのような頻度で2回目以降のアドレナリン投与を実施すべきか？
ECMO導入を待機しているCPR中の乳児および小児に，どのような頻度でアドレナリンを投与すべきか？
代替の圧迫法（咳CPR，拳ペーシング，間欠的腹部圧迫CPR）は，CPRのより効果的な代替になるのか？
CPR中にどのぐらいの頻度でリズムをチェックすべきか？
OHCA時に最適な気道確保方法は何か？バッグマスク換気，声門上器具，気管チューブ？
CPR中に管理する最適なF_{IO_2}はどのくらいか？
高度な気道確保器具の装着の有無を問わず，患者のCPR中の最適な換気回数はどのくらいか？最適な換気回数は年齢に依存するのか？
CPR時の胸骨圧迫の最適なテンポはどのくらいか？胸骨圧迫の最適なテンポは年齢に依存するのか？
CPR中の最適な血圧目標値はいくつか？最適な血圧目標値は年齢に依存するのか？
心エコー法によりCPRの質や心停止の予後を改善できるのか？
OHCAで高度な気道確保器具の留置が有効になる，または有害になる特有の状況が存在するのか？
IHCAで高度な気道確保器具を留置する適切なタイミングとは？
非心臓性の原因によるOHCAおよびIHCAを呈した患者に対するECPRの役割は何か？
VF／無脈性VTに対する除細動の最適なタイミングはどこで，エネルギー量はどのくらいか？
小児のIHCAおよびOHCA蘇生を終了する決定に役立てるために，どのような臨床ツールを用いることができるか？
心拍再開後期間中の最適な血圧目標値はいくつか？
心拍再開後にけいれん発作の予防を実施すべきか？
心拍再開後のけいれん性および非けいれん性発作の治療は，予後を改善するのか？
信頼できる心拍再開後の予後予測の方法は何か？
心拍再開後の予後を改善するために，どのようなリハビリテーション療法とフォローアップを実施すべきか？
アデノシン抵抗性SVTに対する最も有効かつ安全な薬剤は何か？
（1）新生児の蘇生プロトコールから小児の蘇生プロトコールに移行する，および（2）小児の蘇生プロトコールから成人の蘇生プロトコールに移行する適切な年齢と状況は，どのようなものか？

CPR：心肺蘇生，ECMO：体外膜型人工肺，ECPR：体外循環補助を用いた心肺蘇生，F_{IO_2}：吸気酸素濃度，IHCA：院内心停止，IO：骨髄内，IV：静脈内，OHCA：院外心停止，無脈性VT：無脈性心室頻拍，SVT：上室性頻拍，VF：心室細動。

文献情報

アメリカ心臓協会（American Heart Association）は，本書が以下のとおりに引用されることを要請する。Topjian AA, Raymond TT, Atkins D, Chan M, Duff JP, Joyner BL Jr, Lasa JJ, Lavonas EJ, Levy A, Mahgoub M, Meckler GD, Roberts KE, Sutton RM, Schexnayder SM; on behalf of the Pediatric Basic and Advanced Life Support Collaborators. Part 4: pediatric basic and advanced life support: 2020 American Heart Association Guidelines for Cardiopulmonary Resuscitation and Emergency Cardiovascular Care. Circulation. 2020;142(suppl 2):S469-S523. doi: 10.1161/CIR.0000000000000901

謝辞

著者らは，その貢献に対し，以下の方々（「小児一次救命処置と二次救命処置」の協力者）に深く感謝する。Ronald A. Bronicki, MD; Allan R. de Caen, MD; Anne Marie Guerguerian, MD, PhD; Kelly D. Kadlec, MD, MEd; Monica E. Kleinman, MD; Lynda J. Knight, MSN, RN; Taylor N. McCormick, MD, MSc; Ryan W. Morgan, MD, MTR; Joan S. Roberts, MD; Barnaby R. Scholefield, MBBS, PhD; Sarah Tabbutt, MD, PhD; Ravi Thiagarajan, MBBS, MPH; Janice Tijssen, MD, MSc; Brian Walsh, PhD, RRT, RRT-NPS; and Arno Zaritsky, MD.

情報開示

付録 1　執筆グループの情報開示

執筆グループメンバー	所属	研究助成金	その他の研究支援	講演／謝礼金	鑑定人	株式所有	コンサルタント／顧問	その他
Alexis A. Topjian	The Children's Hospital of Philadelphia, University of Pennsylvania School of Medicine Anesthesia and Critical Care	NIH*	なし	なし	Plaintiff*	なし	なし	なし
Dianne L. Atkins	University of Iowa Pediatrics	なし	なし	なし	なし	なし	なし	なし
Melissa Chan	University of British Columbia Pediatrics BC Children's Hospital	なし	なし	なし	なし	なし	なし	なし
Jonathan P. Duff	University of Alberta and Stollery Children's Hospital Pediatrics	なし	なし	なし	なし	なし	なし	なし
Benny L. Joyner Jr	University of North Carolina Pediatrics	なし	なし	なし	なし	なし	なし	なし
Javier J. Lasa	Texas Children's Hospital, Baylor College of Medicine Pediatrics/Critical Care Medicine and Cardiology	なし	なし	なし	なし	なし	なし	なし
Eric J. Lavonas	Denver Health Emergency Medicine	BTG Pharmaceuticals（Denver Health（Lavonas 博士の雇用者）には，BTG Pharmaceuticalsとの研究，コールセンター，コンサルティング，および教育の各契約がある。BTGはジゴキシンの解毒剤（DigiFab）を製造している。Lavonas博士はボーナスやインセンティブ報酬を受け取らず，これらの契約は無関係な製品を対象とする。これらのガイドラインの作成時に，Lavonas博士はジゴキシン中毒に関わる考察に関与しなかった）†	なし	なし	なし	なし	なし	アメリカ心臓協会（上級科学編集者）†
Arielle Levy	University of Montreal Pediatric	なし	なし	なし	なし	なし	なし	なし
Melissa Mahgoub	American Heart Association	なし	なし	なし	なし	なし	なし	なし
Garth D. Meckler	University of British Columbia Pediatrics and Emergency Medicine Ambulatory Care Building, BC Children's	なし	なし	なし	なし	なし	なし	なし
Tia T. Raymond	Medical City Children's Hospital Pediatric Cardiac Intensive Care Unit	なし	なし	なし	なし	なし	なし	なし

（続き）

付録1 続き

執筆グループメンバー	所属	研究助成金	その他の研究支援	講演/謝礼金	鑑定人	株式所有	コンサルタント/顧問	その他
Kathryn E. Roberts	Joe DiMaggio Children's Hospital	なし	なし	なし	なし	なし	なし	なし
Stephen M. Schexnayder	Univ. of Arkansas/ Arkansas Children's Hospital Pediatric Critical Care	なし	なし	なし	なし	なし	なし	なし
Robert M. Sutton	The Children's Hospital of Philadelphia, University of Pennsylvania School of Medicine Anesthesia and Critical Care Medicine	NIH†	なし	なし	Roberts & Durkee, Plantiff, 2019†	なし	なし	なし

この表は，執筆グループの全メンバーに回答および提出が求められる情報開示アンケート（Disclosure Questionnaire）の結果に基づき実在の利益相反または合理的に認定できる利益相反とみなされる可能性のある，執筆グループメンバーの関係を示している。メンバーと該当団体との関係が「顕著」であると考えられるのは，次のいずれかの状況が存在する場合である。（a）当該メンバーが団体から受領する金額が過去いずれの12か月間に＄10,000以上であるか，メンバーの総収入の5％以上である，（b）団体の議決権株式の5％以上，またはその団体の公正市場価値の＄10,000以上を保有している。この定義において「重大」に相当するレベルに満たない場合，その関係は「軽度」とみなされる。

*軽度
†重大

付録2　レビューアーの情報開示

レビューアー	所属	研究助成金	その他の研究支援	講演/謝礼金	鑑定人	株式所有	コンサルタント/顧問	その他
Nandini Calamur	Saint Louis University	なし	なし	なし	なし	なし	なし	なし
Leon Chameides	Connecticut Children's Medical Center	なし	なし	なし	なし	なし	なし	なし
Todd P. Chang	Children's Hospital Los Angeles & Keck School Of Medicine	なし	なし	なし	なし	なし	なし	Oculus from FaceBook†
Ericka L. Fink	Primary Work Children's Hospital of Pittsburgh	NIH†	なし	なし	なし	なし	なし	なし
Monica E. Kleinman	Children's Hospital Boston	なし	なし	なし	なし	なし	International Liaison Committee on Resuscitation*	なし
Michael-Alice Moga	The Hospital for Sick Children, Labatt Family Heart Center and University of Toronto (Canada)	CIHR*，CIHR/ NSERC†	なし	なし	なし	なし	なし	なし
Tara Neubrand	Children's Hospital Colorado, University of Colorado	なし	なし	なし	なし	なし	なし	なし
Ola Didrik Saugstad	University of Oslo (Norway)	なし	なし	なし	なし	なし	なし	なし

この表は，執筆グループの全メンバーに回答および提出が求められる情報開示アンケート（Disclosure Questionnaire）の結果に基づき実在の利益相反または合理的に認定できる利益相反とみなされる可能性のある，執筆グループメンバーの関係を示している。メンバーと該当団体との関係が「顕著」であると考えられるのは，次のいずれかの状況が存在する場合である。（a）当該メンバーが団体から受領する金額が過去いずれの12か月間に＄10,000以上であるか，メンバーの総収入の5％以上である，（b）団体の議決権株式の5％以上，またはその団体の公正市場価値の＄10,000以上を保有している。この定義において「重大」に相当するレベルに満たない場合，その関係は「軽度」とみなされる。

*軽度
†重大

Circulation

第5章：新生児の蘇生
AHA 心肺蘇生と救急心血管治療のためのガイドライン 2020

新生児の救命処置について覚えておくべき10のポイント

1. 新生児蘇生法は，個人およびチームで訓練を受けたプロバイダーによる予測と準備を必要とする。
2. ほとんどの新生児は即時臍帯クランプや蘇生を必要とせず，出生後に母親の胸に直接抱かせている間に評価とモニリングをすることができる。
3. 肺の膨脹と換気は，出生後に補助を必要とする新生児においては優先事項である。
4. 心拍数の上昇は有効な換気と蘇生処置への反応の最も重要な指標である。
5. パルスオキシメトリは酸素療法の指針として酸素飽和度の目標値を達成するために使用される。
6. 適切な換気改善処置（気管挿管を含むことが望ましい）を実施した後に心拍数反応が不良である場合，胸骨圧迫が行われる。
7. 胸骨圧迫および投薬への心拍数反応は心電図検査でモニターする必要がある。
8. 胸骨圧迫への反応が不良である場合，アドレナリン投与が妥当であり，静脈内投与が望ましい。
9. 新生児がアドレナリンに反応せず，既往歴または検査結果が失血と一致する場合，循環血液量を増やすことが必要になる場合がある。
10. 上記の蘇生手順をすべて効果的に完了し，20分経過しても心拍数の反応がない場合，チームおよび家族と処置の方向の調整について話し合う必要がある。

Khalid Aziz, MBBS, MA, MEd（IT）, Chair
Henry C. Lee, MD, Vice Chair
Marilyn B. Escobedo, MD
Amber V. Hoover, RN, MSN
Beena D. Kamath-Rayne, MD, MPH
Vishal S. Kapadia, MD, MSCS
David J. Magid, MD, MPH
Susan Niermeyer, MD, MPH
Georg M. Schmölzer, MD, PhD
Edgardo Szyld, MD, MSc
Gary M. Weiner, MD
Myra H. Wyckoff, MD
Nicole K. Yamada, MD, MS
Jeanette Zaichkin, RN, MN, NNP-BC

前文

新生児の約10％は，生まれてはじめて呼吸をするために助けが必要で[1-3]，約1％は，心肺機能を回復するために積極的な蘇生措置を必要とすると推定されている[4,5]。米国とカナダの新生児死亡率は，1960年代の出生児1,000人あたりほぼ20人[6,7]から，現在の出生児1,000人あたりほぼ4人へと低下している。新生児が適切または自発的な呼吸を確立および維持できない場合，早期死亡につながる可能性が高く，生存しても神経発達に重大な悪影響が及ぶことがある。したがって，出生時の効果的かつ時宜を得た蘇生は，新生児の転帰をさらに改善すると考えられる。

新生児の蘇生の成功は，生存の可能性を最大化できる重要な行動を迅速に連続して行えるかどうかによって決まる。国際蘇生連絡委員会（ILCOR）の生存のための方程式では，良好な蘇生転帰のための3つの重要な要素（健全な蘇生科学に基づくガイドライン，蘇生プロバイダーの効果的な教育，効果的かつ時宜を得た蘇生の実施）を重視している[8]。2020年版の新生児ガイドラインには，利用可能な最良の蘇生科

キーワード：AHA 科学的ステートメント ■ 心肺蘇生 ■ 新生児の蘇生 ■ 新生児

© 2020 American Heart Association, Inc., and American Academy of Pediatrics

https://www.ahajournals.org/journal/circ

学に基づいて，分娩室および新生児期に実行できる最も影響力の強い手順に関する推奨事項が記載されている。また，蘇生プロバイダーのトレーニングと治療システムに関する具体的な推奨事項は，それぞれのガイドラインの各章に記載されている[9,10]。

緒言
ガイドラインの範囲

このガイドラインは，臨床ケアの最新の概要を探している北米の医療従事者，および蘇生科学と現在の知識のギャップに関するより詳細な情報を求めている人々を対象としている。新生児蘇生科学は，羊水で満たされた子宮環境から外気に触れる分娩室環境へ移行する新生児，および出生後数日間の新生児に適用される。移行に変化または障害のある状況では，効果的な新生児蘇生により死亡率と罹患率のリスクが低下する。出生後に正常に呼吸している健康な新生児でさえ，適切な臍帯管理や母親の胸に直接抱かせることによる熱保護など，正常な移行の促進による恩恵を受ける。

2015年版の新生児蘇生アルゴリズム，およびこのアルゴリズムの各セクションに基づく主な概念は，2020年も引き続き参考になる（図）。以下のセクションは特に注意する価値がある。

- 陽圧人工呼吸（PPV）は，新生児蘇生においても介入の中心となる。新生児蘇生のモニタリングやその他の側面を取り巻く科学と実践は進化し続けているが，PPVを取り巻くスキルと実践の開発は強調されるべきである。
- 酸素投与はパルスオキシメトリに基づいて慎重に使用する。
- 低体温の防止は新生児の蘇生において引き続き重要な焦点である。親子の絆の形成，母乳育児，および正常体温を促進する手段として，健康な新生児の場合は母親の胸に直接抱かせることの重要性が強調されている。
- チームトレーニングは，予測，準備，ブリーフィング，報告など，新生児蘇生においても重要な側面である。迅速かつ効果的な反応と実施は，良好な新生児の転帰にとって不可欠である。
- 2015年に満期産児と早期産児の両方で遅延臍帯クランプが推奨された。このガイドラインは以前の推奨事項を支持する。
- 『アメリカ心臓協会（AHA）心肺蘇生（CPR）と救急心血管治療（ECC）のためのガイドラインアップデート 2015』では，元気な新生児にも，羊水が胎便で混濁している状態（meconium-stained amniotic fluid, MSAF）で出生した元気のない新生児にも気管吸引をルーチンで実施することを推奨していない。このガイドラインでは初期処置とPPVが優先事項であるという認識を強化している。

新生児蘇生に関連して，重大な知識不足が存在していることを認識することが重要である。現在の多くの推奨事項は，綿密にデザインされたヒト試験が不足している，薄弱なエビデンスに基づいている。その原因の1つは，分娩室で大規模な無作為化比較試験（RCT）を実施することの難しさにある。そのため現在のガイドラインは，新生児研究における現在の知識不足の概要と，こうした知識不足に対処しうるいくつかの戦略で締めくくっている。

「COVID-19に関するガイダンス」

AHAは，他の専門家団体と協力して，2019年のコロナウイルス感染症（COVID-19）への感染が疑われる，または確認された成人，小児，新生児の一次救命処置および二次救命処置に関する暫定ガイダンスを提供している。COVID-19の状況に関するエビデンスおよびガイダンスは変化し続けているため，この暫定的ガイダンスはECCガイドラインとは分離したままとする。最新のガイダンスについては，AHAウェブサイトを参照されたい[12]。

エビデンス評価とガイドライン作成

次のセクションでは，エビデンスのレビューとガイドラインの作成のプロセスについて簡単に説明する。このプロセスの詳細については，「第2章：エビデンス評価とガイドライン作成」を参照のこと[11]。

執筆委員会の組織

新生児救命処置執筆グループには，臨床医学，教育，研究，公衆衛生の経歴を持つ新生児担当医師および看護師が含まれている。蘇生の専門知識が認められているボランティアが，執筆グループの委員長によって指名され，AHA ECC委員会によって選出される。AHAには，ガイドライン作成における偏見や不適切な影響のリスクを最小限に抑えるための厳格な利益相反方針と手順がある[13]。執筆グループのメンバーと査読者は，任命の前にすべての利害関係とその他の考えうる（知的を含む）利益相反を明らかにした。執筆グループのメンバーの公開情報は，付録1に記載する。

方法論とエビデンスレビュー

これらの2020年版AHA新生児蘇生ガイドラインは，ILCORおよび関連するILCORメンバー評議会と連携して実施された広範なエビデンス評価に基づいている。2020年のプロセスでは，3種類のエビデンスレビュー（体系的レビュー，スコーピングレビュー，エビデンスアップデート）が使用された。これらが個々に文献の説明となり，ガイドライン作成に役立った[14-17]。

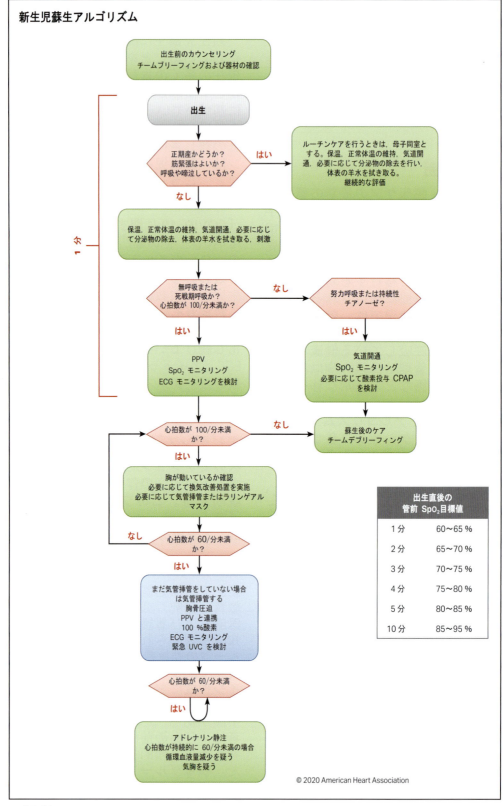

図. 新生児蘇生アルゴリズム
CPAP：持続的気道陽圧法（continuous positive airway pressure），ECG：心電図検査（electrocardiographic），HR：心拍数（heart rate），O_2：酸素，SpO_2：酸素飽和度，UVC：臍帯静脈カテーテル（umbilical venous catheter）

推奨事項のクラスとエビデンスレベル

各 AHA 執筆グループは，現在および関連するすべての『AHA 心肺蘇生と救急心血管治療のためのガイドライン』[18-20] および『2020 年の心肺蘇生と救急心血管治療の科学についての ILCOR 国際コンセンサスと治療推奨（2020 ILCOR International Consensus CPR and ECC Science With Treatment Recommendations）』のエビデンスと推奨事項[21] をレビューし，現在のガイドラインを再確認，改訂，または廃止する必要があるかどうか，または新しい推奨事項が必要かどうかを判断した。次に執筆グループは，推奨事項を

表 患者ケアにおける臨床上の戦略，介入，治療，または診断検査への推奨事項のクラスとエビデンスレベルの適用（2019年5月更新）＊

推奨事項のクラス（強さ）	エビデンスレベル（質）‡
クラス1（強い） 利益＞＞＞リスク 推奨事項文に適した表現例： • 推奨される • 適応／有用／有効／有益である • 実施／投与（など）すべきである • 比較に基づく有効性の表現例†： 　– 治療Bよりも治療／治療戦略Aが推奨される／適応である 　– 治療Bよりも治療Aを選択すべきである	**レベルA** • 複数のRCTから得られた質の高いエビデンス‡ • 質の高いRCTのメタアナリシス • 質の高い症例登録試験によって裏付けられた1件以上のRCT
クラス2a（中等度） 利益＞＞リスク 推奨事項文に適した表現例： • 妥当である • 有用／有効／有益でありうる • 比較に基づく有効性の表現例†： 　– 治療Bよりも治療／治療戦略Aがおそらく推奨される／適応である 　– 治療Bよりも治療Aを選択することが妥当である	**レベルB-R** （無作為化） • 1件以上のRCTから得られた質が中等度のエビデンス‡ • 質が中等度のRCTのメタアナリシス
クラス2b（弱い） 利益≧リスク 推奨事項文に適した表現例： • 妥当としてよい／よいだろう • 考慮してもよい／よいだろう • 有用性／有効性は不明／不明確／不確実である，あるいは十分に確立されていない	**レベルB-NR** （非無作為化） • 1件以上の綿密にデザインされ，適切に実施された非無作為化試験，観察研究，または症例登録試験から得られた質が中等度のエビデンス‡ • そのような試験のメタアナリシス
クラス3：利益なし（中等度） 利益＝リスク （一般にLOE AまたはBの使用に限る） 推奨事項文に適した表現例： • 推奨しない • 適応／有用／有効／有益ではない • 実施／投与（など）すべきでない	**レベルC-LD** （限定的なデータ） • デザインまたは実施に限界がある無作為化または非無作為化観察研究または症例登録試験 • そのような試験のメタアナリシス • ヒトを対象にした生理学的試験または反応機構研究
クラス3：有害（強い） リスク＞利益 推奨事項文に適した表現例： • 有害な可能性がある • 有害となる • 合併症発生率／死亡率の上昇を伴う • 実施／投与（など）すべきでない	**レベルC-EO** （専門家の見解） • 臨床経験に基づく専門家の見解のコンセンサス

CORおよびLOEは個別に決定する（CORとLOEのあらゆる組み合わせが可能）。

LOE Cの推奨事項は，その推奨事項が弱いことを意味するわけではない。ガイドラインが扱っている重要な医療上の問題の多くは，臨床試験の対象となっていない。RCTが行われていなくても，特定の検査あるいは治療法の有用性／有効性について，臨床上非常に明確なコンセンサスが得られている場合がある。

＊ 介入の成果または結果を記述すべきである（臨床転帰の改善，または診断精度の向上，または予後情報の増加）。

† 比較に基づく有効性の推奨事項（COR 1および2a，LOE AおよびBのみ）に関してその推奨事項の裏付けとなる試験は，評価する治療または治療戦略を直接比較しているものでなければならない。

‡ 標準化され，広く用いられていて，望ましくは検証されている複数のエビデンス評価ツールを活用する，システマティックレビューについてはエビデンスレビュー委員会を設けるなど，質を評価する方法は進化している。

COR：推奨事項のクラス（Class of Recommendation），EO：専門家の見解（expert opinion），LD：限定的なデータ（limited data），LOE：エビデンスレベル（Level of Evidence），NR：非無作為化（nonrandomized），R：無作為化（randomized），RCT：無作為化比較試験（randomized controlled trial）。

起草，レビュー，および承認し，それぞれにエビデンスレベル（LOE，つまり品質）と推奨事項のクラス（COR，すなわち強さ）（表）を割り当てた[11]。

ガイドラインの構成

2020年版の各ガイドラインは「知識チャンク」に分けられ，特定のトピックまたは管理の問題に関する個別の情報モジュールにグループ化されている[22]。各モジュール型知識チャンクには，CORとLOEについてAHAの標準的な用語を使用した推奨事項の表が含まれている。簡単な緒言または短い概要は，推奨事項を重要な背景情報や包括的な管理または治療の概念と関連付けて説明するために記載している。推奨事項の解説では，推奨事項を裏付ける理論的根拠と主要な研究データを明確にしている。必要に応じて，フローチャートまたは追加の表を含めた。簡単に参照して確認できるように，ハイパーリンクされた参照資料も記載している。

文書のレビューと承認

各『AHA 心肺蘇生と救急心血管治療のためのガイドライン2020』文書は，匿名の査読のために，AHAが指名した5名の対象分野の専門家に提出した。すべての査読者は，任命の前に業界との関係とその他の考えうる利益相反を明らかにし，その内容をAHAのスタッフがレビューした。査読者からのフィードバックは，草稿形式のガイドラインと最終形式のガイドラインで提供された。すべてのガイドラインは，AHA Science Advisory and Coordinating Committee およ

び AHA Executive Committee によってレビューされ，公開が承認された。査読者の公開情報は，付録 2 に記載する。

参考資料

1. Little MP, Järvelin MR, Neasham DE, Lissauer T, Steer PJ. Factors associated with fall in neonatal intubation rates in the United Kingdom-prospective study. BJOG.2007;114:156–164. doi: 10.1111/j.1471-0528.2006.01188.x
2. Niles DE, Cines C, Insley E, Foglia EE, Elci OU, Skåre C, Olasveengen T, Ades A, Posencheg M, Nadkarni VM, Kramer-Johansen J. Incidence and characteristics of positive pressure ventilation delivered to newborns in a US tertiary academic hospital.Resuscitation.2017;115:102–109. doi: 10.1016/j.resuscitation.2017.03.035
3. Aziz K, Chadwick M, Baker M, Andrews W. Ante- and intra-partum factors that predict increased need for neonatal resuscitation.Resuscitation.2008;79:444–452. doi: 10.1016/j.resuscitation.2008.08.004
4. Perlman JM, Risser R. Cardiopulmonary resuscitation in the delivery room. Associated clinical events. Arch Pediatr Adolesc Med.1995;149:20–25. doi: 10.1001/archpedi.1995.02170130022005
5. Barber CA, Wyckoff MH. Use and efficacy of endotracheal versus intravenous epinephrine during neonatal cardiopulmonary resuscitation in the delivery room.Pediatrics.2006;118:1028–1034. doi: 10.1542/peds.2006-0416
6. MacDorman MF, Rosenberg HM. Trends in infant mortality by cause of death and other characteristics, 1960-88. Vital Health Stat 20. 1993:1–57.
7. Kochanek KD, Murphy SL, Xu JQ, Arias E; Division of Vital Statistics. National Vital Statistics Reports: Deaths: Final Data for 2017 Hyattsville, MD: National Center for Health Statistics; 2019 (68). https://www.cdc.gov/nchs/data/nvsr68/nvsr68_09-508.pdf. Accessed February 28, 2020.
8. Søreide E, Morrison L, Hillman K, Monsieurs K, Sunde K, Zideman D, Eisenberg M, Sterz F, Nadkarni VM, Soar J, Nolan JP; Utstein Formula for Survival Collaborators.The formula for survival in resuscitation.Resuscitation.2013;84:1487–1493. doi: 10.1016/j.resuscitation.2013.07.020
9. Cheng A, Magid DJ, Auerbach M, Bhanji F, Bigham BL, Blewer AL, Dainty KN, Diederich E, Lin Y, Leary M, et al. Part 6: resuscitation education science: 2020 American Heart Association Guidelines for Cardiopulmonary Resuscitation and Emergency Cardiovascular Care.Circulation.2020;142 (suppl 2):S551–S579. doi: 10.1161/CIR.0000000000000903
10. Berg KM, Cheng A, Panchal AR, Topjian AA, Aziz K, Bhanji F, Bigham BL, Hirsch KG, Hoover AV, Kurz MC, et al; on behalf of the Adult Basic and Advanced Life Support, Pediatric Basic and Advanced Life Support, Neonatal Life Support, and Resuscitation Education Science Writing Groups. Part 7: systems of care: 2020 American Heart Association Guidelines for Cardiopulmonary Resuscitation and Emergency Cardiovascular Care.Circulation.2020;142 (suppl 2):S580–S604. doi: 10.1161/CIR.0000000000000899
11. Magid DJ, Aziz K, Cheng A, Hazinski MF, Hoover AV, Mahgoub M, Panchal AR, Sasson C, Topjian AA, Rodriguez AJ, et al. Part 2: evidence evaluation and guidelines development: 2020 American Heart Association Guidelines for Cardiopulmonary Resuscitation and Emergency Cardiovascular Care.Circulation.2020;142 (suppl 2):S358–S365. doi: 10.1161/CIR.0000000000000898
12. American Heart Association. CPR & ECC. https://cpr.heart.org/. Accessed June 19, 2020.
13. American Heart Association.Conflict of interest policy. https://www.heart.org/en/about-us/statements-and-policies/conflict-of-interest-policy. Accessed December 31, 2019.
14. International Liaison Committee on Resuscitation.Continuous evidence evaluation guidance and templates. https://www.ilcor.org/documents/continuous-evidence-evaluation-guidance-and-templates. Accessed December 31, 2019.
15. Institute of Medicine (US) Committee of Standards for Systematic Reviews of Comparative Effectiveness Research.Finding What Works in Health Care: Standards for Systematic Reviews. Eden J, Levit L, Berg A, Morton S, eds. Washington, DC: The National Academies Press; 2011.
16. PRISMA. Preferred Reporting Items for Systematic Reviews and Meta-Analyses (PRISMA) website. http://www.prisma-statement.org/. Accessed December 31, 2019.
17. Tricco AC, Lillie E, Zarin W, O'Brien KK, Colquhoun H, Levac D, Moher D, Peters MDJ, Horsley T, Weeks L, Hempel S, Akl EA, Chang C, McGowan J, Stewart L, Hartling L, Aldcroft A, Wilson MG, Garritty C, Lewin S, Godfrey CM, Macdonald MT, Langlois EV, Soares-Weiser K, Moriarty J, Clifford T, Tunçalp Ö, Straus SE. PRISMA Extension for Scoping Reviews (PRISMA-ScR): Checklist and Explanation. Ann Intern Med.2018;169:467–473. doi: 10.7326/M18-0850
18. Kattwinkel J, Perlman JM, Aziz K, Colby C, Fairchild K, Gallagher J, Hazinski MF, Halamek LP, Kumar P, Little G, et al. Part 15: neonatal resuscitation: 2010 American Heart Association Guidelines for Cardiopulmonary Resuscitation and Emergency Cardiovascular Care.Circulation.2010;122 (suppl 3):S909–S919. doi: 10.1161/CIRCULATIONAHA.110.971119
19. Wyckoff MH, Aziz K, Escobedo MB, Kapadia VS, Kattwinkel J, Perlman JM, Simon WM, Weiner GM, Zaichkin JG.Part 13: neonatal resuscitation: 2015 American Heart Association Guidelines Update for Cardiopulmonary Resuscitation and Emergency Cardiovascular Care.Circulation.2015;132 (suppl 2):S543–S560. doi: 10.1161/CIR.0000000000000267
20. Escobedo MB, Aziz K, Kapadia VS, Lee HC, Niermeyer S, Schmölzer GM, Szyld E, Weiner GM, Wyckoff MH, Yamada NK, Zaichkin JG.2019 American Heart Association Focused Update on Neonatal Resuscitation: An Update to the American Heart Association Guidelines for Cardiopulmonary Resuscitation and Emergency Cardiovascular Care.Circulation.2019;140:e922-e930. doi: 10.1161/CIR.0000000000000729
21. Wyckoff MH, Wyllie J, Aziz K, de Almeida MF, Fabres J, Fawke J, Guinsburg R, Hosono S, Isayama T, Kapadia VS, et al; on behalf of the Neonatal Life Support Collaborators. Neonatal life support: 2020 International Consensus on Cardiopulmonary Resuscitation and Emergency Cardiovascular Care Science With Treatment Recommendations.Circulation.2020;142 (suppl 1):S185–S221. doi: 10.1161/CIR.0000000000000895
22. Levine GN, O'Gara PT, Beckman JA, Al-Khatib SM, Birtcher KK, Cigarroa JE, de Las Fuentes L, Deswal A, Fleisher LA, Gentile F, Goldberger ZD, Hlatky MA, Joglar JA, Piano MR, Wijeysundera DN.Recent Innovations, Modifications, and Evolution of ACC/AHA Clinical Practice Guidelines: An Update for Our Constituencies: A Report of the American College of Cardiology/American Heart Association Task Force on Clinical Practice Guidelines. Circulation.2019;139:e879–e886. doi: 10.1161/CIR.0000000000000651

主要な概念

これらのガイドラインは主に，羊水で満たされた子宮から外気に触れる室内へと移行する「新生児」に適用される。「新生児」期間は，出産から分娩領域での蘇生と安定化の終了までである。ただし，これらのガイドラインの概念は，新生児期（出生から 28 日まで）の新生児に適用される場合がある。

　出生時の新生児ケアの主な目標は，移行を容易にすることである。新生児の生存にとって最も重要な優先事項は，出生後の適切な肺拡張と換気の確立である。したがって，すべての新生児には，PPV を行うスキルがあり機器を備えた要員が 1 名以上付きそう必要がある。その他の重要な目標は，心血管と体温の安定の確立と維持に加えて，母子の絆と母乳育児の促進により，健康な新生児の自然な移行を認識することにある。

　新生児蘇生アルゴリズムは 2015 年から変更されておらず，主要な概念を体系化する枠組みとして，新生児，家族，および周産期介護者を取り巻くチームのニーズを反映している。

予測と準備

移行を容易にするため，すべての健康な新生児に，トレーニングを受け機器を備えた要員を割り当てる必要がある。蘇生の危険因子を特定することで，追加の要員と機器が必要になる場合がある。予測，コミュニケーション，ブリーフィング，機器チェック，役割の割り当てなどの効果的なチーム行動が，チームのパフォーマンスと新生児転帰の改善につながる。

臍帯管理

合併症のない満期産または早産後期の場合，新生児は母親の胸に抱かせ，身体をよく拭き，呼吸，緊張，および活動を評価するまで，臍帯結紮を遅らせるのが合理的である。他の状況では，呼吸，心血管，および温度遷移を評価し，初期処置を実行している間，臍帯結紮と切断を遅らせてもよい。早産では，臍帯結紮を遅らせることには潜在的な利点もある。

最初の行動

可能であれば，健常満期産児は母親の胸に抱かせて管理すべきである。出生後，身体をよく拭き，温かい覆いと正常体温の維持に注意して，母親の胸に直接抱かせる。正常な呼吸移行について，新生児を継続的に評価する必要がある。出生時に蘇生が必要な新生児，特に超早産児や極低出生体重児には，放射加温器やその他の加温補助処置が推奨される。

呼吸努力を促進するために刺激を与えてもよい。気道閉塞が疑われる場合は，吸引を検討してもよい。

心拍数の評価

心拍数は最初に，聴診や触診によって評価する。オキシメトリと心電図検査は，蘇生を必要とする新生児の重要な補助手段である。

陽圧人工呼吸

PPV は依然として，無呼吸，徐脈，または不十分な呼吸努力を示す新生児を支援するための主要な方法である。ほとんどの新生児はこの介入に反応する。心拍数の改善と呼吸または啼泣の開始はすべて，効果的な PPV の徴候である。

酸素療法

PPV は，満期産児および後期早産児では 21 %の酸素で開始し，早産児では最大 30 %の酸素で開始する。オキシメトリは，満期産児の酸素飽和度が自然範囲になることを目的に使用する。

胸骨圧迫

適切な PPV を 30 秒間行っても，心拍数が 60 回/分未満のままである場合は，胸骨圧迫を行う必要がある。推奨される比率は，胸骨圧迫に胸郭包み込み両母指圧迫法を使用して，1 回の換気に3 回の胸骨圧迫を同期させる（1 分あたり 30 回の換気と 90 回の圧迫を行う）ことである。

血管路確保

新生児の血管確保が必要である場合，臍静脈路が望ましい。静脈路の確保が困難な場合は，骨髄路を検討してもよい。

薬物

胸骨圧迫と適切な PPV を 60 秒間行っても心拍数が 60 回/分未満のままである場合は，アドレナリンを投与する。静脈内投与が理想的である。

循環血液増量薬

既往歴や検査に基づいて失血が確認されている，あるいは疑われていて，アドレナリンに反応しない場合は，循環血液増量薬の適応となる。

蘇生の保留と中止

家族や医療従事者が蘇生努力の保留または中止を合理的と判断できる状況を特定できる場合がある。すべての関係者に適切で時宜を得た支援を提供する必要がある。

人的要因およびシステム

新生児蘇生を提供するチームや個人は，効果的な蘇生の実施に必要な知識，スキル，および行動に関して多くの課題に直面している。したがって，新生児蘇生チームには，継続的なブースター訓練，ブリーフィング，およびデブリーフィングが有効である場合がある。

略語

AHA	アメリカ心臓協会（American Heart Association）
COR	推奨事項のクラス（Class of Recommendation）
CPAP	持続的気道陽圧法（continuous positive airway pressure）
ECC	救急心血管治療（emergency cardiovascular care）
ECG	心電図検査（electrocardiogram/electrocardiographic）
H_2O	水
HIE	低酸素性虚血性脳症（hypoxic-ischemic encephalopathy）
ILCOR	国際蘇生連絡委員会（International Liaison Committee on Resuscitation）
LOE	エビデンスレベル（Level of Evidence）
MSAF	胎便性羊水混濁（meconium-stained amniotic fluid）
PEEP	呼気終末陽圧（positive end-expiratory pressure）
PPV	陽圧人工呼吸（positive pressure ventilation）
RCT	無作為化比較試験（randomized controlled trial）
ROSC	自己心拍再開（return of spontaneous circulation）

蘇生の必要性の予測

COR	LOE	推奨事項
1	B-NR	1. 出産では必ず，新生児の蘇生の初期手順を実施しPPVを開始することができる新生児専任担当者が1名以上立ち会うべきである[1-4]。
1	B-NR	2. 出産前には必ず，標準化された危険因子評価ツールを使用して周産期リスクを評価し，このリスクに基づく適格なチームを構成すべきである[5-7]。
1	C-LD	3. 出産前には必ず，標準化された器具チェックリストを使用して，完全な蘇生に必要とされる消耗品および器具類が揃っており，正常に機能することを確認しておくべきである[8,9]。
1	C-LD	4. リスクの高い出産が予測される場合，蘇生前のチームブリーフィングを実施することで，想定される介入法を特定し，役割と責任を割り当てておくべきである[8,10-12]。

「概要」

新生児の約10％は，出生後に呼吸の支援を必要とする[1-3,5,13]。新生児蘇生には，トレーニング，準備，およびチームワークが必要である。蘇生の必要性が予測されていない場合，無呼吸の新生児に対する支援の遅れは死亡リスクを増加させるおそれがある[1,5,13]。したがって，出産時には必ず，新生児を主に担当していてPPVを遅滞なく開始するようトレーニングを受けた人物が少なくとも1名立ち会う必要がある[2-4]。

妊娠および分娩時に存在する危険因子を評価するリスク評価ツールを使用すると，高度な蘇生が必要となる可能性が高い新生児を特定できる。そのような場合は，高度なスキルを持つチームを組織して分娩時に待機させておくことが望ましい[5,7]。リスクの層別化がなされていない場合，PPVを必要とする新生児の最大半数が分娩前に特定されない可能性がある[6,13]。

標準化された器材チェックリストは，ある特定の臨床環境で必要とされる重要な備品や器材の包括的なリストである。分娩環境では，毎回分娩の前に標準チェックリストを使用して，完全な蘇生に必要な備品や器材が揃っていて正常に機能することを確認しておく必要がある[8,9,14,15]。

分娩前にチームブリーフィングを実施してリーダーを決定し，役割と責任を割り当て，考えられる介入について計画を立てる。チームブリーフィングは，効果的なチームワークとコミュニケーションを促進し，患者の安全を支える[8,10-12]。

推奨事項の裏付けとなる解説

1. 大規模な観察研究により，PPVの遅延は死亡と長期入院のリスクを高めることが報告されている[1]。あるシステマティックレビューおよびメタアナリシスによると，新生児蘇生トレーニングは，リソースの乏しい国において死産の減少と新生児の7日生存率の向上をもたらした[3]。ある後ろ向きコホート研究では，新生児蘇生トレーニングを実施した後，高リスク新生児のApgarスコアが改善された[16]。

2. ある多施設症例対照研究において，高度な新生児蘇生の必要性を予測する周産期の危険因子が10個特定された[7]。リスク層別化の使用前に実施された監査研究では，蘇生が予測されたのはPPVを必要とする新生児の半数未満であった[6]。ある前向きコホート研究では，周産期の危険因子に基づいてリスク層別化を行うと，高リスク分娩時に熟練チームが待機している可能性が高くなることが示された[5]。

3. ある多施設品質改善研究では，ブリーフィングと器材チェックリストを含む蘇生バンドル（包括的治療）の使用について，スタッフの高い遵守状況が報告されている[8]。チームブリーフィングと器材チェックリストを含む早産児向けの管理バンドル（包括的管理）は，明確な役割の割り当て，一貫した器材チェック，および体温調節と酸素飽和度の改善をもたらした[9]。

4. ある単一施設RCTでは，チームブリーフィングを実施することで，新生児蘇生のシミュレーション中の役割の混乱が回避され，チームワークスキルが向上した[11]。ある全州的な共同品質イニシアチブでは，チームブリーフィングによってチーム内のコミュニケーションと臨床転帰が改善することが実証された[10]。ある単一施設研究において，チームブリーフィングと器材チェックリストはチーム内のコミュニケーションを改善したが，器材の準備については改善は認められなかった[12]。

参考資料

1. Ersdal HL, Mduma E, Svensen E, Perlman JM. Early initiation of basic resuscitation interventions including face mask ventilation may reduce birth asphyxia related mortality in low-income countries: a prospective descriptive observational study. Resuscitation.2012;83:869-873. doi: 10.1016/j.resuscitation.2011.12.011
2. Dempsey E, Pammi M, Ryan AC, Barrington KJ. Standardised formal resuscitation training programmes for reducing mortality and morbidity in newborn infants. Cochrane Database Syst Rev. 2015:CD009106. doi: 10.1002/14651858.CD009106.pub2
3. Patel A, Khatib MN, Kurhe K, Bhargava S, Bang A. Impact of neonatal resuscitation trainings on neonatal and perinatal mortality: a systematic review and meta-analysis. BMJ Paediatr Open. 2017;1:e000183. doi: 10.1136/bmjpo-2017-000183
4. Wyckoff MH, Aziz K, Escobedo MB, Kapadia VS, Kattwinkel J, Perlman JM, Simon WM, Weiner GM, Zaichkin JG.Part 13: neonatal resuscitation: 2015 American Heart Association Guidelines Update for Cardiopulmonary Resuscitation and Emergency Cardiovascular Care.Circulation.2015;132(suppl 2):S543-S560. doi: 10.1161/CIR.0000000000000267
5. Aziz K, Chadwick M, Baker M, Andrews W. Ante- and intra-partum factors that predict increased need for neonatal resuscitation. Resuscitation.2008;79:444-452. doi: 10.1016/j.resuscitation.2008.08.004
6. Mitchell A, Niday P, Boulton J, Chance G, Dulberg C. A prospective clinical audit of neonatal resuscitation practices in Canada. Adv Neonatal Care.2002;2:316-326. doi: 10.1053/adnc.2002.36831

7. Berazategui JP, Aguilar A, Escobedo M, Dannaway D, Guinsburg R, de Almeida MF, Saker F, Fernández A, Albornoz G, Valera M, Amado D, Puig G, Althabe F, Szyld E; ANR study group. Risk factors for advanced resuscitation in term and near-term infants: a case-control study. Arch Dis Child Fetal Neonatal Ed.2017;102:F44-F50. doi: 10.1136/archdischild-2015-309525
8. Bennett SC, Finer N, Halamek LP, Mickas N, Bennett MV, Nisbet CC, Sharek PJ. Implementing Delivery Room Checklists and Communication Standards in a Multi-Neonatal ICU Quality Improvement Collaborative. Jt Comm J Qual Patient Saf. 2016;42:369-376. doi: 10.1016/s1553-7250(16)42052-0
9. Balakrishnan M, Falk-Smith N, Detman LA, Miladinovic B, Sappenfield WM, Curran JS, Ashmeade TL. Promoting teamwork may improve infant care processes during delivery room management: Florida perinatal quality collaborative's approach. J Perinatol. 2017;37:886-892. doi: 10.1038/jp.2017.27
10. Talati AJ, Scott TA, Barker B, Grubb PH; Tennessee Initiative for Perinatal Quality Care Golden Hour Project Team. Improving neonatal resuscitation in Tennessee: a large-scale, quality improvement project. J Perinatol.2019;39:1676-1683. doi: 10.1038/s41372-019-0461-3
11. Litke-Wager C, Delaney H, Mu T, Sawyer T. Impact of task-oriented role assignment on neonatal resuscitation performance: a simulation-based randomized controlled trial. Am J Perinatol. 2020; doi: 10.1055/s-0039-3402751
12. Katheria A, Rich W, Finer N. Development of a strategic process using checklists to facilitate team preparation and improve communication during neonatal resuscitation. Resuscitation.2013;84:1552-1557. doi: 10.1016/j.resuscitation.2013.06.012
13. Niles DE, Cines C, Insley E, Foglia EE, Elci OU, Skåre C, Olasveengen T, Ades A, Posencheg M, Nadkarni VM, Kramer-Johansen J. Incidence and characteristics of positive pressure ventilation delivered to newborns in a US tertiary academic hospital. Resuscitation.2017;115:102-109. doi: 10.1016/j.resuscitation.2017.03.035
14. Brown T, Tu J, Profit J, Gupta A, Lee HC. Optimal Criteria Survey for Preresuscitation Delivery Room Checklists. Am J Perinatol.2016;33:203-207. doi: 10.1055/s-0035-1564064
15. The Joint Commission. Sentinel Event Alert: Preventing infant death and injury during delivery. 2004. https://www.jointcommission.org/resources/patient-safety-topics/sentinel-event/sentinel-event-alert-newsletters/sentinel-event-alert-issue-30-preventing-infant-death-and-injury-during-delivery/. Accessed February 28, 2020.
16. Patel D, Piotrowski ZH, Nelson MR, Sabich R. Effect of a statewide neonatal resuscitation training program on Apgar scores among high-risk neonates in Illinois. Pediatrics.2001;107:648-655. doi: 10.1542/peds.107.4.648

臍帯管理

臍帯管理に関する推奨事項

COR	LOE	推奨事項
2a	B-R	1. 出生時に蘇生を必要としない早産児の場合、臍帯結紮の時期を30秒以上遅らせることは妥当である[1-8]。
2b	C-LD	2. 出生時に蘇生を必要としない満期産児の場合、臍帯結紮の時期を30秒以上遅らせることは妥当としてよい[9-21]。
2b	C-EO	3. 出生時に蘇生を必要とする満期産児および早産児の場合、臍帯結紮の時期を遅らせるより、早めることを推奨するエビデンスは十分に存在しない[22]。
3：利益なし	B-R	4. 在胎28週未満で出生した新生児には、臍帯ミルキングは推奨されない[23]。

「概要」

合併症のない満期産または後期早産において、臍帯結紮を、乳児を母親の上に置いて呼吸と活動を評価する後まで遅らせることは妥当としてよい。臍帯結紮を早期（30秒以内）に行うと、胎児血が胎盤に留まって新生児の血液循環量が上昇しないため、健常な移行の妨げとなる可能性がある。遅延臍帯結紮は、出生後の高いヘマトクリット値、および幼児期の鉄欠乏の改善と関連性がある[9-21]。発育転帰はまだ十分に評価されていないが、鉄欠乏は運動および認知発達の障害と関連性がある[24-26]。早産児では、臍帯結紮を遅らせると血圧補助と輸血の必要性が減少し、生存率が向上する可能性があるため、臍帯結紮を30秒以上遅らせるのは妥当である[1-8]。

臍帯結紮の前にPPVを必要とする新生児においては、推奨事項を提示できるほど十分な研究は行われていない[22]。早期臍帯結紮は、母親の出血や血行動態不安定、胎盤早期剥離、前置胎盤など、胎盤輸血が行われる可能性が低い場合に検討すべきである[27]。遅延臍帯結紮が早期臍帯結紮と比較して母体に有害であるというエビデンスはない[10-12,28-34]。臍帯ミルキングは、遅延臍帯結紮の代替法として研究されているが、脳損傷と関連性があるため[23]、在胎28週未満の出生児では避けることが望ましい。

推奨事項の裏付けとなる解説

1. 遅延臍帯結紮が実施された早産児は、早期臍帯結紮が実施された早産児と比較して、6件のRCTのメタアナリシスにおいて低血圧の薬物療法を受けた可能性が低く[1-6]、5件のRCTのメタアナリシスにおいて輸血を受けた可能性が低かった[7]。蘇生を必要としない早産児において、遅延臍帯クランプは、早期臍帯クランプよりも高い生存率と関連性がある可能性がある[8]。10件のRCTにおいて、分娩後出血率は遅延臍帯結紮と早期臍帯結紮の間で差はなかった[10-12,28-34]。

2. 遅延臍帯結紮が実施された満期産児は、早期臍帯結紮が実施された満期産児と比較して、それぞれ12件および6件のRCTのメタアナリシスにおいて、出生後24時間のヘモグロビン濃度、および出生後3～6カ月のフェリチン濃度が高かった[9-21]。遅延臍帯結紮が実施された満期産児および後期早産児は、早期臍帯結紮が実施された満期産児および後期早産児と比較して、それぞれ4件[10,13,29,35]、10件[10,12,17,19,21,28,31,34,36,37]、および15件のRCTのメタアナリシスにおいて、死亡率、新生児集中治療室への入院、または光療法につながる高ビリルビン血症について有意差は認められなかった[9,12,14,18-21,28-30,32-34,38,39]。遅延臍帯結紮が実施された満期産児は、早期臍帯結紮が実施された満期産児と比較して、それぞれ13件[10,11,13,14,17,18,21,29,30,33,39-41]および8件のRCT[9,10,13,19,20,28,30,34]のメタアナリシスにおいて、多血症の発生率が高かった。

3. 出生時にPPVを必要とする乳児については，現在のところ，遅延臍帯結紮と早期臍帯結紮のどちらかを推奨できるほど十分なエビデンスはない。
4. ある大規模な多施設RCTにおいて，在胎28週未満で出生した早産児に対する臍帯ミルキングは，脳室内出血の発生率が高かった[23]。

参考資料

1. Dong XY, Sun XF, Li MM, Yu ZB, Han SP. [Influence of delayed cord clamping on preterm infants with a gestational age of <32 weeks]. Zhongguo Dang Dai Er Ke Za Zhi. 2016;18:635-638.
2. Gokmen Z, Ozkiraz S, Tarcan A, Kozanoglu I, Ozcimen EE, Ozbek N. Effects of delayed umbilical cord clamping on peripheral blood hematopoietic stem cells in premature neonates. J Perinat Med. 2011;39:323-329. doi: 10.1515/jpm.2011.021
3. McDonnell M, Henderson-Smart DJ. Delayed umbilical cord clamping in preterm infants: a feasibility study. J Paediatr Child Health. 1997;33:308-310. doi: 10.1111/j.1440-1754.1997.tb01606.x
4. Oh W, Fanaroff A, Carlo WA, Donovan EF, McDonald SA, Poole WK; on behalf of the Eunice Kennedy Shriver National Institute of Child Health and Human Development Neonatal Research Network. Effects of delayed cord clamping in very-low-birth-weight infants. J Perinatol. 2011;31 (suppl 1):S68-71. doi: 10.1038/jp.2010.186
5. Rabe H, Wacker A, Hülskamp G, Hörnig-Franz I, Schulze-Everding A, Harms E, Cirkel U, Louwen F, Witteler R, Schneider HP. A randomised controlled trial of delayed cord clamping in very low birth weight preterm infants. Eur J Pediatr.2000;159:775-777. doi: 10.1007/pl00008345
6. Ruangkit C, Bumrungphuet S, Panburana P, Khositseth A, Nuntnarumit P. A Randomized Controlled Trial of Immediate versus Delayed Umbilical Cord Clamping in Multiple-Birth Infants Born Preterm. Neonatology.2019;115:156-163. doi: 10.1159/000494132
7. Rabe H, Diaz-Rossello JL, Duley L, Dowswell T. Effect of timing of umbilical cord clamping and other strategies to influence placental transfusion at preterm birth on maternal and infant outcomes. Cochrane Database Syst Rev. 2012:CD003248. doi: 10.1002/14651858.CD003248.pub3
8. Fogarty M, Osborn DA, Askie L, Seidler AL, Hunter K, Lui K, Simes J, Tarnow-Mordi W. Delayed vs early umbilical cord clamping for preterm infants: a systematic review and meta-analysis. Am J Obstet Gynecol.2018;218:1-18. doi: 10.1016/j.ajog.2017.10.231
9. Al-Tawil MM, Abdel-Aal MR, Kaddah MA. A randomized controlled trial on delayed cord clamping and iron status at 3-5 months in term neonates held at the level of maternal pelvis. J Neonatal Perinat Med. 2012;5:319-326. doi: 10.3233/NPM-1263112
10. Ceriani Cernadas JM, Carroli G, Pellegrini L, Otaño L, Ferreira M, Ricci C, Casas O, Giordano D, Lardizábal J. The effect of timing of cord clamping on neonatal venous hematocrit values and clinical outcome at term: a randomized, controlled trial. Pediatrics. 2006;117:e779-e786. doi: 10.1542/peds.2005-1156
11. Chaparro CM, Neufeld LM, Tena Alavez G, Eguia-Líz Cedillo R, Dewey KG. Effect of timing of umbilical cord clamping on iron status in Mexican infants: a randomised controlled trial. Lancet.2006;367:1997-2004. doi: 10.1016/S0140-6736(06)68889-2
12. Chen X, Li X, Chang Y, Li W, Cui H. Effect and safety of timing of cord clamping on neonatal hematocrit values and clinical outcomes in term infants: A randomized controlled trial.J Perinatol.2018;38:251-257. doi: 10.1038/s41372-017-0001-y
13. Chopra A, Thakur A, Garg P, Kler N, Gujral K. Early versus delayed cord clamping in small for gestational age infants and iron stores at 3 months of age – a randomized controlled trial. BMC Pediatr. 2018;18:234. doi: 10.1186/s12887-018-1214-8
14. Emhamed MO, van Rheenen P, Brabin BJ. The early effects of delayed cord clamping in term infants born to Libyan mothers. Trop Doct. 2004;34:218-222. doi: 10.1177/004947550403400410
15. Jahazi A, Kordi M, Mirbehbahani NB, Mazloom SR. The effect of early and late umbilical cord clamping on neonatal hematocrit. J Perinatol.2008;28:523-525. doi: 10.1038/jp.2008.55
16. Philip AG. Further observations on placental transfusion. Obstet Gynecol. 1973;42:334-343.
17. Salari Z, Rezapour M, Khalili N. Late umbilical cord clamping, neonatal hematocrit and Apgar scores: a randomized controlled trial. J Neonatal Perinatal Med.2014;7:287-291. doi: 10.3233/NPM-1463913
18. Ultee CA, van der Deure J, Swart J, Lasham C, van Baar AL. Delayed cord clamping in preterm infants delivered at 34 36 weeks' gestation: a randomised controlled trial. Arch Dis Child Fetal Neonatal Ed. 2008;93:F20-F23. doi: 10.1136/adc.2006.100354
19. Vural I, Ozdemir H, Teker G, Yoldemir T, Bilgen H, Ozek E. Delayed cord clamping in term large-for-gestational age infants: A prospective randomised study. J Paediatr Child Health.2019;55:555-560. doi: 10.1111/jpc.14242
20. Yadav AK, Upadhyay A, Gothwal S, Dubey K, Mandal U, Yadav CP. Comparison of three types of intervention to enhance placental redistribution in term newborns: randomized control trial. J Perinatol.2015;35:720-724. doi: 10.1038/jp.2015.65
21. Mercer JS, Erickson-Owens DA, Collins J, Barcelos MO, Parker AB, Padbury JF. Effects of delayed cord clamping on residual placental blood volume, hemoglobin and bilirubin levels in term infants: a randomized controlled trial. J Perinatol.2017;37:260-264. doi: 10.1038/jp.2016.222
22. Wyckoff MH, Aziz K, Escobedo MB, Kapadia VS, Kattwinkel J, Perlman JM, Simon WM, Weiner GM, Zaichkin JG. Part 13: Neonatal Resuscitation: 2015 American Heart Association Guidelines Update for Cardiopulmonary Resuscitation and Emergency Cardiovascular Care (Reprint). Pediatrics. 2015;136 Suppl 2:S196-S218. doi: 10.1542/peds.2015-3373G
23. Katheria A, Reister F, Essers J, Mendler M, Hummler H, Subramaniam A, Carlo W, Tita A, Truong G, Davis-Nelson S, Schmölzer G, Chari R, Kaempf J, Tomlinson M, Yanowitz T, Beck S, Simhan H, Dempsey E, O'Donoghue K, Bhat S, Hoffman M, Faksh A, Arnell K, Rich W, Finer N, Vaucher Y, Khanna P, Meyers M, Varner M, Allman P, Szychowski J, Cutter G. Association of Umbilical Cord Milking vs Delayed Umbilical Cord Clamping With Death or Severe Intraventricular Hemorrhage Among Preterm Infants. JAMA.2019;322:1877-1886. doi: 10.1001/jama.2019.16004
24. Gunnarsson BS, Thorsdottir I, Palsson G, Gretarsson SJ. Iron status at 1 and 6 years versus developmental scores at 6 years in a well-nourished affluent population. Acta Paediatr.2007;96:391-395. doi: 10.1111/j.1651-2227.2007.00086.x
25. Grantham-McGregor S, Ani C. A review of studies on the effect of iron deficiency on cognitive development in children. J Nutr. 2001;131 (2S-2):649S-666S; discussion 666S. doi: 10.1093/jn/131.2.649S
26. Lozoff B, Beard J, Connor J, Barbara F, Georgieff M, Schallert T. Long-lasting neural and behavioral effects of iron deficiency in infancy. Nutr Rev. 2006;64 (5 Pt 2):S34-43; discussion S72. doi: 10.1301/nr.2006.may.s34-s43
27. Committee on Obstetric Practice. Committee opinion no. 684: delayed umbilical cord clamping after birth. Obstet Gynecol.2017;129:e5-e10. doi: 10.1097/aog.0000000000001860
28. Andersson O, Hellström-Westas L, Andersson D, Domellöf M. Effect of delayed versus early umbilical cord clamping on neonatal outcomes and iron status at 4 months: a randomised controlled trial. BMJ.2011;343:d7157. doi: 10.1136/bmj.d7157
29. Backes CH, Huang H, Cua CL, Garg V, Smith CV, Yin H, Galantowicz M, Bauer JA, Hoffman TM. Early versus delayed umbilical cord clamping in infants with congenital heart disease: a pilot, randomized, controlled trial. J Perinatol.2015;35:826-831. doi: 10.1038/jp.2015.89
30. Krishnan U, Rosenzweig EB. Pulmonary hypertension in chronic lung disease of infancy. Curr Opin Pediatr. 2015;27:177-183. doi: 10.1097/MOP.0000000000000205
31. Mohammad K, Tailakh S, Fram K, Creedy D. Effects of early umbilical cord clamping versus delayed clamping on maternal and neonatal outcomes: a Jordanian study. J Matern Fetal Neonatal Med. 2019:1-7. doi: 10.1080/14767058.2019.1602603
32. Oxford Midwives Research Group. A study of the relationship between the delivery to cord clamping interval and the time of cord separation. Midwifery. 1991;7:167-176. doi: 10.1016/s0266-6138 (05)80195-0
33. van Rheenen P, de Moor L, Eschbach S, de Grooth H, Brabin B. Delayed cord clamping and haemoglobin levels in infancy: a randomised controlled trial in term babies. Trop Med Int Health. 2007;12:603-616. doi: 10.1111/j.1365-3156.2007.01835.x
34. Withanathantrige M, Goonewardene I. Effects of early versus delayed umbilical cord clamping during antepartum lower segment caesarean section on placental delivery and postoperative haemorrhage: a randomised controlled trial. Ceylon Med J. 2017;62:5-11. doi: 10.4038/cmj.v62i1.8425
35. Datta BV, Kumar A, Yadav R. A Randomized Controlled Trial to Evaluate the Role of Brief Delay in Cord Clamping in Preterm Neonates (34-36 weeks) on Short-term Neurobehavioural Outcome. J Trop Pediatr. 2017;63:418-424. doi: 10.1093/tropej/fmx004
36. De Paco C, Florido J, Garrido MC, Prados S, Navarrete L. Umbilical cord blood acid-base and gas analysis after early versus delayed cord clamping

37. De Paco C, Herrera J, Garcia C, Corbalán S, Arteaga A, Pertegal M, Checa R, Prieto MT, Nieto A, Delgado JL. Effects of delayed cord clamping on the third stage of labour, maternal haematological parameters and acid-base status in fetuses at term. Eur J Obstet Gynecol Reprod Biol.2016;207:153-156. doi: 10.1016/j.ejogrb.2016.10.031
38. Cavallin F, Galeazzo B, Loretelli V, Madella S, Pizzolato M, Visentin S, Trevisanuto D. Delayed Cord Clamping versus Early Cord Clamping in Elective Cesarean Section: A Randomized Controlled Trial.Neonatology.2019;116:252-259. doi: 10.1159/000500325
39. Salae R, Tanprasertkul C, Somprasit C, Bhamarapravatana K, Suwannarurk K. Efficacy of Delayed versus Immediate Cord Clamping in Late Preterm Newborns following Normal Labor: A Randomized Control Trial. J Med Assoc Thai. 2016;99 Suppl 4:S159-S165.
40. Grajeda R, Pérez-Escamilla R, Dewey KG. Delayed clamping of the umbilical cord improves hematologic status of Guatemalan infants at 2 mo of age. Am J Clin Nutr. 1997;65:425-431. doi: 10.1093/ajcn/65.2.425
41. Saigal S, O'Neill A, Surainder Y, Chua LB, Usher R. Placental transfusion and hyperbilirubinemia in the premature. Pediatrics. 1972;49:406-419.

最初の行動
出生時の体温

COR	LOE	推奨事項
1	B-NR	1. 新生児室入室時の体温はルーチンで記録すべきである[1,2]。
1	C-EO	2. 新生児の体温は，出生後に新生児室に入室して安定するまで，36.5℃〜37.5℃に維持すべきである[2]。
1	B-NR	3. 低体温（体温が36℃未満）は不良転帰のリスクを高めるため，防止すべきである[3-5]。
2a	B-NR	4. 高体温（体温が38℃超）は不良転帰のリスクを高めるため，これを防止することは妥当である[4,6]。

「概要」
出生後に体温を測定および記録し，蘇生の質の指標として監視する必要がある。[1]。新生児の体温は，36.5℃〜37.5℃に維持すべきである[2]。低体温（36℃未満）は，新生児の死亡率と罹患率の増加に関連しているため防止する必要がある。特に超早産児（33週未満）および低出生体重児（1500g未満）では，低体温のリスクが増加する[3-5,7]。また高体温も有害となる可能性があるため，防止することは妥当である[4,6]。

「推奨事項の裏付けとなる解説」
1. 出生後の低体温は世界的に見て多く発生し，在胎期間が短く出生時体重が低い新生児で発生率が高くなっている[3-5]。
2. 新生児のルーチンでの体温管理については，以前から世界的に推奨されている[2]。
3. 早産児（37週未満）と低出生体重児（2500g未満）を対象とした観察研究では，出生後の低体温の存在と程度は，新生児の死亡率と後遺症（または，合併症）の増加と強く関連している[3-5]。
4. 2件の観察研究では，超早産児（質が中等度）および極低出生体重児（質が非常に低い）において，高体温と死亡率と後遺症（または，合併症）の増加との関連が認められた[4,6]。

新生児の体温管理

COR	LOE	推奨事項
2a	B-R	1. 蘇生を必要としない健康な新生児を，生後母親と皮膚接触させることは，授乳の向上，体温コントロール，および血糖値の安定に有効な場合がある[8]。
2a	C-LD	2. 体温調節のための介入を施したうえで，気管挿管，胸骨圧迫，静脈ラインの挿入といったすべての蘇生処置を実施することは妥当である[9]。
2a	B-R	3. 分娩室内で早産児の低体温を防止するため，ラジアントウォーマー，ポリ袋およびプラスチックラップ（キャップ付き）を使用し，室温を上げ，加温および加湿した吸入ガスを使用することは，効果的である可能性がある[10,11]。
2b	B-R	4. 早産児の低体温防止に，発熱性マットレスが効果的である可能性がある[11]。
2b	B-NR	5. 非常に早産の新生児の低体温防止に，さまざまな加温戦略の組み合わせ（「バンドル」とも呼ぶ）は妥当としてよい[12]。
2b	C-LD	6. 医療資源が限られた状況では，低体温を防止するため，新生児の首から下に清潔な食品用ポリ袋をかぶせてくるむ方法は妥当としてよい[13]。

「概要」
健康な新生児は，出生後母親と皮膚接触させるべきである[8]。早産児や低出生体重児，または蘇生が必要な新生児には，加温補助処置（周囲温度を［23℃超に］上げる，母親の胸に直接抱かせる，ラジアントウォーマー，ラップやポリ袋，帽子，毛布，発熱性マットレス，加温および加湿した吸入ガス）[10,11,14]を個々にまたは組み合わせて使用することで，低体温のリスクを減らすことができる。発熱性マットレスは，局所熱傷や高体温を引き起こすことが報告されている[15]。

新生児が病院外や，医療資源が限られた状況，または遠隔地で生まれた場合，母親の胸に直接抱かせる[8]代わりに，清潔な食品用ポリ袋[13]を使用して低体温を防止することは妥当と思われる。

「推奨事項の裏付けとなる解説」
1. 6件のRCTを対象としたシステマティックレビュー（確実性は低から中等度）で，早期に母親の胸に抱かせることは，健康な新生児の正常体温を促進することが認められた[8]。RCTおよび観察研究をレビューした2件のメタアナリシスで，医療資源が限られる一部の状況での初期蘇生および／または安定化後に，より長く母親との皮膚接触の時間をとる方が，早産児および低出生体重児における死亡率低下，授乳の向上，入院期間の短縮，および体重増加の改善が認められた。（中等度の質のエビデンス）[16,17]。
2. 十分な医療資源のある状況では，ほとんどのRCTはリスクのある新生児をラジアントウォーマーに入れた状態でルーチン管理すると考えられる[11]。
3. 加温補助処置を単独または組み合わせて使用したRCTと観察研究では，超早産児および極低出生体重児における低体温の発生率の低下を示した[10,11]。ただし，超早産児または極低出生体重児の低体温を軽減する介入を行ったRCTのメタアナリシスでは，新生児の罹患率または死亡率への影響は認められていない。（確実性が低い）[11]。2件のRCTと専門家の意見は，23℃以上の周囲温度を支持している[2,14,18]。
4. 質が中等度の1件のRCTでは，発熱性マットレスで高体温の発生率が高まった[15]。
5. 多数の非無作為化質改善試験（確実性が非常に低い～低い）は，加温補助処置の「バンドル」使用を支持している[12]。
6. 医療資源が限られた状況での1件のRCTでは，プラスチックの覆いにより低体温の発生率が低下したが，中断なく母親と皮膚接触させた場合との直接的な比較は行われなかった[13]。

新生児の気道開通と触覚刺激

新生児の触覚刺激と気道開通に関する推奨事項		
COR	LOE	推奨事項
3：利益なし	C-LD	1. 新生児の経口吸引，鼻腔内吸引，口咽頭吸引，気管内吸引をルーチンで実施することは推奨されない[7,19]。

「概要」
新生児の即時ケアでは，在胎，呼吸，緊張の初期評価を行う。適切な呼吸や啼泣のある新生児は母親の胸に抱かせる。羊水が胎便で汚れていても，ルーチンの触覚刺激や吸引などの介入は必要ない[7,19]。不必要な吸引を避けることで，気道の吸引の結果として誘発される徐脈のリスクを防ぐことができる。

「推奨事項の裏付けとなる解説」
1. 8件のRCTのメタアナリシス[19]（エビデンスの確実性が低い）は，出生後のルーチン吸引が有益でないことを示唆している[7]。その後，2件の追加研究がこの結論を支持した[7]。

呼吸努力の効果がない新生児の触覚刺激と気道開通に関する推奨事項		
COR	LOE	推奨事項
2a	B-NR	1. 生後，有効な呼吸努力が認められない新生児児に対し，触覚刺激は妥当である[20,21]。
2b	C-EO	2. PPVが必要とされ，気道が閉塞していると見られる場合は吸引を検討できる[20]。

「概要」
出生後に非効果的呼吸または無呼吸が認められる場合，触覚刺激が呼吸を刺激することがある。触覚刺激は，乳児の体を拭いて乾かすことと，背部や足底をこすることに限定すべきである。[21,22] PPVの実施中または実施後に，早産児に繰り返し触覚刺激を与えることは有益な場合もあるが，これについてはさらなる研究が待たれる[23]。初期評価で，気道を塞いでいる液体が目に見える場合，または呼吸が妨げられている懸念がある場合は，口と鼻を吸引してもよい。PPV中に気道閉塞の確証がある場合は，吸引も検討すべきである。

「推奨事項の裏付けとなる解説」
1. 触覚刺激が呼吸努力を改善する可能性を示唆している観察研究は限られている。1件のRCT（エビデンスの確実性が低い）で，触覚刺激を繰り返し受けた早産児における蘇生後の酸素化の改善が示唆されている[23]。
2. PPV中に気道閉塞が疑われる場合の吸引は，専門家の意見に基づくものである[7]。

MSAFの状態で出生した新生児の気道開通に関する推奨事項		
COR	LOE	推奨事項
2a	C-EO	1. MSAFの状態で出生した元気のない新生児に，PPV中に気道閉塞の兆候が認められれば，挿管および気管吸引の実施が有益な場合がある。
3：利益なし	C-LD	2. MSAFの状態で出生した元気のない新生児（無呼吸または非効果的呼吸を呈する）には，気管吸引の有無を問わず，ルーチンの喉頭鏡検査は推奨されない[7]。

「概要」
MSAFの状態で出生した新生児には，直接咽頭鏡検査および気管内吸引のルーチン実施は必要ないが，PPV中に気道閉塞の兆候が認められれば，それらの実施が有益な場合がある[7]。

「推奨事項の裏付けとなる解説」
1. MSAF による明らかな気道閉塞に対する気管内吸引は，専門家の意見に基づくものである。
2. 3件のRCTのメタアナリシス（エビデンスの確実性が低い）と追加1件のRCTは，MSAFの状態で出生した元気のない新生児の転帰（生存，呼吸補助の必要性，神経発達）は，吸引をPPVの前に実施しても後で実施しても同等であることを示唆している。7。

参考資料

1. Perlman JM, Wyllie J, Kattwinkel J, Wyckoff MH, Aziz K, Guinsburg R, Kim HS, Liley HG, Mildenhall L, Simon WM, et al; on behalf of the Neonatal Resuscitation Chapter Collaborators. Part 7: neonatal resuscitation: 2015 International Consensus on Cardiopulmonary Resuscitation and Emergency Cardiovascular Care Science With Treatment Recommendations. Circulation. 2015;132 (suppl 1):S204-S241. doi: 10.1161/CIR.0000000000000276
2. Department of Reproductive Health and Research (RHR) WHO. Thermal Protection of the Newborn: A Practical Guide (WHO/RHT/MSM/97.2) Geneva, Switzerland: World Health Organisation; 1997. https://apps.who.int/iris/bitstream/handle/10665/63986/WHO_RHT_MSM_97.2.pdf;jsessionid=9CF1FA8ABF2E8CE1955D96C1315D9799?sequence=1. Accessed March 1, 2020.
3. Laptook AR, Bell EF, Shankaran S, Boghossian NS, Wyckoff MH, Kandefer S, Walsh M, Saha S, Higgins R; Generic and Moderate Preterm Subcommittees of the NICHD Neonatal Research Network. Admission Temperature and Associated Mortality and Morbidity among Moderately and Extremely Preterm Infants. J Pediatr. 2018;192:53-59.e2. doi: 10.1016/j.jpeds.2017.09.021
4. Lyu Y, Shah PS, Ye XY, Warre R, Piedboeuf B, Deshpandey A, Dunn M, Lee SK; Canadian Neonatal Network. Association between admission temperature and mortality and major morbidity in preterm infants born at fewer than 33 weeks' gestation. JAMA Pediatr.2015;169:e150277. doi: 10.1001/jamapediatrics.2015.0277
5. Lunze K, Bloom DE, Jamison DT, Hamer DH. The global burden of neonatal hypothermia: systematic review of a major challenge for newborn survival. BMC Med. 2013;11:24. doi: 10.1186/1741-7015-11-24
6. Amadi HO, Olateju EK, Alabi P, Kawuwa MB, Ibadin MO, Osibogun AO. Neonatal hyperthermia and thermal stress in low- and middle-income countries: a hidden cause of death in extremely low-birthweight neonates. Paediatr Int Child Health. 2015;35:273-281. doi: 10.1179/2046905515Y.0000000030
7. Wyckoff MH, Wyllie J, Aziz K, de Almeida MF, Fabres J, Fawke J, Guinsburg R, Hosono S, Isayama T, Kapadia VS, et al; on behalf of the Neonatal Life Support Collaborators.Neonatal life support: 2020 International Consensus on Cardiopulmonary Resuscitation and Emergency Cardiovascular Care Science With Treatment Recommendations.Circulation.2020;142 (suppl 1):S185-S221. doi: 10.1161/CIR.0000000000000895
8. Moore ER, Bergman N, Anderson GC, Medley N. Early skin-to-skin contact for mothers and their healthy newborn infants. Cochrane Database Syst Rev. 2016;11:CD003519. doi: 10.1002/14651858.CD003519.pub4
9. Kattwinkel J, Perlman JM, Aziz K, Colby C, Fairchild K, Gallagher J, Hazinski MF, Halamek LP, Kumar P, Little G, et al. Part 15: neonatal resuscitation: 2010 American Heart Association Guidelines for Cardiopulmonary Resuscitation and Emergency Cardiovascular Care.Circulation.2010;122 (suppl 3):S909-S919. doi: 10.1161/CIRCULATIONAHA.110.971119
10. Meyer MP, Owen LS, Te Pas AB. Use of Heated Humidified Gases for Early Stabilization of Preterm Infants: A Meta-Analysis. Front Pediatr. 2018;6:319. doi: 10.3389/fped.2018.00319
11. McCall EM, Alderdice F, Halliday HL, Vohra S, Johnston L. Interventions to prevent hypothermia at birth in preterm and/or low birth weight infants. Cochrane Database Syst Rev. 2018;2:CD004210. doi: 10.1002/14651858.CD004210.pub5
12. Donnellan D, Moore Z, Patton D, O'Connor T, Nugent L. The effect of thermoregulation quality improvement initiatives on the admission temperature of premature/very low birth-weight infants in neonatal intensive care units: a systematic review. J Spec Pediatr Nurs. 2020:e12286. doi: 10.1111/jspn.12286
13. Belsches TC, Tilly AE, Miller TR, Kambeyanda RH, Leadford A, Manasyan A, Chomba E, Ramani M, Ambalavanan N, Carlo WA. Randomized trial of plastic bags to prevent term neonatal hypothermia in a resource-poor setting. Pediatrics.2013;132:e656-e661. doi: 10.1542/peds.2013-0172
14. Duryea EL, Nelson DB, Wyckoff MH, Grant EN, Tao W, Sadana N, Chalak LF, McIntire DD, Leveno KJ. The impact of ambient operating room temperature on neonatal and maternal hypothermia and associated morbidities: a randomized controlled trial. Am J Obstet Gynecol. 2016;214:505.e1-505.e7. doi: 10.1016/j.ajog.2016.01.190
15. McCarthy LK, Molloy EJ, Twomey AR, Murphy JF, O'Donnell CP. A randomized trial of exothermic mattresses for preterm newborns in polyethylene bags. Pediatrics.2013;132:e135-e141. doi: 10.1542/peds.2013-0279
16. Boundy EO, Dastjerdi R, Spiegelman D, Fawzi WW, Missmer SA, Lieberman E, Kajeepeta S, Wall S, Chan GJ. Kangaroo mother care and neonatal outcomes: a meta-analysis. Pediatrics. 2016;137 doi: 10.1542/peds.2015-2238
17. Conde-Agudelo A, Díaz-Rossello JL. Kangaroo mother care to reduce morbidity and mortality in low birthweight infants. Cochrane Database Syst Rev. 2016:CD002771. doi: 10.1002/14651858.CD002771.pub4
18. Jia YS, Lin ZL, Lv H, Li YM, Green R, Lin J. Effect of delivery room temperature on the admission temperature of premature infants: a randomized controlled trial. J Perinatol.2013;33:264-267. doi: 10.1038/jp.2012.100
19. Foster JP, Dawson JA, Davis PG, Dahlen HG. Routine oro/nasopharyngeal suction versus no suction at birth. Cochrane Database Syst Rev. 2017;4:CD010332. doi: 10.1002/14651858.CD010332.pub2
20. Ersdal HL, Mduma E, Svensen E, Perlman JM. Early initiation of basic resuscitation interventions including face mask ventilation may reduce birth asphyxia related mortality in low-income countries: a prospective descriptive observational study.Resuscitation.2012;83:869-873. doi: 10.1016/j.resuscitation.2011.12.011
21. Lee AC, Cousens S, Wall SN, Niermeyer S, Darmstadt GL, Carlo WA, Keenan WJ, Bhutta ZA, Gill C, Lawn JE. Neonatal resuscitation and immediate newborn assessment and stimulation for the prevention of neonatal deaths: a systematic review, meta-analysis and Delphi estimation of mortality effect. BMC Public Health.2011;11 (suppl 3):S12. doi: 10.1186/1471-2458-11-S3-S12
22. World Health Organization. Guidelines on Basic Newborn Resuscitation. Geneva, Switzerland: World Health Organization; 2012. https://apps.who.int/iris/bitstream/handle/10665/75157/9789241503693_eng.pdf;jsessionid=EA13BF490E4D349E12B4DAF16BA64A8D?sequence=1. Accessed March 1, 2020.
23. Dekker J, Hooper SB, Martherus T, Cramer SJE, van Geloven N, Te Pas AB. Repetitive versus standard tactile stimulation of preterm infants at birth – A randomized controlled trial. Resuscitation.2018;127:37-43. doi: 10.1016/j.resuscitation.2018.03.030

新生児蘇生中の心拍数の評価

出生後，新生児の心拍数を使用して，自発呼吸の有効性，介入の必要性，および介入への反応を評価する。また，胸骨圧迫を開始した新生児では，正確で迅速かつ継続的な心拍数の評価が必要である。このため，新生児の蘇生中に，新生児の心拍数を迅速かつ高い信頼性をもって測定できる方法を特定することは，きわめて重要となる。

COR	LOE	推奨事項
2b	C-LD	1. 満期産児と早産児の蘇生中は，新生児の心拍数を迅速かつ正確に測定するために心電図検査（ECG）の使用を妥当としてよい[1-8]。

心拍数の評価に関する推奨事項

「概要」
前胸部の聴診は依然として，心拍数の初期評価のための望ましい診察法である[9]。パルスオキシメトリとECGは，蘇生を必要とする新生児の心拍数を連続評価できる重要な補助手段である。

ECGは，出生時および蘇生中の新生児の心拍数を最も迅速かつ正確に測定する。聴診または触診による心拍数の臨床評価は，信頼性と精度に劣る場合がある[1-4]。パルスオキシメトリは，ECGと比較すると心拍数の検出に時間がかかり，出生後の最初の数分間は不正確になる傾向がある[5,6,10-12]。心拍数の過小評価は，不必要な介入につながる可能性がある。その一方で，新生児が徐脈の状態にある場合の心拍数の過大評価は，必要な介入の遅れにつながる可能性がある。新生児蘇生中のさまざまな心拍数評価のアプローチを他の新生児転帰と比較したデータは限られている。酸素飽和度の評価のためにパルスオキシメトリが必要とされる状況や，酸素投与が必要な状況では，心拍数検出のためのECGはパルスオキシメトリ代替とはならない。

「推奨事項の裏付けとなる解説」

1. 1件のRCTと1件の観察研究では，新生児蘇生中のECGモニタリングに関する技術的な問題は報告されておらず，新生児蘇生中の心拍数のモニタリングツールとしての実現可能性を裏付けている[6,7]。
2. 1件の観察研究では，分娩室でのECGモニタリングの実施前（歴史的コホート）と実施後の新生児転帰を比較している[8]。歴史的コホートの新生児と比較して，ECGモニタリングを行った新生児は気管挿管率が低く，5分間のApgarスコアが高かった。ただし，ECGモニタリングを行っている新生児は，分娩室で胸骨圧迫を受ける割合も高かった。
3. 615例の新生児が登録された8件の非無作為化試験[2,5,6,10,12-15]および2件の小規模RCT[7,16]から得られたきわめて質の低いエビデンスは，出生時の新生児の心拍数評価において，ECGはパルスオキシメトリと比較して迅速かつ信頼性が高いことを示唆している。
4. 2件の非無作為化試験と1件の無作為化試験から得られた非常に質の低いエビデンスは，出生直後の新生児の安定化中の心拍数評価において，聴診はECGほど正確ではないことを示している[2-4]。

心拍数の評価に関する推奨事項

COR	LOE	推奨事項
1	C-EO	1. 胸骨圧迫中は，心拍数を迅速かつ正確に評価するためにECGを使用すべきである[1-7,10,12-16]。

「概要」

胸骨圧迫を開始した場合は，ECGを使用して心拍数を確認する必要がある。ECGの心拍数が60回/分を超え，脈拍を触知できる，または心拍数を聞き取れる場合は，無脈性電気活動が除外される[17-21]。

「推奨事項の裏付けとなる解説」

1. PPVの初期段階でのECGを支持するエビデンスがあることから，専門家の見解は，胸骨圧迫を実施する場合はECGを使用すべきというものである。

参考資料

1. Chitkara R, Rajani AK, Oehlert JW, Lee HC, Epi MS, Halamek LP. The accuracy of human senses in the detection of neonatal heart rate during standardized simulated resuscitation: implications for delivery of care, training and technology design. Resuscitation.2013;84:369-372. doi: 10.1016/j.resuscitation.2012.07.035
2. Kamlin CO, O'Donnell CP, Everest NJ, Davis PG, Morley CJ. Accuracy of clinical assessment of infant heart rate in the delivery room. Resuscitation.2006;71:319-321. doi: 10.1016/j.resuscitation.2006.04.015
3. Owen CJ, Wyllie JP. Determination of heart rate in the baby at birth. Resuscitation.2004;60:213-217. doi: 10.1016/j.resuscitation.2003.10.002
4. Voogdt KG, Morrison AC, Wood FE, van Elburg RM, Wyllie JP. A randomised, simulated study assessing auscultation of heart rate at birth. Resuscitation.2010;81:1000-1003. doi: 10.1016/j.resuscitation.2010.03.021
5. Kamlin CO, Dawson JA, O'Donnell CP, Morley CJ, Donath SM, Sekhon J, Davis PG. Accuracy of pulse oximetry measurement of heart rate of newborn infants in the delivery room. J Pediatr.2008;152:756-760. doi: 10.1016/j.jpeds.2008.01.002
6. Katheria A, Rich W, Finer N. Electrocardiogram provides a continuous heart rate faster than oximetry during neonatal resuscitation. Pediatrics.2012;130:e1177-e1181. doi: 10.1542/peds.2012-0784
7. Katheria A, Arnell K, Brown M, Hassen K, Maldonado M, Rich W, Finer N. A pilot randomized controlled trial of EKG for neonatal resuscitation. PLoS One.2017;12:e0187730. doi: 10.1371/journal.pone.0187730
8. Shah BA, Wlodaver AG, Escobedo MB, Ahmed ST, Blunt MH, Anderson MP, Szyld EG. Impact of electronic cardiac (ECG) monitoring on delivery room resuscitation and neonatal outcomes. Resuscitation.2019;143:10-16. doi: 10.1016/j.resuscitation.2019.07.031
9. Wyckoff MH, Aziz K, Escobedo MB, Kapadia VS, Kattwinkel J, Perlman JM, Simon WM, Weiner GM, Zaichkin JG. Part 13: neonatal resuscitation: 2015 American Heart Association Guidelines Update for Cardiopulmonary Resuscitation and Emergency Cardiovascular Care.Circulation.2015;132(suppl 2):S543-S560. doi: 10.1161/CIR.0000000000000267
10. Mizumoto H, Tomotaki S, Shibata H, Ueda K, Akashi R, Uchio H, Hata D. Electrocardiogram shows reliable heart rates much earlier than pulse oximetry during neonatal resuscitation. Pediatr Int. 2012;54:205-207. doi: 10.1111/j.1442-200X.2011.03506.x
11. Narayen IC, Smit M, van Zwet EW, Dawson JA, Blom NA, te Pas AB. Low signal quality pulse oximetry measurements in newborn infants are reliable for oxygen saturation but underestimate heart rate. Acta Paediatr. 2015;104:e158-e163. doi: 10.1111/apa.12932
12. van Vonderen JJ, Hooper SB, Kroese JK, Roest AA, Narayen IC, van Zwet EW, te Pas AB. Pulse oximetry measures a lower heart rate at birth compared with electrocardiography. J Pediatr.2015;166:49-53. doi: 10.1016/j.jpeds.2014.09.015
13. Dawson JA, Saraswat A, Simionato L, Thio M, Kamlin CO, Owen LS, Schmölzer GM, Davis PG. Comparison of heart rate and oxygen saturation measurements from Masimo and Nellcor pulse oximeters in newly born term infants. Acta Paediatr.2013;102:955-960. doi: 10.1111/apa.12329
14. Gulati R, Zayek M, Eyal F. Presetting ECG electrodes for earlier heart rate detection in the delivery room. Resuscitation.2018;128:83-87. doi: 10.1016/j.resuscitation.2018.03.038
15. Iglesias B, Rodrí Guez MAJ, Aleo E, Criado E, Martí Nez-Orgado J, Arruza L. 3-lead electrocardiogram is more reliable than pulse oximetry to detect bradycardia during stabilisation at birth of very preterm infants. Arch Dis Child Fetal Neonatal Ed. 2018;103:F233-F237. doi: 10.1136/archdischild-2016-311492
16. Murphy MC, De Angelis L, McCarthy LK, O'Donnell CPF. Randomised study comparing heart rate measurement in newly born infants using a monitor incorporating electrocardiogram and pulse oximeter versus pulse oximeter alone. Arch Dis Child Fetal Neonatal Ed.2019;104:F547-F550. doi: 10.1136/archdischild-2017-314366
17. Luong D, Cheung PY, Barrington KJ, Davis PG, Unrau J, Dakshinamurti S, Schmölzer GM. Cardiac arrest with pulseless electrical activity rhythm in newborn infants: a case series. Arch Dis Child Fetal Neonatal Ed.2019;104:F572-F574. doi: 10.1136/archdischild-2018-316087

18. Luong DH, Cheung PY, O'Reilly M, Lee TF, Schmolzer GM. Electrocardiography vs. Auscultation to Assess Heart Rate During Cardiac Arrest With Pulseless Electrical Activity in Newborn Infants. Front Pediatr. 2018;6:366. doi: 10.3389/fped.2018.00366
19. Patel S, Cheung PY, Solevåg AL, Barrington KJ, Kamlin COF, Davis PG, Schmölzer GM. Pulseless electrical activity: a misdiagnosed entity during asphyxia in newborn infants? Arch Dis Child Fetal Neonatal Ed.2019;104:F215-F217. doi: 10.1136/archdischild-2018-314907
20. Sillers L, Handley SC, James JR, Foglia EE. Pulseless Electrical Activity Complicating Neonatal Resuscitation. Neonatology. 2019;115:95-98. doi: 10.1159/000493357
21. Solevåg AL, Luong D, Lee TF, O'Reilly M, Cheung PY, Schmölzer GM. Non-perfusing cardiac rhythms in asphyxiated newborn piglets. PLoS One.2019;14:e0214506. doi: 10.1371/journal.pone.0214506

出生後の換気補助：PPVおよび持続気道陽圧

初期呼吸（PPVを実施するタイミングと実施方法）

体を拭いて乾かし，触覚刺激を与えた後になることもあるが，新生児の大多数は出生後30～60秒以内に自発呼吸を開始する[1]。適切な出生時の初期対応（触覚刺激など）にもかかわらず，出生後最初の60秒以内に呼吸しない，または持続性の徐脈（心拍数が100回/分未満）を呈する新生児は，40～60回/分のテンポでPPVを受ける場合がある[2,3]。新生児の蘇生手順の順序は，小児および成人の蘇生アルゴリズムとは異なる。動物研究から，新生児における一次無呼吸から二次無呼吸への進行は，心不全の発症前の呼吸活動の停止をもたらすことがわかっている[4]。このイベントのサイクルは，呼吸不全と心不全が同時に認められる仮死状態の成人のサイクルとは異なる。そのため，新生児蘇生は胸骨圧迫ではなくPPVから開始する必要がある[2,3]。新生児の換気補助の開始が遅れると，死亡リスクが高まる[1]。

PPVの実施圧に関する推奨事項		
COR	LOE	推奨事項
1	B-NR	1. 適切な出生時の初期対応（触覚刺激など）にもかかわらず，出生後60秒以内に死戦期呼吸または無呼吸になる，または持続性の徐脈（心拍数が100回/分未満）を呈する新生児では，PPVを遅滞なく実施すべきである[1]。
2a	C-LD	2. PPVを必要とする新生児では，ピ最大気道内圧（最大膨張圧）をかけ肺を膨張させ，心拍数を上昇させるのが妥当である。これは通常，20～25 cmH2Oの最大気道内圧（最大膨張圧）で達成できる。場合によっては，これよりも高い最大気道内圧（最大膨張圧）が必要になる[5-14]。
2b	C-LD	3. PPV中の新生児については，呼気終末陽圧（PEEP）の使用を妥当としてよい[15-23]。
3：有害	C-LD	4. 過度な最大気道内圧（最大膨張圧）は有害な可能性があるため，避けること[24,25]。

「概要」

換気の妥当性は，心拍数の上昇および胸郭拡張（信頼性は低い）を判断する。最大気道内圧（最大膨張圧）は，最大で30 cm H_2O（正期産児）および20～25 cm H_2O（早産児）であれば，通常は肺の膨張には十分である[5-7,9,11-14]。ただし場合によっては，より高い最大気道内圧（最大膨張圧）が必要になる[5,7-10]。心拍数の増加および胸郭拡張に必要な圧力よりも高い最大気道内圧（最大膨張圧）または1回換気量は避けること[24,26-28]。

状態の悪い新生児や早産児は，未成熟かつ界面活性物質の欠乏によって，肺胞が虚脱することが多い[15]。PEEPは，呼気時に肺の低圧膨張を提供する。動物実験では，PPV中のPEEPにより肺容量が維持され，それによる肺機能および酸素化の改善が示されている[16]。PEEPは新生児の蘇生において有益である可能性があるが，ヒトを対象とした試験によるエビデンスは限られている。ヒトを対象とした試験では，すべて5 cm H_2OのPEEPレベルが使用されているため，最適なPEEPは特定されていない[18-22]。

「推奨事項の裏付けとなる解説」

1. ある大規模な観察研究では，活気のないほとんどの新生児は，体表刺激およびPPVに反応することが認められた。この研究では，PPVの開始が30秒遅れるごとに，死亡または長期入院のリスクが16%増加することが示されている[1]。
2. 生まれたばかりの哺乳類を対象とした動物実験では，窒息時の心拍数低下が示されている。肺の換気により，心拍数は急速に上昇する[3,4]。ほとんどの満期産児は，30 cm H_2Oの最大気道内圧（最大膨張圧）をPEEPなしで加えることで蘇生できることが，複数の症例集積研究で認められている[5-8]。場合によっては，これよりも高いピーク圧が必要になる[5,7-10]。
3. 早産児を対象とした症例集積研究では，ほとんどの早産児は20～25 cm H_2OのPPV膨張圧を使用することで蘇生できることが認められているが[11-14]，より高い圧力が必要になる場合もある[10,11]。
4. 在胎23～33週の乳児1,962人を対象とした観察研究では，PPVとPEEPを両者を加えた場合は，PEEPを加えなかった場合と比較して，死亡率および慢性肺疾患の発症率が低下することが報告されている[19]。
5. 312人の乳児を対象とした2件の無作為化試験および1件の準無作為化試験（質はきわめて低い）では，Tピースを使用したPPV（PEEPあり）と自己膨張式バック（PEEPなし）を使用したPPVを比較しており，同様の死亡率および慢性肺疾患の発症率が報告されている[20-22]。1件の試験（質はきわめて低い）では，Tピースを使用したPPVにおいて，PEEP 5 cmH2Oの場合とPEEP 0 cmH2Oの場合を比較しており，同様の死亡率および慢性肺疾患の発症率が報告されている[23]。

6. 生まれたばかりの動物を対象とした研究では，PEEP により肺の通気と機能的残気量の蓄積が促進され，末梢気道の虚脱が抑えられるため，肺の表面積とコンプライアンスが増加すること，呼気抵抗が低下すること，界面活性物質が保護されること，および硝子膜の形成，肺胞虚脱，炎症性疾患の発現が低減することが報告されている[16,18]。
7. 新生児を対象とした 1 件の観察研究では，蘇生中の高い 1 回換気量を脳損傷に関連付けている[25]。
8. 複数の動物実験では，未成熟の動物に対する高容量の換気が，肺損傷，ガス交換障害，肺コンプライアンス低下の原因となっていることが認められている[24,26-28]。

PPV 中の呼吸数および吸気時間に関する推奨事項

COR	LOE	推奨事項
2a	C-EO	1. 1 分あたり 40～60 回の吸気回数で PPV を実施することは妥当である。
2a	C-LD	2. 新生児（満期産児および早産児）では，1 秒以下の吸気時間で PPV を開始することは妥当である[2]。
3：有害	B-R	3. 早産の新生児の場合，持続的肺拡張のルーチン使用による蘇生の開始は有害となる可能性があるため，実施すべきでない[29]。

「概要」

適切な最初の行動（触覚刺激など）を取ったにもかかわらず，非効果的呼吸，無呼吸，または持続性の徐脈（心拍数が 100 回/分未満）を呈する新生児に対して，40～60 回/分の回数で PPV を開始することは妥当である[1]。

満期産児および早産児の両方の新生児の自然呼吸のパターンに合わせるため，PPV 実施中の吸気時間は 1 秒未満にすべきである。より長時間の肺拡張を持続した場合の潜在的な有効性について研究した複数の調査が実施されているが，早産児に対して 10 秒を超える拡張時間を持続した場合は，有害となる可能性がある。肺拡張の持続を 1～10 秒とした場合の潜在的な有益性または有害性については不明である[2,29]。

「推奨事項の裏付けとなる解説」

1. 1 分あたり 40～60 回の換気回数での PPV の実施は，専門家の見解に基づいたものである。
2. ILCOR 特別委員会のレビューでは，PPV と持続的吸気の比較に際し，PPV の吸気時間を専門家の見解に基づいて 1 秒以下と定義している。ある観察研究では，新生児（満期産児および早産児）の呼吸における初期パターンとして，吸気時間を約 0.3 秒としている[2]。
3. 早産児を対象とした 2 件のシステマティックレビュー[29,30]（低から中等度の確実性）では，PPV 中の持続的肺拡張による有意な有益性は認められておらず，1 件のレビューでは生後 48 時間以内の死亡リスクが高まることが認められている。1 件の大規模な RCT[31] は，在胎 28 週未満で持続的肺拡張が実施された新生児について，早期死亡率の上昇が認められた時点で早期に中止されている。死亡または気管支肺異形成の主要転帰について，有意な差は認められていない。

持続的気道陽圧法（CPAP）

CPAP の実施に関する推奨事項

COR	LOE	推奨事項
2a	A	1. 実施直後に呼吸補助を必要とする自発呼吸のある早産児に対し，挿管ではなく（マスク・経鼻的）CPAP を使用することは妥当である[32]。

「概要」

自発呼吸のある新生児は，出生後に機能的残気量を確立する必要がある[8]。一部の新生児は呼吸窮迫を発症し，努力呼吸または持続性チアノーゼとして現れる。（マスク・経鼻的）CPAP は呼吸補助の一形態であり，新生児の肺の開存を保持する。（マスク・経鼻的）CPAP は，出生後または蘇生後に呼吸困難を起こしている早産児に対して有用であり[33]，気管内換気と比較して，超早産児の気管支肺異形成リスクを低減できる可能性がある[34-36]。（マスク・経鼻的）CPAP は，挿管および PPV と比べて侵襲性の低い呼吸補助の形態でもある。

「推奨事項の裏付けとなる解説」

1. 4 件の RCT および 1 件のメタアナリシス[32,34-37]（質が高い）では，呼吸窮迫（回避すべき呼吸回数が 25 回）を発症している超早産児（在胎 30 週未満）に対して（マスク・経鼻的）CPAP による治療を開始した場合は，挿管および換気を実施した場合と比較して，死亡および気管支肺異形成を合わせた転帰の減少が示されている。このメタアナリシスでは，死亡率，気管支肺異形成，気胸，脳室内出血，壊死性腸炎，未熟児網膜症それぞれの転帰については，有意な差は報告されていない[32]。

参考資料

1. Ersdal HL, Mduma E, Svensen E, Perlman JM. Early initiation of basic resuscitation interventions including face mask ventilation may reduce birth asphyxia related mortality in low-income countries: a prospective descriptive observational study. Resuscitation. 2012;83:869–873. doi: 10.1016/j.resuscitation.2011.12.011
2. te Pas AB, Wong C, Kamlin CO, Dawson JA, Morley CJ, Davis PG. Breathing patterns in preterm and term infants immediately after birth. Pediatr Res. 2009;65:352-356. doi: 10.1203/PDR.0b013e318193f117
3. Milner AD. Resuscitation of the newborn. Arch Dis Child. 1991;66(1 Spec No):66-69. doi: 10.1136/adc.66.1_spec_no.66
4. Dawes GS, Jacobson HN, Mott JC, Shelley HJ, Stafford A. The treatment of asphyxiated, mature foetal lambs and rhesus monkeys with intravenous glucose and sodium carbonate. J Physiol. 1963;169:167-184. doi: 10.1113/jphysiol.1963.sp007248
5. Hull D. Lung expansion and ventilation during resuscitation of asphyxiated newborn infants. J Pediatr. 1969;75:47-58. doi: 10.1016/s0022-3476(69)80100-9
6. Hoskyns EW, Milner AD, Hopkin IE. A simple method of face mask resuscitation at birth. Arch Dis Child. 1987;62:376-378. doi: 10.1136/adc.62.4.376

7. Field D, Milner AD, Hopkin IE. Efficiency of manual resuscitators at birth. Arch Dis Child. 1986;61:300-302. doi: 10.1136/adc.61.3.300
8. Boon AW, Milner AD, Hopkin IE. Lung expansion, tidal exchange, and formation of the functional residual capacity during resuscitation of asphyxiated neonates. J Pediatr.1979;95:1031–1036. doi: 10.1016/s0022-3476(79)80304-2
9. Vyas H, Milner AD, Hopkin IE, Boon AW. Physiologic responses to prolonged and slow-rise inflation in the resuscitation of the asphyxiated newborn infant. J Pediatr.1981;99:635-639. doi: 10.1016/s0022-3476(81)80279-x
10. Upton CJ, Milner AD. Endotracheal resuscitation of neonates using a rebreathing bag. Arch Dis Child. 1991;66(1 Spec No):39-42. doi: 10.1136/adc.66.1_spec_no.39
11. Hoskyns EW, Milner AD, Boon AW, Vyas H, Hopkin IE. Endotracheal resuscitation of preterm infants at birth. Arch Dis Child.1987;62:663-666. doi: 10.1136/adc.62.7.663
12. Hird MF, Greenough A, Gamsu HR. Inflating pressures for effective resuscitation of preterm infants. Early Hum Dev. 1991;26:69-72. doi: 10.1016/0378-3782(91)90045-5
13. Lindner W, Vossbeck S, Hummler H, Pohlandt F. Delivery room management of extremely low birth weight infants: spontaneous breathing or intubation? Pediatrics. 1999;103(5 Pt 1):961-967. doi: 10.1542/peds.103.5.961
14. Menakaya J, Andersen C, Chirla D, Wolfe R, Watkins A. A randomised comparison of resuscitation with an anaesthetic rebreathing circuit or an infant ventilator in very preterm infants. Arch Dis Child Fetal Neonatal Ed. 2004;89:F494-F496. doi: 10.1136/adc.2003.033340
15. te Pas AB, Davis PG, Hooper SB, Morley CJ. From liquid to air: breathing after birth. J Pediatr. 2008;152:607-611. doi: 10.1016/j.jpeds.2007.10.041
16. Siew ML, Te Pas AB, Wallace MJ, Kitchen MJ, Lewis RA, Fouras A, Morley CJ, Davis PG, Yagi N, Uesugi K, et al. Positive end-expiratory pressure enhances development of a functional residual capacity in preterm rabbits ventilated from birth. J Appl Physiol (1985). 2009;106:1487-1493. doi: 10.1152/japplphysiol.91591.2008
17. Wyckoff MH, Aziz K, Escobedo MB, Kapadia VS, Kattwinkel J, Perlman JM, Simon WM, Weiner GM, Zaichkin JG.Part 13: neonatal resuscitation: 2015 American Heart Association Guidelines Update for Cardiopulmonary Resuscitation and Emergency Cardiovascular Care.Circulation.2015;132(suppl 2):S543-S560. doi: 10.1161/CIR.0000000000000267
18. Probyn ME, Hooper SB, Dargaville PA, McCallion N, Crossley K, Harding R, Morley CJ. Positive end expiratory pressure during resuscitation of premature lambs rapidly improves blood gases without adversely affecting arterial pressure. Pediatr Res.2004;56:198-204. doi: 10.1203/01.PDR.0000132752.94155.13
19. Guinsburg R, de Almeida MFB, de Castro JS, Gonçalves-Ferri WA, Marques PF, Caldas JPS, Krebs VLJ, Souza Rugolo LMS, de Almeida JHCL, Luz JH, Procianoy RS, Duarte JLMB, Penido MG, Ferreira DMLM, Alves Filho N, Diniz EMA, Santos JP, Acquesta AL, Santos CND, Gonzalez MRC, da Silva RPVC, Meneses J, Lopes JMA, Martinez FE. T-piece versus self-inflating bag ventilation in preterm neonates at birth. Arch Dis Child Fetal Neonatal Ed.2018;103:F49-F55. doi: 10.1136/archdischild-2016-312360
20. Dawson JA, Schmölzer GM, Kamlin CO, Te Pas AB, O'Donnell CP, Donath SM, Davis PG, Morley CJ. Oxygenation with T-piece versus self-inflating bag for ventilation of extremely preterm infants at birth: a randomized controlled trial. J Pediatr. 2011;158:912-918.e1-e2 doi: 10.1016/j.jpeds.2010.12.003
21. Szyld E, Aguilar A, Musante GA, Vain N, Prudent L, Fabres J, Carlo WA; Delivery Room Ventilation Devices Trial Group. Comparison of devices for newborn ventilation in the delivery room. J Pediatr. 2014;165:234-239.e3. doi: 10.1016/j.jpeds.2014.02.035
22. Thakur A, Saluja S, Modi M, Kler N, Garg P, Soni A, Kaur A, Chetri S. T-piece or self inflating bag for positive pressure ventilation during delivery room resuscitation: an RCT. Resuscitation. 2015;90:21-24. doi: 10.1016/j.resuscitation.2015.01.021
23. Finer NN, Carlo WA, Duara S, Fanaroff AA, Donovan EF, Wright LL, Kandefer S, Poole WK; National Institute of Child Health and Human Development Neonatal Research Network. Delivery room continuous positive airway pressure/positive end-expiratory pressure in extremely low birth weight infants: a feasibility trial. Pediatrics.2004;114:651-657. doi: 10.1542/peds.2004-0394
24. Hillman NH, Moss TJ, Kallapur SG, Bachurski C, Pillow JJ, Polglase GR, Nitsos I, Kramer BW, Jobe AH. Brief, large tidal volume ventilation initiates lung injury and a systemic response in fetal sheep. Am J Respir Crit Care Med. 2007;176:575-581. doi: 10.1164/rccm.200701-051OC
25. Mian Q, Cheung PY, O'Reilly M, Barton SK, Polglase GR, Schmölzer GM. Impact of delivered tidal volume on the occurrence of intraventricular haemorrhage in preterm infants during positive pressure ventilation in the delivery room. Arch Dis Child Fetal Neonatal Ed. 2019;104:F57-F62. doi: 10.1136/archdischild-2017-313864
26. Björklund LJ, Ingimarsson J, Curstedt T, John J, Robertson B, Werner O, Vilstrup CT. Manual ventilation with a few large breaths at birth compromises the therapeutic effect of subsequent surfactant replacement in immature lambs. Pediatr Res. 1997;42:348-355. doi: 10.1203/00006450-199709000-00016
27. Björklund LJ, Ingimarsson J, Curstedt T, Larsson A, Robertson B, Werner O. Lung recruitment at birth does not improve lung function in immature lambs receiving surfactant. Acta Anaesthesiol Scand. 2001;45:986-993. doi: 10.1034/j.1399-6576.2001.450811.x
28. Wada K, Jobe AH, Ikegami M. Tidal volume effects on surfactant treatment responses with the initiation of ventilation in preterm lambs. J Appl Physiol (1985). 1997;83:1054-1061. doi: 10.1152/jappl.1997.83.4.1054
29. Wyckoff MH, Wyllie J, Aziz K, de Almeida MF, Fabres J, Fawke J, Guinsburg R, Hosono S, Isayama T, Kapadia VS, et al; on behalf of the Neonatal Life Support Collaborators. Neonatal life support: 2020 International Consensus on Cardiopulmonary Resuscitation and Emergency Cardiovascular Care Science With Treatment Recommendations. Circulation. 2020;142(suppl 1):S185-S221. doi: 10.1161/CIR.0000000000000895
30. Foglia EE, Te Pas AB, Kirpalani H, Davis PG, Owen LS, van Kaam AH, Onland W, Keszler M, Schmölzer GM, Hummler H, et al. Sustained inflation vs standard resuscitation for preterm infants: a systematic review and meta-analysis. JAMA Pediatr. 2020:e195897. doi: 10.1001/jamapediatrics.2019.5897
31. Kirpalani H, Ratcliffe SJ, Keszler M, Davis PG, Foglia EE, Te Pas A, Fernando M, Chaudhary A, Localio R, van Kaam AH, Onland W, Owen LS, Schmölzer GM, Katheria A, Hummler H, Lista G, Abbasi S, Klotz D, Simma B, Nadkarni V, Poulain FR, Donn SM, Kim HS, Park WS, Cadet C, Kong JY, Smith A, Guillen U, Liley HG, Hopper AO, Tamura M; on behalf of the SAIL Site Investigators. Effect of Sustained Inflations vs Intermittent Positive Pressure Ventilation on Bronchopulmonary Dysplasia or Death Among Extremely Preterm Infants: The SAIL Randomized Clinical Trial. JAMA.2019;321:1165-1175. doi: 10.1001/jama.2019.1660
32. Schmölzer GM, Kumar M, Pichler G, Aziz K, O'Reilly M, Cheung PY. Non-invasive versus invasive respiratory support in preterm infants at birth: systematic review and meta-analysis. BMJ. 2013;347:f5980. doi: 10.1136/bmj.f5980
33. Hooper SB, Polglase GR, Roehr CC. Cardiopulmonary changes with aeration of the newborn lung. Paediatr Respir Rev. 2015;16:147-150. doi: 10.1016/j.prrv.2015.03.003
34. Dunn MS, Kaempf J, de Klerk A, de Klerk R, Reilly M, Howard D, Ferrelli K, O'Conor J, Soll RF; Vermont Oxford Network DRM Study Group. Randomized trial comparing 3 approaches to the initial respiratory management of preterm neonates. Pediatrics. 2011;128:e1069-e1076. doi: 10.1542/peds.2010-3848
35. Morley CJ, Davis PG, Doyle LW, Brion LP, Hascoet JM, Carlin JB; COIN Trial Investigators. Nasal CPAP or intubation at birth for very preterm infants. N Engl J Med.2008;358:700-708. doi: 10.1056/NEJMoa072788
36. SUPPORT Study Group of the Eunice Kennedy Shriver NICHD Neonatal Research Network. Early CPAP versus surfactant in extremely preterm infants. N Engl J Med.2010;362:1970-1979. doi: 10.1056/NEJMoa0911783
37. Sandri F, Plavka R, Ancora G, Simeoni U, Stranak Z, Martinelli S, Mosca F, Nona J, Thomson M, Verder H, Fabbri L, Halliday H; CURPAP Study Group. Prophylactic or early selective surfactant combined with nCPAP in very preterm infants. Pediatrics.2010;125:e1402-e1409. doi: 10.1542/peds.2009-2131

酸素投与

新生児の蘇生中に実施する酸素投与に関する推奨事項

COR	LOE	推奨事項
2a	B-R	1. 出生時に呼吸補助を受ける満期産児および後期早産児（在胎 35 週以上）に対しては，21 %の初期酸素濃度の使用が妥当である[1]。
2b	C-LD	2. 出生時に呼吸補助を受ける早産新生児（在胎 35 週未満）に対しては，21 %～30 %の濃度から酸素投与を始め，その後はパルスオキシメータに基づいて酸素濃度を調節することを妥当としてよい[2,3]。
3：有害	B-R	3. 出生時に呼吸補助を受ける満期産児および後期早産児（在胎 35 週以上）に対しては，死亡率の上昇と関連があるため，100 %の酸素を投与しないこと[1]。

「概要」

合併症のない分娩では，胎児から新生児への移行に伴い，子宮内の低酸素環境から大気（酸素濃度21％）への遷移が発生するため，数分で血中酸素濃度が上昇する。蘇生中は，不十分な酸素供給（低酸素血症）による害を防止する目的で酸素を投与できる[4]。ただし，過剰な酸素暴露（高酸素症）は，有害となる可能性がある[5]。

満期産児および後期早産児の蘇生中に，21％の酸素濃度（大気）で呼吸補助を開始した場合は，100％の酸素濃度で開始した場合と比較して，短期死亡率が低下している[1]。生存者の神経発達に関する転帰について，差は認められていない[1]。蘇生中は，経腟分娩の健常満期産児の酸素飽和度（海抜0メートル）をモニタリングする目的でパルスオキシメトリを使用できる[3]。

在胎期間が短い早産児の場合は，死亡率などの重要な転帰について，低酸素濃度（50％以下）で呼吸補助を開始した場合と，高酸素濃度（50％超）で開始した場合との差は見られなかった[2]。高酸素症による有害性を考慮すると，21％〜30％の酸素濃度から開始することは妥当といえる。このような集団では，酸素濃度の目標値を設定したパルスオキシメトリが推奨される[3]。

「推奨事項の裏付けとなる解説」

1. 満期産児および後期早産児が登録した5件の無作為化試験および準無作為化試験のメタアナリシスでは，低酸素性虚血性脳症（HIE）の発症率に差は見られなかった。同様に，2件の準無作為化試験のメタアナリシスでは，新生児の時点で21％の濃度で酸素投与した患者と，100％の濃度で投与した患者を比較した場合[1]，1〜3歳時点での中等度〜重度の神経発達障害について差は見られなかった[1]。
2. 早産児が登録した10件の無作為化試験のメタアナリシス（7件の試験のサブアナリシスを含む）で報告されている在胎28週以下の新生児の転帰では，低酸素濃度で呼吸補助を開始した場合と高酸素濃度で開始した場合との間に差は見られなかった[2]。対象となる試験での低酸素濃度は一般的に21％〜30％で，高酸素濃度は常に60％〜100％であった。さらに，長期死亡率，神経発達に関する転帰，未熟児網膜症，気管支肺異形成，壊死性腸炎，脳内の大きな出血についても差は見られなかった[2]。共介入として酸素飽和度目標を使用した8件の試験のシステマティックレビューでは，21％の酸素濃度（大気）で呼吸補助を開始したすべての早産児が，事前に決められた酸素飽和度の目標値に到達するために，酸素の追加投与を必要とした[2]。低酸素濃度で呼吸補助を開始するという推奨事項は，早産児に対する過剰な酸素暴露（あらかじめ決めた酸素飽和度の目標値に到達するために必要な濃度を超える）を回避することの優位性を反映したものであり，重要な転帰に対する高酸素濃度の有益性を示すエビデンスがないためである[3]。
3. 満期産児および後期早産児が登録した7件の無作為化試験および準無作為化試験のメタアナリシスでは，分娩室での蘇生の際に21％の酸素濃度を使用した場合，100％の酸素濃度を使用した場合と比較して短期死亡率の低下が認められた[1]。その中間の酸素濃度（22％〜99％）で呼吸補助を開始した場合について調べた研究は存在しない。

参考資料

1. Welsford M, Nishiyama C, Shortt C, Isayama T, Dawson JA, Weiner G, Roehr CC, Wyckoff MH, Rabi Y; on behalf of the International Liaison Committee on Resuscitation Neonatal Life Support Task Force. Room air for initiating term newborn resuscitation: a systematic review with meta-analysis. Pediatrics. 2019;143. doi: 10.1542/peds.2018-1825
2. Welsford M, Nishiyama C, Shortt C, Weiner G, Roehr CC, Isayama T, Dawson JA, Wyckoff MH, Rabi Y; on behalf of the International Liaison Committee on Resuscitation Neonatal Life Support Task Force. Initial oxygen use for preterm newborn resuscitation: a systematic review with meta-analysis. Pediatrics. 2019;143 doi: 10.1542/peds.2018-1828
3. Escobedo MB, Aziz K, Kapadia VS, Lee HC, Niermeyer S, Schmölzer GM, Szyld E, Weiner GM, Wyckoff MH, Yamada NK, Zaichkin JG. 2019 American Heart Association Focused Update on Neonatal Resuscitation: An Update to the American Heart Association Guidelines for Cardiopulmonary Resuscitation and Emergency Cardiovascular Care. Circulation.2019;140:e922-e930. doi: 10.1161/CIR.0000000000000729
4. Saugstad OD. Resuscitation of newborn infants: from oxygen to room air. Lancet.2010;376:1970-1971. doi: 10.1016/S0140-6736(10)60543-0
5. Weinberger B, Laskin DL, Heck DE, Laskin JD. Oxygen toxicity in premature infants. Toxicol Appl Pharmacol. 2002;181:60-67. doi: 10.1006/taap.2002.9387

胸骨圧迫
CPRのタイミング

CPRの開始に関する推奨事項		
COR	LOE	推奨事項
2a	C-EO	1. 適切な換気を30秒以上実施しても，出生後の心拍数が60回/分未満の場合，胸骨圧迫の開始は妥当である[1,2]。
2b	C-EO	2. 胸骨圧迫中の換気について，21％（大気）または他の酸素濃度と比較した100％酸素濃度の有益性は不明である。胸骨圧迫中は，高い酸素濃度の使用を妥当としてよい[1,2]。

「概要」

出生時に無呼吸または非効果的呼吸を呈しているほとんどの新生児は，新生児蘇生の初期手順（気道確保のための体位，分泌物の除去，乾燥，触覚刺激），または効果的なPPVに反応し，心拍数の上昇と呼吸を改善する。このような介入を行っても心拍数が60回/分未満の場合は，心拍数が上昇するまで，胸骨圧迫を実施することで酸素を含んだ血液を脳に供給することができる。可能であれば気管挿管により，胸骨圧迫の

開始前に換気を最適化する必要がある。適切なPPVを30秒以上実施しても心拍数が60回/分未満の場合は，胸骨圧迫を開始する必要がある[1]。

臓器機能にとって酸素は不可欠であるが，蘇生中の過度の酸素吸入は，有害になる可能性がある。現行のガイドラインでは，胸骨圧迫を実施しながら100%の酸素を供給することを推奨しているが，大気（21%）を含め，他の酸素濃度と比較した100%酸素の有益性は，どの研究でも認められていない。ただし，低酸素濃度によるPPVに対する反応が見られない場合は，吸入酸素濃度を100%に高めることを妥当としてよい。自己心拍再開（ROSC）が認められたら，高酸素症に関連するリスクを低減するため，パルスオキシメトリに基づき，生理学的なレベルを目標として，投与する酸素濃度を引き下げることができる[1,2]。

「推奨事項の裏付けとなる解説」

1. 心拍数が60回/分未満の新生児に対する胸骨圧迫の開始は，専門家の見解に基づくものであり，この問題に取り組んでいるヒトを対象とした臨床的または生理学的研究は行われていない。
2. 胸骨圧迫中に濃度100%の酸素を供給した場合について調査した8件の動物実験（動物323例）のメタアナリシス（質はきわめて低い）では，曖昧な結果が示されている[3]。2件の動物実験（質はきわめて低い）では，大気（21%）と100%の酸素濃度の場合について，組織の酸化ストレスまたは損傷を比較しており，脳または肺の炎症マーカーにおける差は報告されていない[3]。そのため，胸骨圧迫中の100%酸素の使用は，専門家の見解に基づくものである。

胸骨圧迫と人工呼吸の比率および手技（新生児）

COR	LOE	推奨事項
2b	C-EO	1. 新生児に対して胸骨圧迫を実施する場合は，3回の圧迫に続けて肺拡張を行う方法（3：1の比率）の繰り返しを妥当としてよい[4-8]。
2b	C-LD	2. 新生児に対して胸骨圧迫を実施する場合は，2本指法ではなく胸郭包み込み両母指圧迫法を選択することを妥当としてよい。これは，胸郭包み込み両母指圧迫法が，血圧の改善と救助者の疲労軽減に関連するためである[9,10]。

「概要」

満期産新生児に対する胸骨圧迫はまれなイベントであるが（約0.1%），早産新生児の場合は実施頻度が高くなる[11]。新生児に対して胸骨圧迫を実施する場合は，換気の前または後に3回の圧迫を実施することを妥当としてよい。つまり，1分あたり30回の換気と90回の圧迫を実施することになる（比率は3：1で，1分あたり120回の合計イベント数）。

新生児期以外の場合は，3：1以外の胸骨圧迫と人工呼吸の比率や非同期のPPV（胸骨圧迫と同調しない肺拡張を患者に実施する）がルーチンに使用されているが，新生児に推奨されるのは3：1の比率で同調して実施する方法である。胸骨圧迫については，胸骨圧迫を実施しながら肺拡張を維持する新しい手法（持続的肺拡張）が調査中であるが，現時点では研究プロトコール以外で推奨することはできない[12,13]。

新生児に対して胸骨圧迫を実施する場合は，血圧の上昇と救助者の疲労軽減という観点から，2本指法よりも胸郭包み込み両母指圧迫法のほうが有益である可能性がある。胸郭包み込み両母指圧迫法によって胸骨圧迫を実施する場合は，両方の親指を使って胸骨を押し込みながら，両手の指で乳児の胸郭を包み込む[1,2]。胸郭包み込み両母指圧迫法は，乳児の場合は側部から，新生児の場合は頭部の上方から実施できる[1]。頭部の上方から胸郭包み込み両母指圧迫法を実施することで，臍帯静脈カテーテルを留置しやすくなる。

「推奨事項の裏付けとなる解説」

1. 動物実験（質はきわめて低い）では，3：1以外の胸骨圧迫と肺拡張の比率（2：1，4：1，5：1，9：3，15：2，および非同期PPVを伴う継続的な胸骨圧迫）を使用した場合でも，同様のROSCおよび死亡率になるとされている[4-8]。
2. 留置カテーテルを挿入した少数の新生児（2例）では，2本指法と比較して，胸郭包み込み両母指圧迫法のほうが，高い収縮期血圧および平均血圧を生み出している[9]。
3. 1件のマネキンを用いた小規模な研究（質はきわめて低い）では，60秒間の中断のない胸骨圧迫という条件下で，胸郭包み込み両母指圧迫法と2本指法を比較した。その結果，2本指法よりも胸郭包み込み両母指圧迫法のほうが，深い圧迫，疲労の軽減，変動の低減が達成されている[10]。

参考資料

1. Wyckoff MH, Aziz K, Escobedo MB, Kapadia VS, Kattwinkel J, Perlman JM, Simon WM, Weiner GM, Zaichkin JG. Part 13: neonatal resuscitation: 2015 American Heart Association Guidelines Update for Cardiopulmonary Resuscitation and Emergency Cardiovascular Care. Circulation. 2015;132(suppl 2):S543-S560. doi: 10.1161/CIR.0000000000000267
2. Perlman JM, Wyllie J, Kattwinkel J, Wyckoff MH, Aziz K, Guinsburg R, Kim HS, Liley HG, Mildenhall L, Simon WM, et al; on behalf of the Neonatal Resuscitation Chapter Collaborators. Part 7: neonatal resuscitation: 2015 International Consensus on Cardiopulmonary Resuscitation and Emergency Cardiovascular Care Science With Treatment Recommendations. Circulation. 2015;132(suppl 1):S204-S241. doi: 10.1161/CIR.0000000000000276
3. Garcia-Hidalgo C, Cheung PY, Solevåg AL, Vento M, O'Reilly M, Saugstad O, Schmölzer GM. A Review of Oxygen Use During Chest Compressions in Newborns-A Meta-Analysis of Animal Data. Front Pediatr. 2018;6:400. doi: 10.3389/fped.2018.00400
4. Solevåg AL, Schmölzer GM, O'Reilly M, Lu M, Lee TF, Hornberger LK, Nakstad B, Cheung PY. Myocardial perfusion and oxidative stress after 21% vs. 100% oxygen ventilation and uninterrupted chest compressions in severely

asphyxiated piglets. Resuscitation. 2016;106:7-13. doi: 10.1016/j.resuscitation.2016.06.014
5. Schmölzer GM, O'Reilly M, Labossiere J, Lee TF, Cowan S, Nicoll J, Bigam DL, Cheung PY. 3:1 compression to ventilation ratio versus continuous chest compression with asynchronous ventilation in a porcine model of neonatal resuscitation. Resuscitation.2014;85:270-275. doi: 10.1016/j.resuscitation.2013.10.011
6. Solevåg AL, Dannevig I, Wyckoff M, Saugstad OD, Nakstad B. Extended series of cardiac compressions during CPR in a swine model of perinatal asphyxia. Resuscitation.2010;81:1571-1576. doi: 10.1016/j.resuscitation.2010.06.007
7. Solevag AL, Dannevig I, Wyckoff M, Saugstad OD, Nakstad B. Return of spontaneous circulation with a compression:ventilation ratio of 15:2 versus 3:1 in newborn pigs with cardiac arrest due to asphyxia. Arch Dis Child Fetal Neonatal Ed. 2011;96:F417-F421. doi: 10.1136/adc.2010.200386
8. Pasquin MP, Cheung PY, Patel S, Lu M, Lee TF, Wagner M, O'Reilly M, Schmolzer GM. Comparison of Different Compression to Ventilation Ratios (2: 1, 3: 1, and 4: 1) during Cardiopulmonary Resuscitation in a Porcine Model of Neonatal Asphyxia. Neonatology. 2018;114:37-45. doi: 10.1159/000487988
9. David R. Closed chest cardiac massage in the newborn infant. Pediatrics. 1988;81:552-554.
10. Christman C, Hemway RJ, Wyckoff MH, Perlman JM. The two-thumb is superior to the two-finger method for administering chest compressions in a manikin model of neonatal resuscitation. Arch Dis Child Fetal Neonatal Ed. 2011;96:F99-F101. doi: 10.1136/adc.2009.180406
11. Handley SC, Sun Y, Wyckoff MH, Lee HC. Outcomes of extremely preterm infants after delivery room cardiopulmonary resuscitation in a population-based cohort. J Perinatol.2015;35:379-383. doi: 10.1038/jp.2014.222
12. Schmölzer GM, M OR, Fray C, van Os S, Cheung PY. Chest compression during sustained inflation versus 3:1 chest compression:ventilation ratio during neonatal cardiopulmonary resuscitation: a randomised feasibility trial. Arch Dis Child Fetal Neonatal Ed. 2018;103:F455-F460. doi: 10.1136/archdischild-2017-313037
13. Schmölzer GM, O'Reilly M, Labossiere J, Lee TF, Cowan S, Qin S, Bigam DL, Cheung PY. Cardiopulmonary resuscitation with chest compressions during sustained inflations: a new technique of neonatal resuscitation that improves recovery and survival in a neonatal porcine model. Circulation.2013;128:2495-2503. doi: 10.1161/circulationaha.113.002289

血管路の確保

COR	LOE	推奨事項
1	C-EO	1. 出生時に血管路の確保が必要な新生児については，アクセスルートとして臍静脈が推奨される[1]。
2b	C-EO	2. 静脈路を確保できない場合は，骨髄路の使用を妥当としてよい[1]。

「概要」
新生児が PPV および胸骨圧迫に反応しない場合は，アドレナリンおよび／または血漿増量剤投与のための血管路確保が必要となる。分娩室環境では，血管路確保の主要な方法は臍静脈カテーテル挿入である。分娩室以外，または静脈路の確保が不可能な場合は，代替として骨髄路の使用を妥当としてよいが，現地での器具の入手可能性や，救助者のトレーニングおよび経験に応じて判断する。

「推奨事項の裏付けとなる解説」
1. 臍静脈カテーテル挿入は，分娩室環境では数十年にわたり標準的な血管路確保の方法として採用されている[2]。臍静脈カテーテル挿入を他の血管路に優先することを支持するために，ヒトの新生児を対象として研究が行われたことはない[1]。
2. 骨髄針の挿入に伴う局所合併症が示唆される症例は，6 例報告されている[3-8]。
3. 分娩室以外の環境で臍静脈カテーテル挿入が不可能な場合は，骨髄路を使用して血管路を確保してもよい。

参考資料
1. Wyckoff MH, Wyllie J, Aziz K, de Almeida MF, Fabres J, Fawke J, Guinsburg R, Hosono S, Isayama T, Kapadia VS, et al; on behalf of the Neonatal Life Support Collaborators.Neonatal life support: 2020 International Consensus on Cardiopulmonary Resuscitation and Emergency Cardiovascular Care Science With Treatment Recommendations.Circulation.2020;142 (suppl 1):S185-S221. doi: 10.1161/CIR.0000000000000895
2. Niermeyer S, Kattwinkel J, Van Reempts P, Nadkarni V, Phillips B, Zideman D, Azzopardi D, Berg R, Boyle D, Boyle R, Burchfield D, Carlo W, Chameides L, Denson S, Fallat M, Gerardi M, Gunn A, Hazinski MF, Keenan W, Knaebel S, Milner A, Perlman J, Saugstad OD, Schleien C, Solimano A, Speer M, Toce S, Wiswell T, Zaritsky A. International Guidelines for Neonatal Resuscitation: An excerpt from the Guidelines 2000 for Cardiopulmonary Resuscitation and Emergency Cardiovascular Care: International Consensus on Science. Contributors and Reviewers for the Neonatal Resuscitation Guidelines. Pediatrics.2000;106:E29. doi: 10.1542/peds.106.3.e29
3. Vidal R, Kissoon N, Gayle M. Compartment syndrome following intraosseous infusion. Pediatrics.1993;91:1201-1202.
4. Katz DS, Wojtowycz AR. Tibial fracture: a complication of intraosseous infusion. Am J Emerg Med.1994;12:258-259. doi: 10.1016/0735-6757 (94)90261-5
5. Ellemunter H, Simma B, Trawöger R, Maurer H. Intraosseous lines in preterm and full term neonates. Arch Dis Child Fetal Neonatal Ed. 1999;80:F74-F75. doi: 10.1136/fn.80.1.f74
6. Carreras-González E, Brió-Sanagustín S, Guimerá I, Crespo C. Complication of the intraosseous route in a newborn infant [in Spanish]. Med Intensiva. 2012;36:233-234. doi: 10.1016/j.medin.2011.05.004
7. Oesterlie GE, Petersen KK, Knudsen L, Henriksen TB. Crural amputation of a newborn as a consequence of intraosseous needle insertion and calcium infusion. Pediatr Emerg Care.2014;30:413-414. doi: 10.1097/PEC.0000000000000150
8. Suominen PK, Nurmi E, Lauerma K. Intraosseous access in neonates and infants: risk of severe complications – a case report. Acta Anaesthesiol Scand.2015;59:1389-1393. doi: 10.1111/aas.12602

新生児の蘇生における投薬（アドレナリン）

COR	LOE	推奨事項
2b	C-LD	1. 人工呼吸および胸骨圧迫を最適化しても心拍数が 60 回/分以上まで上昇しない場合は，アドレナリンの血管内* 投与（0.01～0.03 mg/kg）を妥当としてよい[1-3]。
2b	C-LD	2. 血管路を確保している間は，高用量のアドレナリン（0.05～0.1 mg/kg）の気管内投与を妥当としてよい[1-3]。
2b	C-LD	3. 血管路の確保前にアドレナリンを気管内投与し，反応が不十分な場合は，間隔にかかわらず，血管路を確保でき次第，血管内* の投与を妥当としてよい[1,2]。
2b	C-LD	4. 心拍数が 60 回/分未満の状態が続く場合は，3～5 分ごとに，追加のアドレナリン投与（血管内* 投与が望ましい）を妥当としてよい[2,3]。

*この状況での「血管内」とは，「静脈内」または「骨髄内」を意味する。アドレナリンの動脈内投与は推奨されない。

「概要」

新生児の心拍数が低いのは，一般的に胎内での非常に低い酸素濃度，または出生後の不十分な肺拡張が原因であるため，蘇生中に投薬が必要になることはまれである。低心拍数の改善で最も重要な手順は，換気の確立である。ただし，100 %酸素の投与による換気（気管チューブの使用が望ましい）と胸骨圧迫を行っても心拍数が 60 回/分未満の状態が続く場合は，アドレナリン投与の適応となる。

低位臍帯静脈カテーテルを通じたアドレナリンの投与が，最も迅速かつ信頼性の高い薬剤送達を実現する。静脈内投与によるアドレナリンの用量は 0.01～0.03 mg/kg で，生理食塩液で後押し投与する[4]。臍静脈路を確保できていない場合は，0.05～0.1 mg/kg の用量でアドレナリンを気管内投与できる。心拍数が 60 回/分未満の状態が続く場合は，3～5 分の間隔でアドレナリンを投与するが，アドレナリンを気管内投与しても十分な反応を得られない場合は，臍静脈路を確保でき次第，静脈内投与できる。

「推奨事項の裏付けとなる解説」

1. ヒトの新生児を対象とした非常に限定的な観察研究によるエビデンスでは，気管内または静脈内のアドレナリン投与のどちらのほうが有効性に優れているのかは示されていないが，ほとんどの新生児は，ROSC の前に少なくとも 1 回の静注内投与を受けていた[1,2]。満期産の子羊を使用した心停止の周産期モデル（呼吸原性の心肺停止を伴って移行期を迎える）では，中心静脈路からアドレナリンを投与した場合のほうが，気管内にアドレナリンを投与した場合よりも，ROSC までの時間が短縮されること，および ROSC 率が高くなることにつながると認められた[3]。アドレナリンの静脈内投与に続けて生理食塩液で後押し投与することで，有効に薬剤を投与できる。[4]

2. 1 件の非常に限定的な観察研究（ヒト）では，気管内の用量として 0.03 mg/kg では不十分であることが示されている[1]。動物を使った心停止の周産期モデルでは，中心静脈路または低位臍帯静脈カテーテルから投与した場合，気管内投与と比較して，用量を低くしたにもかかわらず（静脈内投与は 0.03 mg/kg，気管内投与は 0.1 mg/kg），アドレナリンの最高血漿濃度は高くなり，その到達速度も速くなっている[3]。

3. 1 件の非常に限定的な観察研究では，気管内投与を受けたほとんどの新生児は，それ以降に静脈内投与を受けた後で ROSC に至っている。[2] 臍静脈路を確保でき次第，アドレナリンをただちに静脈内投与することで迅速な反応を得ることができるが，気管内投与を繰り返し行ったり，静脈内投与の用量を高くしたりすると，有害となり得る血漿濃度に達し，高血圧や頻拍につながる可能性がある[5-8]。

4. 1 件の非常に限定的な観察研究では，多くの新生児が，ROSC に至る前に複数回のアドレナリン投与を受けていた[2]。心停止の周産期モデルでは，静脈内投与から 1 分後のアドレナリンの最高血漿濃度は記録されているが，気管内投与については，投与後 5 分までの記録が行われていない[3]。

参考資料

1. Barber CA, Wyckoff MH.Use and efficacy of endotracheal versus intravenous epinephrine during neonatal cardiopulmonary resuscitation in the delivery room.Pediatrics.2006;118:1028-1034. doi: 10.1542/peds.2006-0416
2. Halling C, Sparks JE, Christie L, Wyckoff MH. Efficacy of Intravenous and Endotracheal Epinephrine during Neonatal Cardiopulmonary Resuscitation in the Delivery Room. J Pediatr.2017;185:232-236. doi: 10.1016/j.jpeds.2017.02.024
3. Vali P, Chandrasekharan P, Rawat M, Gugino S, Koenigsknecht C, Helman J, Jusko WJ, Mathew B, Berkelhamer S, Nair J, et al. Evaluation of timing and route of epinephrine in a neonatal model of asphyxial arrest. J Am Heart Assoc. 2017;6:e004402. doi: 10.1161/JAHA.116.004402
4. Vali P, Sankaran D, Rawat M, Berkelhamer S, Lakshminrusimha S. Epinephrine in neonatal resuscitation. Children (Basel). 2019;6:E51. doi: 10.3390/children6040051
5. Perondi MB, Reis AG, Paiva EF, Nadkarni VM, Berg RA. A comparison of high-dose and standard-dose epinephrine in children with cardiac arrest. N Engl J Med.2004;350:1722-1730. doi: 10.1056/NEJMoa032440
6. Vandycke C, Martens P. High dose versus standard dose epinephrine in cardiac arrest – a meta-analysis. Resuscitation.2000;45:161-166. doi: 10.1016/s0300-9572(00)00188-x
7. Berg RA, Otto CW, Kern KB, Hilwig RW, Sanders AB, Henry CP, Ewy GA. A randomized, blinded trial of high-dose epinephrine versus standard-dose epinephrine in a swine model of pediatric asphyxial cardiac arrest. Crit Care Med.1996;24:1695-1700. doi: 10.1097/00003246-199610000-00016
8. Burchfield DJ, Preziosi MP, Lucas VW, Fan J. Effects of graded doses of epinephrine during asphxia-induced bradycardia in newborn lambs. Resuscitation.1993;25:235-244. doi: 10.1016/0300-9572(93)90120-f

血液量補充

輸液蘇生法に関する推奨事項

COR	LOE	推奨事項
2b	C-EO	1. 病歴および身体診察から循環血液量減少が疑われ，換気や胸骨圧迫，アドレナリン投与を行っても徐脈（心拍数が 60 回/分未満）の状態が続く新生児については，血漿増量剤の投与を妥当としてよい[1-3]。
2b	C-EO	2. 10～20 mL/kg の生理食塩液（0.9 %塩化ナトリウム）または血液を用いて循環血液量を増やすことを妥当としてよい[4,5]。

「概要」

失血性ショックを呈している新生児は，換気，胸骨圧迫，アドレナリン投与による初期の蘇生措置に対する反応が低い場合がある。病歴および身体診察の所見から示唆される失血の症状としては，青白い見た目，弱い脈拍，持続的な徐脈（心拍数が 60 回/分未満）などが挙げられる。血液は胎盤から母体の血液循環へと失われる場合や，臍帯または新生児から失われる場合がある。

失血が疑われ，蘇生措置（換気，胸骨圧迫，アドレナリン投与）に対する反応が低い新生児については，血漿増量剤の即時投与を妥当としてよい。晶質液としては，生理食塩液（0.9％塩化ナトリウム）が最適な選択肢である。失血量が大きい場合は，未交差O型，Rh-の血液（ただちに入手できる場合は，交差適合試験済みの血液）が推奨される[4,5]。初期輸液量としては，5～10分で10 mL/kgを妥当としてよい。また，反応が不十分な場合は，これを繰り返してもよい。推奨される血液路は静脈路であるが，代替として骨髄路を使用できる。

「推奨事項の裏付けとなる解説」

1. 分娩時の輸液蘇生法の使用を支持する無作為化試験のエビデンスは存在しない。ある大規模な後ろ向き調査によると，分娩室環境で輸液蘇生法を受けた新生児は0.04％であり，比較的まれなイベントであることが確認されている[1]。このような，分娩室環境で輸液蘇生法を受けた新生児は，新生児集中治療室への入室時の血圧が，入室しなかった新生児と比較して低く，失血以外の因子が重要である可能性を示唆している。[1]
2. 新生児の蘇生において，どのような種類の血漿増量剤（晶質液または血液）の有益性が高いのかを裏付ける臨床的エビデンスは不十分である。出生直後の低血圧新生児の研究[6-8]，および動物（子豚）の研究からの推定により，アルブミンよりも晶質液の増量剤を使用することが支持され[5]，晶質液よりも血液を使用することが支持される[4]。あるレビューでは，血漿増量剤の使用に関する推奨事項について議論された[2]。

参考資料

1. Wyckoff MH, Perlman JM, Laptook AR. Use of volume expansion during delivery room resuscitation in near-term and term infants. Pediatrics.2005;115:950–955. doi: 10.1542/peds.2004-0913
2. Finn D, Roehr CC, Ryan CA, Dempsey EM. Optimising intravenous volume resuscitation of the newborn in the delivery room: practical considerations and gaps in knowledge. Neonatology.2017;112:163–171. doi: 10.1159/000475456
3. Conway-Orgel M. Management of hypotension in the very low-birth-weight infant during the golden hour. Adv Neonatal Care. 2010;10:241-5; quiz 246. doi: 10.1097/ANC.0b013e3181f0891c
4. Mendler MR, Schwarz S, Hechenrieder L, Kurth S, Weber B, Hofler S, Kalbitz M, Mayer B, Hummler HD. Successful resuscitation in a model of asphyxia and hemorrhage to test different volume resuscitation strategies. a study in newborn piglets after transition. Front Pediatr. 2018;6:192. doi: 10.3389/fped.2018.00192
5. Wyckoff M, Garcia D, Margraf L, Perlman J, Laptook A. Randomized trial of volume infusion during resuscitation of asphyxiated neonatal piglets. Pediatr Res.2007;61:415-420. doi: 10.1203/pdr.0b013e3180332c45
6. Niermeyer S. Volume resuscitation: crystalloid versus colloid. Clin Perinatol. 2006;33:133-140. doi: 10.1016/j.clp.2005.12.002
7. Shalish W, Olivier F, Aly H, Sant'Anna G. Uses and misuses of albumin during resuscitation and in the neonatal intensive care unit. Semin Fetal Neonatal Med. 2017;22:328-335. doi: 10.1016/j.siny.2017.07.009
8. Keir AK, Karam O, Hodyl N, Stark MJ, Liley HG, Shah PS, Stanworth SJ; NeoBolus Study Group. International, multicentre, observational study of fluid bolus therapy in neonates. J Paediatr Child Health. 2019;55:632–639. doi: 10.1111/jpc.14260

蘇生後管理

COR	LOE	推奨事項
1	A	1. 推定在胎期間36週以上で出生し，中等症～重症の低酸素性虚血性脳症（HIE）に至る可能性がある新生児には，明確に定義されたプロトコールに従って低体温療法を実施する必要がある[1]。
1	C-EO	2. 長時間にわたるPPV，または高度な蘇生処置（挿管，胸骨圧迫，アドレナリン投与）を受けている新生児は，厳密なモニタリングを提供できる環境を維持するか，そのような環境に転送すべきである[2-7]。
1	C-LD	3. 高度な蘇生処置後は，実施可能な状況になり次第，適応の治療とともに血糖値をモニタリングする必要がある[8-14]。
2b	C-LD	4. 蘇生処置後に意図せず低体温となった新生児（体温が36℃未満）については，急速に（0.5℃/時）または徐々に（0.5℃/時未満）復温することを妥当としてよい[15-19]。

「概要」

長時間にわたるPPV，または高度な蘇生処置（挿管，胸骨圧迫，（±）-アドレナリン投与）を受けている新生児は，さらに悪化するリスクを伴うため，新生児集中治療室または監視下にあるトリアージエリアで安定化したら，厳密にモニタリングする必要がある。

在胎36週以上と推定され，高度な蘇生処置を受けた新生児は，低体温療法の適応となるか判断するために，HIEの兆候がないか検査する必要がある。低体温療法は，公表されている臨床試験で使用されるものと同様に定義されたプロトコール下で，複数の専門分野にわたるケアと長期的な追跡調査が可能な施設において実施しなければならない。在胎36週未満でHIEを発症している新生児に対する低体温療法の影響は不明であり，現在進行中の研究試験の対象となっている。

高度な蘇生処置を受けた新生児は低血糖になることが多く，転帰不良に関連付けられる[8]。このような新生児は，低血糖を起こしていないかモニタリングを行い，適切に治療する必要がある。

安定化後ただちに，意図しない低体温（体温が36℃未満）になっている新生児は，低体温に関連する合併症（死亡率の上昇，脳損傷，低血糖，呼吸窮迫など）を回避するため，復温する必要がある。加温は急速に（0.5℃/時）行っても，徐々に（0.5℃/時未満）行っても，転帰に有意な差が見られないことがエビデンスによって示されている[15-19]。過熱状態を避けるよう注意を払う必要がある。

「推奨事項の裏付けとなる解説」

1. 中等度〜重度の脳症を持ち，分娩時に仮死状態であったエビデンスのある 1344 人の満期産児および後期早産児を対象とした 8 件の RCT のメタアナリシスでは，低体温療法によって，18 ヵ月までの死亡率または神経発達学的障害を合わせた転帰が有意に減少している（オッズ比：0.75，95％ CI：0.68〜0.83）[1]。
2. 高度な蘇生処置を必要とした新生児は，中等度〜重度の HIE[2-4] など，疾病を発症するリスクが高い[5-7]。
3. 血糖値に異常がある（低血糖および高血糖）新生児は，低酸素性虚血性発作の後に脳損傷や有害な転帰をもたらすリスクが高い[8-14]。
4. 分娩室での安定化後に低体温となった新生児を対象とした 2 件の小規模な RCT[16,19] および 4 件の観察研究[15,17,18,20] では，急速に復温した場合と徐々に復温した場合の死亡率，[15,17] けいれん／ひきつけ[19]，脳室内出血または肺出血，[15,17,19,20] 低血糖，[16,17,19] 無呼吸の転帰について，有意な差は認められていない[16,17,19]。ある観察研究では，徐々に復温した新生児のほうが呼吸窮迫の発症率が低いことが認められている一方で[18]，別の研究では，急速に復温した新生児のほうが呼吸窮迫症候群の発症率が低くなるとされている[17]。

参考資料

1. Jacobs SE, Berg M, Hunt R, Tarnow-Mordi WO, Inder TE, Davis PG. Cooling for newborns with hypoxic ischaemic encephalopathy. Cochrane Database Syst Rev. 2013;CD003311. doi: 10.1002/14651858.CD003311.pub3
2. Laptook AR, Shankaran S, Ambalavanan N, Carlo WA, McDonald SA, Higgins RD, Das A; Hypothermia Subcommittee of the NICHD Neonatal Research Network. Outcome of term infants using apgar scores at 10 minutes following hypoxic-ischemic encephalopathy. Pediatrics. 2009;124:1619-1626. doi: 10.1542/peds.2009-0934
3. Ayrapetyan M, Talekar K, Schwabenbauer K, Carola D, Solarin K, McElwee D, Adeniyi-Jones S, Greenspan J, Aghai ZH. Apgar scores at 10 minutes and outcomes in term and late preterm neonates with hypoxic-ischemic encephalopathy in the cooling era. Am J Perinatol. 2019;36:545-554. doi: 10.1055/s-0038-1670637
4. Kasdorf E, Laptook A, Azzopardi D, Jacobs S, Perlman JM. Improving infant outcome with a 10 min Apgar of 0. Arch Dis Child Fetal Neonatal Ed. 2015;100:F102-F105. doi: 10.1136/archdischild-2014-306687
5. Barber CA, Wyckoff MH. Use and efficacy of endotracheal versus intravenous epinephrine during neonatal cardiopulmonary resuscitation in the delivery room. Pediatrics. 2006;118:1028-1034. doi: 10.1542/peds.2006-0416
6. Harrington DJ, Redman CW, Moulden M, Greenwood CE. The long-term outcome in surviving infants with Apgar zero at 10 minutes: a systematic review of the literature and hospital-based cohort. Am J Obstet Gynecol. 2007;196:463.e1-463.e5. doi: 10.1016/j.ajog.2006.10.877
7. Wyckoff MH, Salhab WA, Heyne RJ, Kendrick DE, Stoll BJ, Laptook AR; National Institute of Child Health and Human Development Neonatal Research Network. Outcome of extremely low birth weight infants who received delivery room cardiopulmonary resuscitation. J Pediatr. 2012;160:239-244.e2. doi: 10.1016/j.jpeds.2011.07.041
8. Salhab WA, Wyckoff MH, Laptook AR, Perlman JM. Initial hypoglycemia and neonatal brain injury in term infants with severe fetal acidemia. Pediatrics. 2004;114:361-366. doi: 10.1542/peds.114.2.361
9. Castrodale V, Rinehart S. The golden hour: improving the stabilization of the very low birth-weight infant. Adv Neonatal Care. 2014;14:9-14; quiz 15. doi: 10.1097/ANC.0b013e31828b0289
10. Nadeem M, Murray DM, Boylan GB, Dempsey EM, Ryan CA. Early blood glucose profile and neurodevelopmental outcome at two years in neonatal hypoxic-ischaemic encephalopathy. BMC Pediatr. 2011;11:10. doi: 10.1186/1471-2431-11-10
11. McKinlay CJ, Alsweiler JM, Ansell JM, Anstice NS, Chase JG, Gamble GD, Harris DL, Jacobs RJ, Jiang Y, Paudel N, Signal M, Thompson B, Wouldes TA, Yu TY, Harding JE; CHYLD Study Group. Neonatal Glycemia and Neurodevelopmental Outcomes at 2 Years. N Engl J Med.2015;373:1507-1518. doi: 10.1056/NEJMoa1504909
12. Tan JKG, Minutillo C, McMichael J, Rao S. Impact of hypoglycaemia on neurodevelopmental outcomes in hypoxic ischaemic encephalopathy: a retrospective cohort study. BMJ Paediatr Open. 2017;1:e000175. doi: 10.1136/bmjpo-2017-000175
13. Shah BR, Sharifi F. Perinatal outcomes for untreated women with gestational diabetes by IADPSG criteria: a population-based study. BJOG. 2020;127:116-122. doi: 10.1111/1471-0528.15964
14. Pinchefsky EF, Hahn CD, Kamino D, Chau V, Brant R, Moore AM, Tam EWY. Hyperglycemia and Glucose Variability Are Associated with Worse Brain Function and Seizures in Neonatal Encephalopathy: A Prospective Cohort Study. J Pediatr.2019;209:23-32. doi: 10.1016/j.jpeds.2019.02.027
15. Feldman A, De Benedictis B, Alpan G, La Gamma EF, Kase J. Morbidity and mortality associated with rewarming hypothermic very low birth weight infants. J Neonatal Perinatal Med. 2016;9:295-302. doi: 10.3233/NPM-16915143
16. Motil KJ, Blackburn MG, Pleasure JR. The effects of four different radiant warmer temperature set-points used for rewarming neonates. J Pediatr.1974;85:546-550. doi: 10.1016/s0022-3476(74)80467-1
17. Rech Morassutti F, Cavallin F, Zaramella P, Bortolus R, Parotto M, Trevisanuto D. Association of Rewarming Rate on Neonatal Outcomes in Extremely Low Birth Weight Infants with Hypothermia. J Pediatr.2015;167:557-61.e1. doi: 10.1016/j.jpeds.2015.06.008
18. Sofer S, Yagupsky P, Hershkowits J, Bearman JE. Improved outcome of hypothermic infants. Pediatr Emerg Care.1986;2:211-214. doi: 10.1097/00006565-198612000-00001
19. Tafari N, Gentz J. Aspects of rewarming newborn infants with severe accidental hypothermia. Acta Paediatr Scand. 1974;63:595-600. doi: 10.1111/j.1651-2227.1974.tb04853.x
20. Racine J, Jarjoui E. Severe hypothermia in infants. Helv Paediatr Acta. 1982;37:317-322.

蘇生の保留と中止

蘇生の保留と中止に関する推奨事項

COR	LOE	推奨事項
1	C-EO	1. 蘇生を開始しないことと，蘇生途中または蘇生後に生命維持治療を中止することは倫理上同等に検討する必要がある[1,2]。
1	C-LD	2. 蘇生中の新生児の心拍数を検知できず，蘇生の全手順を実施した場合は，蘇生努力の中止について医療チームおよび家族と協議する。このような治療目標の変更を行うのに妥当な時間は，出生後約 20 分である[3]。
2a	C-EO	3. 生育力が下限の状態，または早期死亡あるいは重篤な疾病につながる可能性が高い状態で出生した場合は，専門家との相談および家族も参加した意思決定のうえで，新生児の蘇生処置を開始しないこと，または制限を設けることは妥当である[1,2,4,5]。

「概要」

新生児および生命倫理学の専門家委員会は，特定の臨床状態においては，新生児および家族への支持療法の実施を継続することを条件として，生命維持努力を開始しない，または継続しないことを妥当とすることに同意している[1,2,4]。

心拍数が依然として検知されず，蘇生手順をすべて完了した場合は，治療目標の変更を妥当としてよい。症例集積研究では，少数ではあるが，心拍数を検知できなくなってから 20 分経過した後に無障害で生存した患者も認められている。蘇生努力の継続または中止は個別に判断し，出生後約 20 分の時点で検討する必要がある。考慮すべきこととして，その蘇生が最適と考えられるか，低体温療法などの高度な新生児治療の利用可能性，分娩前の特異的な環境，および家族の希望が挙げられる[3,6]。

一部の新生児は病状が悪い，または未成熟なために，新生児の蘇生処置や集中治療を施しても生存の可能性が低い場合がある。また，病状が重篤な場合は，疾病および治療の負担が，生存または健康転帰の可能性を大幅に上回る。このような状態を分娩時または分娩前に特定できる場合，蘇生努力を開始しないことは妥当である。このような状況では，専門家との相談や家族も参加した意思決定，さらに適応となる場合は緩和ケアの計画が有益である[1,2,4-6]。

「推奨事項の裏付けとなる解説」

1. 該当する状況であることが確認された場合は，蘇生処置を開始しない，または蘇生処置を中止することを妥当とする状況が存在することは，米国内の医師会の専門家による見解である[1,2,4,5]。
2. 低体温療法を実施できる環境における無作為化比較試験および観察研究（エビデンスの確実性はきわめて低い）では，蘇生処置を継続しても，10 分以上経過してから ROSC に至った新生児が中等症〜重症の障害なく生存する確率にはばらつきがあるとしている。このような研究の中で，障害を残さない生存率が非常に低くなる生後 20 分を超えて蘇生処置を行った場合の転帰を評価しているものはない。これらの研究は不均一が大きすぎるため，メタアナリシスに適していない[3]。
3. 蘇生処置を開始しない，または中止することを検討する条件としては，極端な早産や特定の重篤な先天性異常などが挙げられる。米国全国ガイドライン（National Guideline）では，社会的な要因のほか，母体や胎児／新生児の要因に基づき，家族への告知を行ったうえで個別に判断することを推奨している[1,2,4]。システマティックレビューでは，在胎 22〜24 週の生存性については，各国のガイドラインで説明にばらつきがあることを示している[7]。

参考資料

1. American Academy of Pediatrics Committee on Fetus and Newborn, Bell EF. Noninitiation or withdrawal of intensive care for high-risk newborns. Pediatrics. 2007;119:401-403. doi: 10.1542/peds.2006-3180
2. Cummings J; and the Committee on Fetus and Newborn. Antenatal Counseling Regarding Resuscitation and Intensive Care Before 25 Weeks of Gestation. Pediatrics.2015;136:588-595. doi: 10.1542/peds.2015-2336
3. Wyckoff MH, Wyllie J, Aziz K, de Almeida MF, Fabres J, Fawke J, Guinsburg R, Hosono S, Isayama T, Kapadia VS, et al; on behalf of the Neonatal Life Support Collaborators. Neonatal life support: 2020 International Consensus on Cardiopulmonary Resuscitation and Emergency Cardiovascular Care Science With Treatment Recommendations.Circulation.2020;142(suppl 1):S185-S221. doi: 10.1161/CIR.0000000000000895
4. American College of Obstetricians and Gynecologists; Society for Maternal-Fetal M. Obstetric Care Consensus No. 6: periviable birth. Obstet Gynecol. 2017;130:e187-e199. doi: 10.1097/AOG.0000000000002352
5. Lemyre B, Moore G. Counselling and management for anticipated extremely preterm birth. Paediatr Child Health. 2017;22:334-341. doi: 10.1093/pch/pxx058
6. Wyckoff MH, Aziz K, Escobedo MB, Kapadia VS, Kattwinkel J, Perlman JM, Simon WM, Weiner GM, Zaichkin JG.Part 13: neonatal resuscitation: 2015 American Heart Association Guidelines Update for Cardiopulmonary Resuscitation and Emergency Cardiovascular Care.Circulation.2015;132(suppl 2):S543-S560. doi: 10.1161/CIR.0000000000000267
7. Guillén Ú, Weiss EM, Munson D, Maton P, Jefferies A, Norman M, Naulaers G, Mendes J, Justo da Silva L, Zoban P, Hansen TW, Hallman M, Delivoria-Papadopoulos M, Hosono S, Albersheim SG, Williams C, Boyle E, Lui K, Darlow B, Kirpalani H. Guidelines for the Management of Extremely Premature Deliveries: A Systematic Review. Pediatrics.2015;136:343-350. doi: 10.1542/peds.2015-0542

個人およびシステム

トレーニングの頻度

トレーニングの頻度に関する推奨事項		
COR	LOE	推奨事項
1	C-LD	1. 新生児蘇生の訓練を受けた参加者には，獲得した知識，スキル，および行動の維持をサポートできる頻度（少なくとも 2 年ごと）で，個別またはチームでのブースター訓練を実施するべきである[1-5]。

「概要」

新生児の蘇生を効果的に実施するには，必要な知識，スキル，行動について，個別のプロバイダーおよびチームでトレーニングを受ける必要がある。これまで，繰り返しのトレーニングは 2 年ごとに行われてきた[6-9]。しかし，成人，小児，および新生児の研究では，練習を行わなかった場合，CPR に関する知識とスキルは，トレーニング後 3〜12 カ月[10-12] 以内に低下することが示唆されている。短時間の練習を頻繁に実施することで（ブースター訓練），新生児の蘇生転帰が改善することが示されている[5]。知識とスキルを維持できる十分な頻度の個人およびチームのトレーニングを確実に実施できるように，教育プログラムおよび周産期施設において戦略を策定する必要がある。

「推奨事項の裏付けとなる解説」

1. 無作為化比較シミュレーション試験では，ブースター訓練を受けた医学生は，ブースター訓練を受けなかった医学生と比較して，新生児に対する挿管スキルの改善が 6 週間にわたり維持された。ブースター訓練を 4 週間にわたり週 1 回受けた場合と，4 日間連続で毎日受けた場合の比較では，新生児に対する挿管パフォーマンスに差は見られなかった[1]。

無作為化比較シミュレーション試験では，新生児蘇生プログラムコースの初回受講から 9 カ月後にブースター訓練を受けた

小児／家庭医は，16 カ月時点でのフォローアップ評価において，ブースター訓練を受けなかった集団よりも優れた施術スキルおよびチームワーク行動を示した[2]。

ある前向きコホート研究では，新生児の呼吸補助に関するトレーニングを受けた医師および看護師は，トレーニングの 1 カ月後までに蘇生スキルが急速に失われることが示されている。1 カ月に 1 回の練習セッションを受講した対象者は，より低い頻度で練習を行った対象者と比較して，客観的臨床能力試験の合格率が高かった[3]。

ある前向き観察研究では，新生児の呼吸補助に関する終日トレーニングコースの受講後に，新生児の呼吸補助に関する簡潔なシミュレーショントレーニングを週 1 回実施した場合，新生児の刺激頻度が高くなることと，バッグマスク換気の頻度が低くなること，および新生児の 24 時間死亡率が低くなることが示されている[4]。

参考資料

1. Ernst KD, Cline WL, Dannaway DC, Davis EM, Anderson MP, Atchley CB, Thompson BM.Weekly and consecutive day neonatal intubation training: comparable on a pediatrics clerkship.Acad Med.2014;89:505–510. doi: 10.1097/ACM.0000000000000150
2. Bender J, Kennally K, Shields R, Overly F. Does simulation booster impact retention of resuscitation procedural skills and teamwork? J Perinatol.2014;34:664–668. doi: 10.1038/jp.2014.72
3. Tabangin ME, Josyula S, Taylor KK, Vasquez JC, Kamath-Rayne BD.Resuscitation skills after Helping Babies Breathe training: a comparison of varying practice frequency and impact on retention of skills in different types of providers.Int Health.2018;10:163–171. doi: 10.1093/inthealth/ihy017
4. Mduma E, Ersdal H, Svensen E, Kidanto H, Auestad B, Perlman J. Frequent brief on-site simulation training and reduction in 24-h neonatal mortality-an educational intervention study.Resuscitation.2015;93:1–7. doi: 10.1016/j.resuscitation.2015.04.019
5. Reisman J, Arlington L, Jensen L, Louis H, Suarez-Rebling D, Nelson BD. Newborn resuscitation training in resource-limited settings: a systematic literature review. Pediatrics. 2016;138:e20154490. doi: 10.1542/peds.2015-4490
6. American Academy of Pediatrics and American Heart Association. Textbook of Neonatal Resuscitation (NRP) 7th ed. Elk Grove Village, IL: American Academy of Pediatrics; 2016.
7. American Heart Association. Basic Life Support Provider Manual. Dallas, TX: American Heart Association; 2016.
8. American Heart Association. Pediatric Advanced Life Support Provider Manual. Dallas, TX: American Heart Association; 2016.
9. American Heart Association. Advanced Cardiovascular Life Support Provider Manual. Dallas, TX: American Heart Association; 2016.
10. Soar J, Mancini ME, Bhanji F, Billi JE, Dennett J, Finn J, Ma MH, Perkins GD, Rodgers DL, Hazinski MF, et al; on behalf of the Education, Implementation, and Teams Chapter Collaborators. Part 12: education, implementation, and teams: 2010 International Consensus on Cardiopulmonary Resuscitation and Emergency Cardiovascular Care Science with Treatment Recommendations. Resuscitation. 2010;81 (suppl 1):e288–e330. doi: 10.1016/j.resuscitation.2010.08.030
11. Bang A, Patel A, Bellad R, Gisore P, Goudar SS, Esamai F, Liechty EA, Meleth S, Goco N, Niermeyer S, Keenan W, Kamath-Rayne BD, Little GA, Clarke SB, Flanagan VA, Bucher S, Jain M, Mujawar N, Jain V, Rukunga J, Mahantshetti N, Dhaded S, Bhandankar M, McClure EM, Carlo WA, Wright LL, Hibberd PL. Helping Babies Breathe (HBB) training: What happens to knowledge and skills over time? BMC Pregnancy Childbirth. 2016;16:364. doi: 10.1186/s12884-016-1141-3
12. Arlington L, Kairuki AK, Isangula KG, Meda RA, Thomas E, Temu A, Mponzi V, Bishanga D, Msemo G, Azayo M, et al. Implementation of "Helping Babies Breathe": a 3-year experience in Tanzania. Pediatrics.2017;139:e20162132. doi: 10.1542/peds.2016-2132

ブリーフィングおよびデブリーフィング

COR	LOE	推奨事項
トレーニングの頻度に関する推奨事項		
2b	C-LD	1. 新生児の蘇生プロバイダーについては，分娩前にブリーフィングを行い，新生児の蘇生後にデブリーフィングを行うことを妥当としてよい[1-3]。

「概要」

ブリーフィングとは，「失敗や有害な事象が発生するリスクを低減するために，これから起こるイベントについて議論し，それに携わる人員の準備を整えること」と定義されている[4]。デブリーフィングとは，「内省的学習を促進し，臨床パフォーマンスを向上させるために，イベント後に行動や思考の過程について議論すること」[5] または「進行役によって進められる，学習とパフォーマンスの向上に重点を置いた議論」と定義されている[6]。2010 年以降，新生児の蘇生トレーニングにおいては，ブリーフィングおよびデブリーフィングの実施が推奨されており[7]，新生児，小児，成人を対象としたシミュレーションベースの研究および臨床研究では，教育および臨床のさまざまな点で成果が向上することが示されている。長期的な転帰および臨床的に関するブリーフィングおよびデブリーフィングの効果は，まだ不明である。

「推奨事項の裏付けとなる解説」

ブリーフィングまたはデブリーフィングと蘇生チームのパフォーマンスについて調査した複数の臨床研究およびシミュレーション研究では，知識またはスキルの向上が示されている[8-12]。

1. 前向き介入臨床研究では，ビデオを使用した新生児蘇生のデブリーフィングの実施が，新生児蘇生アルゴリズムの初期手順への準備態勢と順守の向上，PPV の質の向上，チームの機能およびコミュニケーションの改善に関連付けられている[1]。

2　件の品質改善前／品質改善後イニシアチブでは，チームブリーフィング，デブリーフィング，分娩前チェックリストの使用が，分娩室でのチームのコミュニケーションと短期的な臨床転帰の改善（分娩室での挿管頻度の低下，新生児集中治療室への移送時に正常体温であった頻度の向上など）に関連付けられている。気管支肺異形成，壊死性腸炎，未熟児網膜症，脳室内出血，入院期間など，その他の院内臨床転帰については有意な影響は見られなかった[2,3]。

参考資料

1. Skåre C, Calisch TE, Saeter E, Rajka T, Boldingh AM, Nakstad B, Niles DE, Kramer-Johansen J, Olasveengen TM. Implementation and effectiveness of a video-based debriefing programme for neonatal resuscitation. Acta Anaesthesiol Scand.2018;62:394–403. doi: 10.1111/aas.13050

2. Sauer CW, Boutin MA, Fatayerji AN, Proudfoot JA, Fatayerji NI, Golembeski DJ. Delivery Room Quality Improvement Project Improved Compliance with Best Practices for a Community NICU. Sci Rep. 2016;6:37397. doi: 10.1038/srep37397
3. Katheria A, Rich W, Finer N. Development of a strategic process using checklists to facilitate team preparation and improve communication during neonatal resuscitation.Resuscitation.2013;84:1552–1557. doi: 10.1016/j.resuscitation.2013.06.012
4. Halamek LP, Cady RAH, Sterling MR. Using briefing, simulation and debriefing to improve human and system performance. Semin Perinatol. 2019;43:151178. doi: 10.1053/j.semperi.2019.08.007
5. Mullan PC, Kessler DO, Cheng A. Educational opportunities with postevent debriefing. JAMA. 2014;312:2333–2334. doi: 10.1001/jama.2014.15741
6. Sawyer T, Loren D, Halamek LP. Post-event debriefings during neonatal care: why are we not doing them, and how can we start? J Perinatol.2016;36:415–419. doi: 10.1038/jp.2016.42
7. Kattwinkel J, Perlman JM, Aziz K, Colby C, Fairchild K, Gallagher J, Hazinski MF, Halamek LP, Kumar P, Little G, et al.Part 15: neonatal resuscitation: 2010 American Heart Association Guidelines for Cardiopulmonary Resuscitation and Emergency Cardiovascular Care.Circulation.2010;122 (suppl 3):S909–S919. doi: 10.1161/CIRCULATIONAHA.110.971119
8. Savoldelli GL, Naik VN, Park J, Joo HS, Chow R, Hamstra SJ. Value of debriefing during simulated crisis management: oral versus video-assisted oral feedback. Anesthesiology.2006;105:279–285. doi: 10.1097/00000542-200608000-00010
9. Edelson DP, Litzinger B, Arora V, Walsh D, Kim S, Lauderdale DS, Vanden Hoek TL, Becker LB, Abella BS. Improving in-hospital cardiac arrest process and outcomes with performance debriefing.Arch Intern Med.2008;168:1063–1069. doi: 10.1001/archinte.168.10.1063
10. Morgan PJ, Tarshis J, LeBlanc V, Cleave-Hogg D, DeSousa S, Haley MF, Herold-McIlroy J, Law JA. Efficacy of high-fidelity simulation debriefing on the performance of practicing anaesthetists in simulated scenarios. Br J Anaesth. 2009;103:531–537. doi: 10.1093/bja/aep222
11. Dine CJ, Gersh RE, Leary M, Riegel BJ, Bellini LM, Abella BS. Improving cardiopulmonary resuscitation quality and resuscitation training by combining audiovisual feedback and debriefing. Crit Care Med. 2008;36:2817-2822. doi: 10.1097/CCM.0b013e318186fe37
12. Wolfe H, Zebuhr C, Topjian AA, Nishisaki A, Niles DE, Meaney PA, Boyle L, Giordano RT, Davis D, Priestley M, Apkon M, Berg RA, Nadkarni VM, Sutton RM. Interdisciplinary ICU cardiac arrest debriefing improves survival outcomes*. Crit Care Med.2014;42:1688–1695. doi: 10.1097/CCM.0000000000000327

今後の課題

新生児の蘇生科学は過去30年ほどで飛躍的に発展し，研究室，分娩室，およびその他の臨床環境で多数の研究者が功績を挙げている。こうした研究により，新生児蘇生アルゴリズムは大幅に改良されたが，早産児および満期産児の蘇生を最適化するためにまだ学ぶべき事があることも浮き彫りとなった。新生児に対する臨床研究への熱が高まる中，新たなエビデンスの出現に伴い，新生児蘇生アルゴリズムを構成する各要素は進化し続けている。

現在のガイドラインは，各手順に最も適した器具についてではなく，蘇生アルゴリズムで説明されている臨床活動に焦点を当てている。2021年以降のレビューでは，器具や支援ツールの選択を検証する予定であるが，これには換気（Tピース，自動膨張型バッグ，流量膨張型バッグ），換気インタフェース（フェイスマスク，ラリンゲアルマスク），吸引（バルブシリンジ，胎便吸引器），モニタリング（呼吸機能モニター，心拍数モニタリング，近赤外分光法），フィードバック，および文書化に必要とされる器具や支援ツール等が含まれる。

今回の改訂で多量な知識をレビューしたことで，エビデンスが脆弱または不確実であったり，あるいは欠落している多数の疑問と慣行が特定された。以下に述べる今後の課題には，さらなる研究が必要である。

蘇生の準備

- 新生児の蘇生に関する知識，技術領域および行動領域のスキルの定着を的確に支援するブースター訓練または再トレーニングの頻度と形式
- チームパフォーマンスに対するブリーフィングおよびデブリーフィングの効果

分娩中および分娩直後

- 活気のない新生児，先天性の心疾患または肺疾患を持つ新生児など，多様な集団に対する最適な臍帯管理戦略
- MSAFの状態で出生した活気のない新生児の最適な管理

早期蘇生

- PPVの実施に最も効果的な器具とインタフェース
- 新生児の蘇生中にECGをルーチン使用することの蘇生への影響
- 心拍数を迅速に測定するための新技術（電気器具，超音波装置，光学装置など）の実行可能性および有効性
- 蘇生中および蘇生後の最適な酸素管理

高度な蘇生

- 持続的肺拡張を伴う胸骨圧迫など，CPRを効果的に実施するための新手法
- アドレナリンまたはその他の血管作動薬を投与するための最適なタイミング，用量，投与間隔，投与経路（極端に活気のない新生児に対する早期使用も含む）
- 投与量の増加に対する適応，ならびに最適な用量，タイミング，投与量の種類
- 無脈性電気活動の管理

特定集団

- 蘇生中および蘇生後の早産児の管理
- 蘇生中および蘇生後の，心臓および肺の先天性異常の管理
- 新生児処置室における新生児期後の新生児の蘇生
- その他の状況での日齢28日までの新生児の蘇生

蘇生後管理

- 侵襲性の低い投与手技も含め、リスクのある新生児へのサーファクタント投与の最適な用量、投与経路、およびタイミング
- 軽度の HIE を持つ新生児、および在胎 36 週未満で出生した新生児に対する低体温療法の適応
- 低体温療法の補助的療法
- 最適な血糖管理
- 意図的でない低体温の新生児に対する最適な復温戦略

これらすべての課題に対し、医療従事者および新生児の家族によってクリティカルまたは重要とみなされる転帰についての情報が得られていることは重要である。

研究団体は、高度な確実性を有する転帰を実現するための教育研究の不足に対処する必要がある。内的妥当性は、明確に定義された主要転帰、適切なサンプルサイズ、関連性のある適時の介入と管理、および実施研究での時系列解析によって適切に対処できる可能性がある。外的妥当性は、学習者の成果だけに研究を限定するのではなく、関連する学習者またはプロバイダー集団について研究し、患者とシステムの重要な転帰に対する影響を測定することによって向上する可能性がある。

こうした課題を研究する研究者は、実用的研究のデザインや、新たな同意取得プロセスなど、臨床試験のデザインにおけるイノベーションを考慮する必要があるだろう。医療提供における生物医学的発展と改良により、死亡率と重篤な疾病率が低下しているため、従来的な個々の患者による無作為化試験を使用していくつかの臨床的な問題に対応する十分な力が損なわれている。もう一つの障壁は、分娩室での臨床試験に対する出産前の同意取得が困難であることである。活気のない新生児に見られる MSAF への最適な対処法など、いくつかの問題には、適応試験、比較有効性デザイン、およびクラスター無作為化を使用した試験が適する可能性がある。大規模集団を対象とした高品質の観察研究も、エビデンスに加えられる可能性がある。実施が可能であれば、綿密にデザインされた多施設無作為化臨床試験は依然として、最も質の高いエビデンスを得るために最適である。

最後に、蘇生プロセスに携わる主要な関係者、家族、およびチームにとっての価値および優先順位に対処することの重要性を強調したい。認識されているものか現実のものかにかかわらず、この領域の課題は研究活動、教育活動、および臨床活動のすべての段階で対処すべきである。

文献情報

アメリカ心臓協会は、本書を以下のとおりに引用するよう要請する。Aziz K, Lee HC, Escobedo MB, Hoover AV, Kamath-Rayne BD, Kapadia VS, Magid DJ, Niermeyer S, Schmölzer GM, Szyld E, Weiner GM, Wyckoff MH, Yamada NK, Zaichkin J. Part 5: neonatal resuscitation: 2020 American Heart Association Guidelines for Cardiopulmonary Resuscitation and Emergency Cardiovascular Care.循環. 2020;142 (suppl 2):S524-S550. doi: 10.1161/CIR.0000000000000902

この文献は『Pediatrics』で共同出版されたものである。

謝辞

私たちは Abhrajit Ganguly 医師に、原稿作成の準備を支援していただいたことに感謝する。

情報開示

付録 1　執筆グループの情報開示

執筆グループメンバー	所属	研究助成金	その他の研究支援	講演／謝礼金	鑑定人	株式所有	コンサルタント／顧問	その他
Khalid Aziz	University of Alberta Pediatrics	なし	なし	なし	なし	なし	なし	給与：アルバータ大学†
Henry C. Lee	Stanford University	NICHD（きわめて早い在胎期間で出生した新生児の集中治療を研究するための R01 グラントの PI）*	なし	なし	なし	なし	なし	なし
Marilyn B Escobedo	University of Oklahoma Medical School Pediatrics	なし	なし	なし	なし	なし	なし	なし
Amber V. Hoover	American Heart Association	なし	なし	なし	なし	なし	なし	なし
Beena D. Kamath-Rayne	American Academy of Pediatrics	なし	なし	なし	なし	なし	なし	なし
Vishal S. Kapadia	UT Southwestern Pediatrics	NIH，NICHD†	なし	なし	なし	なし	なし	なし

（続き）

付録 1（続き）

執筆グループメンバー	所属	研究助成金	その他の研究支援	講演／謝礼金	鑑定人	株式所有	コンサルタント／顧問	その他
David J. Magid	University of Colorado	NIH†，NHLBI†，CMS†，AHA†	なし	なし	なし	なし	なし	アメリカ心臓協会（上級科学編集者）†
Susan Niermeyer	University of Colorado Pediatrics	なし	なし	なし	なし	なし	なし	なし
Georg M. Schmölzer	University of Alberta Pediatrics	カナダ心肺蘇生基金（Heart and Stroke Foundation Canada）*：カナダ保険研究機構（Canadian Institute of Health Research）*，THRASHER基金（THRASHER Foundation）*：カナダ保険研究機構*	なし	なし	なし	RETAIN LABS Medical Inc オーナー*	なし	なし
Edgardo Szyld	University of Oklahoma	なし	なし	なし	なし	なし	なし	なし
Gary M. Weiner	University of Michigan Pediatrics-Neonatology	なし	なし	なし	なし	なし	なし	なし
Myra H. Wyckoff	UT Southwestern Pediatrics	なし	なし	なし	なし	なし	なし	なし
Nicole K. Yamada	Stanford University	AHRQ†	なし	なし	なし	なし	なし	なし
Jeanette Zaichkin	自営	なし	なし	なし	なし	なし	米国小児科学会新生児蘇生プログラム（American Academy of Pediatrics Neonatal Resuscitation Program）†	なし

この表は，執筆グループの全メンバーに回答および提出が求められる情報開示アンケート（Disclosure Questionnaire）の結果に基づき実在の利益相反または合理的に認定できる利益相反とみなされる可能性のある，執筆グループメンバーの関係を示している。メンバーと該当団体との関係が「顕著」であると考えられるのは，次のいずれかの状況が存在する場合である。(a) 当該メンバーが団体から受領する金額が過去いずれの 12 か月間に $10,000 以上であるか，メンバーの総収入の 5 ％以上である。(b) 団体の議決権株式の 5 ％以上，またはその団体の公正市場価値の $10,000 以上を保有している。この定義において「重大」に相当するレベルに満たない場合，その関係は「軽度」とみなされる。
*軽度
†重大

付録 2　レビューアーの情報開示

レビューアー	所属	研究助成金	その他の研究支援	講演／謝礼金	鑑定人	株式所有	コンサルタント／顧問	その他
Christoph Bührer	Charite University Medical Center	なし	なし	テュービンゲン大学*	なし	なし	なし	なし
Praveen Chandrasekharan	SUNY Buffalo	なし	なし	なし	なし	なし	なし	なし
Krithika Lingappan	Baylor College of Medicine	なし	なし	なし	なし	なし	なし	なし
Ju-Lee Oei	Royal Hospital for Women	なし	なし	なし	なし	なし	なし	なし
Birju A. Shah	The University of Oklahoma	なし	なし	なし	なし	なし	なし	なし

この表は，執筆グループの全メンバーに回答および提出が求められる情報開示アンケート（Disclosure Questionnaire）の結果に基づき実在の利益相反または合理的に認定できる利益相反とみなされる可能性のある，執筆グループメンバーの関係を示している。メンバーと該当団体との関係が「顕著」であると考えられるのは，次のいずれかの状況が存在する場合である。(a) 当該メンバーが団体から受領する金額が過去いずれの 12 か月間に $10,000 以上であるか，メンバーの総収入の 5 ％以上である。(b) 団体の議決権株式の 5 ％以上，またはその団体の公正市場価値の $10,000 以上を保有している。この定義において「重大」に相当するレベルに満たない場合，その関係は「軽度」とみなされる。
*軽度
†重大

Circulation

第6章：蘇生教育科学
AHA 心肺蘇生と救急心血管治療のためのガイドライン 2020

覚えておくべき 10 のポイント

1. 効果的な教育は，心停止からの生存転帰改善における不可欠な寄与因子である。
2. 蘇生トレーニング中に集中的な練習および完全習得学習モデルを使用することで，多くの重要タスクのスキルの習得および維持が改善する。
3. 蘇生コースでのブースター訓練の実施は，長期にわたる心肺蘇生（CPR）スキルの維持の改善および新生児の転帰の改善に関連している。
4. 蘇生トレーニングで反復学習アプローチを採用すると，集中学習と比較して臨床パフォーマンスと技術的スキルが向上する。
5. 蘇生トレーニング中に CPR フィードバック器具を使用すると，CPR スキルの習得と維持が改善する。
6. チームワークとリーダーシップのトレーニング，忠実度の高いマネキン，現場でのトレーニング，ゲーム方式の学習，バーチャルリアリティは，蘇生トレーニングを強化する機会となり，学習成果を向上させる可能性がある。
7. 自主学習による CPR トレーニングは，市民救助者にとって，インストラクターが指導する CPR トレーニングの合理的な代替手段となる。
8. 中高生には，質の高い CPR の実施方法を教えるべきである。これにより，地域に根差した，トレーニングを受けた市民救助者となる集団を育てることができる。
9. バイスタンダーによる CPR 率を上げるには，社会経済的地位の低い地域や特定の人種および民族のコミュニティなど，現在トレーニングの機会が不足している場所に合わせて CPR トレーニングを調整する必要がある。
10. 将来の蘇生教育研究には，臨床的に関連性のある成果を含めること，トレーニングにおける成果と患者転帰との関係を確立すること，介入の費用対効果を説明すること，教授システム学（インストラクショナル・デザイン）を特定のスキルに合わせて調整する方法を探ることが必要とされる。

Adam Cheng, MD, Chair
David J. Magid, MD, MPH
Marc Auerbach, MD, MSCE
Farhan Bhanji, MD, MEd
Blair L. Bigham, MD, MSc
Audrey L. Blewer, PhD, MPH
Katie N. Dainty, MSc, PhD
Emily Diederich, MD, MS
Yiqun Lin, MD, MHSc, PhD
Marion Leary, RN, MSN, MPH
Melissa Mahgoub, PhD
Mary E. Mancini, RN, PhD
Kenneth Navarro, PhD(c)
Aaron Donoghue, MD, MSCE, Vice Chair

前文

毎年，何百万人ものプロバイダーが，心停止からの患者転帰を改善することを目的として，一次救命処置および二次救命処置のトレーニングを受けている[1]。蘇生トレーニングプログラムは，エビデンスに基づく内容を取り入れながら，学習者が個人およびチームベースの臨床環境で救命スキルを実践する機会を提供している。蘇生トレーニングは広く行われているものの，学習者は望ましい学習成果を達成できない結果，実際の

キーワード：AHA 科学的ステートメント ■ 心肺蘇生 ■ 教育 ■ 蘇生 ■ トレーニング

© 2020 American Heart Association, Inc.

https://www.ahajournals.org/journal/circ

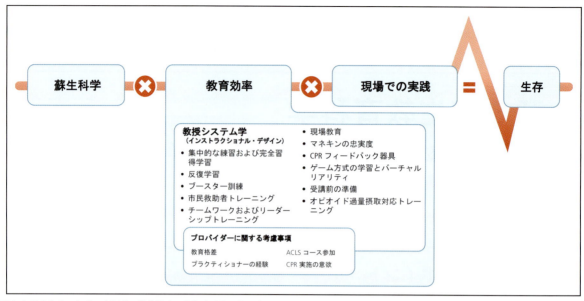

図. 蘇生における生存のための方程式：教育効率に寄与する主要な要素。
ACLS：二次救命処置（advanced cardiovascular life support），CPR：心肺蘇生（cardiopulmonary resuscitation）。

患者の臨床ケアにスキルをつなげられないことが頻繁に起こっている[1,2]。

国際蘇生連絡委員会の生存のための方程式（図）では，心停止からの生存転帰に影響を与える3つの重要な要素（現在の蘇生科学に基づくガイドライン，蘇生プロバイダーの効果的な教育，患者ケアにおける地域レベルでのガイドラインの実施）を重視している[3]。効果的な教育に重点を置くことで，プロバイダーのパフォーマンスが向上し，地域でのガイドラインの実施が促進され，心停止からの生存率が高まると考えられる。

これらのガイドラインには，市民救助者および医療従事者向けの蘇生トレーニングのデザインと提供に関する推奨事項が記載されている。教育の効果的な提供は，教育プログラムの教授システム学（インストラクショナル・デザイン）に大きく左右される。内容が学習者にどのように届くかは教授システム学（インストラクショナル・デザイン）によって決まるためである。この章では，エビデンスが示すさまざまな教授システム学（インストラクショナル・デザイン）上の要素を取り上げ，健康の社会的決定要因（社会経済的地位［SES］，人種など）と個々の要因（医療者の経験など）が臨床パフォーマンスと患者転帰にどのように影響するかについて説明する。

参考資料

1. Cheng A, Nadkarni VM, Mancini MB, Hunt EA, Sinz EH, Merchant RM, Donoghue A, Duff JP, Eppich W, Auerbach M, Bigham BL, Blewer AL, Chan PS, Bhanji F; American Heart Association Education Science Investigators; and on behalf of the American Heart Association Education Science and Programs Committee, Council on Cardiopulmonary, Critical Care, Perioperative and Resuscitation; Council on Cardiovascular and Stroke Nursing; and Council on Quality of Care and Outcomes Research.Resuscitation education science: educational strategies to improve outcomes from cardiac arrest: a scientific statement from the American Heart Association. Circulation.2018;138:e82-e122. doi: 10.1161/CIR.0000000000000583
2. Bhanji F, Donoghue AJ, Wolff MS, Flores GE, Halamek LP, Berman JM, Sinz EH, Cheng A. Part 14: education: 2015 American Heart Association Guidelines Update for Cardiopulmonary Resuscitation and Emergency Cardiovascular Care.Circulation.2015;132(suppl 2):S561-e573. doi: 10.1161/CIR.0000000000000268
3. Søreide E, Morrison L, Hillman K, Monsieurs K, Sunde K, Zideman D, Eisenberg M, Sterz F, Nadkarni VM, Soar J, Nolan JP; Utstein Formula for Survival Collaborators.The formula for survival in resuscitation.Resuscitation.2013;84:1487-1493. doi: 10.1016/j.resuscitation.2013.07.020

緒言
ガイドラインの範囲

心停止は依然として公衆衛生上の大きな問題であり，米国では年間60万件以上の心停止が発生している[1,2]。心停止患者の生存率は，蘇生科学の進歩にもかかわらず低いままである[3]。毎年，何百万人ものプロバイダーが，心停止患者に提供されるケアの質を向上させることを目的に，一次救命処置および二次救命処置のトレーニングを受けている[4]。蘇生トレーニングプログラムは，エビデンスに基づく内容を伝達し，学習者（蘇生トレーニングプログラムに登録している人）が知識を応用して重要なスキルを実践できる機会を提供するように設計されている。しかしこれらのプログラムは，望ましい学習結果（知識とスキルの習得など）を達成できないことが頻繁にあるため，パフォーマンスを実世界の臨床環境に反映できない場合がある[4,5]。例えば，一次救命処置（BLS）トレーニングの直後に習得できていた心肺蘇生（CPR）スキルは，3か月という短期間で衰退することが多く，その結果，BLSトレーニングを受けた多くの医療従事者（医師，看護師，呼吸療法士などの医療専門家）は，シミュレートした心停止や実際の心停止で，ガイドラインに準拠したCPRを実行するのに苦労する[6-14]。また，市民救助者のCPRトレーニングに関する最新の調査には，バイスタンダーが心停止を認識して，CPRを開始し，自動体外式除細動器を適切に使用できるようにする最適なトレーニング方法を説明するエビデンスが不足している[15-17]。心停止した患者をケアする際に，トレーニングで習得した知識とスキルを確実に使用できるようにするには，教授システ

ム学（インストラクショナル・デザイン）に重点を置くことが不可欠である[4]。

心停止からの生存率の向上は，蘇生ケアの質に大きく左右される。心停止の迅速な認識，CPR の患者転帰の改善を目的とした蘇生トレーニングの要素次第で，早期開始，早期除細動，質の高い胸骨圧迫など，生存を決定する重要な要因が変化する。教授システム学（インストラクショナル・デザイン）上の要素は，内容が学習者にどのように届くかを決定する，蘇生トレーニングプログラムの重要な要素，つまり「有効因子」である[18]。教授システム学（インストラクショナル・デザイン）上の要素が学習成果に与える影響を深く理解することで，指導者は心停止時の卓越した臨床パフォーマンスにつながるトレーニングプログラムを設計できるようになる。さらに，健康の社会的決定要因（SES，人種など）と個々の要因（医師の経験など）が蘇生教育の行く末にどのような影響を及ぼすかを理解することは，将来の方針戦略や実施戦略の策定に役立つ。この章では，エビデンスに裏付けられた蘇生教育の重要な要素について説明し，学習成果と心停止からの患者転帰を改善することを目的とした推奨事項を提示する。

次のセクションでは，エビデンスのレビューとガイドラインの作成のプロセスについて簡単に説明する。このプロセスの詳細については，「第 2 章：エビデンス評価とガイドライン作成」を参照のこと[19]。

蘇生教育科学執筆グループの組織

蘇生教育科学執筆グループは，蘇生教育，臨床医学（小児科，集中治療，救急医療），看護，病院前治療，医療サービス，および教育研究の経歴を持つ多様な専門家チームで構成された。執筆グループのメンバーは，蘇生法に関心があり，専門知識が認められているアメリカ心臓協会（AHA）のボランティアで，AHA 救急心血管治療（ECC）委員会によって選出される。AHA には，ガイドライン作成における偏見や不適切な影響のリスクを最小限に抑えるための厳格な利益相反方針と手順がある[20]。執筆グループのメンバーと査読者は，任命の前にすべての利害関係とその他の考えうる（知的を含む）利益相反を明らかにした。執筆グループのメンバーの公開情報は，付録 1 に記載する。

方法論とエビデンスレビュー

『AHA 心肺蘇生と救急心血管治療のためのガイドライン 2020』のこの章 は，国際蘇生連絡委員会および国際蘇生連絡委員会の関連するメンバー評議会と連携して実施された広範なエビデンス評価に基づいている。2020 年のプロセスでは，3 種類のエビデンスレビュー（体系的レビュー，スコーピングレビュー，エビデンスアップデート）が使用された。これらが個々に文献の説明となり，ガイドライン作成に役立った[21-25]。レビューは蘇生教育の科学文献に限定されていたが，レビューされた概念の多くは他の分野（医学教育，心理学など）を起源としている。

推奨事項のクラスとエビデンスレベル

AHA 蘇生教育科学執筆グループは，現在および関連するすべての『AHA 心肺蘇生と救急心血管治療のためのガイドライン』[5,26-37]および関連する『2020 年の心肺蘇生と救急心血管治療の科学についての国際コンセンサスと治療推奨（2020 International Consensus CPR and ECC Science With Treatment Recommendations）』[27] をレビューし，現在のガイドラインを再確認，改訂，または廃止する必要があるかどうか，および新しい推奨事項が必要かどうかを判断した。次に執筆グループは，推奨事項を起草，レビュー，および承認し（メンバー間の多数決により），それぞれにエビデンスレベル（LOE，つまり品質）と推奨事項のクラス（COR，すなわち強さ，詳細は，表 1，患者ケアにおける臨床上の戦略，介入，治療，または診断検査への COR と LOE の適用を参照）を割り当てた。

重要なことは，推奨判定，開発，評価の格付（GRADE）[38] の教育研究への適用は，臨床研究への適用よりも大きな課題が生じることである。教育成果（例えば，シミュレートされた患者環境で改善された「転帰」または総括的評価ツールで改善されたパフォーマンス）を伴う研究に関する特定の考慮事項は，GRADE 方法論では提供されない。執筆グループは，研究の質に関する通常のレビュー，教育科学の文脈において認識された基本的な構成の重要性，および（可能な場合）類似の臨床現象への所見の外挿（例えば，シミュレートされたものとは対照的な実際の患者転帰）の組み合わせに従って，これらの研究に LOE を頻繁に割り当てた。

ガイドラインの構成

2020 年版の各ガイドラインは知識チャンク（大きな塊）に分けられ，特定のトピックまたは管理の問題に関する個別の情報モジュールにグループ化されている[39]。各モジュール型の知識チャンクには，COR と LOE について AHA の標準的な用語を使用した推奨事項の表が含まれている。簡単な緒言または短い概要では，推奨事項を重要な背景情報や包括的な管理または治療の概念と関連付けて説明している。推奨事項の裏付けとなる解説では，推奨事項を裏付ける理論的根拠と主要な研究データを明確にしている。簡単に参照して確認できるように，ハイパーリンクされた参照資料も記載している。

文書のレビューと承認

3つのガイドラインは，匿名の査読のために，AHA が指名した対象分野の専門家に提出した。査読者からのフィードバックは，草稿形式のガイドラインと最終形式のガイドラインで提供された。ガイドラインは，AHA Science Advisory and Coordinating Committee および AHA Executive Committee がレビューし，公開を承認した。査読者の公開情報は，付録2に記載する。

略語

略語	意味／表現例
ACLS	二次救命処置（advanced cardiovascular life support）
AHA	American Heart Association
B-CPR	バイスタンダーによる心肺蘇生（bystander cardiopulmonary resuscitation）
BLS	一次救命処置（basic life support）
COR	推奨事項のクラス（Class of Recommendation）
CPR	心肺蘇生（cardiopulmonary resuscitation）
ECC	救急心血管治療
EMS	救急医療サービス（emergency medical services）
EO	専門家の見解（expert opinion）
LD	限定的なデータ（limited data）
LOE	エビデンスレベル（Level of Evidence）
NR	非無作為化（nonrandomized）
OHCA	院外心停止（out-of-hospital cardiac arrest）
PALS	小児の二次救命処置（pediatric advanced life support）
RCT	無作為化比較試験（randomized controlled trial）
ROSC	自己心拍再開（return of spontaneous circulation）
SES	社会経済的地位（socioeconomic status）
VR	バーチャルリアリティ（virtual reality）

参考資料

1. Andersen LW, Holmberg MJ, Berg KM, Donnino MW, Granfeldt A. In-hospital cardiac arrest: a review.JAMA.2019;321:1200-1210. doi: 10.1001/jama.2019.1696
2. Benjamin EJ, Muntner P, Alonso A, Bittencourt MS, Callaway CW, Carson AP, Chamberlain AM, Chang AR, Cheng S, Das SR, et al; on behalf of the American Heart Association Council on Epidemiology and Prevention Statistics Committee and Stroke Statistics Subcommittee.Heart disease and stroke statistics-2019 update: a report from the American Heart Association. Circulation.2019;139:e56-e528. doi: 10.1161/CIR.0000000000000659
3. Meaney PA, Bobrow BJ, Mancini ME, Christenson J, de Caen AR, Bhanji F, Abella BS, Kleinman ME, Edelson DP, Berg RA, et al; CPR Quality Summit Investigators, the American Heart Association Emergency Cardiovascular Care Committee, and the Council on Cardiopulmonary, Critical Care, Perioperative and Resuscitation.Cardiopulmonary resuscitation quality: [corrected] improving cardiac resuscitation outcomes both inside and outside the hospital: a consensus statement from the American Heart Association.Circulation.2013;128:417-435. doi: 10.1161/CIR.0b013e31829d8654
4. Cheng A, Nadkarni VM, Mancini MB, Hunt EA, Sinz EH, Merchant RM, Donoghue A, Duff JP, Eppich W, Auerbach M, et al; American Heart Association Education Science Investigators; on behalf of the American Heart Association Education Science and Programs Committee, Council on Cardiopulmonary, Critical Care, Perioperative and Resuscitation; Council on Cardiovascular and Stroke Nursing; and Council on Quality of Care and Outcomes Research.Resuscitation education science: educational strategies to improve outcomes from cardiac arrest: a scientific statement from the American Heart Association.Circulation.2018;138:e82-e122. doi: 10.1161/CIR.0000000000000583
5. Bhanji F, Donoghue AJ, Wolff MS, Flores GE, Halamek LP, Berman JM, Sinz EH, Cheng A. Part 14: education: 2015 American Heart Association Guidelines Update for Cardiopulmonary Resuscitation and Emergency Cardiovascular Care.Circulation.2015;132 (suppl 2):S561-573. doi: 10.1161/CIR.0000000000000268
6. Lin Y, Cheng A, Grant VJ, Currie GR, Hecker KG.Improving CPR quality with distributed practice and real-time feedback in pediatric healthcare providers – a randomized controlled trial.Resuscitation.2018;130:6-12. doi: 10.1016/j.resuscitation.2018.06.025
7. Anderson R, Sebaldt A, Lin Y, Cheng A. Optimal training frequency for acquisition and retention of high-quality CPR skills: a randomized trial.Resuscitation.2019;135:153-161. doi: 10.1016/j.resuscitation.2018.10.033
8. Sutton RM, Case E, Brown SP, Atkins DL, Nadkarni VM, Kaltman J, Callaway C, Idris A, Nichol G, Hutchison J, et al; ROC Investigators.A quantitative analysis of out-of-hospital pediatric and adolescent resuscitation quality-a report from the ROC epistry-cardiac arrest.Resuscitation.2015;93:150-157. doi: 10.1016/j.resuscitation.2015.04.010
9. Sutton RM, Niles D, French B, Maltese MR, Leffelman J, Eilevstjonn J, Wolfe H, Nishisaki A, Meaney PA, Berg RA, et al.First quantitative analysis of cardiopulmonary resuscitation quality during in-hospital cardiac arrests of young children.Resuscitation.2014;85:70-74. doi: 10.1016/j.resuscitation.2013.08.014
10. Sutton RM, Niles D, Nysaether J, Abella BS, Arbogast KB, Nishisaki A, Maltese MR, Donoghue A, Bishnoi R, Helfaer MA, et al.Quantitative analysis of CPR quality during in-hospital resuscitation of older children and adolescents.Pediatrics.2009;124:494-499. doi: 10.1542/peds.2008-1930
11. Stiell IG, Brown SP, Christenson J, Cheskes S, Nichol G, Powell J, Bigham B, Morrison LJ, Larsen J, Hess E, et al; Resuscitation Outcomes Consortium (ROC) Investigators.What is the role of chest compression depth during out-of-hospital cardiac arrest resuscitation? Crit Care Med.2012;40:1192-1198. doi: 10.1097/CCM.0b013e31823bc8bb
12. Wik L, Steen PA, Bircher NG.Quality of bystander cardiopulmonary resuscitation influences outcome after prehospital cardiac arrest.Resuscitation.1994;28:195-203. doi: 10.1016/0300-9572 (94)90064-7
13. Idris AH, Guffey D, Aufderheide TP, Brown S, Morrison LJ, Nichols P, Powell J, Daya M, Bigham BL, Atkins DL, et al; Resuscitation Outcomes Consortium (ROC) Investigators.Relationship between chest compression rates and outcomes from cardiac arrest.Circulation.2012;125:3004-3012. doi: 10.1161/CIRCULATIONAHA.111.059535
14. Cheng A, Hunt EA, Grant D, Lin Y, Grant V, Duff JP, White ML, Peterson DT, Zhong J, Gottesman R, et al; International Network for Simulation-based Pediatric Innovation, Research, and Education CPR Investigators.Variability in quality of chest compressions provided during simulated cardiac arrest across nine pediatric institutions.Resuscitation.2015;97:13-19. doi: 10.1016/j.resuscitation.2015.08.024
15. Plant N, Taylor K. How best to teach CPR to schoolchildren: a systematic review.Resuscitation.2013;84:415-421. doi: 10.1016/j.resuscitation.2012.12.008
16. Todd KH, Heron SL, Thompson M, Dennis R, O'Connor J, Kellermann AL.Simple CPR: a randomized, controlled trial of video self-instructional cardiopulmonary resuscitation training in an African American church congregation.Ann Emerg Med.1999;34:730-737. doi: 10.1016/s0196-0644(99)70098-3
17. Castrén M, Nurmi J, Laakso JP, Kinnunen A, Backman R, Niemi-Murola L. Teaching public access defibrillation to lay volunteers-a professional health care provider is not a more effective instructor than a trained lay person. Resuscitation.2004;63:305-310. doi: 10.1016/j.resuscitation.2004.06.011
18. Cook DA, Hamstra SJ, Brydges R, Zendejas B, Szostek JH, Wang AT, Erwin PJ, Hatala R. Comparative effectiveness of instructional design features in simulation-based education: systematic review and meta-analysis.Med Teach.2013;35:e867-898. doi: 10.3109/0142159X.2012.714886
19. Magid DJ, Aziz K, Cheng A, Hazinski MF, Hoover AV, Mahgoub M, Panchal AR, Sasson C, Topjian AA, Rodriguez AJ, et al.Part 2: evidence evaluation and guidelines development: 2020 American Heart Association Guidelines for Cardiopulmonary Resuscitation and Emergency Cardiovascular Care.Circulation.2020;142:(suppl 2):S358-S365. doi: 10.1161/CIR.0000000000000903
20. American Heart Association.Conflict of interest policy.https://www.heart.org/en/about-us/statements-and-policies/conflict-of-interest-policy.Accessed December 31, 2019.
21. Tricco AC, Lillie E, Zarin W, O'Brien KK, Colquhoun H, Levac D, Moher D, Peters MDJ, Horsley T, Weeks L, et al.PRISMA Extension for Scoping Reviews (PRISMAScR): checklist and explanation.Ann Intern Med.2018;169:467-473. doi: 10.7326/M18-0850

表1. 患者ケアにおける臨床上の戦略，介入，治療，または診断検査への推奨事項のクラスとエビデンスレベルの適用（2019年5月更新）*

推奨事項のクラス（強さ）

クラス1（強い） 利益＞＞＞リスク

推奨事項文に適した表現例：
- 推奨される
- 適応／有用／有効／有益である
- 実施／投与（など）すべきである
- 比較に基づく有効性の表現例†：
  – 治療Bよりも治療／治療戦略Aが推奨される／適応である
  – 治療Bよりも治療Aを選択すべきである

クラス2a（中等度） 利益＞＞リスク

推奨事項文に適した表現例：
- 妥当である
- 有用／有効／有益でありうる
- 比較に基づく有効性の表現例†：
  – 治療Bよりも治療／治療戦略Aがおそらく推奨される／適応である
  – 治療Bよりも治療Aを選択することが妥当である

クラス2b（弱い） 利益≧リスク

推奨事項文に適した表現例：
- 妥当としてよい／よいだろう
- 考慮してもよい／よいだろう
- 有用性／有効性は不明／不明確／不確実である，あるいは十分に確立されていない

クラス3：利益なし（中等度） 利益＝リスク
（一般にLOE AまたはBの使用に限る）

推奨事項文に適した表現例：
- 推奨しない
- 適応／有用／有効／有益ではない
- 実施／投与（など）すべきでない

クラス3：有害（強い） リスク＞利益

推奨事項文に適した表現例：
- 有害な可能性がある
- 有害となる
- 合併症発生率／死亡率の上昇を伴う
- 実施／投与（など）すべきでない

エビデンスレベル（質）‡

レベルA
- 複数のRCTから得られた質の高いエビデンス‡
- 質の高いRCTのメタアナリシス
- 質の高い症例登録試験によって裏付けられた1件以上のRCT

レベルB-R （無作為化）
- 1件以上のRCTから得られた質が中等度のエビデンス‡
- 質が中等度のRCTのメタアナリシス

レベルB-NR （非無作為化）
- 1件以上の綿密にデザインされ，適切に実施された非無作為化試験，観察研究，または症例登録試験から得られた質が中等度のエビデンス‡
- そのような試験のメタアナリシス

レベルC-LD （限定的なデータ）
- デザインまたは実施に限界がある無作為化または非無作為化観察研究または症例登録試験
- そのような試験のメタアナリシス
- ヒトを対象にした生理学的試験または反応機構研究

レベルC-EO （専門家の見解）
- 臨床経験に基づく専門家の見解のコンセンサス

CORおよびLOEは個別に決定する（CORとLOEのあらゆる組み合わせが可能）。

LOE Cの推奨事項は，その推奨事項が弱いことを意味するわけではない。ガイドラインが扱っている重要な医療上の問題の多くは，臨床試験の対象となっていない。RCTが行われていなくても，特定の検査あるいは治療法の有用性／有効性について，臨床上非常に明確なコンセンサスが得られている場合がある。

* 介入の成果または結果を記述すべきである（臨床転帰の改善，または診断精度の向上，または予後情報の増加）。

† 比較に基づく有効性の推奨事項（COR 1 および 2a，LOE A および B のみ）に関してその推奨事項の裏付けとなる試験は，評価する治療または治療戦略を直接比較しているものでなければならない。

‡ 標準化され，広く用いられていて，望ましくは検証されている複数のエビデンス評価ツールを活用する，システマティックレビューについてはエビデンスレビュー委員会を設けるなど，質を評価する方法は進化している。

COR：推奨事項のクラス（Class of Recommendation），EO：専門家の見解（expert opinion），LD：限定的なデータ（limited data），LOE：エビデンスレベル（Level of Evidence），NR：非無作為化（nonrandomized），R：無作為化（randomized），RCT：無作為化比較試験（randomized controlled trial）。

---

22. International Liaison Committee on Resuscitation.Continuous evidence evaluation guidance and templates.https://www.ilcor.org/documents/continuous-evidence-evaluation-guidance-and-templates.Accessed December 31, 2019.
23. Institute of Medicine (US) Committee of Standards for Systematic Reviews of Comparative Effectiveness Research.Finding What Works in Health Care: Standards for Systematic Reviews.Eden J, Levit L, Berg A, Morton S, eds. Washington, DC: The National Academies Press; 2011.
24. PRISMA. PRISMA for scoping reviews.http://www.prisma-statement.org/Extensions/ScopingReviews.Accessed December 31, 2019.
25. International Liaison Committee on Resuscitation website.Continuous evidence evaluation guidance and templates: 2020 evidence update process final.https://www.ilcor.org/documents/continuous-evidence-evaluation-guidance-and-templates.Accessed December 31, 2019.
26. Bhanji F, Mancini ME, Sinz E, Rodgers DL, McNeil MA, Hoadley TA, Meeks RA, Hamilton MF, Meaney PA, Hunt EA, et al.Part 16: education, implementation, and teams: 2010 American Heart Association Guidelines for Cardiopulmonary Resuscitation and Emergency Cardiovascular Care.Circulation.2010;122 (suppl 3):S920-S933. doi: 10.1161/CIRCULATIONAHA.110.971135
27. Greif R, Bhanji F, Bigham BL, Bray J, Breckwoldt J, Cheng A, Duff JP, Gilfoyle E, Hsieh M-J, Iwami T, et al; on behalf of the Education, Implementation, and Teams Collaborators.Education, implementation, and teams: 2020 International Consensus on Cardiopulmonary Resuscitation and Emergency Cardiovascular Care Science With Treatment Recommendations.Circulation.2020;142(suppl 1):S222-S283. doi: 10.1161/CIR.0000000000000896
28. Atkins DL, de Caen AR, Berger S, Samson RA, Schexnayder SM, Joyner BL Jr, Bigham BL, Niles DE, Duff JP, Hunt EA, et al.2017 American Heart Association focused update on pediatric basic life support and cardiopulmonary resuscitation quality: an update to the American Heart Association Guidelines for Cardiopulmonary Resuscitation and Emergency Cardiovascular Care. Circulation.2018;137:e1-e6. doi: 10.1161/CIR.0000000000000540

29. Kleinman ME, Goldberger ZD, Rea T, Swor RA, Bobrow BJ, Brennan EE, Terry M, Hemphill R, Gazmuri RJ, Hazinski MF, et al.2017 American Heart Association focused update on adult basic life support and cardiopulmonary resuscitation quality: an update to the American Heart Association Guidelines for Cardiopulmonary Resuscitation and Emergency Cardiovascular Care. Circulation.2018;137:e7–e13. doi: 10.1161/CIR.0000000000000539
30. Panchal AR, Berg KM, Hirsch KG, Kudenchuk PJ, Del Rios M, Cabañas JG, Link MS, Kurz MC, Chan PS, Morley PT, et al.2019 American Heart Association focused update on advanced cardiovascular life support: use of advanced airways, vasopressors, and extracorporeal cardiopulmonary resuscitation during cardiac arrest: an update to the American Heart Association Guidelines for Cardiopulmonary Resuscitation and Emergency Cardiovascular Care.Circulation.2019;140:e881–e894. doi: 10.1161/CIR.0000000000000732
31. Panchal AR, Berg KM, Cabañas JG, Kurz MC, Link MS, Del Rios M, Hirsch KG, Chan PS, Hazinski MF, Morley PT, et al.2019 American Heart Association focused update on systems of care: dispatcher-assisted cardiopulmonary resuscitation and cardiac arrest centers: an update to the American Heart Association Guidelines for Cardiopulmonary Resuscitation and Emergency Cardiovascular Care.Circulation.2019;140:e895–e903. doi: 10.1161/CIR.0000000000000733
32. Panchal AR, Berg KM, Kudenchuk PJ, Del Rios M, Hirsch KG, Link MS, Kurz MC, Chan PS, Cabañas JG, Morley PT, et al.2018 American Heart Association focused update on advanced cardiovascular life support use of antiarrhythmic drugs during and immediately after cardiac arrest: an update to the American Heart Association Guidelines for Cardiopulmonary Resuscitation and Emergency Cardiovascular Care.Circulation.2018;138:e740–e749. doi: 10.1161/CIR.0000000000000613
33. Duff JP, Topjian A, Berg MD, Chan M, Haskell SE, Joyner BL Jr, Lasa JJ, Ley SJ, Raymond TT, Sutton RM, et al.2018 American Heart Association focused update on pediatric advanced life support: an update to the American Heart Association Guidelines for Cardiopulmonary Resuscitation and Emergency Cardiovascular Care.Circulation.2018;138:e731–e739. doi: 10.1161/CIR.0000000000000612
34. Escobedo MB, Aziz K, Kapadia VS, Lee HC, Niermeyer S, Schmölzer GM, Szyld E, Weiner GM, Wyckoff MH, Yamada NK, et al.2019 American Heart Association focused update on neonatal resuscitation: an update to the American Heart Association Guidelines for Cardiopulmonary Resuscitation and Emergency Cardiovascular Care.Circulation.2019;140:e922–e930. doi: 10.1161/CIR.0000000000000729
35. Charlton NP, Pellegrino JL, Kule A, Slater TM, Epstein JL, Flores GE, Goolsby CA, Orkin AM, Singletary EM, Swain JM.2019 American Heart Association and American Red Cross focused update for first aid: presyncope: an update to the American Heart Association and American Red Cross Guidelines for First Aid.Circulation.2019;140:e931–e938. doi: 10.1161/CIR.0000000000000730
36. Duff JP, Topjian AA, Berg MD, Chan M, Haskell SE, Joyner BL Jr, Lasa JJ, Ley SJ, Raymond TT, Sutton RM, et al.2019 American Heart Association focused update on pediatric advanced life support: an update to the American Heart Association Guidelines for Cardiopulmonary Resuscitation and Emergency Cardiovascular Care.Circulation.2019;140:e904–e914. doi: 10.1161/CIR.0000000000000731
37. Duff JP, Topjian AA, Berg MD, Chan M, Haskell SE, Joyner BL Jr, Lasa JJ, Ley SJ, Raymond TT, Sutton RM, et al.2019 American Heart Association focused update on pediatric basic life support: an update to the American Heart Association guidelines for cardiopulmonary resuscitation and emergency cardiovascular care.Circulation.2019;140:e915–e921. doi: 10.1161/CIR.0000000000000736
38. GRADE Working Group.5.2.1.Study limitations (risk of bias).In: Schunemann HJ, Brożek J, Guyatt G, Oxman A, eds.GRADE Handbook.2013. https://gdt.gradepro.org/app/handbook/handbook.html.Updated October 2013.Accessed December 31, 2019.
39. Levine GN, O'Gara PT, Beckman JA, Al-Khatib SM, Birtcher KK, Cigarroa JE, de Las Fuentes L, Deswal A, Fleisher LA, Gentile F, et al.Recent innovations, modifications, and evolution of ACC/AHA clinical practice guidelines: an update for our constituencies: a report of the American College of Cardiology/American Heart Association Task Force on Clinical Practice Guidelines. Circulation.2019;139:e879–e886. doi: 10.1161/CIR.0000000000000651

主要な概念

2018年，AHAは「Resuscitation Education Science: Educational Strategies to Improve Outcomes From Cardiac Arrest（蘇生教育科学：心停止の予後を改善するための教育戦略）」[1]という科学的ステートメントを発表し，蘇生に関する最良の教育実践を裏付けるエビデンスを包括的に集約した。このステートメントで取り上げたトピックは，「蘇生における生存のための方程式」という図に図式化されている[2]。この図は，蘇生科学（ガイドラインの質），教育効率（教育の質と影響），および現場での実践（ガイドラインの理解と採用）が心停止からの生存転帰の改善に寄与することを示したものである。本ガイドラインでは，上記の科学的ステートメントを補うため，科学の最新のレビューを提供し，エビデンスに基づく蘇生教育の変化に応じた具体的な推奨事項を強調している。

本ガイドラインは，主に教授システム学（インストラクショナル・デザイン），プロバイダーに関する考慮事項，今後の課題とさらなる研究の3つのセクションで構成されている。蘇生トレーニングプログラムでは，1つの主要な教授システム学（インストラクショナル・デザイン）上の要素を組み込むか，学習成果を最適化するためにそれらを融合させることができる。最良の教授システム学（インストラクショナル・デザイン）は，具体的な学習目的，学習者の種類，および学習の文脈に合わせて個別に調整されている。ここでは，集中的な練習および完全習得学習，ブースター訓練および反復学習，市民救助者トレーニング，チームワークおよびリーダーシップトレーニング，現場教育，マネキンの忠実度，トレーニングにおけるCPRフィードバック器具，ゲーム方式の学習とバーチャルリアリティ（VR），二次救命処置コースの受講前の準備，およびオピオイド過量投与の管理におけるトレーニングの考慮事項に関連する推奨事項を提示する。上記の図で強調されているように，生存のための方程式において教授システム学（インストラクショナル・デザイン）上の要素は教育効率に寄与する。

2つ目のセクションでは，プロバイダーに関する特定の考慮事項が教育の全体的影響にどのように作用するかについて説明する。例えば，蘇生教育機会の格差（SES，人種など）やプロバイダーの過去の経験は，学習成果にプラスまたはマイナス方向に寄与する可能性がある。プロバイダーの中には，AHAのACLS（二次救命処置）コースを受講する者もいれば，しない者もいる。これは患者転帰にどのように影響するのであろうか。これらすべての考慮事項が教授システム学（インストラクショナル・デザイン）の潜在的影響に作用し，最終的に生存のための方程式（図）の教育効率の要素に影響を及ぼす。

本ガイドラインの内容をレビューするにあたり，執筆グループは，蘇生教育に関連する数多くの重要なトピック（学習における認知的負荷の役割，拡張現実，ブログ，およびポッドキャストの教育ツールとしての利用，学習者の評価，リソースの乏しい環境でのトレーニング，蘇生指導者のトレーニングにおけるファカルティ・ディベロップメントの役割など）を特定し，それらについて議論した。これらを含む

いくつかのトピックは関心の高い領域ではあるものの，それぞれの概念が蘇生教育にどのように影響するかについて検討した，推奨事項策定の裏付けとなるエビデンスは不足している。関心のある読者は，AHA の科学的ステートメント「Resuscitation Education Science: Educational Strategies to Improve Outcomes From Cardiac Arrest（蘇生教育科学：心停止の予後を改善するための教育戦略）」でこれらの概念の説明を参照されたい[1]。これらの問題を今後の AHA ガイドラインの改訂に組み込むためには，もっと多くの文献が必要である。最後に，本章の締めくくりとして，蘇生教育科学の今後の課題をまとめ，蘇生トレーニングプログラムの影響を最適化するための今後の方向性について考察する。

参考資料

1. Cheng A, Nadkarni VM, Mancini MB, Hunt EA, Sinz EH, Merchant RM, Donoghue A, Duff JP, Eppich W, Auerbach M, Bigham BL, Blewer AL, Chan PS, Bhanji F; American Heart Association Education Science Investigators; and on behalf of the American Heart Association Education Science and Programs Committee, Council on Cardiopulmonary, Critical Care, Perioperative and Resuscitation; Council on Cardiovascular and Stroke Nursing; and Council on Quality of Care and Outcomes Research.Resuscitation Education Science: Educational Strategies to Improve Outcomes From Cardiac Arrest: A Scientific Statement From the American Heart Association. Circulation.2018;138:e82–e122. doi: 10.1161/CIR.0000000000000583
2. Søreide E, Morrison L, Hillman K, Monsieurs K, Sunde K, Zideman D, Eisenberg M, Sterz F, Nadkarni VM, Soar J, Nolan JP; Utstein Formula for Survival Collaborators.The formula for survival in resuscitation.Resuscitation.2013;84:1487–1493. doi: 10.1016/j.resuscitation.2013.07.020

教授システム学（インストラクショナル・デザイン）上の要素

集中的な練習および完全習得学習

集中的な練習および完全習得学習に関する推奨事項		
COR	LOE	推奨事項
2b	B-NR	1. スキル習得およびパフォーマンスの向上のため，一次または二次救命処置コースに集中的な練習および完全習得学習モデルを組み込むことを検討してよい[1-12]。

「概要」

集中的な練習 は，受講者に（1）個別の達成目標を与え，（2）パフォーマンスに対するフィードバックを即座に提供し，（3）パフォーマンスを改善するための反復の時間を十分に取るトレーニングアプローチである[13,14]。完全習得学習 は，集中的な練習によるトレーニングと，学習するタスクの完全な習得を意味する基準（具体的な到達基準など）を用いたテストを使用することと定義される[15]。集中的な練習と完全習得学習を蘇生トレーニングにどのように組み込めるかを十分に理解すれば，トレーニングの強化と患者転帰の改善につながる。蘇生トレーニングにおける集中的な練習および／または完全習得学習の影響を調査した研究がこれまで 12 件実施されている[1-12]。そのうち 8 件の研究では，集中的な練習と完全習得学習によって受講者のパフォーマンス（臨床評価のスコア，介入までの時間など）が向上したが[1,2,5-10]，残りの研究では学習成果に差は見られなかった[3,4,11,12]。これらの研究の大部分で肯定的な結果が報告されていることから，集中的な練習および完全習得学習を一次および二次救命処置トレーニングに組み込むことを推奨する。具体的には，2人1組での反復と，評価に基づくカスタマイズされたフィードバックの提供，弱点を克服するための具体的な練習の指定，および受講者が特定のスキルの最低到達基準に達するように十分な時間を与えることを推奨する。今後の研究では，集中的な練習と完全習得学習の定義を一貫させ，明確に定義された適切な比較群を使用して集中的な練習と完全習得学習の効果を分離することが求められる。

「推奨事項の裏付けとなる解説」

1. 4 件の無作為化比較試験（RCT）のうち 2 件で，集中的な練習を行った受講者はシミュレーション患者において臨床パフォーマンスが向上し，重要な介入を行うまでの時間（換気までの時間，アドレナリン投与までの時間など）が短縮された[1,2]。4 件の RCT のうち 2 件では，集中的な練習は従来のトレーニングと比較して学習成果に有意差はなかった[3,4]。

  8 件の観察研究のうち 6 件で，シミュレーション患者において集中的な練習および完全習得学習とパフォーマンス評価基準（圧迫までの時間，除細動までの時間，チェックリストのスコアなど）との間に関連性が見られた[5-10]。市民救助者に関する 2 件の研究（1 件は RCT，もう 1 件は観察研究）では，集中的な練習および完全習得学習に関連するパフォーマンスの向上は見られなかった[4,11]。

  スキルの低下が 5 件の研究で測定された[5,9-12]。そのうち 4 件では，集中的な練習および完全習得学習の後最長 6 カ月間，有意な低下は認められず[9-12]，残り 1 件では，トレーニング後 6 カ月の時点でパフォーマンスの有意な線形の低下が見られた（P = 0.039）[5]。1 件の研究において，集中的な練習および完全習得学習モデルの蘇生トレーニングへの組み込みに伴う 1 回限りのコストは従来のトレーニングより高かったが，インストラクターの関与が減少したため，繰り返し発生するコストは低下した[12]。今後の研究で，より大人数の受講者グループのトレーニングにおいて集中的な練習および完全習得学習が長期的なコストの削減に寄与するかどうかを調べることが望まれる。

参考資料

1. Magee MJ, Farkouh-Karoleski C, Rosen TS.Improvement of Immediate Performance in Neonatal Resuscitation Through Rapid Cycle Deliberate Practice Training.J Grad Med Educ.2018;10:192-197. doi: 10.4300/JGME-D-17-00467.1
2. Diederich E, Lineberry M, Blomquist M, Schott V, Reilly C, Murray M, Nazaran P, Rourk M, Werner R, Broski J. Balancing Deliberate Practice and Reflection: A Randomized Comparison Trial of Instructional Designs for Simulation-Based Training in Cardiopulmonary Resuscitation Skills.Simul Healthc.2019;14:175-181. doi: 10.1097/SIH.0000000000000375
3. Lemke DS, Fielder EK, Hsu DC, Doughty CB.Improved Team Performance During Pediatric Resuscitations After Rapid Cycle Deliberate

Practice Compared With Traditional Debriefing: A Pilot Study.Pediatr Emerg Care.2019;35:480-486. doi: 10.1097/PEC.0000000000000940
4. Madou T, Iserbyt P. Mastery versus self-directed blended learning in basic life support: a randomised controlled trial.Acta Cardiol.2019:1-7. doi: 10.1080/00015385.2019.1677374
5. Braun L, Sawyer T, Smith K, Hsu A, Behrens M, Chan D, Hutchinson J, Lu D, Singh R, Reyes J, Lopreiato J. Retention of pediatric resuscitation performance after a simulation-based mastery learning session: a multicenter randomized trial.Pediatr Crit Care Med.2015;16:131-138. doi: 10.1097/PCC.0000000000000315
6. Cordero L, Hart BJ, Hardin R, Mahan JD, Nankervis CA.Deliberate practice improves pediatric residents' skills and team behaviors during simulated neonatal resuscitation.Clin Pediatr (Phila).2013;52:747-752. doi: 10.1177/0009922813488646
7. Hunt EA, Duval-Arnould JM, Chime NO, Jones K, Rosen M, Hollingsworth M, Aksamit D, Twilley M, Camacho C, Nogee DP, Jung J, Nelson-McMillan K, Shilkofski N, Perretta JS.Integration of in-hospital cardiac arrest contextual curriculum into a basic life support course: a randomized, controlled simulation study.Resuscitation.2017;114:127-132. doi: 10.1016/j.resuscitation.2017.03.014
8. Hunt EA, Duval-Arnould JM, Nelson-McMillan KL, Bradshaw JH, Diener-West M, Perretta JS, Shilkofski NA.Pediatric resident resuscitation skills improve after "rapid cycle deliberate practice" training.Resuscitation.2014;85:945-951. doi: 10.1016/j.resuscitation.2014.02.025
9. Jeffers J, Eppich W, Trainor J, Mobley B, Adler M. Development and Evaluation of a Learning Intervention Targeting First-Year Resident Defibrillation Skills.Pediatr Emerg Care.2016;32:210-216. doi: 10.1097/PEC.0000000000000765
10. Reed T, Pirotte M, McHugh M, Oh L, Lovett S, Hoyt AE, Quinones D, Adams W, Gruener G, McGaghie WC.Simulation-Based Mastery Learning Improves Medical Student Performance and Retention of Core Clinical Skills.Simul Healthc.2016;11:173-180. doi: 10.1097/SIH.0000000000000154
11. Boet S, Bould MD, Pigford AA, Rössler B, Nambyiah P, Li Q, Bunting A, Schebesta K. Retention of Basic Life Support in Laypeople: Mastery Learning vs. Time-based Education.Prehosp Emerg Care.2017;21:362-377. doi: 10.1080/10903127.2016.1258096
12. Devine LA, Donkers J, Brydges R, Perelman V, Cavalcanti RB, Issenberg SB.An Equivalence Trial Comparing Instructor-Regulated With Directed Self-Regulated Mastery Learning of Advanced Cardiac Life Support Skills. Simul Healthc.2015;10:202-209. doi: 10.1097/SIH.0000000000000095
13. Ericsson KA.Deliberate practice and the acquisition and maintenance of expert performance in medicine and related domains.Acad Med.2004;79 (suppl):S70-81. doi: 10.1097/00001888-200410001-00022
14. Ericsson KA, Krampe RT, Tesch-Romer.The role of deliberate practice in the acquisition of expert performance.Psychol Rev. 1993;100:363-406. doi: 10.1037/0033-295X.100.3.363
15. McGaghie WC.When I say … mastery learning.Med Educ.2015;49:558-559. doi: 10.1111/medu.12679

ブースター訓練および反復学習

現行のほとんどの蘇生コースでは，集中学習アプローチ（数時間または数日続く単一のトレーニングイベントを実施し，1～2年ごとに再トレーニングする）が採用されている[1]。残りの蘇生コースでは，反復学習が採用されている。つまり，トレーニングを数分から数時間の複数のセッションに分割し，数週間から数カ月の間隔を開けて各セッションを実施する[2-5]。個々の反復セッションでは，新しい内容を学習するか，以前のセッションの内容を反復する。その両方を行うこともある。ブースター訓練は，これとは別の教授システム学（インストラクショナル・デザイン）上の要素であり，初期の集中学習コースで学んだ内容の反復に重点を置いた短いセッションを毎週または毎月実施する[6-18]。

高頻度のブースター訓練（1～6カ月間隔）はCPRスキルの向上と関連性があった[6-9,14,16,18]。週1回の新生児トレーニングの追加セッションを実施した後，死亡率が低下したことが報告されている[13]。ある研究によると，追加セッションの頻度を増やすと受講者はすべてのセッションに参加しなくなり，受講者の減少が最も高かったのは月1回練習を行う群であった[6]。PALS（小児二次救命処置）またはACLSコースのブースター訓練について評価した研究はまだない。小児蘇生トレーニングにおいて，反復学習コースは集中学習コースと比較して同等またはそれ以上の効果がある[3-5]。BLS，新生児（新生児蘇生プログラムなど），またはACLSコースで反復学習と集中学習を比較した研究はまだない。蘇生トレーニングプログラムに集中学習アプローチを使用する場合は，追加セッションを実施することを推奨する。また，集中学習の代わりに反復学習コースの実施を検討することも推奨する。今後の研究により，コストを最小限に抑えながら受講者の継続的な参加を維持できる最適なトレーニング間隔を特定することが求められる。

ブースター訓練に関する推奨事項		
COR	LOE	推奨事項
1	B-R	1. 蘇生トレーニングに集中学習アプローチを用いる場合は，追加セッションの実施が推奨される[6-18]。

「推奨事項の裏付けとなる解説」

1. 1～6カ月間隔の追加CPRトレーニングをブースター訓練なしの場合と比較した7件のRCTでは，CPRパフォーマンスの向上が認められた[6-9,14,16,18]。看護師を頻度の異なるCPRブースター訓練に無作為に割り付けた1件のRCTでは，1年後時点のCPRスキルはトレーニングの回数に応じて向上した（12カ月時点で総合的に優秀なCPRスキルを示した看護師の割合：ブースター訓練の頻度が1カ月に1回の場合は58％，3カ月に1回の場合は26％，6カ月に1回の場合は21％，12カ月に1回の場合は15％）[6]。ただし，1カ月に1回の群は，すべてのセッションに参加した看護師の割合が最も低かった。別のRCTでは，1カ月に1回のCPRブースター訓練に無作為に割り付けられた救急部のスタッフは，ブースター訓練を受けなかったスタッフと比較して，12カ月の時点で優秀なCPRスキルを示した割合が高かった（成人マネキンで優秀なCPRスキルを示したスタッフの割合：54.3％対14.6％，P＜0.001，乳児マネキンの場合：71.7％対19.5％，P＜0.001）[14]。その他のRCTでは，以下の結果が得られている。1カ月，3カ月，および6カ月の時点で30分のブースター訓練を実施した後，知識とCPRスキルの向上が認められた[7]。6分のブースター訓練を1カ月に1回実施した後，換気と圧迫のスキルが向上した[8,16]。さらに，2カ月，3カ月，または6カ月ごとに15分のブースター訓練を実施した後，圧迫および除細動を開始するまでの時間が短縮された[18]。

3件のRCTで，新生児蘇生プログラムの高頻度のブースター訓練（週1回から9カ月に1回まで）は経時的なスキルパフォーマンスの向上と関連性があることが認められた[10-12]。また，1件の観察研究において，3～5分のブースター訓練を週1回実施した後，臨床パフォーマンスの向上と乳児死亡率の低下が見られた（トレーニング前：11.1/1,000，トレーニング後：7.2/1,000，P＝0.04）[13]。

反復学習に関する推奨事項		
COR	LOE	推奨事項
2a	B-R	1. 蘇生トレーニングには，集中学習アプローチの代わりに反復学習アプローチを用いることが妥当である[3-5]。

「推奨事項の裏付けとなる解説」

1. 2件のRCTと1件の観察研究で，小児蘇生トレーニングにおける反復学習と集中学習が比較された。[3-5] 1件のRCTでは，救急医療サービス（EMS）のスタッフが反復学習（週1回3.5時間のセッションを4回）または集中学習（7時間のトレーニングを2日連続）に無作為に割り付けられた。[3] 反復学習群は，集中学習群と比較して，3カ月時点での乳児バッグマスク換気スキルと乳児骨髄内挿入スキルについては定着が高かったが，胸骨圧迫スキルについては差はなかった。知識の低下は，集中学習群では認められたが，反復学習群では認められなかった。[3]

   もう1件のRCTでは，小児科の看護師と呼吸療法士が，PALS再認定のための反復学習（30分のセッションを6カ月間に6回）または集中学習（7.5時間のトレーニングを1日）に無作為に割り付けられた。[5] 反復学習群では，臨床パフォーマンススコアが向上した。コース修了時に測定されたチームワークについては，どちらの群も同じような改善を示した。

   観察研究では，医学生が小児蘇生スキルの反復学習（週1回1.25時間のセッションを4回）または集中学習（5時間のセッションを1回）を受けた。コース修了から4週間後に測定されたスキル（バッグマスク換気，骨髄内挿入，胸骨圧迫）の知識または全般的評価において，両群の間に差はなかった。[4]

参考資料

1. Cheng A, Nadkarni VM, Mancini MB, Hunt EA, Sinz EH, Merchant RM, Donoghue A, Duff JP, Eppich W, Auerbach M, Bigham BL, Blewer AL, Chan PS, Bhanji F; American Heart Association Education Science Investigators; and on behalf of the American Heart Association Education Science and Programs Committee, Council on Cardiopulmonary, Critical Care, Perioperative and Resuscitation; Council on Cardiovascular and Stroke Nursing; and Council on Quality of Care and Outcomes Research.Resuscitation Education Science: Educational Strategies to Improve Outcomes From Cardiac Arrest: A Scientific Statement From the American Heart Association. Circulation.2018;138:e82-e122. doi: 10.1161/CIR.0000000000000583
2. Greif R, Bhanji F, Bigham BL, Bray J, Breckwoldt J, Cheng A, Duff JP, Gilfoyle E, Hsieh M-J, Iwami T, et al; on behalf of the Education, Implementation, and Teams Collaborators.Education, implementation, and teams: 2020 International Consensus on Cardiopulmonary Resuscitation and Emergency Cardiovascular Care Science With Treatment Recommendations.Circulation.2020;142(suppl 1):S222-S283. doi: 10.1161/CIR.0000000000000896
3. Patocka C, Cheng A, Sibbald M, Duff JP, Lai A, Lee-Nobbee P, Levin H, Varshney T, Weber B, Bhanji F. A randomized education trial of spaced versus massed instruction to improve acquisition and retention of paediatric resuscitation skills in emergency medical service (EMS) providers.Resuscitation.2019;141:73-80. doi: 10.1016/j.resuscitation.2019.06.010
4. Patocka C, Khan F, Dubrovsky AS, Brody D, Bank I, Bhanji F. Pediatric resuscitation training–instruction all at once or spaced over time? Resuscitation.2015;88:6-11. doi: 10.1016/j.resuscitation.2014.12.003
5. Kurosawa H, Ikeyama T, Achuff P, Perkel M, Watson C, Monachino A, Remy D, Deutsch E, Buchanan N, Anderson J, Berg RA, Nadkarni VM, Nishisaki A. A randomized, controlled trial of in situ pediatric advanced life support recertification ("pediatric advanced life support reconstructed") compared with standard pediatric advanced life support recertification for ICU frontline providers*.Crit Care Med.2014;42:610-618. doi: 10.1097/CCM.0000000000000024
6. Anderson R, Sebaldt A, Lin Y, Cheng A. Optimal training frequency for acquisition and retention of high-quality CPR skills: A randomized trial.Resuscitation.2019;135:153-161. doi: 10.1016/j.resuscitation.2018.10.033
7. O'Donnell CM, Skinner AC.An evaluation of a short course in resuscitation training in a district general hospital.Resuscitation.1993;26:193-201. doi: 10.1016/0300-9572(93)90179-t
8. Oermann MH, Kardong-Edgren SE, Odom-Maryon T. Effects of monthly practice on nursing students' CPR psychomotor skill performance.Resuscitation.2011;82:447-453. doi: 10.1016/j.resuscitation.2010.11.022
9. Nishiyama C, Iwami T, Murakami Y, Kitamura T, Okamoto Y, Marukawa S, Sakamoto T, Kawamura T. Effectiveness of simplified 15-min refresher BLS training program: a randomized controlled trial.Resuscitation.2015;90:56-60. doi: 10.1016/j.resuscitation.2015.02.015
10. Tabangin ME, Josyula S, Taylor KK, Vasquez JC, Kamath-Rayne BD.Resuscitation skills after Helping Babies Breathe training: a comparison of varying practice frequency and impact on retention of skills in different types of providers.Int Health.2018;10:163-171. doi: 10.1093/inthealth/ihy017
11. Bender J, Kennally K, Shields R, Overly F. Does simulation booster impact retention of resuscitation procedural skills and teamwork? J Perinatol.2014;34:664-668. doi: 10.1038/jp.2014.72
12. Ernst KD, Cline WL, Dannaway DC, Davis EM, Anderson MP, Atchley CB, Thompson BM.Weekly and consecutive day neonatal intubation training: comparable on a pediatrics clerkship.Acad Med.2014;89:505-510. doi: 10.1097/ACM.0000000000000150
13. Mduma E, Ersdal H, Svensen E, Kidanto H, Auestad B, Perlman J. Frequent brief on-site simulation training and reduction in 24-h neonatal mortality-an educational intervention study.Resuscitation.2015;93:1-7. doi: 10.1016/j.resuscitation.2015.04.019
14. Lin Y, Cheng A, Grant VJ, Currie GR, Hecker KG.Improving CPR quality with distributed practice and real-time feedback in pediatric healthcare providers – A randomized controlled trial.Resuscitation.2018;130:6-12. doi: 10.1016/j.resuscitation.2018.06.025
15. Montgomery C, Kardong-Edgren SE, Oermann MH, Odom-Maryon T. Student satisfaction and self report of CPR competency: HeartCode BLS courses, instructor-led CPR courses, and monthly voice advisory manikin practice for CPR skill maintenance.Int J Nurs Educ Scholarsh.2012;9. doi: 10.1515/1548-923X.2361
16. Kardong-Edgren S, Oermann MH, Odom-Maryon T. Findings from a nursing student CPR study: implications for staff development educators.J Nurses Staff Dev.2012;28:9-15. doi: 10.1097/NND.0b013e318240a6ad
17. Cepeda Brito JR, Hughes PG, Firestone KS, Ortiz Figueroa F, Johnson K, Ruthenburg T, McKinney R, Gothard MD, Ahmed R. Neonatal Resuscitation Program Rolling Refresher: Maintaining Chest Compression Proficiency Through the Use of Simulation-Based Education.Adv Neonatal Care.2017;17:354-361. doi: 10.1097/ANC.0000000000000384
18. Sullivan NJ, Duval-Arnould J, Twilley M, Smith SP, Aksamit D, Boone-Guercio P, Jeffries PR, Hunt EA.Simulation exercise to improve retention of cardiopulmonary resuscitation priorities for in-hospital cardiac arrests: A randomized controlled trial.Resuscitation.2015;86:6-13. doi: 10.1016/j.resuscitation.2014.10.021

市民救助者トレーニング

COR	LOE	推奨事項
1	C-LD	1. 自主学習と実践トレーニングを伴うインストラクターが指導するコースとの組み合わせは、市民救助者向けの従来のインストラクターが指導するコースに代わるものとして推奨される。インストラクターが指導するトレーニングが利用できない場合、市民救助者には自主学習トレーニングが推奨される[1-9]。
1	C-LD	2. 中高生には、質の高いCPRを実施するトレーニングを行うことが推奨される[10-18]。
2a	C-LD	3. 地域社会において、従来のCPRトレーニングに代わるものとして、成人の院外心停止(OHCA)に対する胸骨圧迫のみのCPRトレーニングをバイスタンダーに実施することは妥当である[19-25]。
2a	C-LD	4. 高リスク患者の主介護者および/または家族に対してCPRトレーニングを実施することは妥当である[26-39]。
2a	A	5. フィードバック器具を使用すると、市民救助者トレーニング中にCPRのパフォーマンスを向上する効果が得られる[40-47]。
2b	B-R	6. フィードバック器具を使用できない場合は、胸骨圧迫のテンポに関する推奨事項の遵守を改善する目的にのみ、音によるガイド(メトロノーム、音楽など)の使用を検討してもよい[48-52]。
2b	C-LD	7. 心停止に遭遇する可能性の高い市民救助者に対して、2年に1回以上の頻度でCPRの再トレーニングを実施することは妥当としてよい[4,53-57]。

「概要」

迅速なCPRは、心停止後の生存率を2～3倍高める可能性がある[58,59]。市民救助者(医療従事者でない人)に対する蘇生トレーニングの主要な目標は、OHCAに遭遇したときの即時バイスタンダーCPR(B-CPR)の実施率、自動体外式除細動器の使用、および救急対応システムへの適時の通報を増加させることである。この集団のCPR実施の意欲を高めることは、OHCAの生存率に直接的な影響を与える可能性がある[60]。このモジュール知識チャンク(大きな塊)では、「市民救助者において、どのようなCPRトレーニングの特性および/またはトレーニングの文脈が、実際の蘇生現場でCPRを実施しようという意欲、スキルパフォーマンスの質、および患者転帰に影響を及ぼすか」という論点に目を向ける。

レビューしたエビデンスは、市民救助者がCPRスキルを向上させるためには、リアルタイムのフィードバックまたは遅延フィードバックを伴うインストラクター主導および/または自主学習方式のCPRトレーニングセッションを受けることが望ましいことを示唆している[1-4]。トレーニングセッションでは、CPRスキルの定着を強化するように設計されたスキル固有のトレーニング戦略を組み合わせて使用するのがよい[54-57]。知識ではなくスキルと自信に重点を置いた復習トレーニングを定期的に実施すべきであるが、最適な周期についてはさらなる研究が待たれる[4,53-57]。地域社会においては、市民救助者に対して従来の換気と胸骨圧迫のCPRよりも胸骨圧迫のみのCPRのトレーニングを行うほうが妥当である[19,20]。質の高いCPRは生存率の向上と関連性があるが、これまでのところ、マネキンで評価されたCPRパフォーマンスを実際の患者転帰に直接関連付けた研究はない。

「推奨事項の裏付けとなる解説」

1. インストラクターが関与しない自主学習とインストラクターが指導するコースを比較した4件の研究において、両者に有意差は認められなかった[1-4]。短いビデオによる指導は、トレーニングを受けていない場合と比較して圧迫のテンポを改善した[5,6]。ただし、圧迫の深さと手の位置の改善、および中断の最小化については、インストラクター主導のトレーニングのほうが若干優れていた[6-9]。

2. 複数の研究から、中高生には質の高いCPRスキルを学習し、それを思い出す能力があることが明らかになっている[10-18]。中学および高校での早期トレーニングは、自信を植え付け、実際の心停止現場で積極的に対応する姿勢を浸透させる可能性がある。

3. 市民救助者を対象として従来のCPRプログラムと胸骨圧迫のみのCPRプログラムを比較したいくつかの研究において、受講者による適切な胸骨圧迫の回数は、胸骨圧迫のみのCPRプログラムのほうが多かった[19,20]。調査に応じた市民救助者は、胸骨圧迫のみのCPRのほうが換気補助を伴う従来のCPRよりも積極的に行おうという気持ちになると報告した[21-23]。州全体で市民救助者に対する教育キャンペーンを実施した後に発表された2件の研究によると、総合的なB-CPRと胸骨圧迫のみのCPRの実施率はどちらも時間とともに増加したが、患者生存率に対する効果は認められなかった[24,25]。

4. 多くの研究で、心停止リスクの高い患者の家族および/または介護者に対するBLSトレーニングの有効性が評価されている。アウトカムには、家族によってCPRが実施された頻度；知識、スキル、および実施の妥当性；および家族からCPRを受けた心停止傷病者の生存率が使用された。トレーニングを受けた市民救助者の大部分はBLSスキルを適切に遂行でき、これらのスキルを使用する意欲があると報告していて、大きな不安は感じていなかった[26-39]。多くの研究でOHCAの件数の少なさと追跡調査不能の割合の高さが報告されているため、明確な利点を立証するためにはさらに多くの研究が必要となる。

5. CPRトレーニング中に修正フィードバックを提供する器具を使用した市民救助者は、フィードバック器具を使用せずにCPRを実施した受講者に比べて、圧迫のテンポ、圧迫の深さ、および胸郭の戻りが改善した[40-44]。フィードバック器具がCPRスキルの定着に及ぼす効果に関するエビデンスは少なく、4件の研究のうち1件で定着の向上が示されている[41,45-47]。

6. 3 件の無作為化試験で，市民救助者に対するトレーニング中に音によるガイド（メトロノームや音楽）を使用して CPR 手技を指導する方法が検討された[48-50]。どの試験でも，音によるガイドを使用した場合は胸骨圧迫のテンポが改善されたが，1 件の試験で圧迫の深さに対する悪影響が報告されている。流行歌によるガイドを使用したトレーニングでは，胸骨圧迫テンポの経時的な悪化が防止された[48,51,52]。

7. いくつかの試験で，市民救助者の CPR スキルは初回トレーニングから早ければ 3 カ月後に低下することが明らかになっている[4,53]。より短時間のトレーニングセッションを高頻度で行うと，知識と胸骨圧迫能力がわずかに向上し，除細動までの時間が短縮された[54-57]。

参考資料

1. Reder S, Cummings P, Quan L. Comparison of three instructional methods for teaching cardiopulmonary resuscitation and use of an automatic external defibrillator to high school students.Resuscitation.2006;69:443-453. doi: 10.1016/j.resuscitation.2005.08.020
2. Roppolo LP, Pepe PE, Campbell L, Ohman K, Kulkarni H, Miller R, Idris A, Bean L, Bettes TN, Idris AH.Prospective, randomized trial of the effectiveness and retention of 30-min layperson training for cardiopulmonary resuscitation and automated external defibrillators: The American Airlines Study. Resuscitation.2007;74:276-285. doi: 10.1016/j.resuscitation.2006.12.017
3. de Vries W, Turner NM, Monsieurs KG, Bierens JJ, Koster RW.Comparison of instructor-led automated external defibrillation training and three alternative DVD-based training methods.Resuscitation.2010;81:1004-1009. doi: 10.1016/j.resuscitation.2010.04.006
4. Saraç L, Ok A. The effects of different instructional methods on students' acquisition and retention of cardiopulmonary resuscitation skills.Resuscitation.2010;81:555-561. doi: 10.1016/j.resuscitation.2009.08.030
5. Bobrow BJ, Vadeboncoeur TF, Spaite DW, Potts J, Denninghoff K, Chikani V, Brazil PR, Ramsey B, Abella BS.The effectiveness of ultrabrief and brief educational videos for training lay responders in hands-only cardiopulmonary resuscitation: implications for the future of citizen cardiopulmonary resuscitation training.Circ Cardiovasc Qual Outcomes.2011;4:220-226. doi: 10.1161/CIRCOUTCOMES.110.959353
6. Panchal AR, Meziab O, Stolz U, Anderson W, Bartlett M, Spaite DW, Bobrow BJ, Kern KB.The impact of ultra-brief chest compression-only CPR video training on responsiveness, compression rate, and hands-off time interval among bystanders in a shopping mall.Resuscitation.2014;85:1287-1290. doi: 10.1016/j.resuscitation.2014.06.013
7. Chung CH, Siu AY, Po LL, Lam CY, Wong PC.Comparing the effectiveness of video self-instruction versus traditional classroom instruction targeted at cardiopulmonary resuscitation skills for laypersons: a prospective randomised controlled trial.Hong Kong Med J. 2010;16:165-170.
8. Jones I, Handley AJ, Whitfield R, Newcombe R, Chamberlain D. A preliminary feasibility study of a short DVD-based distance-learning package for basic life support.Resuscitation.2007;75:350-356. doi: 10.1016/j.resuscitation.2007.04.030
9. Beskind DL, Stolz U, Thiede R, Hoyer R, Robertson W, Brown J, Ludgate M, Tiutan T, Shane R, McMorrow D, Pleasants M, Kern KB, Panchal AR.Viewing an ultra-brief chest compression only video improves some measures of bystander CPR performance and responsiveness at a mass gathering event. Resuscitation.2017;118:96-100. doi: 10.1016/j.resuscitation.2017.07.011
10. Zeleke BG, Biswas ES, Biswas M. Teaching Cardiopulmonary Resuscitation to Young Children (<12 Years Old).Am J Cardiol.2019;123:1626-1627. doi: 10.1016/j.amjcard.2019.02.011
11. Schmid KM, García RQ, Fernandez MM, Mould-Millman NK, Lowenstein SR.Teaching Hands-Only CPR in Schools: A Program Evaluation in San José, Costa Rica.Ann Glob Health.2018;84:612-617. doi: 10.9204/aogh.2367
12. Li H, Shen X, Xu X, Wang Y, Chu L, Zhao J, Wang Y, Wang H, Xie G, Cheng B, et al.Bystander cardiopulmonary resuscitation training in primary and secondary school children in China and the impact of neighborhood socioeconomic status: A prospective controlled trial.Medicine (Baltimore).2018;97:e12673. doi: 10.1097/MD.0000000000012673
13. Paglino M, Contri E, Baggiani M, Tonani M, Costantini G, Bonomo MC, Baldi E. A video-based training to effectively teach CPR with long-term retention: the ScuolaSalvaVita.it ("SchoolSavesLives.it") project.Intern Emerg Med.2019;14:275-279. doi: 10.1007/s11739-018-1946-3
14. Magid KH, Heard D, Sasson C. Addressing Gaps in Cardiopulmonary Resuscitation Education: Training Middle School Students in Hands-Only Cardiopulmonary Resuscitation.J Sch Health.2018;88:524-530. doi: 10.1111/josh.12634
15. Andrews T, Price L, Mills B, Holmes L. Young adults' perception of mandatory CPR training in Australian high schools: a qualitative investigation.Austr J Paramedicine.2018;15. doi: 10.33151/ajp.15.2.577
16. Aloush S, Tubaishat A, ALBashtawy M, Suliman M, Alrimawi I, Al Sabah A, Banikhaled Y. Effectiveness of Basic Life Support Training for Middle School Students.J Sch Nurs.2019;35:262-267. doi: 10.1177/1059840517753879
17. Gabriel IO, Aluko JO.Theoretical knowledge and psychomotor skill acquisition of basic life support training programme among secondary school students.World J Emerg Med.2019;10:81-87. doi: 10.5847/wjem.j.1920-8642.2019.02.003
18. Brown LE, Carroll T, Lynes C, Tripathi A, Halperin H, Dillon WC.CPR skill retention in 795 high school students following a 45-minute course with psychomotor practice.Am J Emerg Med.2018;36:1110-1112. doi: 10.1016/j.ajem.2017.10.026
19. Nishiyama C, Iwami T, Kawamura T, Ando M, Yonemoto N, Hiraide A, Nonogi H. Effectiveness of simplified chest compression-only CPR training for the general public: a randomized controlled trial.Resuscitation.2008;79:90-96. doi: 10.1016/j.resuscitation.2008.05.009
20. Heidenreich JW, Sanders AB, Higdon TA, Kern KB, Berg RA, Ewy GA.Uninterrupted chest compression CPR is easier to perform and remember than standard CPR.Resuscitation.2004;63:123-130. doi: 10.1016/j.resuscitation.2004.04.011
21. Hawkes CA, Brown TP, Booth S, Fothergill RT, Siriwardena N, Zakaria S, Askew S, Williams J, Rees N, Ji C, et al.Attitudes to cardiopulmonary resuscitation and defibrillator use: a survey of UK adults in 2017.J Am Heart Assoc.2019;8:e008267. doi: 10.1161/JAHA.117.008267
22. Cheskes L, Morrison LJ, Beaton D, Parsons J, Dainty KN.Are Canadians more willing to provide chest-compression-only cardiopulmonary resuscitation (CPR)?-a nation-wide public survey.CJEM.2016;18:253-263. doi: 10.1017/cem.2015.113
23. Cho GC, Sohn YD, Kang KH, Lee WW, Lim KS, Kim W, Oh BJ, Choi DH, Yeom SR, Lim H. The effect of basic life support education on laypersons' willingness in performing bystander hands only cardiopulmonary resuscitation. Resuscitation.2010;81:691-694. doi: 10.1016/j.resuscitation.2010.02.021
24. Bobrow BJ, Spaite DW, Berg RA, Stolz U, Sanders AB, Kern KB, Vadeboncoeur TF, Clark LL, Gallagher JV, Stapczynski JS, LoVecchio F, Mullins TJ, Humble WO, Ewy GA.Chest compression-only CPR by lay rescuers and survival from out-of-hospital cardiac arrest.JAMA.2010;304:1447-1454. doi: 10.1001/jama.2010.1392
25. Panchal AR, Bobrow BJ, Spaite DW, Berg RA, Stolz U, Vadeboncoeur TF, Sanders AB, Kern KB, Ewy GA.Chest compression-only cardiopulmonary resuscitation performed by lay rescuers for adult out-of-hospital cardiac arrest due to non-cardiac aetiologies.Resuscitation.2013;84:435-439. doi: 10.1016/j.resuscitation.2012.07.038
26. González-Salvado V, Abelairas-Gómez C, Gude F, Peña-Gil C, Neiro-Rey C, González-Juanatey JR, Rodriguez-Núñez A. Targeting relatives: Impact of a cardiac rehabilitation programme including basic life support training on their skills and attitudes.Eur J Prev Cardiol.2019;26:795-805. doi: 10.1177/2047487319830190
27. Blewer AL, Leary M, Esposito EC, Gonzalez M, Riegel B, Bobrow BJ, Abella BS.Continuous chest compression cardiopulmonary resuscitation training promotes rescuer self-confidence and increased secondary training: a hospital-based randomized controlled trial*.Crit Care Med.2012;40:787-792. doi: 10.1097/CCM.0b013e318236f2ca
28. Dracup K, Guzy PM, Taylor SE, Barry J. Cardiopulmonary resuscitation (CPR) training.Consequences for family members of high-risk cardiac patients. Arch Intern Med.1986;146:1757-1761. doi: 10.1001/archinte.146.9.1757
29. Dracup K, Moser DK, Doering LV, Guzy PM, Juarbe T. A controlled trial of cardiopulmonary resuscitation training for ethnically diverse parents of infants at high risk for cardiopulmonary arrest.Crit Care Med.2000;28:3289-3295. doi: 10.1097/00003246-200009000-00029

30. Moser DK, Dracup K, Doering LV.Effect of cardiopulmonary resuscitation training for parents of high-risk neonates on perceived anxiety, control, and burden.Heart Lung.1999;28:326-333. doi: 10.1053/hl.1999.v28.a101053
31. Haugk M, Robak O, Sterz F, Uray T, Kliegel A, Losert H, Holzer M, Herkner H, Laggner AN, Domanovits H. High acceptance of a home AED programme by survivors of sudden cardiac arrest and their families.Resuscitation.2006;70:263-274. doi: 10.1016/j.resuscitation.2006.03.010
32. Kliegel A, Scheinecker W, Sterz F, Eisenburger P, Holzer M, Laggner AN.The attitudes of cardiac arrest survivors and their family members towards CPR courses.Resuscitation.2000;47:147-154. doi: 10.1016/s0300-9572(00)00214-8
33. Knight LJ, Wintch S, Nichols A, Arnolde V, Schroeder AR.Saving a life after discharge: CPR training for parents of high-risk children.J Healthc Qual.2013;35:9-16; quiz17. doi: 10.1111/j.1945-1474.2012.00221.x
34. Tomatis Souverbielle C, González-Martínez F, González-Sánchez MI, Carrón M, Guerra Miguez L, Butragueño L, Gonzalo H, Villalba T, Perez Moreno J, Toledo B, Rodríguez-Fernández R. Strengthening the Chain of Survival: Cardiopulmonary Resuscitation Workshop for Caregivers of Children at Risk.Pediatr Qual Saf.2019;4:e141. doi: 10.1097/pq9.0000000000000141
35. Dracup K, Moser DK, Doering LV, Guzy PM.Comparison of cardiopulmonary resuscitation training methods for parents of infants at high risk for cardiopulmonary arrest.Ann Emerg Med.1998;32:170-177. doi: 10.1016/s0196-0644(98)70133-7
36. Dracup K, Moser DK, Guzy PM, Taylor SE, Marsden C. Is cardiopulmonary resuscitation training deleterious for family members of cardiac patients? Am J Public Health.1994;6:1184-118. doi: 10.2105/ajph.84.1.116
37. Higgins SS, Hardy CE, Higashino SM.Should parents of children with congenital heart disease and life-threatening dysrhythmias be taught cardiopulmonary resuscitation? Pediatrics.1989;84:1102-1104.
38. McLauchlan CA, Ward A, Murphy NM, Griffith MJ, Skinner DV, Camm AJ.Resuscitation training for cardiac patients and their relatives-its effect on anxiety.Resuscitation.1992;24:7-11. doi: 10.1016/0300-9572(92)90168-c
39. Pierick TA, Van Waning N, Patel SS, Atkins DL.Self-instructional CPR training for parents of high risk infants.Resuscitation.2012;83:1140-1144. doi: 10.1016/j.resuscitation.2012.02.007
40. Renshaw AA, Mena-Allauca M, Gould EW, Sirintrapun SJ.Synoptic Reporting: Evidence-Based Review and Future Directions.JCO Clin Cancer Inform.2018;2:1-9. doi: 10.1200/CCI.17.00088
41. Baldi E, Cornara S, Contri E, Epis F, Fina D, Zelaschi B, Dossena C, Fichtner F, Tonani M, Di Maggio M, Zambaiti E, Somaschini A. Real-time visual feedback during training improves laypersons' CPR quality: a randomized controlled manikin study.CJEM.2017;19:480-487. doi: 10.1017/cem.2016.410
42. Saraç L. Effects of augmented feedback on cardiopulmonary resuscitation skill acquisition: concurrent versus terminal.Eurasian J Educ Res.2017;72:83-106.
43. Yeung J, Davies R, Gao F, Perkins GD.A randomised control trial of prompt and feedback devices and their impact on quality of chest compressions—a simulation study.Resuscitation.2014;85:553-559. doi: 10.1016/j.resuscitation.2014.01.015
44. Mpotos N, Yde L, Calle P, Deschepper E, Valcke M, Peersman W, Herregods L, Monsieurs K. Retraining basic life support skills using video, voice feedback or both: a randomised controlled trial.Resuscitation.2013;84:72-77. doi: 10.1016/j.resuscitation.2012.08.320
45. Zhou XL, Wang J, Jin XQ, Zhao Y, Liu RL, Jiang C. Quality retention of chest compression after repetitive practices with or without feedback devices: A randomized manikin study.Am J Emerg Med.2020;38:73-78. doi: 10.1016/j.ajem.2019.04.025
46. Wik L, Myklebust H, Auestad BH, Steen PA.Retention of basic life support skills 6 months after training with an automated voice advisory manikin system without instructor involvement.Resuscitation.2002;52:273-279. doi: 10.1016/s0300-9572(01)00476-2
47. Williamson LJ, Larsen PD, Tzeng YC, Galletly DC.Effect of automatic external defibrillator audio prompts on cardiopulmonary resuscitation performance.Emerg Med J. 2005;22:140-143. doi: 10.1136/emj.2004.016444
48. Rawlins L, Woollard M, Williams J, Hallam P. Effect of listening to Nellie the Elephant during CPR training on performance of chest compressions by lay people: randomised crossover trial.BMJ.2009;339:b4707. doi: 10.1136/bmj.b4707
49. Woollard M, Poposki J, McWhinnie B, Rawlins L, Munro G, O'Meara P. Achy breaky makey wakey heart? A randomised crossover trial of musical prompts. Emerg Med J. 2012;29:290-294. doi: 10.1136/emermed-2011-200187
50. Oh JH, Lee SJ, Kim SE, Lee KJ, Choe JW, Kim CW.Effects of audio tone guidance on performance of CPR in simulated cardiac arrest with an advanced airway.Resuscitation.2008;79:273-277. doi: 10.1016/j.resuscitation.2008.06.022
51. Hafner JW, Jou AC, Wang H, Bleess BB, Tham SK.Death before disco: the effectiveness of a musical metronome in layperson cardiopulmonary resuscitation training.J Emerg Med.2015;48:43-52. doi: 10.1016/j.jemermed.2014.07.048
52. Hong CK, Hwang SY, Lee KY, Kim YS, Ha YR, Park SO.Metronome vs. popular song: a comparison of long-term retention of chest compression skills after layperson training for cardiopulmonary resuscitation.Hong Kong J Emerg Med.2016;32:145-152.
53. Papadimitriou L, Xanthos T, Bassiakou E, Stroumpoulis K, Barouxis D, Iacovidou N. Distribution of pre-course BLS/AED manuals does not influence skill acquisition and retention in lay rescuers: a randomised study.Resuscitation.2010;81:348-352. doi: 10.1016/j.resuscitation.2009.11.020
54. Hsieh MJ, Chiang WC, Jan CF, Lin HY, Yang CW, Ma MH.The effect of different retraining intervals on the skill performance of cardiopulmonary resuscitation in laypeople–A three-armed randomized control study.Resuscitation.2018;128:151-157. doi: 10.1016/j.resuscitation.2018.05.010
55. Niles D, Sutton RM, Donoghue A, Kalsi MS, Roberts K, Boyle L, Nishisaki A, Arbogast KB, Helfaer M, Nadkarni V. "Rolling Refreshers": a novel approach to maintain CPR psychomotor skill competence.Resuscitation.2009;80:909-912. doi: 10.1016/j.resuscitation.2009.04.021
56. Woollard M, Whitfield R, Newcombe RG, Colquhoun M, Vetter N, Chamberlain D. Optimal refresher training intervals for AED and CPR skills: a randomised controlled trial.Resuscitation.2006;71:237-247. doi: 10.1016/j.resuscitation.2006.04.005
57. Chamberlain D, Smith A, Woollard M, Colquhoun M, Handley AJ, Leaves S, Kern KB.Trials of teaching methods in basic life support (3): comparison of simulated CPR performance after first training and at 6 months, with a note on the value of re-training.Resuscitation.2002;53:179-187. doi: 10.1016/s0300-9572(02)00025-4
58. Naim MY, Burke RV, McNally BF, Song L, Griffis HM, Berg RA, Vellano K, Markenson D, Bradley RN, Rossano JW.Association of Bystander Cardiopulmonary Resuscitation With Overall and Neurologically Favorable Survival After Pediatric Out-of-Hospital Cardiac Arrest in the United States: A Report From the Cardiac Arrest Registry to Enhance Survival Surveillance Registry. JAMA Pediatr.2017;171:133-141. doi: 10.1001/jamapediatrics.2016.3643
59. Swor RA, Jackson RE, Cynar M, Sadler E, Basse E, Boji B, Rivera-Rivera EJ, Maher A, Grubb W, Jacobson R. Bystander CPR, ventricular fibrillation, and survival in witnessed, unmonitored out-of-hospital cardiac arrest.Ann Emerg Med.1995;25:780-784. doi: 10.1016/s0196-0644(95)70207-5
60. McCarthy JJ, Carr B, Sasson C, Bobrow BJ, Callaway CW, Neumar RW, Ferrer JME, Garvey JL, Ornato JP, Gonzales L, Granger CB, Kleinman ME, Bjerke C, Nichol G; American Heart Association Emergency Cardiovascular Care Committee; Council on Cardiopulmonary, Critical Care, Perioperative and Resuscitation; and the Mission: Lifeline Resuscitation Subcommittee.Out-of-Hospital Cardiac Arrest Resuscitation Systems of Care: A Scientific Statement From the American Heart Association.Circulation.2018;137:e645-e660. doi: 10.1161/CIR.0000000000000557

チームワークおよびリーダーシップトレーニング

COR	LOE	推奨事項
2a	B-NR	1. 特定のチームおよびリーダーシップトレーニングを医療従事者向けの二次救命処置トレーニングに組み込むことは妥当である[1-15]。

「概要」

心停止患者の蘇生を行うには，複数のプロバイダーが連携して一刻を争う治療を施す必要がある。そのため，チームワークとリーダーシップは最適なケアを提供するために不可欠な要素である[16-18]。チームを協調的なユニットとして機能させるために必要なコミュニケーションおよび対人能力に焦点を合わせたトレーニングは，患者転帰に潜在的な影響を及ぼす可能性がある[19-21]。チームおよびリーダーシップトレーニングを医療従事者向けの二次救命処置トレーニ

ングに組み込んだ場合の効果を評価した研究では，心停止のシミュレーションおよび実際の心停止現場においてプロバイダーのスキルに良い影響を与えることがわかった[1-15,22]。これらの研究では，幅広い教育戦略（ビデオモジュール，シミュレーションなど）とアウトカム評価項目（コミュニケーションの質，推奨される二次救命処置方法の遵守など）が用いられた。エビデンスの質は低から中等度ではあるが，チームおよびリーダーシップトレーニングを医療従事者向けの二次救命処置トレーニングに組み込むことを推奨する。チームおよびリーダーシップトレーニングの潜在的有益性は潜在的リスクを大きく上回るため，この推奨は妥当である。チームおよびリーダーシップトレーニングの最適な教育戦略を定義するため，およびプロバイダースキルと患者転帰に対するチームトレーニング，リーダーシップトレーニング，スキルトレーニング間の相互作用や相対的有益性を理解するために，さらなる研究が必要である。

「推奨事項の裏付けとなる解説」

1. いくつかの研究で，チームまたはリーダーシップトレーニングが実際の心停止現場での患者転帰またはプロバイダースキルに及ぼす影響が検討されている。1件の前向き観察研究において，病院全体での正式なモックコード（模擬学習）チームトレーニングプログラムを実施した後1年間で小児の心停止からの生存率が33％から約50％に上昇したことが報告されている（P = 0.00）[1]。シミュレーションベースのリーダーシップトレーニングについて調べた1件のRCTでは，患者の蘇生処置中のCPRの質に対する効果は認められなかった[6]。4件の観察研究において，チームワークとCPRの質，コミュニケーション，および機械的器具の適用時間の改善を図る介入の間に関連性が見られた[2-5]。

   7件のRCTと1件の多施設前向き介入研究で，チームおよびリーダーシップトレーニングが蘇生シミュレーションにおける臨床タスクのパフォーマンスに及ぼす影響が，コース修了時と3～15カ月後のフォローアップの時点に評価された[7-14]。それぞれの研究で1つ以上のパフォーマンスの側面の改善が認められたが，改善はすべての評価基準にわたって普遍的なものではなかった。改善は，臨床ケアの特定の側面（CPRの開始までの時間，除細動までの時間など）[7-13]とACLSガイドラインの遵守[12-14]の両方で見られた。10件のRCTで，チームまたはリーダーシップトレーニングは，蘇生シミュレーション中のチームワークおよびリーダーシップ評価基準の改善と関連性があった。具体的には，リーダーの発声の頻度[8,10,14]，特定のチームスキルの頻度[7,11,13,23]，および各種チームワーク評価スケールのスコアの改善に関連していた[9,11,12,15]。

参考資料

1. Andreatta P, Saxton E, Thompson M, Annich G. Simulation-based mock codes significantly correlate with improved pediatric patient cardiopulmonary arrest survival rates.Pediatr Crit Care Med.2011;12:33-38. doi: 10.1097/PCC.0b013e3181e89270
2. Nadler I, Sanderson PM, Van Dyken CR, Davis PG, Liley HG.Presenting video recordings of newborn resuscitations in debriefings for teamwork training. BMJ Qual Saf.2011;20:163-169. doi: 10.1136/bmjqs.2010.043547
3. Ong ME, Quah JL, Annathurai A, Noor NM, Koh ZX, Tan KB, Pothiawala S, Poh AH, Loy CK, Fook-Chong S. Improving the quality of cardiopulmonary resuscitation by training dedicated cardiac arrest teams incorporating a mechanical load-distributing device at the emergency department.Resuscitation.2013;84:508-514. doi: 10.1016/j.resuscitation.2012.07.033
4. Su L, Spaeder MC, Jones MB, Sinha P, Nath DS, Jain PN, Berger JT, Williams L, Shankar V. Implementation of an extracorporeal cardiopulmonary resuscitation simulation program reduces extracorporeal cardiopulmonary resuscitation times in real patients.Pediatr Crit Care Med.2014;15:856-860. doi: 10.1097/PCC.0000000000000234
5. Spitzer CR, Evans K, Buehler J, Ali NA, Besecker BY.Code blue pit crew model: A novel approach to in-hospital cardiac arrest resuscitation.Resuscitation.2019;143:158-164. doi: 10.1016/j.resuscitation.2019.06.290
6. Weidman EK, Bell G, Walsh D, Small S, Edelson DP.Assessing the impact of immersive simulation on clinical performance during actual in-hospital cardiac arrest with CPR-sensing technology: A randomized feasibility study.Resuscitation.2010;81:1556-1561. doi: 10.1016/j.resuscitation.2010.05.021
7. Thomas EJ, Williams AL, Reichman EF, Lasky RE, Crandell S, Taggart WR.Team training in the neonatal resuscitation program for interns: teamwork and quality of resuscitations.Pediatrics.2010;125:539-546. doi: 10.1542/peds.2009-1635
8. Hunziker S, Bühlmann C, Tschan F, Balestra G, Legeret C, Schumacher C, Semmer NK, Hunziker P, Marsch S. Brief leadership instructions improve cardiopulmonary resuscitation in a high-fidelity simulation: a randomized controlled trial.Crit Care Med.2010;38:1086-1091. doi: 10.1097/CCM.0b013e3181cf7383
9. Blackwood J, Duff JP, Nettel-Aguirre A, Djogovic D, Joynt C. Does teaching crisis resource management skills improve resuscitation performance in pediatric residents?*.Pediatr Crit Care Med.2014;15:e168-e174. doi: 10.1097/PCC.0000000000000100
10. Fernandez Castelao E, Russo SG, Cremer S, Strack M, Kaminski L, Eich C, Timmermann A, Boos M. Positive impact of crisis resource management training on no-flow time and team member verbalisations during simulated cardiopulmonary resuscitation: a randomised controlled trial.Resuscitation.2011;82:1338-1343. doi: 10.1016/j.resuscitation.2011.05.009
11. Haffner L, Mahling M, Muench A, Castan C, Schubert P, Naumann A, Reddersen S, Herrmann-Werner A, Reutershan J, Riessen R, Celebi N. Improved recognition of ineffective chest compressions after a brief Crew Resource Management (CRM) training: a prospective, randomised simulation study. BMC Emerg Med.2017;17:7. doi: 10.1186/s12873-017-0117-6
12. Gilfoyle E, Koot DA, Annear JC, Bhanji F, Cheng A, Duff JP, Grant VJ, St George-Hyslop CE, Delaloye NJ, Kotsakis A, McCoy CD, Ramsay CE, Weiss MJ, Gottesman RD; Teams4Kids Investigators and the Canadian Critical Care Trials Group.Improved Clinical Performance and Teamwork of Pediatric Interprofessional Resuscitation Teams With a Simulation-Based Educational Intervention.Pediatr Crit Care Med.2017;18:e62-e69. doi: 10.1097/PCC.0000000000001025
13. Jankouskas TS, Haidet KK, Hupcey JE, Kolanowski A, Murray WB.Targeted crisis resource management training improves performance among randomized nursing and medical students.Simul Healthc.2011;6:316-326. doi: 10.1097/SIH.0b013e31822bc676
14. Fernandez Castelao E, Boos M, Ringer C, Eich C, Russo SG.Effect of CRM team leader training on team performance and leadership behavior in simulated cardiac arrest scenarios: a prospective, randomized, controlled study. BMC Med Educ.2015;15:116. doi: 10.1186/s12909-015-0389-z
15. Cooper S. Developing leaders for advanced life support: evaluation of a training programme.Resuscitation.2001;49:33-38. doi: 10.1016/s0300-9572(00)00345-2
16. Bhanji F, Finn JC, Lockey A, Monsieurs K, Frengley R, Iwami T, Lang E, Ma MH, Mancini ME, McNeil MA, et al; on behalf of the Education, Implementation, and Teams Chapter Collaborators.Part 8: education, implementation, and teams: 2015 International Consensus on Cardiopulmonary Resuscitation and Emergency Cardiovascular Care Science With Treatment Recommendations.Circulation.2015;132 (suppl 1):S242-S268. doi: 10.1161/CIR.0000000000000277
17. Bhanji F, Donoghue AJ, Wolff MS, Flores GE, Halamek LP, Berman JM, Sinz EH, Cheng A. Part 14: education: 2015 American Heart Association Guidelines Update for Cardiopulmonary Resuscitation and Emergency Cardiovascular Care.Circulation.2015;132 (suppl 2):S561-573. doi: 10.1161/CIR.0000000000000268

18. Cheng A, Donoghue A, Gilfoyle E, Eppich W. Simulation-based crisis resource management training for pediatric critical care medicine: a review for instructors.Pediatr Crit Care Med.2012;13:197–203. doi: 10.1097/PCC.0b013e3182192832
19. Rosen MA, DiazGranados D, Dietz AS, Benishek LE, Thompson D, Pronovost PJ, Weaver SJ.Teamwork in healthcare: Key discoveries enabling safer, high-quality care.Am Psychol.2018;73:433–450. doi: 10.1037/amp0000298
20. Salas E, DiazGranados D, Weaver SJ, King H. Does team training work? Principles for health care.Acad Emerg Med.2008;15:1002–1009. doi: 10.1111/j.1553-2712.2008.00254.x
21. Marlow SL, Hughes AM, Sonesh SC, Gregory ME, Lacerenza CN, Benishek LE, Woods AL, Hernandez C, Salas E. A Systematic Review of Team Training in Health Care: Ten Questions.Jt Comm J Qual Patient Saf.2017;43:197–204. doi: 10.1016/j.jcjq.2016.12.004
22. Greif R, Bhanji F, Bigham BL, Bray J, Breckwoldt J, Cheng A, Duff JP, Gilfoyle E, Hsieh M-J, Iwami T, et al; on behalf of the Education, Implementation, and Teams Collaborators.Education, implementation, and teams: 2020 International Consensus on Cardiopulmonary Resuscitation and Emergency Cardiovascular Care Science With Treatment Recommendations.Circulation.2020;142(suppl 1):S222–S283. doi: 10.1161/CIR.0000000000000896
23. Thomas EJ, Taggart B, Crandell S, Lasky RE, Williams AL, Love LJ, Sexton JB, Tyson JE, Helmreich RL.Teaching teamwork during the Neonatal Resuscitation Program: a randomized trial.J Perinatol.2007;27:409–414. doi: 10.1038/sj.jp.7211771

現場教育

現場教育に関する推奨事項		
COR	LOE	推奨事項
2a	C-LD	1. 従来のトレーニングに加えて、現場でのシミュレーションに基づく蘇生トレーニングを実施することは妥当である[1-12]。
2b	B-R	2. 従来のトレーニングの代わりに、現場でのシミュレーションに基づく蘇生トレーニングを実施することが妥当な場合がある[13-15]。

「概要」

現場シミュレーションとは、シミュレーショントレーニングのひとつで、実際の患者治療エリア（実際の臨床環境）で行うシミュレーションのことである[16]。現場シミュレーションは、個人および／または医療チームをトレーニングする戦略として使用できる[17,18]。現場トレーニングは、プロバイダー個人の技術的スキルまたはチームベースのスキル（コミュニケーション、リーダーシップ、役割の割り当て、状況認識など）を目的とすることができる[17,18]。現場トレーニングの明白な利点のひとつは、より現実に近いトレーニング環境を学習者に提供することである。本レビューでは、現場シミュレーションに基づく医療従事者向けの蘇生トレーニングが学習、パフォーマンス、および／または患者転帰の向上につながるかどうかを検討した。

現場トレーニングと従来のトレーニング教室または実習室ベースのトレーニングを比較した研究では、学習成果に有意差はなかった[13-15]。介入なしと比較した場合、他の教育戦略に追加した現場トレーニングは、学習成果（チームパフォーマンスの向上、重要タスクまでの時間の短縮など）[2,7-12]、実際の臨床環境での行動の変化（チームパフォーマンスの向上、悪化しつつある患者の認識など）[2-4]、および患者転帰（生存率の向上、神経学的転帰など）に良い影響を与えた[1,4-6]。現場トレーニングの利点は、潜在的リスクと比較検討する必要がある。このようなリスクには、臨床現場でのトレーニングの実施に伴うロジスティクス上の課題や、トレーニングリソースを実際の臨床リソースと混同するリスク（シミュレーション用の薬剤や輸液と実際の薬剤や輸液との混同など）が挙げられる[19,20]。

「推奨事項の裏付けとなる解説」

1. 3件の観察研究で、定期的な現場シミュレーショントレーニングを他の教育戦略（BLS／PALSの再教育トレーニング、コードチームの導入、分散練習）と組み合わせた場合、チームパフォーマンスの向上、および悪化しつつある患者を認識するまでの時間の短縮という点で効果的であることが実証されている[2-4]。現場トレーニングを含むバンドル介入を評価した別の4件の観察研究では、心停止生存率の有意な改善が認められた[1,4-6]。これらの研究では、現場トレーニングはバンドル介入の一部として評価されたため、現場トレーニング単独の貢献度は明確に判断できない。

  2件のRCTにおいて、現場での心停止トレーニングと反復学習の組み合わせは、教室で集中学習の形式で実施されたトレーニングと比較して、学習成果が高かった（臨床パフォーマンスの向上、圧迫および除細動を開始するまでの時間の短縮）[8,9]。1件のRCTと4件の前向き観察研究で、現場シミュレーショントレーニングはシミュレーション環境において臨床パフォーマンスを向上させることが示された[2,7,10-12]。ほとんどの観察研究は、並行対照群の欠如、裏付けとなる妥当性エビデンスを伴うパフォーマンス評価基準の欠如、および潜在的な交絡因子により、限界がある。

2. 現場シミュレーショントレーニングの学習成果（チームパフォーマンス、技術的スキル）を標準的な教室トレーニングまたは検査室ベースのトレーニング環境と比較した2件のRCTと1件の観察研究では、2つの環境の間に有意差は認められなかった[13-15]。

参考資料

1. Andreatta P, Saxton E, Thompson M, Annich G. Simulation-based mock codes significantly correlate with improved pediatric patient cardiopulmonary arrest survival rates.Pediatr Crit Care Med.2011;12:33–38. doi: 10.1097/PCC.0b013e3181e89270
2. Steinemann S, Berg B, Skinner A, DiTulio A, Anzelon K, Terada K, Oliver C, Ho HC, Speck C. In situ, multidisciplinary, simulation-based teamwork training improves early trauma care.J Surg Educ.2011;68:472–477. doi: 10.1016/j.jsurg.2011.05.009
3. Theilen U, Leonard P, Jones P, Ardill R, Weitz J, Agrawal D, Simpson D. Regular in situ simulation training of paediatric medical emergency team improves hospital response to deteriorating patients.Resuscitation.2013;84:218–222. doi: 10.1016/j.resuscitation.2012.06.027

4. Knight LJ, Gabhart JM, Earnest KS, Leong KM, Anglemyer A, Franzon D. Improving code team performance and survival outcomes: implementation of pediatric resuscitation team training.Crit Care Med.2014;42:243-251. doi: 10.1097/CCM.0b013e3182a6439d
5. Sodhi K, Singla MK, Shrivastava A. Institutional resuscitation protocols: do they affect cardiopulmonary resuscitation outcomes? A 6-year study in a single tertiary-care centre.J Anesth.2015;29:87-95. doi: 10.1007/s00540-014-1873-z
6. Josey K, Smith ML, Kayani AS, Young G, Kasperski MD, Farrer P, Gerkin R, Theodorou A, Raschke RA.Hospitals with more-active participation in conducting standardized in-situ mock codes have improved survival after in-hospital cardiopulmonary arrest.Resuscitation.2018;133:47-52. doi: 10.1016/j.resuscitation.2018.09.020
7. Clarke SO, Julie IM, Yao AP, Bang H, Barton JD, Alsomali SM, Kiefer MV, Al Khulaif AH, Aljahany M, Venugopal S, Bair AE.Longitudinal exploration of in situ mock code events and the performance of cardiac arrest skills.BMJ Simul Technol Enhanc Learn.2019;5:29-33. doi: 10.1136/bmjstel-2017-000255
8. Kurosawa H, Ikeyama T, Achuff P, Perkel M, Watson C, Monachino A, Remy D, Deutsch E, Buchanan N, Anderson J, Berg RA, Nadkarni VM, Nishisaki A. A randomized, controlled trial of in situ pediatric advanced life support recertification ("pediatric advanced life support reconstructed") compared with standard pediatric advanced life support recertification for ICU frontline providers*.Crit Care Med.2014;42:610-618. doi: 10.1097/CCM.0000000000000024
9. Sullivan NJ, Duval-Arnould J, Twilley M, Smith SP, Aksamit D, Boone-Guercio P, Jeffries PR, Hunt EA.Simulation exercise to improve retention of cardiopulmonary resuscitation priorities for in-hospital cardiac arrests: A randomized controlled trial.Resuscitation.2015;86:6-13. doi: 10.1016/j.resuscitation.2014.10.021
10. Rubio-Gurung S, Putet G, Touzet S, Gauthier-Moulinier H, Jordan I, Beissel A, Labaune JM, Blanc S, Amamra N, Balandras C, Rudigoz RC, Colin C, Picaud JC.In situ simulation training for neonatal resuscitation: an RCT. Pediatrics.2014;134:e790-e797. doi: 10.1542/peds.2013-3988
11. Saqe-Rockoff A, Ciardiello AV, Schubert FD.Low-Fidelity, In-Situ Pediatric Resuscitation Simulation Improves RN Competence and Self-Efficacy.J Emerg Nurs.2019;45:538-544.e1. doi: 10.1016/j.jen.2019.02.003
12. Katznelson JH, Wang J, Stevens MW, Mills WA.Improving Pediatric Preparedness in Critical Access Hospital Emergency Departments: Impact of a Longitudinal In Situ Simulation Program.Pediatr Emerg Care.2018;34:17-20. doi: 10.1097/PEC.0000000000001366
13. Crofts JF, Ellis D, Draycott TJ, Winter C, Hunt LP, Akande VA.Change in knowledge of midwives and obstetricians following obstetric emergency training: a randomised controlled trial of local hospital, simulation centre and teamwork training.BJOG.2007;114:1534-1541. doi: 10.1111/j.1471-0528.2007.01493.x
14. Ellis D, Crofts JF, Hunt LP, Read M, Fox R, James M. Hospital, simulation center, and teamwork training for eclampsia management: a randomized controlled trial.Obstet Gynecol.2008;111:723-731. doi: 10.1097/AOG.0b013e3181637a82
15. Couto TB, Kerrey BT, Taylor RG, FitzGerald M, Geis GL.Teamwork skills in actual, in situ, and in-center pediatric emergencies: performance levels across settings and perceptions of comparative educational impact.Simul Healthc.2015;10:76-84. doi: 10.1097/SIH.0000000000000081
16. Kurup V, Matei V, Ray J. Role of in-situ simulation for training in healthcare: opportunities and challenges.Curr Opin Anaesthesiol.2017;30:755-760. doi: 10.1097/ACO.0000000000000514
17. Goldshtein D, Krensky C, Doshi S, Perelman VS.In situ simulation and its effects on patient outcomes: a systematic review.BMJ Simulation and Technology Enhanced Learning.2020;6:3-9. doi: 10.1136/bmjstel-2018-000387
18. Rosen MA, Hunt EA, Pronovost PJ, Federowicz MA, Weaver SJ.In situ simulation in continuing education for the health care professions: a systematic review.J Contin Educ Health Prof. 2012;32:243-254. doi: 10.1002/chp.21152
19. U.S. Food and Drug Administration.Simulated IV solutions from Wallcur: CDER statement—FDA's investigation into patients being injected.2015. https://www.fdanews.com/ext/resources/files/01-15/01-15-2015-Saline-Safety-Warning.pdf?152088501.Accessed February 11, 2020.
20. Petrosoniak A, Auerbach M, Wong AH, Hicks CM.In situ simulation in emergency medicine: Moving beyond the simulation lab.Emerg Med Australas.2017;29:83-88. doi: 10.1111/1742-6723.12705

マネキンの忠実度

COR	LOE	推奨事項
2a	B-R	1. 忠実度の高いマネキンを二次救命処置トレーニングに使用することは，運用基盤と人員が整っているトレーニングセンターでは受講者に有益となりうる[1-4]。
2b	C-LD	2. コスト，人員，入手可能性，その他の問題によって忠実度の高いマネキンを使用できないトレーニングセンターでは，忠実度の低いマネキンを二次救命処置トレーニングに使用することを検討してもよい[1,3]。
2b	C-EO	3. インストラクターが，学習目的を個々の受講者グループのニーズに合わせるため，それに即した方法でマネキンおよびマネキン機能を使用することは妥当としてよい[1,5,6]。

「概要」

蘇生教育における学習者の学びへの集中は，トレーニング経験の現実感を高めることで強化される[1]。忠実度（現実性）の分類として，（a）概念的な忠実度（シミュレーションで表現される概念と関係），（b）精神的な忠実度（シミュレーションの全人的な経験），（c）物理的な忠実度（マネキンの特性と環境）の3つが論じられている[7]。マネキンは，患者の身体の全体または一部を模したものである[8]。「マネキンの忠実度」という用語は，蘇生患者をより忠実に再現した模擬的な身体的特徴の存在を意味するために使われている[2]。高度な身体的特徴を備えた忠実度の高いマネキンは，幅広い年齢群（新生児，乳児，小児，成人など）の患者の生理的状態（外傷性負傷，妊娠，心停止など）のシミュレーションを可能とする。忠実度の高いマネキンを使用すると，理論上，シナリオベースの学習において学習者の集中や関与が向上する可能性がある。忠実度の高いマネキンの欠点としては，購入によるコストの増加，マネキンを扱うトレーニングを受けた人員の必要性，および継続的な保守の必要性が挙げられる[1]。

忠実度の高いマネキンが蘇生教育に及ぼす影響について調べた研究は，結果が一貫していない。最近のシステマティックレビューによると，忠実度の高いマネキンを蘇生トレーニングに使用した場合，コース修了時のスキル習得は向上したが，長期的なスキルまたは知識に対する影響は認められなかった[2]。今回ガイドラインを改訂するにあたり，受講者の知識と精神運動領域のスキルに対するマネキン忠実度の影響を調べたRCTが2件見つかったが，結果は一貫していない[3,4]。患者転帰に対するマネキン忠実度の影響を評価した研究はまだない。忠実度の高いマネキンの使用は，入手可能性や運用基盤によってその使用が許される場合には有益となる可能性がある。この推奨は，コストとマネキン操作者のトレーニング要件，およびマネキンの特徴を学習目的と正確に一致させる必要性との間でバランスをとる必要がある。

「推奨事項の裏付けとなる解説」
1. 忠実度の高いマネキンが蘇生教育に及ぼす影響を評価した研究のメタアナリシスによると，コース修了時のスキルパフォーマンスについては適度の有益性が認められたが，長期的なスキルまたは知識に対する影響はなかった[2]。このレビューでは，コストの増加と，忠実度の高いマネキンを扱うトレーニングを受けた人員の必要性が認められた。1件のPALSトレーニングに関する非無作為化試験で，忠実度の高い乳児マネキンを使用し医療介入を訓練した受講者と，標準マネキンを操作し訓練した受講者の間で，知識（試験スコア）およびスキル（タスク実施時間）が比較された。コース修了時の知識またはスキルには差は見られなかったが，コース修了後6カ月時点の知識は高忠実度群のほうが高かった[4]。
2. 新生児蘇生プログラムのトレーニングを受けた医学生のRCTにおいて，忠実度の高いマネキン（バイタルサイン，チアノーゼ，四肢の動き，および呼吸音を観察できるマネキン）を使用した介入群受講者と，このような機能のない簡易的なマネキンを使用した対照群受講者の間で知識（試験スコア）およびスキル（メガコードスコア）が比較された。コース修了時または3カ月時点のスキルまたは知識について，医療介入を訓練した群と操作する訓練をした群の間に有意差は見られなかった[3]。
3. マネキン（身体的特徴）をシナリオおよび受講者の実習範囲のニーズに合わせて選択すると，受講者の学びへの集中を高めるために必要な身体的特徴が確実に用意される[6]。

参考資料
1. Cheng A, Nadkarni VM, Mancini MB, Hunt EA, Sinz EH, Merchant RM, Donoghue A, Duff JP, Eppich W, Auerbach M, Bigham BL, Blewer AL, Chan PS, Bhanji F; American Heart Association Education Science Investigators; and on behalf of the American Heart Association Education Science and Programs Committee, Council on Cardiopulmonary, Critical Care, Perioperative and Resuscitation; Council on Cardiovascular and Stroke Nursing; and Council on Quality of Care and Outcomes Research.Resuscitation Education Science: Educational Strategies to Improve Outcomes From Cardiac Arrest: A Scientific Statement From the American Heart Association. Circulation.2018;138:e82-e122. doi: 10.1161/CIR.0000000000000583
2. Cheng A, Lockey A, Bhanji F, Lin Y, Hunt EA, Lang E. The use of high-fidelity manikins for advanced life support training-A systematic review and meta-analysis.Resuscitation.2015;93:142-149. doi: 10.1016/j.resuscitation.2015.04.004
3. Nimbalkar A, Patel D, Kungwani A, Phatak A, Vasa R, Nimbalkar S. Randomized control trial of high fidelity vs low fidelity simulation for training undergraduate students in neonatal resuscitation.BMC Res Notes.2015;8:636. doi: 10.1186/s13104-015-1623-9
4. Stellflug SM, Lowe NK.The Effect of High Fidelity Simulators on Knowledge Retention and Skill Self Efficacy in Pediatric Advanced Life Support Courses in a Rural State.J Pediatr Nurs.2018;39:21-26. doi: 10.1016/j.pedn.2017.12.006
5. Donoghue AJ, Durbin DR, Nadel FM, Stryjewski GR, Kost SI, Nadkarni VM.Perception of realism during mock resuscitations by pediatric housestaff: the impact of simulated physical features.Simul Healthc.2010;5:16-20. doi: 10.1097/SIH.0b013e3181a46aa1
6. Hamstra SJ, Brydges R, Hatala R, Zendejas B, Cook DA. Reconsidering fidelity in simulation-based training. Acad Med. 2014;89:387-392. doi: 10.1097/ACM.0000000000000130
7. Rudolph JW, Simon R, Raemer DB. Which reality matters? Questions on the path to high engagement in healthcare simulation. Simul Healthc. 2007;2:161-163. doi: 10.1097/SIH.0b013e31813d1035
8. Lopreiato JO. Heatlhcare Simulation Dictionary. Rockville, MD: Agency for Healthcare Research and Quality; 2016. https://www.ahrq.gov/sites/default/files/publications/files/sim-dictionary.pdf.Accessed April 27, 2020.

トレーニングにおけるCPRフィードバック器具

トレーニングにおけるCPRフィードバック器具に関する推奨事項		
COR	LOE	推奨事項
2a	B-R	1. トレーニング中にフィードバック器具を使用すると，CPRのパフォーマンスを向上する効果が得られる[1-10]。

「概要」
CPRスキルの正確な評価は，学習者がパフォーマンスを向上させるために不可欠である[11]。これまでの研究から，目視によるCPRの質の評価は信頼できず不正確であることが明らかになっており，インストラクターがCPRトレーニング中にどのようにして意味のあるフィードバックを一貫して提供するかが課題となっている[12-15]。フィードバック器具は，実習中に客観的なフィードバックを学習者とインストラクターに提供することで，この問題を解決する。CPRフィードバック器具は，修正フィードバック器具（深さの視覚的表示など）と，学習者が追従すべき音を発する指示器（メトロノームなど）の2種類に分けられる。本レビューでは，トレーニング中にCPRフィードバック器具を使用した場合に，CPRフィードバック器具を使用しない場合と比較してCPRスキル，臨床パフォーマンス，および患者転帰が改善するかどうかを評価した[16]。

トレーニング中のCPRフィードバック器具の使用について調べた研究は結果が一貫しておらず，8件中6件でトレーニング終了時のCPRスキルパフォーマンスの向上が報告されている[1-6,17,18]。トレーニング中にコレクティブフィードバック器具を使用した場合，初期トレーニング後7日から3カ月の時点でのスキル定着は，フィードバック器具を使用しなかった場合よりも高かった[2,6-10,19]。トレーニング中のフィードバック器具の使用の費用対効果，または臨床環境における医療従事者のパフォーマンスと患者転帰に対する影響について報告した研究はまだない。トレーニング中のフィードバック器具の使用については，その利点と，フィードバック器具のコスト，およびCPRトレーニング中の学習者に生じる認知処理の増加との間のバランスをとる必要がある。

「推奨事項の裏付けとなる解説」
1. 7件のRCTと1件の観察研究で，トレーニング中にフィードバック器具を使用した場合とトレーニング中またはインストラクター主導トレーニング中にフィードバック器具を使用しない場合が比較されている[1-6,17,18]。そのうち6件の研究では，コース修了時のCPRスキルはトレーニング中にフィードバック器具を使用した場合

のほうが有意に高かったが[1-6]，残り2件では，CPRフィードバック器具の使用について有益性は認められなかった[17,18]。5件のRCTと2件の観察研究において，トレーニング中のフィードバック器具の使用は7日から3カ月後の時点のCPRスキル定着の有意な向上と関連性があった[2,6-10,19]。

これらのうち一部の研究では，市民救助者，年少受講者，または医学生が母集団とされており，得られた結果を実際の医療従事者に一般化するには限界がある[2,3,5,9,10,17-19]。その他に，リアルタイムのフィードバックを他の教育戦略と組み合わせた研究もあるが[6,19]，フィードバック器具の使用が及ぼす真の影響を分離することは難しい。今後，トレーニング中のCPRフィードバック器具の使用を実際の患者転帰や医療従事者の臨床パフォーマンスに結び付ける研究や，トレーニング中のフィードバック器具の使用の費用対効果について調べる研究が必要となる。

参考資料

1. Cheng A, Brown LL, Duff JP, Davidson J, Overly F, Tofil NM, Peterson DT, White ML, Bhanji F, Bank I, et al; on behalf of the International Network for Simulation-Based Pediatric Innovation, Research, & Education (INSPIRE) CPR Investigators.Improving cardiopulmonary resuscitation with a CPR feedback device and refresher simulations (CPR CARES Study): a randomized clinical trial.JAMA Pediatr.2015;169:137-144. doi: 10.1001/jamapediatrics.2014.2616
2. Katipoglu B, Madziala MA, Evrin T, Gawlowski P, Szarpak A, Dabrowska A, Bialka S, Ladny JR, Szarpak L, Konert A, et al.How should we teach cardiopulmonary resuscitation? Randomized multi-center study.Cardiol J. 2019:Epub ahead of print. doi: 10.5603/CJ.a2019.0092
3. McCoy CE, Rahman A, Rendon JC, Anderson CL, Langdorf MI, Lotfipour S, Chakravarthy B. Randomized controlled trial of simulation vs. standard training for teaching medical students high-quality cardiopulmonary resuscitation.West J Emerg Med.2019;20:15-22. doi: 10.5811/westjem.2018.11.39040
4. Navarro-Patón R, Freire-Tellado M, Basanta-Camiño S, Barcala-Furelos R, Arufe-Giraldez V, Rodriguez-Fernández JE.Effect of 3basic life support training programs in future primary school teachers.A quasi-experimental design.Med Intensiva.2018;42:207-215. doi: 10.1016/j.medin.2017.06.005
5. Wagner M, Bibl K, Hrdliczka E, Steinbauer P, Stiller M, Gröpel P, Goeral K, Salzer-Muhar U, Berger A, Schmölzer GM, et al.Effects of feedback on chest compression quality: a randomized simulation study. Pediatrics.2019;143:e20182441. doi: 10.1542/peds.2018-2441
6. Lin Y, Cheng A, Grant VJ, Currie GR, Hecker KG.Improving CPR quality with distributed practice and real-time feedback in pediatric healthcare providers – A randomized controlled trial.Resuscitation.2018;130:6-12. doi: 10.1016/j.resuscitation.2018.06.025
7. Niles DE, Nishisaki A, Sutton RM, Elci OU, Meaney PA, O'Connor KA, Leffelman J, Kramer-Johansen J, Berg RA, Nadkarni V. Improved Retention of Chest Compression Psychomotor Skills With Brief "Rolling Refresher" Training.Simul Healthc.2017;12:213-219. doi: 10.1097/SIH.0000000000000228
8. Smart JR, Kranz K, Carmona F, Lindner TW, Newton A. Does real-time objective feedback and competition improve performance and quality in manikin CPR training-a prospective observational study from several European EMS.Scand J Trauma Resusc Emerg Med.2015;23:79. doi: 10.1186/s13049-015-0160-9
9. Smereka J, Szarpak L, Czekajlo M, Abelson A, Zwolinski P, Plusa T, Dunder D, Dabrowski M, Wiesniewska Z, Robak O, et al.The TrueCPR device in the process of teaching cardiopulmonary resuscitation: a randomized simulation trial.Medicine (Baltimore).2019;98:e15995. doi: 10.1097/MD.0000000000015995
10. Zhou XL, Wang J, Jin XQ, Zhao Y, Liu RL, Jiang C. Quality retention of chest compression after repetitive practices with or without feedback devices: A randomized manikin study.Am J Emerg Med.2020;38:73-78. doi: 10.1016/j.ajem.2019.04.025
11. Ende J. Feedback in clinical medical education.JAMA.1983;250:777-781.
12. Jones A, Lin Y, Nettel-Aguirre A, Gilfoyle E, Cheng A. Visual assessment of CPR quality during pediatric cardiac arrest: does point of view matter? Resuscitation.2015;90:50-55. doi: 10.1016/j.resuscitation.2015.01.036
13. Cheng A, Overly F, Kessler D, Nadkarni VM, Lin Y, Doan Q, Duff JP, Tofil NM, Bhanji F, Adler M, Charnovich A, Hunt EA, Brown LL; International Network for Simulation-based Pediatric Innovation, Research, Education (INSPIRE) CPR Investigators.Perception of CPR quality: Influence of CPR feedback, Just-in-Time CPR training and provider role.Resuscitation.2015;87:44-50. doi: 10.1016/j.resuscitation.2014.11.015
14. Hansen C, Bang C, Stærk M, Krogh K, Løfgren B. Certified Basic Life Support Instructors Identify Improper Cardiopulmonary Resuscitation Skills Poorly: Instructor Assessments Versus Resuscitation Manikin Data.Simul Healthc.2019;14:281-286. doi: 10.1097/SIH.0000000000000386
15. Cheng A, Kessler D, Lin Y, Tofil NM, Hunt EA, Davidson J, Chatfield J, Duff JP; International Network for Simulation-based Pediatric Innovation, Research and Education (INSPIRE) CPR Investigators.Influence of Cardiopulmonary Resuscitation Coaching and Provider Role on Perception of Cardiopulmonary Resuscitation Quality During Simulated Pediatric Cardiac Arrest.Pediatr Crit Care Med.2019;20:e191-e198. doi: 10.1097/PCC.0000000000001871
16. Greif R, Bhanji F, Bigham BL, Bray J, Breckwoldt J, Cheng A, Duff JP, Gilfoyle E, Hsieh M-J, Iwami T, et al; on behalf of the Education, Implementation, and Teams Collaborators.Education, implementation, and teams: 2020 International Consensus on Cardiopulmonary Resuscitation and Emergency Cardiovascular Care Science With Treatment Recommendations.Circulation.2020;142 (suppl 1):S222-S283. doi: 10.1161/CIR.0000000000000896
17. Min MK, Yeom SR, Ryu JH, Kim YI, Park MR, Han SK, Lee SH, Park SW, Park SC.Comparison between an instructor-led course and training using a voice advisory manikin in initial cardiopulmonary resuscitation skill acquisition.Clin Exp Emerg Med.2016;3:158-164. doi: 10.15441/ceem.15.114
18. Pavo N, Goliasch G, Nierscher FJ, Stumpf D, Haugk M, Breckwoldt J, Ruetzler K, Greif R, Fischer H. Short structured feedback training is equivalent to a mechanical feedback device in two-rescuer BLS: a randomised simulation study.Scand J Trauma Resusc Emerg Med.2016;24:70. doi: 10.1186/s13049-016-0265-9
19. Cortegiani A, Russotto V, Montalto F, Iozzo P, Meschis R, Pugliesi M, Mariano D, Benenati V, Raineri SM, Gregoretti C, Giarratano A. Use of a Real-Time Training Software (Laerdal QCPR®) Compared to Instructor-Based Feedback for High-Quality Chest Compressions Acquisition in Secondary School Students: A Randomized Trial.PLoS One.2017;12:e0169591. doi: 10.1371/journal.pone.0169591

ゲーム方式の学習とVR

ゲーム方式の学習とVRに関する推奨事項		
COR	LOE	推奨事項
2b	B-R	1. 市民救助者や医療従事者を対象とした一次または二次救命処置トレーニングには，ゲーム方式の学習の利用を検討してもよい[1-6]。
2b	B-NR	2. 市民救助者や医療従事者を対象とした一次または二次救命処置トレーニングには，VRの利用を検討してもよい[7-10]。

「概要」

市民救助者や医療従事者のトレーニングにゲーム方式の学習とVRの利用を検討する事例がますます増えている[11,12]。ゲーム方式の学習には，リーダーボードとシリアスゲームがある。リーダーボードは，受講者の間に競争の要素を取り入れることで練習の頻度を増やすことを目的とする。それに対して，シリアスゲームは，ボードゲームやコンピュータゲームといった娯楽の形を通して蘇生などの深刻な問題に向き合うために特別に設計されている[6,13]。VRとは，ユーザーがコンピュータによって作り出された3次元世界で物体の空間的な存在を認識し，それらとやり取りできるコンピュータインタフェースである[14,15]。

ゲーム方式の学習とVRに関する文献のレビューは，結果が一貫していないことを示しており，これらの学習方法で知識の習得，知識の保持，およびCPRスキルの改善を報告している研究もあれば[1-5,7,16]，有益性がまったく認められていない研究もある[6,8-10,17,18]。学習に対する悪影響を示した研究はない。ゲーム方式の学習とVRが実際の心停止現場でのパフォーマンスまたは患者転帰に及ぼす効果は不明である。ゲーム方式の学習およびVRを蘇生プログラムに組み込む場合は，機器や関連ソフトウェアの購入に伴う立上げ費用を考慮する必要がある。拡張現実（コンピュータによって生成されたホログラフィ像を現実環境に重ね合わせる技術）は関連する研究が不足しているため，今回のレビューからは除外した。

「推奨事項の裏付けとなる解説」

1. ゲーム方式の学習の効果を評価したいくつかの研究で，知識の習得，知識の保持，およびCPRスキルの改善が認められている[2-5]。学習に対する悪影響または顕著な有害作用を示した研究はない。リーダーボードの使用についても同様に結果は一貫しておらず，1件の研究でCPRパフォーマンスの向上が報告されているものの[1]，他の研究ではCPRの練習頻度またはCPRスキルの有意な向上は示されていない[6]。

2. CPRトレーニングでのVRを評価した研究のうち，1件の無作為化試験と1件の横断的観察研究で，VRは市民救助者と医療従事者の両方で知識とスキルパフォーマンスを向上させたと報告されている[7,8]。1件の無作為化試験では，医療従事者を対象としたフィードバックを伴うACLSトレーニングと比較して差は認められず[9]，別の1件の無作為化試験では，VRを使用した場合，バイスタンダー対応指標（自動体外式除細動器の要請など）は改善されたものの，胸骨圧迫の深さは浅くなった。ただし，どちらの群も胸骨圧迫の深さはガイドラインの基準を満たしていなかった[10]。

参考資料

1. MacKinnon RJ, Stoeter R, Doherty C, Fullwood C, Cheng A, Nadkarni V, Stenfors-Hayes T, Chang TP.Self-motivated learning with gamification improves infant CPR performance, a randomised controlled trial.BMJ Stel 2015;1:71-76.
2. Boada I, Rodriguez-Benitez A, Garcia-Gonzalez JM, Olivet J, Carreras V, Sbert M. Using a serious game to complement CPR instruction in a nurse faculty.Comput Methods Programs Biomed.2015;122:282-291. doi: 10.1016/j.cmpb.2015.08.006
3. Desailly V, Hajage D, Pasquier P, Brun P, Iglesias P, Huet J, Masseran C, Claudon A, Ebeyer C, Truong T, et al.The use of the serious game Stayingalive® at school improves basic life support performed by secondary pupils: a randomized controlled study: proceedings of Réanimation 2017, the French Intensive Care Society International Congress.Ann Intensive Care.2017;7:P49.
4. Otero-Agra M, Barcala-Furelos R, Besada-Saavedra I, Peixoto-Pino L, Martínez-Isasi S, Rodríguez-Núñez A. Let the kids play: gamification as a CPR training methodology in secondary school students.A quasi-experimental manikin simulation study.Emerg Med J. 2019;36:653-659. doi: 10.1136/emermed-2018-208108
5. Semeraro F, Frisoli A, Loconsole C, Mastronicola N, Stroppa F, Ristagno G, Scapigliati A, Marchetti L, Cerchiari E. Kids (learn how to) save lives in the school with the serious game Relive.Resuscitation.2017;116:27-32. doi: 10.1016/j.resuscitation.2017.04.038
6. Chang TP, Raymond T, Dewan M, MacKinnon R, Whitfill T, Harwayne-Gidansky I, Doughty C, Frisell K, Kessler D, Wolfe H, Auerbach M, Rutledge C, Mitchell D, Jani P, Walsh CM; INSPIRE In-Hospital QCPR Leaderboard Investigators.The effect of an International competitive leaderboard on self-motivated simulation-based CPR practice among healthcare professionals: A randomized control trial.Resuscitation.2019;138:273-281. doi: 10.1016/j.resuscitation.2019.02.050
7. Semeraro F, Frisoli A, Loconsole C, Bannò F, Tammaro G, Imbriaco G, Marchetti L, Cerchiari EL.Motion detection technology as a tool for cardiopulmonary resuscitation (CPR) quality training: a randomised crossover mannequin pilot study.Resuscitation.2013;84:501-507. doi: 10.1016/j.resuscitation.2012.12.006
8. Espinoza ED.Virtual reality in cardiopulmonary resuscitation training: a randomized trial [in Spanish].Emergencias.2019:43.
9. Khanal P, Vankipuram A, Ashby A, Vankipuram M, Gupta A, Drumm-Gurnee D, Josey K, Tinker L, Smith M. Collaborative virtual reality based advanced cardiac life support training simulator using virtual reality principles.J Biomed Inform.2014;51:49-59. doi: 10.1016/j.jbi.2014.04.005
10. Leary M, McGovern SK, Chaudhary Z, Patel J, Abella BS, Blewer AL.Comparing bystander response to a sudden cardiac arrest using a virtual reality CPR training mobile app versus a standard CPR training mobile app.Resuscitation.2019;139:167-173. doi: 10.1016/j.resuscitation.2019.04.017
11. Cheng A, Nadkarni VM, Mancini MB, Hunt EA, Sinz EH, Merchant RM, Donoghue A, Duff JP, Eppich W, Auerbach M, Bigham BL, Blewer AL, Chan PS, Bhanji F; American Heart Association Education Science Investigators; and on behalf of the American Heart Association Education Science and Programs Committee, Council on Cardiopulmonary, Critical Care, Perioperative and Resuscitation; Council on Cardiovascular and Stroke Nursing; and Council on Quality of Care and Outcomes Research.Resuscitation Education Science: Educational Strategies to Improve Outcomes From Cardiac Arrest: A Scientific Statement From the American Heart Association. Circulation.2018;138:e82-e122. doi: 10.1161/CIR.0000000000000583
12. Rumsfeld JS, Brooks SC, Aufderheide TP, Leary M, Bradley SM, Nkonde-Price C, Schwamm LH, Jessup M, Ferrer JM, Merchant RM; American Heart Association Emergency Cardiovascular Care Committee; Council on Cardiopulmonary, Critical Care, Perioperative and Resuscitation; Council on Quality of Care and Outcomes Research; Council on Cardiovascular and Stroke Nursing; and Council on Epidemiology and Prevention.Use of Mobile Devices, Social Media, and Crowdsourcing as Digital Strategies to Improve Emergency Cardiovascular Care: A Scientific Statement From the American Heart Association.Circulation.2016;134:e87-e108. doi: 10.1161/CIR.0000000000000428
13. Graafland M, Schraagen JM, Schijven MP.Systematic review of serious games for medical education and surgical skills training.Br J Surg.2012;99:1322-1330. doi: 10.1002/bjs.8819
14. Lopreiato JO.Heatlhcare Simulation Dictionary.Rockville, MD: Agency for Healthcare Research and Quality; 2016.https://www.ahrq.gov/sites/default/files/publications/files/sim-dictionary.pdf.Accessed April 27, 2020.
15. Giraldi G, Silva R, de Oliveira JC.Introduction to virtual reality. https://www.lncc.br/~jauvane/papers/RelatorioTecnicoLNCC-0603.pdf.Accessed February 14, 2020.
16. Ghoman SK, Patel SD, Cutumisu M, von Hauff P, Jeffery T, Brown MRG, Schmölzer GM.Serious games, a game changer in teaching neonatal resuscitation? A review.Arch Dis Child Fetal Neonatal Ed.2020;105:98-107. doi: 10.1136/archdischild-2019-317011
17. Drummond D, Delval P, Abdenouri S, Truchot J, Ceccaldi PF, Plaisance P, Hadchouel A, Tesnière A. Serious game versus online course for pretraining medical students before a simulation-based mastery learning course on cardiopulmonary resuscitation: A randomised controlled study.Eur J Anaesthesiol.2017;34:836-844. doi: 10.1097/EJA.0000000000000675
18. Yeung J, Kovic I, Vidacic M, Skilton E, Higgins D, Melody T, Lockey A. The school Lifesavers study–A randomised controlled trial comparing the impact of Lifesaver only, face-to-face training only, and Lifesaver with face-to-face training on CPR knowledge, skills and attitudes in UK school children.Resuscitation.2017;120:138-145. doi: 10.1016/j.resuscitation.2017.08.010

二次救命処置コースの受講前の準備

COR	LOE	推奨事項
2b	C-LD	1. 既存の二次救命処置コースに受講前eラーニングを組み込むことは妥当としてよい[1,2]。

「概要」

二次救命処置コースの受講者は，受講前に十分な準備を行うことで，学習機会を最大限に活かすことができる[3]。そのため，受講者は指定された受講前学習を行うか，開講前にコース教材に目を通すことができる。受講前の準備（画面ベースのシミュレーションなど）が課されたコースでは[1,2]，インストラクターは教室でのすべての時間を費やして，新しく習得した知識と，学習成果を高めるために必要な技術的スキルおよびチームワークの実習を融合させることができる。この文献レビューでは，受講前の準備が，インストラクターが指導する従来の二次救命処置トレーニングを補助する手段として効果的であるかどうかを判断した[4]。この課題に取り組んだRCTは2件あり，そのうち1件でいくつかの独立したCPRパフォーマンス変数についてパフォーマンスの向上が見られたが，どちらの試験でも全体的な合格率の向上は示されなかった[1,2]。文献検索により，従来の2日間の二次救命処置コースの1日目を受講前の準備に当てた研究が3件見つかったが，これらの研究は今回のレビューから除外した。有益性は不確かであるが，リスクは低いことから，可能な場合に受講前学習を組み込むことは妥当としてよい。今後の研究で，受講前学習のさまざまな実施方法の有効性を比較検討することが望まれる。

「推奨事項の裏付けとなる解説」

1. システマティックレビューにより，この研究課題に取り組んだRCTが2件見つかった[1,2]。どちらの試験でも，コース開講の2～4週間前にコンピュータベースのシミュレーションプログラムへのアクセス権が受講者に与えられた。1件のRCTでは，受講前の準備は，心室細動の除細動までの時間の短縮（112秒対149.9秒，P＜0.05），および症候性徐脈のペーシングまでの時間の短縮（95.1秒対154.9秒，P＜0.05）と関連性があったが，コース合格率は向上しなかった[1]。もう1件のRCTでは，画面ベースの学習による受講前準備を追加しても臨床パフォーマンスと知識の向上は見られなかった[2]。どちらの試験もすべての受講者に受講前プログラムのアクセス権を与えていたが，受講者が実際にシミュレーションプログラムを実施したかどうかを主観的にモニタリングしていたのは1件だけだったため，受講前準備の影響を十分に理解することは難しい[2]。その試験では，受講者の3分の1が受講前シミュレーションを行わずにコースに参加した。シミュレーションを行った受講者の平均所要時間は2時間であった。

参考資料

1. Nacca N, Holliday J, Ko PY. Randomized trial of a novel ACLS teaching tool: does it improve student performance? West J Emerg Med. 2014;15:913-918. doi: 10.5811/westjem.2014.9.20149
2. Perkins GD, Fullerton JN, Davis-Gomez N, Davies RP, Baldock C, Stevens H, Bullock I, Lockey AS. The effect of pre-course e-learning prior to advanced life support training: a randomised controlled trial. Resuscitation. 2010;81:877-881. doi: 10.1016/j.resuscitation.2010.03.019
3. Bhanji F, Donoghue AJ, Wolff MS, Flores GE, Halamek LP, Berman JM, Sinz EH, Cheng A. Part 14: education: 2015 American Heart Association Guidelines Update for Cardiopulmonary Resuscitation and Emergency Cardiovascular Care. Circulation. 2015;132(suppl 2):S561-573. doi: 10.1161/CIR.0000000000000268
4. Greif R, Bhanji F, Bigham BL, Bray J, Breckwoldt J, Cheng A, Duff JP, Gilfoyle E, Hsieh M-J, Iwami T, et al; on behalf of the Education, Implementation, and Teams Collaborators. Education, implementation, and teams: 2020 International Consensus on Cardiopulmonary Resuscitation and Emergency Cardiovascular Care Science With Treatment Recommendations. Circulation. 2020;142(suppl 1):S222-S283. doi: 10.1161/CIR.0000000000000896

市民救助者向けのオピオイド過量摂取対応トレーニング

COR	LOE	推奨事項
2a	C-LD	1. 市民救助者が，ナロキソン投与を含むオピオイド過量摂取対応トレーニングを受けることは妥当である[1-8]。

「概要」

アメリカ疾病予防管理センターによると，米国でのオピオイド過量摂取による死亡者数は過去10年間で倍増している（2007年は18,515人，2017年は47,600人）[9]。オピオイド過量摂取の認識を広め，市民救助者によるナロキソン投与の意欲とその能力を高めることは，転帰の改善につながる可能性がある。対象を絞った蘇生およびナロキソントレーニングがオピオイド使用者およびオピオイド過量摂取に遭遇する可能性のある市民救助者に及ぼす影響を明らかにするために，スコーピングレビューが実施された[10]。教育的介入としては，オピオイド使用者の家族を対象としたトレーニングプログラム（ナロキソン配付を含む），オピオイド使用者のコンピュータベースのトレーニング，仲間同士のトレーニング（オピオイド使用者が別のオピオイド使用者を指導する），および救急部スタッフによる短時間のカウンセリングが用いられた[1-8]。

オピオイド使用者[5,7]，その友人や家族[1]，および密接な関係にある人[5]に対する教育は，ナロキソン投与の意欲とその能力，リスク認識，過量摂取に関する知識の認識，およびEMSへの通報の心構えを高める[3,10]。オピオイド使用者またはオピオイド過量摂取を目撃する可能性のある人

は，ナロキソン投与を含むオピオイド過量摂取対応トレーニングを受けることを提案する。集団レベルの介入を個々の患者転帰に結び付けることができないことから，レビューしたデータは限られている。学習成果と患者転帰の両方を評価することで最も有益性の高い教育的介入を特定するために，さらなる研究が求められる。

「推奨事項の裏付けとなる解説」

1. 8件の研究（1件のRCTと7件の観察研究）[1-8]で，オピオイドトレーニングの影響が比較群を用いて評価されている。これらの研究は，オピオイド使用者，友人，および家族を対象とする短時間の教育コースの影響を評価したものである。アウトカムは研究によって異なり，リスクの知識，過量摂取の特定，過量摂取対応の知識とスキル，および処置の実施または通報の意欲であった[1,3-8]。

    1件のRCTで，直近の3カ月以内にトレーニングを受けた個人によるオピオイド過量摂取の目撃例のうち60％で応急処置および／またはナロキソン投与が行われた。比較群で応急処置またはナロキソン投与が行われたケースはゼロであった[1]。ある観察研究では，教育を受けた後12カ月以内に過量摂取を目撃した参加者の40％がナロキソンを投与した[5]。別の研究では，オピオイドトレーニングを受けた人のほうが受けなかった人よりもナロキソン投与率が高かった（32％対0％）[4]。9-1-1への通報率または補助呼吸の実施率については，2つの群の間に差はなかった[4]。別の研究では，処置の実施についてトレーニングを受けた救助者と受けていない救助者の間に差は見られなかった[2]。スキル実習（ナロキソン投与）を含む介入は，スキル実習なしの介入と比較して，臨床パフォーマンスの向上につながる可能性が高かった[1,11-22]。

参考資料

1. Williams AV, Marsden J, Strang J. Training family members to manage heroin overdose and administer naloxone: randomized trial of effects on knowledge and attitudes.Addiction.2014;109:250-259. doi: 10.1111/add.12360
2. Doe-Simkins M, Quinn E, Xuan Z, Sorensen-Alawad A, Hackman H, Ozonoff A, Walley AY.Overdose rescues by trained and untrained participants and change in opioid use among substance-using participants in overdose education and naloxone distribution programs: a retrospective cohort study.BMC Public Health.2014;14:297. doi: 10.1186/1471-2458-14-297
3. Dunn KE, Yepez-Laubach C, Nuzzo PA, Fingerhood M, Kelly A, Berman S, Bigelow GE.Randomized controlled trial of a computerized opioid overdose education intervention.Drug Alcohol Depend.2017;173 Suppl 1:S39-S47. doi: 10.1016/j.drugalcdep.2016.12.003
4. Dwyer K, Walley AY, Langlois BK, Mitchell PM, Nelson KP, Cromwell J, Bernstein E. Opioid education and nasal naloxone rescue kits in the emergency department.West J Emerg Med.2015;16:381-384. doi: 10.5811/westjem.2015.2.24909
5. Espelt A, Bosque-Prous M, Folch C, Sarasa-Renedo A, Majó X, Casabona J, Brugal MT; REDAN Group.Is systematic training in opioid overdose prevention effective? PLoS One.2017;12:e0186833. doi: 10.1371/journal.pone.0186833
6. Franko TS II, Distefano D, Lewis L. A novel naloxone training compared with current recommended training in an overdose simulation.J Am Pharm Assoc (2003).2019;59:375-378. doi: 10.1016/j.japh.2018.12.022
7. Jones JD, Roux P, Stancliff S, Matthews W, Comer SD.Brief overdose education can significantly increase accurate recognition of opioid overdose among heroin users.Int J Drug Policy.2014;25:166-170. doi: 10.1016/j.drugpo.2013.05.006
8. Lott DC, Rhodes J. Opioid overdose and naloxone education in a substance use disorder treatment program.Am J Addict.2016;25:221-226. doi: 10.1111/ajad.12364
9. National Institute on Drug Abuse.Overdose death rates.2020.https://www.drugabuse.gov/related-topics/trends-statistics/overdose-death-rates.Updated March 2020.Accessed March 18, 2020.
10. Greif R, Bhanji F, Bigham BL, Bray J, Breckwoldt J, Cheng A, Duff JP, Gilfoyle E, Hsieh M-J, Iwami T, et al; on behalf of the Education, Implementation, and Teams Collaborators.Education, implementation, and teams: 2020 International Consensus on Cardiopulmonary Resuscitation and Emergency Cardiovascular Care Science With Treatment Recommendations.Circulation.2020;142(suppl 1):S222-S283.DOI: 10.1161/CIR.0000000000000896
11. Pietrusza LM, Puskar KR, Ren D, Mitchell AM.Evaluation of an Opiate Overdose Educational Intervention and Naloxone Prescribing Program in Homeless Adults Who Use Opiates.J Addict Nurs.2018;29:188-195. doi: 10.1097/JAN.0000000000000235
12. Katzman JG, Greenberg NH, Takeda MY, Moya Balasch M. Characteristics of Patients With Opioid Use Disorder Associated With Performing Overdose Reversals in the Community: An Opioid Treatment Program Analysis.J Addict Med.2019;13:131-138. doi: 10.1097/ADM.0000000000000461
13. Piper TM, Stancliff S, Rudenstine S, Sherman S, Nandi V, Clear A, Galea S. Evaluation of a naloxone distribution and administration program in New York City.Subst Use Misuse.2008;43:858-870. doi: 10.1080/10826080701801261
14. Walley AY, Doe-Simkins M, Quinn E, Pierce C, Xuan Z, Ozonoff A. Opioid overdose prevention with intranasal naloxone among people who take methadone.J Subst Abuse Treat.2013;44:241-247. doi: 10.1016/j.jsat.2012.07.004
15. Walley AY, Xuan Z, Hackman HH, Quinn E, Doe-Simkins M, Sorensen-Alawad A, Ruiz S, Ozonoff A. Opioid overdose rates and implementation of overdose education and nasal naloxone distribution in Massachusetts: interrupted time series analysis.BMJ.2013;346:f174. doi: 10.1136/bmj.f174
16. Wagner KD, Bovet LJ, Haynes B, Joshua A, Davidson PJ.Training law enforcement to respond to opioid overdose with naloxone: Impact on knowledge, attitudes, and interactions with community members.Drug Alcohol Depend.2016;165:22-28. doi: 10.1016/j.drugalcdep.2016.05.008
17. Dahlem CHG, King L, Anderson G, Marr A, Waddell JE, Scalera M. Beyond rescue: Implementation and evaluation of revised naloxone training for law enforcement officers.Public Health Nurs.2017;34:516-521. doi: 10.1111/phn.12365
18. Panther SG, Bray BS, White JR.The implementation of a naloxone rescue program in university students.J Am Pharm Assoc (2003).2017;57:S107-S112 e102. doi: 10.1016/j.japh.2016.11.002
19. Mcauley A, Lindsay G, Woods M, Louttit D. Responsible management and use of a personal take-home naloxone supply: a pilot project.Drugs: Education, Prevention and Policy.2010;17:388-399.
20. Seal KH, Thawley R, Gee L, Bamberger J, Kral AH, Ciccarone D, Downing M, Edlin BR.Naloxone distribution and cardiopulmonary resuscitation training for injection drug users to prevent heroin overdose death: a pilot intervention study.J Urban Health.2005;82:303-311. doi: 10.1093/jurban/jti053
21. Tobin KE, Sherman SG, Beilenson P, Welsh C, Latkin CA.Evaluation of the Staying Alive programme: training injection drug users to properly administer naloxone and save lives.Int J Drug Policy.2009;20:131-136. doi: 10.1016/j.drugpo.2008.03.002
22. Lankenau SE, Wagner KD, Silva K, Kecojevic A, Iverson E, McNeely M, Kral AH.Injection drug users trained by overdose prevention programs: responses to witnessed overdoses.J Community Health.2013;38:133-141. doi: 10.1007/s10900-012-9591-7

プロバイダーに関する考慮事項
教育格差

COR	LOE	推奨事項
1	B-NR	1. 米国では，市民救助者へのCPRトレーニングを，特定の人種および民族の集団や地区を対象として，ターゲットに合わせて調整することが推奨される[1-10]。
1	B-NR	2. SESが低い集団や地区を市民救助者へのCPRトレーニングおよび認識向上の取り組みの対象とすることが推奨される[11-20]。
2a	C-LD	3. 教育的トレーニングおよび一般市民の認識向上の取り組みを通じて女性へのB-CPRに対する障壁に対処することは妥当である[21-24]。

「概要」

医療格差は，人種，民族，SES，性別などの社会的決定因子を理由として医療から体系的に阻害されてきた集団に悪影響を及ぼす[25]。AHAでは，人種および民族集団を，不公平や偏見を歴史的に経験してきた個人および地区（黒人やヒスパニック系の人，英語力が乏しい言語的に隔離された地域社会など）と定義している。SESは，自己認識された所得と教育によって個人または地区ごとに特徴付けられる。性別は，自己認識または医師によって同定された男性または女性として個人レベルで定義されている。ここでは，このような集団を対象としたトレーニングが妥当かどうかを判断するため，人種，民族，SES，および性別とB-CPRの実施率またはCPRトレーニングの受講率の低さとの関連性を調べた[1-24]。黒人，ヒスパニック系，および低SESが圧倒的に多い地区は，B-CPRの実施率およびCPRトレーニングの受講率が低い[3-5,16]。言語障壁は，CPRトレーニングの受講率の低さと関連性がある[9,10]。女性はB-CPRを受ける可能性が低い。これは，バイスタンダーが女性を負傷させたり，不適切な接触を訴えられることを恐れていることに起因する可能性がある[22,23]。特定の人種，民族，およびSESが低い集団を対象としたCPR教育や，性差に対処することを目的とした教育内容の修正により，CPRトレーニングおよびB-CPRの格差を取り除き，これらの集団における心停止の転帰を改善できる可能性がある。このような重要な問題の理解を前進させるため，B-CPRおよびCPR教育に対する人種的，社会経済的，および性別的な障壁に関する研究を今後さらに進めることが重要である。

「推奨事項の裏付けとなる解説」

1. 4件の後ろ向きコホート研究と1件の横断的研究から，黒人およびヒスパニック系地区の住民はB-CPRを受ける可能性が低く，黒人住民はCPRトレーニングを受講している可能性が低いことがわかっている[1-5]。ある記述的研究によると，スペイン語集団向けの質の高いCPR教育リソースはほとんどない[6]。さまざまな質的研究により，言語障壁，金銭的問題，および情報不足は，言語的に隔離された地域社会でのB-CPRの実施率の低さと関連性があることが示されている[6-10]。

2. いくつかの後ろ向きコホート研究で，低いSESはB-CPRを受ける可能性が低いことと関連性があった[11-16]。さらに，最近の横断的研究によると，低いSESはCPRトレーニングを受講する可能性が低いこととも関連性がある[17,18]。これに対処するため，いくつかの後ろ向き研究で，地域マッピングを使用してトレーニングの対象となる社会的経済地位が低い地区を特定することの実行可能性が実証された[19,20]。

3. B-CPRの実施における性差について調べた最近の研究では，公共の場でB-CPRを受ける可能性は男性のほうが女性よりも高かった[21]。いくつかの横断的調査研究によると，市民救助者は，B-CPRを必要とする女性への不適切な接触，性的暴行，および傷害によって訴えられることを恐れている[22,23]。ある無作為化シミュレーション試験において，被験者が衣類を脱がせる可能性は，女性マネキンのほうが男性マネキンよりも低かった[24]。

参考資料

1. Brookoff D, Kellermann AL, Hackman BB, Somes G, Dobyns P. Do blacks get bystander cardiopulmonary resuscitation as often as whites? Ann Emerg Med.1994;24:1147-1150. doi: 10.1016/s0196-0644(94)70246-2
2. Vadeboncoeur TF, Richman PB, Darkoh M, Chikani V, Clark L, Bobrow BJ.Bystander cardiopulmonary resuscitation for out-of-hospital cardiac arrest in the Hispanic vs the non-Hispanic populations.Am J Emerg Med.2008;26:655-660. doi: 10.1016/j.ajem.2007.10.002
3. Anderson ML, Cox M, Al-Khatib SM, Nichol G, Thomas KL, Chan PS, Saha-Chaudhuri P, Fosbol EL, Eigel B, Clendenen B, Peterson ED.Rates of cardiopulmonary resuscitation training in the United States.JAMA Intern Med.2014;174:194-201. doi: 10.1001/jamainternmed.2013.11320
4. Fosbøl EL, Dupre ME, Strauss B, Swanson DR, Myers B, McNally BF, Anderson ML, Bagai A, Monk L, Garvey JL, Bitner M, Jollis JG, Granger CB.Association of neighborhood characteristics with incidence of out-of-hospital cardiac arrest and rates of bystander-initiated CPR: implications for community-based education intervention.Resuscitation.2014;85:1512-1517. doi: 10.1016/j.resuscitation.2014.08.013
5. Blewer AL, Schmicker RH, Morrison LJ, Aufderheide TP, Daya M, Starks MA, May S, Idris AH, Callaway CW, Kudenchuk PJ, Vilke GM, Abella BS; Resuscitation Outcomes Consortium Investigators.Variation in Bystander Cardiopulmonary Resuscitation Delivery and Subsequent Survival From Out-of-Hospital Cardiac Arrest Based on Neighborhood-Level Ethnic Characteristics.Circulation.2020;141:34-41. doi: 10.1161/CIRCULATIONAHA.119.041541
6. Liu KY, Haukoos JS, Sasson C. Availability and quality of cardiopulmonary resuscitation information for Spanish-speaking population on the Internet. Resuscitation.2014;85:131-137. doi: 10.1016/j.resuscitation.2013.08.274
7. Yip MP, Ong B, Tu SP, Chavez D, Ike B, Painter I, Lam I, Bradley SM, Coronado GD, Meischke HW.Diffusion of cardiopulmonary resuscitation training to Chinese immigrants with limited English proficiency.Emerg Med Int. 2011;2011:685249. doi: 10.1155/2011/685249
8. Meischke H, Taylor V, Calhoun R, Liu Q, Sos C, Tu SP, Yip MP, Eisenberg D. Preparedness for cardiac emergencies among Cambodians with limited English proficiency.J Community Health.2012;37:176-180. doi: 10.1007/s10900-011-9433-z
9. Sasson C, Haukoos JS, Bond C, Rabe M, Colbert SH, King R, Sayre M, Heisler M. Barriers and facilitators to learning and performing cardiopulmonary resuscitation in neighborhoods with low bystander cardiopulmonary resuscitation prevalence and high rates of cardiac arrest in Columbus, OH.Circ Cardiovasc Qual Outcomes.2013;6:550-558. doi: 10.1161/CIRCOUTCOMES.111.000097

10. Sasson C, Haukoos JS, Ben-Youssef L, Ramirez L, Bull S, Eigel B, Magid DJ, Padilla R. Barriers to calling 911 and learning and performing cardiopulmonary resuscitation for residents of primarily Latino, high-risk neighborhoods in Denver, Colorado.Ann Emerg Med.2015;65:545-552.e2. doi: 10.1016/j.annemergmed.2014.10.028

11. Mitchell MJ, Stubbs BA, Eisenberg MS.Socioeconomic status is associated with provision of bystander cardiopulmonary resuscitation.Prehosp Emerg Care.2009;13:478-486. doi: 10.1080/10903120903144833

12. Vaillancourt C, Lui A, De Maio VJ, Wells GA, Stiell IG.Socioeconomic status influences bystander CPR and survival rates for out-of-hospital cardiac arrest victims.Resuscitation.2008;79:417-423. doi: 10.1016/j.resuscitation.2008.07.012

13. Chiang WC, Ko PC, Chang AM, Chen WT, Liu SS, Huang YS, Chen SY, Lin CH, Cheng MT, Chong KM, Wang HC, Yang CW, Liao MW, Wang CH, Chien YC, Lin CH, Liu YP, Lee BC, Chien KL, Lai MS, Ma MH.Bystander-initiated CPR in an Asian metropolitan: does the socioeconomic status matter? Resuscitation.2014;85:53-58. doi: 10.1016/j.resuscitation.2013.07.033

14. Moncur L, Ainsborough N, Ghose R, Kendal SP, Salvatori M, Wright J. Does the level of socioeconomic deprivation at the location of cardiac arrest in an English region influence the likelihood of receiving bystander-initiated cardiopulmonary resuscitation? Emerg Med J. 2016;33:105-108. doi: 10.1136/emermed-2015-204643

15. Dahan B, Jabre P, Karam N, Misslin R, Tafflet M, Bougouin W, Jost D, Beganton F, Marijon E, Jouven X. Impact of neighbourhood socio-economic status on bystander cardiopulmonary resuscitation in Paris.Resuscitation.2017;110:107-113. doi: 10.1016/j.resuscitation.2016.10.028

16. Brown TP, Booth S, Hawkes CA, Soar J, Mark J, Mapstone J, Fothergill RT, Black S, Pocock H, Bichmann A, Gunson I, Perkins GD.Characteristics of neighbourhoods with high incidence of out-of-hospital cardiac arrest and low bystander cardiopulmonary resuscitation rates in England.Eur Heart J Qual Care Clin Outcomes.2019;5:51-62. doi: 10.1093/ehjqcco/qcy026

17. Blewer AL, Ibrahim SA, Leary M, Dutwin D, McNally B, Anderson ML, Morrison LJ, Aufderheide TP, Daya M, Idris AH, et al.Cardiopulmonary resuscitation training disparities in the United States J Am Heart Assoc.2017;6:e006124. doi: 10.1161/JAHA.117.006124

18. Abdulhay NM, Totolos K, McGovern S, Hewitt N, Bhardwaj A, Buckler DG, Leary M, Abella BS.Socioeconomic disparities in layperson CPR training within a large U.S. city.Resuscitation.2019;141:13-18. doi: 10.1016/j.resuscitation.2019.05.038

19. Sasson C, Keirns CC, Smith DM, Sayre MR, Macy ML, Meurer WJ, McNally BF, Kellermann AL, Iwashyna TJ.Examining the contextual effects of neighborhood on out-of-hospital cardiac arrest and the provision of bystander cardiopulmonary resuscitation.Resuscitation.2011;82:674-679. doi: 10.1016/j.resuscitation.2011.02.002

20. Root ED, Gonzales L, Persse DE, Hinchey PR, McNally B, Sasson C. A tale of two cities: the role of neighborhood socioeconomic status in spatial clustering of bystander CPR in Austin and Houston.Resuscitation.2013;84:752-759. doi: 10.1016/j.resuscitation.2013.01.007

21. Blewer AL, McGovern SK, Schmicker RH, May S, Morrison LJ, Aufderheide TP, Daya M, Idris AH, Callaway CW, Kudenchuk PJ, Vilke GM, Abella BS; Resuscitation Outcomes Consortium (ROC) Investigators.Gender Disparities Among Adult Recipients of Bystander Cardiopulmonary Resuscitation in the Public.Circ Cardiovasc Qual Outcomes.2018;11:e004710. doi: 10.1161/CIRCOUTCOMES.118.004710

22. Becker TK, Gul SS, Cohen SA, Maciel CB, Baron-Lee J, Murphy TW, Youn TS, Tyndall JA, Gibbons C, Hart L, Alviar CL; Florida Cardiac Arrest Resource Team.Public perception towards bystander cardiopulmonary resuscitation. Emerg Med J. 2019;36:660-665. doi: 10.1136/emermed-2018-208234

23. Perman SM, Shelton SK, Knoepke C, Rappaport K, Matlock DD, Adelgais K, Havranek EP, Daugherty SL.Public Perceptions on Why Women Receive Less Bystander Cardiopulmonary Resuscitation Than Men in Out-of-Hospital Cardiac Arrest.Circulation.2019;139:1060-1068. doi: 10.1161/CIRCULATIONAHA.118.037692

24. Kramer CE, Wilkins MS, Davies JM, Caird JK, Hallihan GM.Does the sex of a simulated patient affect CPR? Resuscitation.2015;86:82-87. doi: 10.1016/j.resuscitation.2014.10.016

25. LaVeist TA.Race, Ethnicity, and Health: A Public Health Reader.Hoboken, NJ: John Wiley & Sons, Inc; 2002.

EMSプラクティショナーの経験およびOHCAの体験

EMSプラクティショナーの経験およびOHCAの体験に関する推奨事項

COR	LOE	推奨事項
2a	C-LD	1. EMSシステムが臨床スタッフによる蘇生の体験をモニタリングし、心停止症例に対応する能力を有するメンバーを治療担当チームに入れることは妥当である。スタッフ配置やトレーニング戦略を通じてチームの能力をサポートしてもよい[1-6]。

「概要」

病院搬送前の蘇生治療を適切に実施することは、OHCAの転帰を決定するうえで重要な要素である[7]。継続的な体験（実際の心停止患者への対応）または一般的な経験（勤務期間）がOHCAの患者転帰に及ぼす影響を理解しておくと、適切なスタッフ配置やトレーニング戦略の実施に役立つ可能性がある。システマティックレビューによると、EMSプロバイダーの体験（これまでに対応した心停止症例の数と、直近（6カ月未満）の心停止の体験の両方）は、自己心拍再開（ROSC）の改善[2,3]、および生存退院率の改善と関連性がある[1,8]。個々の研究の結果は一貫していないが、既知の生存予測因子について調整された質の高い研究では、生存転帰はEMSプロバイダーの体験が多いほど高かった[1]。EMSプロバイダーの経験（勤務年数）は、生存退院率の改善との関連性はなかった[1]。

EMSシステムがプロバイダーによる蘇生の体験をモニタリングし、体験の少なさを考慮してトレーニング戦略を実施すること、または最近心停止症例に対応したメンバーを治療担当チームに入れることは妥当である。スタッフ配置の調整またはシミュレーションベースのトレーニングによる体験不足の埋め合わせは、他の有益な質改善活動を犠牲にする可能性があるため、その利点とスケジューリングの現実性およびトレーニングの追加コストを比較検討する必要がある。小児心停止患者の治療に必要な体験については、推奨事項を提示することはできない。

「推奨事項の裏付けとなる解説」

1. システマティックレビューの結果、プロバイダーの体験の影響を評価した観察研究が2件見つかった[1,3]。調整後の結果を報告している規模の大きい方の研究では、チームの体験数（直前3年間の心停止症例数）が多いほど生存退院率は高かった。生存の可能性は、体験数が6以下のチームと比較して、体験数が6超11以下の群（調整後オッズ比：1.26、95％CI：1.04〜1.54）、が11超17以下の群（調整後オッズ比：1.29、95％CI：1.04〜1.59）、および17超の群（調整後オッズ比：1.50、95％CI：1.22〜1.86）のほうが高く、体験数との間に「用量反応」関係があることを示している[1]。未調整の結果を報告しているもう

1 件の観察研究では，体験と生存退院率の間に関連性は認められていない。

1 件の観察研究で，直前の 6 カ月間に心停止症例を体験していないチームによって治療を受けた患者は，最近（直前の 1 カ月未満）心停止症例を体験したチームによって治療を受けた患者と比較して，生存退院率が低かった（調整後オッズ比：0.70，95 ％ CI：0.54～0.91）[1]。その他の研究では，チームリーダーの心停止症例の体験とイベント生存率との関連性[3]，および EMS プロバイダーまたは EMS チームの臨床経験年数と生存退院率との関連性はなかった[1,4,9]。2 件の研究で，一次治療を担当した救急医療チームの体験数が多いほど ROSC が高いことが報告されている[2,3]。

参考資料

1. Dyson K, Bray JE, Smith K, Bernard S, Straney L, Finn J. Paramedic Exposure to Out-of-Hospital Cardiac Arrest Resuscitation Is Associated With Patient Survival.Circ Cardiovasc Qual Outcomes.2016;9:154-160. doi: 10.1161/CIRCOUTCOMES.115.002317
2. Tuttle JE, Hubble MW.Paramedic out-of-hospital cardiac arrest case volume is a predictor of return of spontaneous circulation West J Emerg Med.2018;19:654-659. doi: 10.5811/westjem.2018.3.37051
3. Weiss N, Ross E, Cooley C, Polk J, Velasquez C, Harper S, Walrath B, Redman T, Mapp J, Wampler D. Does Experience Matter? Paramedic Cardiac Resuscitation Experience Effect on Out-of-Hospital Cardiac Arrest Outcomes.Prehosp Emerg Care.2018;22:332-337. doi: 10.1080/10903127.2017.1392665
4. Gold LS, Eisenberg MS.The effect of paramedic experience on survival from cardiac arrest.Prehosp Emerg Care.2009;13:341-344. doi: 10.1080/10903120902935389
5. Soo LH, Gray D, Young T, Skene A, Hampton JR.Influence of ambulance crew's length of experience on the outcome of out-of-hospital cardiac arrest.Eur Heart J. 1999;20:535-540.
6. Bjornsson HM, Marelsson S, Magnusson V, Sigurdsson G, Thorgeirsson G. Physician experience in addition to ACLS training does not significantly affect the outcome of prehospital cardiac arrest.Eur J Emerg Med.2011;18:64-67. doi: 10.1097/MEJ.0b013e32833c6642
7. Perkins GD, Jacobs IG, Nadkarni VM, Berg RA, Bhanji F, Biarent D, Bossaert LL, Brett SJ, Chamberlain D, de Caen AR, Deakin CD, Finn JC, Gräsner JT, Hazinski MF, Iwami T, Koster RW, Lim SH, Huei-Ming Ma M, McNally BF, Morley PT, Morrison LJ,Monsieurs KG, Montgomery W, Nichol G, Okada K, Eng Hock Ong M,Travers AH, Nolan JP; Utstein Collaborators.Cardiac arrest and cardiopulmonary resuscitation outcome reports: update of the Utstein Resuscitation Registry Templates for Out-of-Hospital Cardiac Arrest: a statement for healthcare professionals from a task force of the International Liaison Committee on Resuscitation (American Heart Association, European Resuscitation Council, Australian and New Zealand Council on Resuscitation, Heart and Stroke Foundation of Canada, InterAmerican Heart Foundation, Resuscitation Council of Southern Africa, Resuscitation Council of Asia); and the American Heart Association Emergency Cardiovascular Care Committee and the Council on Cardiopulmonary, Critical Care, Perioperative and Resuscitation.Circulation.2015;132:1286–1300. doi: 10.1161/CIR.0000000000000144
8. Greif R, Bhanji F, Bigham BL, Bray J, Breckwoldt J, Cheng A, Duff JP, Gilfoyle E, Hsieh M-J, Iwami T, et al; on behalf of the Education, Implementation, and Teams Collaborators.Education, implementation, and teams: 2020 International Consensus on Cardiopulmonary Resuscitation and Emergency Cardiovascular Care Science With Treatment Recommendations.Circulation.2020;142 (suppl 1):S222–S283. doi: 10.1161/CIR.0000000000000896
9. Lukić A, Lulić I, Lulić D, Ognjanović Z, Cerovečki D, Telebar S, Mašić I. Analysis of out-of-hospital cardiac arrest in Croatia—survival, bystander cardiopulmonary resuscitation, and impact of physician's experience on cardiac arrest management: a single center observational study. Croat Med J. 2016;57:591-600. doi: 10.3325/cmj.2016.57.591

ACLS コース参加

ACLS コース参加に関する推奨事項		
COR	LOE	推奨事項
2a	C-LD	1. 医療従事者が成人の ACLS コースまたは同等のトレーニングを受けることは妥当である[1-9]。

「概要」

蘇生協議会はこれまで 30 年以上にわたって成人の二次救命処置コース（AHA による ACLS，欧州蘇生協議会による二次救命処置コースなど）を開講し，危篤状態にある成人患者の認識と治療に必要な知識やスキルを提供してきた[10]。このコースは，心停止した成人患者に対応する可能性のある医療従事者を対象としている。ACLS コースの内容と教授システム学（インストラクショナル・デザイン）は，最新の蘇生ガイドラインを反映するために 5 年ごとに更新されており，最新版はシミュレーションベースのトレーニングによる多職種連携のチーム医療に焦点を合わせている[10-12]。関連する研究のメタアナリシスによると，過去に ACLS コースを受講したチームメンバーが 1 名以上いる蘇生チームは，ROSC，生存退院率，30 日生存率などの患者転帰が良好である[9,13]。そのため，成人心停止患者の治療に参加する可能性のある医療従事者はすべて，ACLS コースまたは同等のトレーニングを受けることを推奨する。

特にリソースの乏しい環境では，ACLS を受講することで他の有益な介入が犠牲になる可能性があるため，コース参加の利点と受講にかかるコストを比較検討する必要がある。新生児および小児科の医療従事者については，患者転帰を PALS および新生児蘇生プログラムコースと関連付けて評価したエビデンスが不足しているため，推奨事項を提示することはできない。

「推奨事項の裏付けとなる解説」

1. 最近実施された 6 件の観察研究[3-8]のシステマティックレビューから，登録された 1,461 名の患者において，成人の院内心停止患者の ROSC 率は，メンバーの少なくとも 1 人が認定 ACLS コースを修了している蘇生チームの治療を受けたほうが，過去に ACLS トレーニングを受けたメンバーがいないチームの治療を受けた場合よりも高いことがわかった（オッズ比：1.64，95 ％ CI：1.12～2.41）[9]。また，7 件の観察研究[1-3,5-8]のシステマティックレビューから，登録された 1,507 名の成人院内心停止患者において，生存退院率または 30 日生存率は，メンバーの少なくとも 1 人が認定 ACLS コースを修了しているチームの治療を受けたほうが高いこともわかった（オッズ比：2.43，95 ％ CI：1.04～5.70）[9]。2 件の観察研究[5,6]の統合データでは，登録された 455 名の患者において，1 年生存率と ACLS トレーニングの間に有意な関連性はなかった[9]。

ACLS トレーニングのその他の利点としては，ROSC までの時間の短縮[5]，治療ミス（心リズムの誤った評価など）の減少[4]，およびトレーニング受講済みのチームメンバーの人数とROSC の向上との関連性[5]が挙げられる。

神経学的な障害を残さない生存率に対する ACLS トレーニングの影響，または患者転帰に対するコースの構成要素の影響を報告した研究はない。レビューされた研究の間で，調査対象集団の差異による選択バイアスの高いリスクがあった。ほとんどの研究は 2010 年より前に実施されており，現在の標準治療と現行の ACLS コース設計（チーム医療とシミュレーションベースの学習に重点が置かれている）を正確に反映していない可能性がある。

参考資料

1. Camp BN, Parish DC, Andrews RH.Effect of advanced cardiac life support training on resuscitation efforts and survival in a rural hospital.Ann Emerg Med.1997;29:529-533. doi: 10.1016/s0196-0644 (97)70228-2
2. Dane FC, Russell-Lindgren KS, Parish DC, Durham MD, Brown TD.In-hospital resuscitation: association between ACLS training and survival to discharge. Resuscitation.2000;47:83-87. doi: 10.1016/s0300-9572 (00)00210-0
3. Lowenstein SR, Sabyan EM, Lassen CF, Kern DC.Benefits of training physicians in advanced cardiac life support.Chest.1986;89:512-516. doi: 10.1378/chest.89.4.512
4. Makker R, Gray-Siracusa K, Evers M. Evaluation of advanced cardiac life support in a community teaching hospital by use of actual cardiac arrests. Heart Lung.1995;6:1124-120. doi: 10.1016/s0147-9563 (05)80005-6
5. Moretti MA, Cesar LA, Nusbacher A, Kern KB, Timerman S, Ramires JA.Advanced cardiac life support training improves long-term survival from in-hospital cardiac arrest.Resuscitation.2007;72:458-465. doi: 10.1016/j.resuscitation.2006.06.039
6. Pottle A, Brant S. Does resuscitation training affect outcome from cardiac arrest? Accid Emerg Nurs.2000;8:46-51. doi: 10.1054/aaen.1999.0089
7. Sanders AB, Berg RA, Burress M, Genova RT, Kern KB, Ewy GA.The efficacy of an ACLS training program for resuscitation from cardiac arrest in a rural community.Ann Emerg Med.1994;23:56-59. doi: 10.1016/s0196-0644 (94)70009-5
8. Sodhi K, Singla MK, Shrivastava A. Impact of advanced cardiac life support training program on the outcome of cardiopulmonary resuscitation in a tertiary care hospital.Indian J Crit Care Med.2011;15:209-212. doi: 10.4103/0972-5229.92070
9. Lockey A, Lin Y, Cheng A. Impact of adult advanced cardiac life support course participation on patient outcomes-A systematic review and meta-analysis.Resuscitation.2018;129:48-54. doi: 10.1016/j.resuscitation.2018.05.034
10. Bhanji F, Donoghue AJ, Wolff MS, Flores GE, Halamek LP, Berman JM, Sinz EH, Cheng A. Part 14: education: 2015 American Heart Association Guidelines Update for Cardiopulmonary Resuscitation and Emergency Cardiovascular Care.Circulation.2015;132 (suppl 2):S561-573. doi: 10.1161/CIR.0000000000000268
11. Cheng A, Lockey A, Bhanji F, Lin Y, Hunt EA, Lang E. The use of high-fidelity manikins for advanced life support training-A systematic review and meta-analysis.Resuscitation.2015;93:142-149. doi: 10.1016/j.resuscitation.2015.04.004
12. Cheng A, Nadkarni VM, Mancini MB, Hunt EA, Sinz EH, Merchant RM, Donoghue A, Duff JP, Eppich W, Auerbach M, Bigham BL, Blewer AL, Chan PS, Bhanji F; American Heart Association Education Science Investigators; and on behalf of the American Heart Association Education Science and Programs Committee, Council on Cardiopulmonary, Critical Care, Perioperative and Resuscitation; Council on Cardiovascular and Stroke Nursing; and Council on Quality of Care and Outcomes Research.Resuscitation Education Science: Educational Strategies to Improve Outcomes From Cardiac Arrest: A Scientific Statement From the American Heart Association. Circulation.2018;138:e82-e122. doi: 10.1161/CIR.0000000000000583
13. Greif R, Bhanji F, Bigham BL, Bray J, Breckwoldt J, Cheng A, Duff JP, Gilfoyle E, Hsieh M-J, Iwami T, et al; on behalf of the Education, Implementation, and Teams Collaborators.Education, implementation, and teams: 2020 International Consensus on Cardiopulmonary Resuscitation and Emergency Cardiovascular Care Science With Treatment Recommendations.Circulation.2020;142 (suppl1):S222-S283. doi: 10.1161/CIR.0000000000000896

B-CPR の自主的な実施

COR	LOE	推奨事項
2a	C-LD	1. バイスタンダーによる自主的な CPR を，CPR トレーニング，集団 CPR トレーニング，CPR 認識向上の取り組み，およびハンズオンリー CPR のプロモーションを通じて高めることは妥当である[1-4]。
2b	C-LD	2. 市民救助者向けの CPR トレーニングプログラムにおいて，バイスタンダーによる CPR 実施の意欲に影響を与える可能性のある物理的障壁の認識を高めることは妥当としてよい[2,5-11]。
2b	C-LD	3. 市民救助者向けの CPR トレーニングプログラムにおいて，バイスタンダーによる CPR 実施の意欲に影響を与える可能性のある精神的障壁に対処することは妥当としてよい[3,6,12]。

「概要」

B-CPR を迅速に実施すると，突然の心停止からの生存の可能性は 2 倍に高まるが，多くの地域社会において，B-CPR を受ける心停止傷病者の割合は 40 ％未満である[13,14]。B-CPR の実施率が比較的低いことを考えると，B-CPR 実施の促進要因と障壁を評価することは妥当である。B-CPR の自主的な実施を高める個人レベルの促進要因には，過去の CPR トレーニング，年齢の若さ，および心停止患者との家族関係がある[2,12,15,16]。地域社会レベルの促進要因には，ハンズオンリー CPR トレーニング，集団 CPR トレーニング（多人数のトレーニング），およびバイスタンダー CPR の実施を増やす CPR 認識向上の取り組みがある[1-4]。バイスタンダーの CPR 開始を妨げる障壁には，個人レベルの精神的障壁（恐怖，パニック，自信の欠如，傷病者を負傷させるかもしれないという不安など）[3,8,12]，傷病者の物理的特性の知覚（吐物，血液，女性という性別，状況の無益性の認識，患者の体位など）[2,5,7-11]，および地域社会レベルの低い SES と人種構成がある[16-21]。バイスタンダーによる CPR 実施の意欲を，集団 CPR トレーニング，CPR 認識向上の取り組み，およびハンズオンリー CPR のプロモーションを通じて高めることを提案する。また，市民救助者向けの CPR トレーニングプログラムにおいて，バイスタンダーによる CPR 実施の妨げとなる物理的障壁および精神的障壁に対処することも提案する。このような努力は，バイスタンダーによる CPR の開始を改善し，こうした既知の障壁を打破できるよう今後の取り組みを調整するための手段となる可能性がある。

「推奨事項の裏付けとなる解説」

1. あるコホート研究において，過去に CPR トレーニングを受けたバイスタンダーは，CPR を実施する可能性が 3 倍高かった[2]。5,500

名以上の大学生に対する40分間の集団ハンズオンリーCPRトレーニングは、B-CPRを促進することがわかった[3]。地域社会レベルでのハンズオンリーCPRトレーニングのプロモーションは、B-CPRの増加、および良好な神経学的転帰を伴う生存率の向上と関連性があった[1]。CPRを認識している住民、過去にCPRトレーニングを受けたことがある住民、および自己効力感が高い住民の比率が高い地域社会は、B-CPRの可能性が高いことと関連性があった[4]。測定項目が過去のCPRトレーニングおよび生態学的な地域社会レベルの事項であったことから、一部の研究には限界があった。

2. バイスタンダーへのインタビューに基づくいくつかの研究では、吐物、傷病者の呼気中のアルコール、および血液の視認がCPR開始の妨げとなる物理的障壁とされた[5,6]。通信指令員の指示によるCPRの録音テープの分析では、患者を硬く平らな面に移動できないことが、CPR実施率の低下と関連性があった[7,8]。4件の後ろ向きコホート研究において、女性は男性よりもB-CPRを受ける可能性が低かった[2,9-11]。

3. いくつかの観察研究では、パニック、自信の欠如、無益性の認識、および負傷させるかもしれないという恐怖がCPR開始の妨げとなる精神的障壁であった[6,12]。大学生へのアンケートでは、責任の重圧と心停止を判断する難しさが追加の障壁として挙げられた[3]。これらの研究は、こうした精神的障壁を打破できるようCPRトレーニングを調整すること、およびこのような障壁を広く認識させることで、バイスタンダーによるCPR実施の意欲が高まる可能性があることを示唆する。

参考資料

1. Iwami T, Kitamura T, Kiyohara K, Kawamura T. Dissemination of Chest Compression–Only Cardiopulmonary Resuscitation and Survival After Out-of-Hospital Cardiac Arrest.Circulation.2015;132:415–422. doi: 10.1161/CIRCULATIONAHA.114.014905
2. Tanigawa K, Iwami T, Nishiyama C, Nonogi H, Kawamura T. Are trained individuals more likely to perform bystander CPR? An observational study. Resuscitation.2011;82:523–528. doi: 10.1016/j.resuscitation.2011.01.027
3. Nishiyama C, Sato R, Baba M, Kuroki H, Kawamura T, Kiguchi T, Kobayashi D, Shimamoto T, Koike K, Tanaka S, Naito C, Iwami T. Actual resuscitation actions after the training of chest compression-only CPR and AED use among new university students.Resuscitation.2019;141:63–68. doi: 10.1016/j.resuscitation.2019.05.040
4. Ro YS, Shin SD, Song KJ, Hong SO, Kim YT, Lee DW, Cho SI.Public awareness and self-efficacy of cardiopulmonary resuscitation in communities and outcomes of out-of-hospital cardiac arrest: A multi-level analysis.Resuscitation.2016;102:17–24. doi: 10.1016/j.resuscitation.2016.02.004
5. McCormack AP, Damon SK, Eisenberg MS.Disagreeable physical characteristics affecting bystander CPR.Ann Emerg Med.1989;18:283–285. doi: 10.1016/s0196-0644(89)80415-9
6. Axelsson A, Herlitz J, Ekström L, Holmberg S. Bystander-initiated cardiopulmonary resuscitation out-of-hospital.A first description of the bystanders and their experiences.Resuscitation.1996;33:3–11. doi: 10.1016/s0300-9572(96)00993-8
7. Langlais BT, Panczyk M, Sutter J, Fukushima H, Wu Z, Iwami T, Spaite D, Bobrow B. Barriers to patient positioning for telephone cardiopulmonary resuscitation in out-of-hospital cardiac arrest.Resuscitation.2017;115:163–168. doi: 10.1016/j.resuscitation.2017.03.034
8. Case R, Cartledge S, Siedenburg J, Smith K, Straney L, Barger B, Finn J, Bray JE.Identifying barriers to the provision of bystander cardiopulmonary resuscitation (CPR) in high-risk regions: A qualitative review of emergency calls. Resuscitation.2018;129:43–47. doi: 10.1016/j.resuscitation.2018.06.001
9. Blewer AL, McGovern SK, Schmicker RH, May S, Morrison LJ, Aufderheide TP, Daya M, Idris AH, Callaway CW, Kudenchuk PJ, Vilke GM, Abella BS; Resuscitation Outcomes Consortium (ROC) Investigators.Gender Disparities Among Adult Recipients of Bystander Cardiopulmonary Resuscitation in the Public.Circ Cardiovasc Qual Outcomes.2018;11:e004710. doi: 10.1161/CIRCOUTCOMES.118.004710
10. Matsuyama T, Okubo M, Kiyohara K, Kiguchi T, Kobayashi D, Nishiyama C, Okabayashi S, Shimamoto T, Izawa J, Komukai S, Gibo K, Ohta B, Kitamura T, Kawamura T, Iwami T. Sex-Based Disparities in Receiving Bystander Cardiopulmonary Resuscitation by Location of Cardiac Arrest in Japan.Mayo Clin Proc.2019;94:577–587. doi: 10.1016/j.mayocp.2018.12.028
11. Matsui S, Kitamura T, Kiyohara K, Sado J, Ayusawa M, Nitta M, Iwami T, Nakata K, Kitamura Y, Sobue T; SPIRITS Investigators.Sex Disparities in Receipt of Bystander Interventions for Students Who Experienced Cardiac Arrest in Japan.JAMA Netw Open.2019;2:e195111. doi: 10.1001/jamanetworkopen.2019.5111
12. Swor R, Khan I, Domeier R, Honeycutt L, Chu K, Compton S. CPR training and CPR performance: do CPR-trained bystanders perform CPR? Acad Emerg Med.2006;13:596–601. doi: 10.1197/j.aem.2005.12.021
13. Girotra S, van Diepen S, Nallamothu BK, Carrel M, Vellano K, Anderson ML, McNally B, Abella BS, Sasson C, Chan PS; CARES Surveillance Group and the HeartRescue Project.Regional Variation in Out-of-Hospital Cardiac Arrest Survival in the United States.Circulation.2016;133:2159–2168. doi: 10.1161/CIRCULATIONAHA.115.018175
14. Iwami T, Nichol G, Hiraide A, Hayashi Y, Nishiuchi T, Kajino K, Morita H, Yukioka H, Ikeuchi H, Sugimoto H, Nonogi H, Kawamura T. Continuous improvements in "chain of survival" increased survival after out-of-hospital cardiac arrests: a large-scale population-based study.Circulation.2009;119:728–734. doi: 10.1161/CIRCULATIONAHA.108.802058
15. Greif R, Bhanji F, Bigham BL, Bray J, Breckwoldt J, Cheng A, Duff JP, Gilfoyle E, Hsieh M-J, Iwami T, et al; on behalf of the Education, Implementation, and Teams Collaborators.Education, implementation, and teams: 2020 International Consensus on Cardiopulmonary Resuscitation and Emergency Cardiovascular Care Science With Treatment Recommendations.Circulation.2020;142(suppl 1):S222–S283. doi: 10.1161/CIR.0000000000000896
16. Chang I, Kwak YH, Shin SD, Ro YS, Kim DK.Characteristics of bystander cardiopulmonary resuscitation for paediatric out-of-hospital cardiac arrests: A national observational study from 2012 to 2014.Resuscitation.2017;111:26–33. doi: 10.1016/j.resuscitation.2016.11.007
17. Chiang WC, Ko PC, Chang AM, Chen WT, Liu SS, Huang YS, Chen SY, Lin CH, Cheng MT, Chong KM, Wang HC, Yang CW, Liao MW, Wang CH, Chien YC, Lin CH, Liu YP, Lee BC, Chien KL, Lai MS, Ma MH.Bystander-initiated CPR in an Asian metropolitan: does the socioeconomic status matter? Resuscitation.2014;85:53–58. doi: 10.1016/j.resuscitation.2013.07.033
18. Dahan B, Jabre P, Karam N, Misslin R, Tafflet M, Bougouin W, Jost D, Beganton F, Marijon E, Jouven X. Impact of neighbourhood socio-economic status on bystander cardiopulmonary resuscitation in Paris.Resuscitation.2017;110:107–113. doi: 10.1016/j.resuscitation.2016.10.028
19. Moncur L, Ainsborough N, Ghose R, Kendal SP, Salvatori M, Wright J. Does the level of socioeconomic deprivation at the location of cardiac arrest in an English region influence the likelihood of receiving bystander-initiated cardiopulmonary resuscitation? Emerg Med J. 2016;33:105–108. doi: 10.1136/emermed-2015-204643
20. Vaillancourt C, Lui A, De Maio VJ, Wells GA, Stiell IG.Socioeconomic status influences bystander CPR and survival rates for out-of-hospital cardiac arrest victims.Resuscitation.2008;79:417–423. doi: 10.1016/j.resuscitation.2008.07.012
21. Sasson C, Magid DJ, Chan P, Root ED, McNally BF, Kellermann AL, Haukoos JS; CARES Surveillance Group.Association of neighborhood characteristics with bystander-initiated CPR.N Engl J Med.2012;367:1607–1615. doi: 10.1056/NEJMoa1110700

今後の課題とさらなる研究

蘇生教育を実施する最適な手段を規定するには、重要な課題を扱うしっかりとデザインされた研究が必要となる。蘇生教育研究には固有の限界があり、臨床蘇生研究と比べて進展が阻まれている。これは、本章で提示されている推奨事項のほとんどが「弱」に分類され、GRADE基準で「低」に分類されたエビデンスレベルに基づいていることから容易に理解できる[1]。これは、部分的には、教育研究の評価にGRADEを使用することに伴う固有の限界を表していると考えられる。今回レビューした研究の多くは検出力が不十分な単一施設研究であり、そこから関心のある介入の真の影響を明らかにすることは難しい。多施設研究という形で多くの施設が協力し合えば、この問題の解決に役立つ[2]。教育研究ネットワークは、メンター

表2. 蘇生教育における今後の全般的な課題

トピック領域	研究課題の例
アウトカムの関連性	トレーニングの教育成果（知識とスキル），臨床パフォーマンス，および患者転帰の間に関連性はあるか。
患者転帰	教育的介入および／または特定の教授システム学（インストラクショナル・デザイン）上の要素は患者転帰にどのような影響を及ぼすか。
報告の標準化	研究間の不均一性をなくすために蘇生教育研究のアウトカムをどのように標準化できるか。
費用対効果	各種教育的介入の費用対効果はどの程度か。
教授システム学（インストラクショナル・デザイン）の最適化	教授システム学（インストラクショナル・デザイン）上の要素を組み合わせて学習成果と患者転帰を最適化するにはどうすればよいか。
教授システム学（インストラクショナル・デザイン）の調整	それぞれの教授システム学（インストラクショナル・デザイン）の要素に最も適している蘇生スキル／能力はどれか。
学習曲線とスキル定着	主要な蘇生スキルの学習曲線はどのようなもので，スキルの長期的な定着を最適化するにはトレーニングをどのように構成すればよいか。

シップ，助成金申請，研究のデザインと実施，および知識普及を支えるために必要な基盤を提供する[2,3]。蘇生教育研究の間に広がっているもう1つの全般的な問題は，アウトカムの選択である[4,5]。他の科学分野とはかなり異なるやり方で，シミュレーション環境におけるプロバイダーのパフォーマンスを実際の患者治療時のパフォーマンス（または患者転帰）に直接結び付けることは，依然として難しい。過去数年の間，教育的介入を実際の患者イベント後の臨床転帰にうまく結び付けた研究はほんの一握りであり[6-10]，ほとんどの教育研究は，学習者の知識とシミュレーション環境でのスキルパフォーマンスという代理アウトカムを検討している。蘇生研究者は，教育的介入に由来する臨床転帰を報告したいと望んでいる（表2）。患者転帰の選択が不可能な場合，教育研究者には，心停止からの臨床転帰の改善との関連性がすでに認められている定量的な評価基準（胸骨圧迫の深さなど）を選択することを勧める。そうすることで，研究者は，シミュレーションベースの研究と臨床研究で同じように報告されているアウトカムの間の因果関係を確立できる[11]。

今回の文献レビューで見つかった介入やアウトカム評価基準の種類は一貫しておらず，主要トピックの多くについてメタアナリシスを行うのは難しい。多くの研究の間で共通しているアウトカムでさえ（CPRの深さなど），アウトカム評価基準の種類は多岐にわたった（CPRの深さの平均，30秒ごとのCPRの深さの遵守率，イベントあたりのCPRの深さの遵守率など）。蘇生教育研究におけるアウトカムの報告について標準化されたガイドラインが確立されれば，この問題は解決し，今後主要な問題のメタアナリシスが可能となる（表2）。このような欠点を認めてもなお，教育研究には，他の蘇生科学の分野と同じように，さらなる調査を必要とする基本的な知識の格差がある。

いくつかの一般的な課題は，今後の蘇生教育研究にとって不可欠な検討事項として特筆に値する。教育的介入を患者転帰に結び付けた研究は非常に少ないため，教育成果と心停止からの生存率との関係，および既知の生存寄与因子である他の中間的な臨床転帰（質の高いCPR，除細動までの時間，CPR開始までの時間など）からの生存率との関係を調べるためにさらなる研究が必要とされる。知識やスキルをアウトカムとする研究の中で，それらのアウトカムをコース終了直後の単一時点にのみ評価しているものが非常に多い。特に，一部の教育戦略は短期的には良好な改善を示すものの長期的な学習成果は低いという事実を考え合わせると，今後の研究では，コース終了時点だけでなく長期にわたる知識やスキルの定着に重点を置く必要がある。今回特定された研究の多くは，ある特定の教授システム学（インストラクショナル・デザイン）上の要素を単独で検討していたか，関心変数を適切に分離できない研究デザインを実施していた。今後の研究は，潜在的交絡変数（同時教育機会，過去の経験，評価者盲検化など）を制御するようデザインするか，関心変数について調整を行う統計解析を含めるようにデザインするのが望ましい。さらに，複数の教授システム学（インストラクショナル・デザイン）上の要素を特定の蘇生スキルに適用する場合は，それらの要素の複合効果を深く理解すると，将来的に学習成果の向上に役立つ。

蘇生教育の経済的評価に関して，大きな課題が存在する。経済的評価とは，少なくとも2つの選択肢（CPRフィードバック器具を使用したBLSトレーニングと使用しないBLSトレーニングなど）をコストと結果の両面から調べる研究様式である[12]。最新の文献から，ある特定の教授システム学（インストラクショナル・デザイン）上の要素の有効性を裏付けるエビデンスが得られてはいるが，それでも，教育プログラムにおいてあるトレーニング方法を採用するかどうかを決定する際には潜在的有益性とコストのバランスをとる必要がある。費用対効果分析を適切に実施することで，このような決断を下すことができる。今後の教育研究では，トレーニングの有効性と関連コストの両方を探求することが求められる（表2）。これは，ある特定の教授システム学（インストラクショナル・デザイン）の実践を促進するだけでなく，限られたリソースで学習成果を最大限に高める方法についてのエビデンスを確立するためにも役立つ。

執筆グループは，明白な課題がある主要分野をいくつか特定した。学習を推進する評価はAHAの中心的な教育概念のひとつであるが，蘇生教育における評価の慣行について報告する研究は比較的少ない[5]。今後のコース設計に活かすため，フィードバックの提供元（インストラクター，マネキン，器具），タイミング，および構造を検討する研究が求められる。発表されている文献で

表3. 蘇生教育におけるトピック別の今後の具体的な課題

トピック領域	研究課題の例
完全習得学習	各種蘇生スキルの最低到達基準はどのようなもので、それらの基準をトレーニングの完全習得学習モデルに組み込むことはスキルの習得と定着の向上につながるか。
ブースター訓練	主要な蘇生スキルの、経時的なスキル低下を防ぐ最適なブースター訓練の間隔はどの程度か。
市民救助者トレーニング	バイスタンダーCPR実施率、CPRの質、および患者転帰の向上を実現するために市民救助者トレーニングを最適化するにはどうすればよいか。
チームワークおよびリーダーシップトレーニング	パフォーマンスを強化するために蘇生チームの構成をどのように変更できるか（CPR指導者の追加など）。また、そのような新しい構成でのトレーニングによって成果は向上するか。
フィードバックとデブリーフィング	蘇生トレーニング中のフィードバックとデブリーフィングの提供元、頻度、構造、内容、およびタイミングは成果にどのように影響するか。
トレーニングにおける技術	蘇生の実施や患者転帰を改善するために新しい技術（VR、拡張現実、アイトラッキング、人工知能など）をどのように利用できるか。
教育格差	蘇生教育において人種的、民族的、社会経済的、および性別的な格差に対処する最適な方法はどのようなものか。
ファカルティ・ディベロップメント	拡張性と効果を兼ね備えた、蘇生インストラクターの最良のトレーニング方法はどのようなものか。
学習者の評価	蘇生トレーニング中の最も効果的な評価戦略はどのようなものか。
トレーニングにおける認知支援ツール	学習を支援するために認知支援ツールを蘇生トレーニングプログラムに効果的に組み込むにはどうすればよいか。

CPR：心肺蘇生（cardiopulmonary resuscitation），VR：バーチャルリアリティ（virtual reality）。

は、蘇生コース受講者の形成的および累積的評価を行うためにさまざまな手段が用いられており、その数は増え続けている[4]。医療従事者の評価は、臨床知識、技術的スキル、およびチームワークの領域にわたる。特定の領域に適した手段を選択することは、トレーニングプログラムの評価戦略の一部である。このような目的のために設計された手段は、信頼性と一般化可能性について厳しくテストする必要がある。評価者トレーニングの戦略について定義し、これらの手段の使用を異なる学習者グループや環境にわたって広く標準化すれば、今後の研究に役立つ（表3）。

蘇生指導者にファカルティ・ディベロップメントの機会を与えると、蘇生トレーニングプログラムを効果的に実施できるようになる。医学教育における効果的なファカルティ・ディベロップメントの重要な特徴について記述した文献はあるが[13]、蘇生指導者のトレーニングに適用するには研究がまだ不足している。最後に、トレーニング中の認知支援ツールの使用、ハイブリッドコース設計（eラーニングとその他の学習方法の組み合わせなど）、人工知能、拡張現実などのトピックは、興味深いテーマではあるものの、今後の実践に関する推奨事項を提示するためにはもっと多くのエビデンスが必要である（表3）。

本ガイドラインではVRやゲーム方式の学習といった新しい教育戦略を取り上げたが、反復学習、ブースター訓練、集中的な練習、フィードバックなどの基本的な構成要素にも引き続き目を向けていく必要がある。これらすべての領域で、重要な課題（とそれに伴う今後の研究の余地）が残っている（表3）。AHAは資金提供機関に対して、心停止の転帰を改善するうえでの蘇生教育の重要な役割を認識し、蘇生教育の研究に的を絞った資金援助の機会を提供するよう求めている。適切な資金提供があれば、研究者はより新しい事象を探求でき、従来からある蘇生教育のパラダイムを引き続き評価することもできる。このアプローチにより、AHAは今後も教育効率の向上と心停止からの転帰の改善を推進していく。

参考資料

1. Magid DJ, Aziz K, Cheng A, Hazinski MF, Hoover AV, Mahgoub M, Panchal AR, Sasson C, Topjian AA, Rodriguez AJ, et al.Part 2: evidence evaluation and guidelines development: 2020 American Heart Association Guidelines for Cardiopulmonary Resuscitation and Emergency Cardiovascular Care.Circulation.2020;142 (suppl 2):S358-S365. doi: 10.1161/CIR.0000000000000898

2. Schwartz A, Young R, Hicks PJ, Appd L. Medical education practice-based research networks: Facilitating collaborative research.Med Teach.2016;38:64-74. doi: 10.3109/0142159X.2014.970991

3. Cheng A, Auerbach M, Calhoun A, Mackinnon R, Chang TP, Nadkarni V, Hunt EA, Duval-Arnould J, Peiris N, Kessler DatII.Building a community of practice for researchers: the international network for simulation-based pediatric innovation, research and education.Simul Healthc.2018;13(suppl 1):S28-S34. doi: 10.1097/SIH.0000000000000269

4. Cheng A, Nadkarni VM, Mancini MB, Hunt EA, Sinz EH, Merchant RM, Donoghue A, Duff JP, Eppich W, Auerbach M, Bigham BL, Blewer AL, Chan PS, Bhanji F; American Heart Association Education Science Investigators; and on behalf of the American Heart Association Education Science and Programs Committee, Council on Cardiopulmonary, Critical Care, Perioperative and Resuscitation; Council on Cardiovascular and Stroke Nursing; and Council on Quality of Care and Outcomes Research.Resuscitation Education Science: Educational Strategies to Improve Outcomes From Cardiac Arrest: A Scientific Statement From the American Heart Association.Circulation.2018;138:e82-e122. doi: 10.1161/CIR.0000000000000583

5. Bhanji F, Donoghue AJ, Wolff MS, Flores GE, Halamek LP, Berman JM, Sinz EH, Cheng A. Part 14: education: 2015 American Heart Association Guidelines Update for Cardiopulmonary Resuscitation and Emergency Cardiovascular Care.Circulation.2015;132(suppl 2):S561-573. doi: 10.1161/CIR.0000000000000268

6. Wayne DB, Didwania A, Feinglass J, Fudala MJ, Barsuk JH, McGaghie WC.Simulation-based education improves quality of care during cardiac arrest team responses at an academic teaching hospital: a case-control study. Chest.2008;133:56-61. doi: 10.1378/chest.07-0131

7. Edelson DP, Litzinger B, Arora V, Walsh D, Kim S, Lauderdale DS, Vanden Hoek TL, Becker LB, Abella BS.Improving in-hospital cardiac arrest process and outcomes with performance debriefing.Arch Intern Med.2008;168:1063-1069. doi: 10.1001/archinte.168.10.1063

8. Wolfe H, Zebuhr C, Topjian AA, Nishisaki A, Niles DE, Meaney PA, Boyle L, Giordano RT, Davis D, Priestley M, Apkon M, Berg RA, Nadkarni VM, Sutton RM.Interdisciplinary ICU cardiac arrest debriefing improves survival outcomes*.Crit Care Med.2014;42:1688-1695. doi: 10.1097/CCM.0000000000000327

9. Bobrow BJ, Spaite DW, Vadeboncoeur TF, Hu C, Mullins T, Tormala W, Dameff C, Gallagher J, Smith G, Panczyk M. Implementation of a Regional Telephone Cardiopulmonary Resuscitation Program and Outcomes After Out-of-Hospital Cardiac Arrest.JAMA Cardiol.2016;1:294-302. doi: 10.1001/jamacardio.2016.0251

10. Morrison LJ, Brooks SC, Dainty KN, Dorian P, Needham DM, Ferguson ND, Rubenfeld GD, Slutsky AS, Wax RS, Zwarenstein M, Thorpe K, Zhan C, Scales DC; Strategies for Post-Arrest Care Network.Improving use of targeted temperature management after out-of-hospital cardiac arrest: a stepped wedge cluster randomized controlled trial.Crit Care Med.2015;43:954-964. doi: 10.1097/CCM.0000000000000864
11. Cook DA, West CP.Perspective: reconsidering the focus on "outcomes research" in medical education: a cautionary note.Acad Med.2013;88:162-167. doi: 10.1097/ACM.0b013e31827c3d78
12. Lin Y, Cheng A, Hecker K, Grant V, Currie GR.Implementing economic evaluation in simulation-based medical education: challenges and opportunities.Med Educ.2018;52:150-160. doi: 10.1111/medu.13411
13. Steinert Y, Mann K, Anderson B, Barnett BM, Centeno A, Naismith L, Prideaux D, Spencer J, Tullo E, Viggiano T, Ward H, Dolmans D. A systematic review of faculty development initiatives designed to enhance teaching effectiveness: A 10-year update: BEME Guide No. 40.Med Teach.2016;38:769-786. doi: 10.1080/0142159X.2016.1181851

文献情報

アメリカ心臓協会は，本書を以下のとおりに引用するよう要請する。Cheng A, Magid DJ, Auerbach M, Bhanji F, Bigham BL, Blewer AL, Dainty KN, Diederich E, Lin Y, Leary M, Mahgoub M, Mancini ME, Navarro K, Donoghue A. Part 6: resuscitation education science: 2020 American Heart Association Guidelines for Cardiopulmonary Resuscitation and Emergency Cardiovascular Care.循環.2020;142 (suppl 2):S551-S579. doi: 10.1161/CIR.0000000000000903

情報開示

付録 1.　執筆グループの情報開示

執筆グループメンバー	所属	研究助成金	その他の研究支援	講演／謝礼金	鑑定人	株式所有	コンサルタント／顧問	その他
Adam Cheng	University of Calgary	なし	なし	なし	なし	なし	なし	なし
Aaron Donoghue	The Children's Hospital of Philadelphia, University of Pennsylvania School of Medicine	なし	なし	なし	Atkinson, Haskins, Nellis, Brittingham, Gladd & Fiasco*	なし	なし	なし
Marc Auerbach	Yale University	なし	なし	なし	なし	なし	なし	なし
Farhan Bhanji	McGill University	なし	なし	なし	なし	なし	なし	なし
Blair L. Bigham	McMaster University Emergency Medicine	なし	なし	なし	なし	なし	なし	なし
Audrey L. Blewer	Duke University	なし	なし	なし	なし	なし	なし	なし
Katie N. Dainty	North York General Hospital Research and Innovation	なし	なし	なし	なし	なし	なし	なし
Emily Diederich	University of Kansas Medical Center Internal Medicine	なし	なし	なし	なし	なし	なし	なし
Marion Leary	Center for Resuscitation Science	なし	なし	なし	なし	なし	なし	なし
Yiqun Lin	Alberta Children's Hospital KidSIM Simulation Research Program	なし	なし	なし	なし	なし	なし	なし
David J. Magid	University of Colorado	NIH†，NHLBI†，CMS†，AHA†	なし	なし	なし	なし	なし	アメリカ心臓協会（上級科学編集者）†
Melissa Mahgoub	American Heart Association	なし	なし	なし	なし	なし	なし	なし
Mary E. Mancini	The University of Texas at Arlington College of Nursing and Health Innovation	なし	なし	Stryker*	なし	なし	なし	なし
Kenneth Navarro	The University of Texas Southwestern Medical Center at Dallas Emergency Medicine	なし	なし	なし	なし	なし	なし	なし

　この表は，執筆グループの全メンバーに回答および提出が求められる情報開示アンケート（Disclosure Questionnaire）の結果に基づき実在の利益相反または合理的に認定できる利益相反とみなされる可能性のある，執筆グループメンバーの関係を示している。メンバーと該当団体との関係が「顕著」であると考えられるのは，次のいずれかの状況が存在する場合である。（a）当該メンバーが団体から受領する金額が過去いずれの 12 か月間に $10,000 以上であるか，メンバーの総収入の 5％以上である，（b）団体の議決権株式の 5％以上，またはその団体の公正市場価値の $10,000 以上を保有している。この定義において「重大」に相当するレベルに満たない場合，その関係は「軽度」とみなされる。
　*軽度
　†重大

付録 2. レビューアーの情報開示

レビューアー	所属	研究助成金	その他の研究支援	講演／謝礼金	鑑定人	株式所有	コンサルタント／顧問	その他
Jeffrey M. Berman	UNC Hospitals	なし	なし	なし	なし	なし	なし	なし
Aaron W. Calhoun	University of Louisville	なし	なし	なし	なし	なし	なし	なし
Maia Dorsett	University of Rochester Medical Center	なし	なし	なし	なし	なし	なし	なし
Joyce Foresman-Capuzzi	Lankenau Medical Center	なし	なし	なし	なし	なし	なし	なし
Louis P. Halamek	Stanford University	なし	なし	なし	なし	なし	なし	なし
Mary Ann McNeil	University of Minnesota	なし	なし	なし	なし	なし	なし	なし
Catherine Patocka	University of Calgary（カナダ）	なし	なし	なし	なし	なし	なし	なし
David L. Rodgers	Penn State	なし	なし	なし	なし	なし	なし	なし

この表は，執筆グループの全メンバーに回答および提出が求められる情報開示アンケート（Disclosure Questionnaire）の結果に基づき実在の利益相反または合理的に認定できる利益相反とみなされる可能性のある，執筆グループメンバーの関係を示している。メンバーと該当団体との関係が「顕著」であると考えられるのは，次のいずれかの状況が存在する場合である。（a）当該メンバーが団体から受領する金額が過去いずれの 12 か月間に $10,000 以上であるか，メンバーの総収入の 5％以上である，（b）団体の議決権株式の 5％以上，またはその団体の公正市場価値の $10,000 以上を保有している。この定義において「重大」に相当するレベルに満たない場合，その関係は「軽度」とみなされる。

*軽度
†重大

Circulation

第7章：治療システム
AHA 心肺蘇生と救急心血管治療のためのガイドライン2020

抄録：心停止後の生存には，共通の目標を目指して連携する人，訓練，機器，および組織の統合されたシステムが必要である。『アメリカ心臓協会（AHA）心肺蘇生と救急心血管治療のためのガイドライン2020（2020 American Heart Association (AHA) Guidelines for Cardiopulmonary Resuscitation and Emergency Cardiovascular Care）』の第7章は，治療システムに焦点を当て，さまざまな蘇生状況に関連する要素に注目する。過去の治療システムガイドラインでは，心停止の予防と早期認識に始まり，蘇生から心拍再開後の治療にいたるまでの救命の連鎖を明らかにした。この概念は，心停止からの生存にとって重要な一段階として，回復を加えることによって強化される。デブリーフィングとその他の質向上戦略については以前から言及されており，現在も協調されている。特に院外心停止について，心停止の認識を推進する地域の取り組み，心肺蘇生法，市民による電気ショック（除細動），第1救助者を招集する携帯電話のテクノロジー，救急テレコミュニケーターの役割強化に関する推奨事項を扱う。院内心停止と密接に関係するのは，心停止に陥るにリスクのある院内患者の認識と安定化についての推奨事項である。この章では，臨床デブリーフィング，専門の心停止治療センターへの搬送，臓器提供，一連の蘇生状況を通してのパフォーマンス測定に関する推奨事項も取り上げる。

Katherine M. Berg, MD, Chair
Adam Cheng, MD
Ashish R. Panchal, MD, PhD
Alexis A. Topjian, MD, MSCE
Khalid Aziz, MBBS, MA, MEd（IT）
Farhan Bhanji, MD, MSc（Ed）
Blair L. Bigham, MD, MSc
Karen G. Hirsch, MD
Amber V. Hoover, RN, MSN
Michael C. Kurz, MD, MS
Arielle Levy, MD, MEd
Yiqun Lin, MD, MHSc, PhD
David J. Magid, MD, MPH
Melissa Mahgoub, PhD
Mary Ann Peberdy, MD
Amber J. Rodriguez, PhD
Comilla Sasson, MD, PhD
Eric J. Lavonas, MD, MS
成人一次救命処置と二次救命処置，小児一次救命処置と二次救命処置，新生児救命処置，蘇生教育科学執筆グループを代表して

キーワード：AHA による科学的提言
■ 心肺蘇生 ■ ヘルスケアの提供
■ 救急サービスの通信指令員
■ 院内の迅速対応チーム ■ 臓器移植 ■ 患者治療チーム ■ 質向上

© 2020 American Heart Association, Inc.

https://www.ahajournals.org/journal/circ

覚えておくべき重要な事項（10項目）：治療システム

1. 回復は蘇生における救命の連鎖の重要な要素である。
2. 一般市民が心肺蘇生（CPR）を実施し自動体外式除細動器（AED）を使用する能力および意欲をサポートする取り組みが，地域における蘇生の転帰を改善する。
3. CPRを要するイベントの発生を，訓練を受けた市民救助者に通知する，携帯電話技術を用いる新しい方法は都市部では有望であり，さらなる研究が求められる。
4. 救急システムのテレコミュニケーターは，成人のハンズオンリーCPRを実施するよう，バイスタンダーに指示することができる。No-No-Goの枠組みは有効である。
5. 早期警告スコアシステムおよび迅速対応チームは，小児および成人いずれの病院でも心停止を防ぐことができるが，これらのシステムのどの要素が利益に関連するのかについては，文献によって異なり理解が難しい。
6. 認知支援ツールにより，訓練を受けていない市民救助者による蘇生の実施は改善する可能性があるが，CPRの開始が遅延する。これらのシステムが完全に支持されるには，さらなる開発と研究が必要である。
7. 救急医療サービス（EMS）または病院ベースの蘇生チームのパフォーマンスに対する認知支援の影響については，驚くべきことにほとんどわかっていない。
8. 専門の心停止治療センターでは，すべての病院では実施できないプロトコルとテクノロジーが提供されるが，文献による蘇生の転帰への影響は一貫していない。
9. チームのフィードバックは重要である。体系的なデブリーフィングプロトコルにより，その後の蘇生活動における蘇生チームのパフォーマンスが改善する。
10. システム全体のフィードバックは重要である。体系的なデータ収集およびレビューを実施することにより，院内および院外のいずれの蘇生プロセスと生存も改善する。

前文

蘇生の成功には，訓練を受けたプロバイダーが体系化された枠組みの中でそれぞれに重要な役割を果たし，迅速かつ協調した行動をとる必要がある。意欲のあるバイスタンダー，自動体外式除細動器（AED）を維持管理する所有者，救急サービスのテレコミュニケーター（通信指令員または通報対応オペレーターとも呼ばれる），および救急医療サービス（EMS）システム内の一次救命処置（BLS）および二次救命処置（ALS）プロバイダーのすべてが，院外心停止（OHCA）からの蘇生成功に寄与している。病院内では，医師，看護師，呼吸療法士，薬剤師，および他の多くのスタッフの努力が蘇生の転帰を支える。また，蘇生の成功は，機器メーカー，製薬会社，心肺蘇生インストラクター，インストラクターの指導者，ガイドライン作成者，その他多くの人々にも依心肺存している。心停止後の長期的な回復には家族と専門介護者のサポートが必要であり，それには多くの場合，認知面，身体面，そして心理面でのリハビリテーションおよび回復の専門家が含まれる。心停止後の良好な転帰を達成するためには，予防から認識や治療まで，ケアのあらゆるレベルで，システム全体として学習し前進するといったアプローチが不可欠である。

このような治療システムのガイドラインは，あらゆる年齢層に幅広く適用できるさまざまな蘇生の側面に重点を置く。ガイドラインが強調するのは，一連のケアの各手順で心停止からの生存を改善する戦略である。迅速な心肺蘇生（CPR）と早期の除細動を受けるOHCA患者の割合を増加させること，院内心停止（IHCA）を予防すること，蘇生チームのパフォーマンスを改善する認知支援ツールの利用や，専門の心停止治療センターの役割，臓器提供，蘇生チームのパフォーマンス向上と蘇生の転帰改善の手段を検討することなどが挙げられる。

概要

ガイドラインの範囲

このガイドラインは主に臨床ケアの概要や蘇生システムのデザインとオペレーションに関する最新のサマリーを求めている北米の医療従事者に向けて作成されているが，蘇生科学に関してさらに詳細な情報を得て現在の知識とのギャップを埋めたい人にも役立つ。『AHA心肺蘇生と救急心血管治療のためのガイドライン2020 (2020 American Heart Association (AHA) Guidelines for CPR and Emergency Cardiovascular Care (ECC))』のこの章では，救命の連鎖に寄与するさまざまな人（救急のテレコミュニケーターや訓練を受けていない市民救助者など）の連携にかかわるケアの各要素，異なる集団の蘇生に共通する要素（地域社会のCPR訓練と一般市民による除細動，IHCAを予防するための早期介入），蘇生チームとシステムのパフォーマンスを改善する手段を主に取り上げる。

推奨事項の一部は，市民救助者に直接関係するものである。市民救助者には，CPRの訓練を受けた人と受けていない人がおり，蘇生器具をほとんど利用しないあるいはまったく利用しない人がいる。また，高度な蘇生訓練を受け，場合によって蘇生薬や蘇生器具を使用し，院内または院外で活動する人に関連する推奨事項も提示する。EMSの到着前に指示を与える救急テレコミュニケーターの行動についての推奨事項も記載する。治療に関する推奨事項の中には，自己心拍再開（ROSC）後または蘇生が不成功であった後の医療処置と意思決定にかかわるものがある。重要なこととして，将来の蘇生成功率を

表 1. 患者ケアにおける臨床上の戦略，介入，治療，または診断検査への推奨事項のクラスとエビデンスレベルの適用（2019 年 5 月更新）*

推奨事項のクラス（強さ）

クラス 1（強い）　　　　　　　　　　　　　　利益＞＞＞リスク

推奨事項文に適した表現例：
- 推奨される
- 適応／有用／有効／有益である
- 実施／投与（など）すべきである
- 比較に基づく有効性の表現例†：
  - 治療 B よりも治療／治療戦略 A が推奨される／適応である
  - 治療 B よりも治療 A を選択すべきである

クラス 2a（中等度）　　　　　　　　　　　　　利益＞＞リスク

推奨事項文に適した表現例：
- 妥当である
- 有用／有効／有益でありうる
- 比較に基づく有効性の表現例†：
  - 治療 B よりも治療／治療戦略 A がおそらく推奨される／適応である
  - 治療 B よりも治療 A を選択することが妥当である

クラス 2b（弱い）　　　　　　　　　　　　　　利益≧リスク

推奨事項文に適した表現例：
- 妥当としてよい／よいだろう
- 考慮してもよい／よいだろう
- 有用性／有効性は不明／不明確／不確実である，あるいは十分に確立されていない

クラス 3：利益なし（中等度）　　　　　　　　　利益＝リスク
（一般に LOE A または B の使用に限る）

推奨事項文に適した表現例：
- 推奨しない
- 適応／有用／有効／有益ではない
- 実施／投与（など）すべきでない

クラス 3：有害（強い）　　　　　　　　　　　　リスク＞利益

推奨事項文に適した表現例：
- 有害な可能性がある
- 有害となる
- 合併症発生率／死亡率の上昇を伴う
- 実施／投与（など）すべきでない

エビデンスレベル（質）‡

レベル A
- 複数の RCT から得られた質の高いエビデンス‡
- 質の高い RCT のメタアナリシス
- 質の高い症例登録試験によって裏付けられた 1 件以上の RCT

レベル B-R　　　　　　　　　　　　　　　　　（無作為化）
- 1 件以上の RCT から得られた質が中等度のエビデンス‡
- 質が中等度の RCT のメタアナリシス

レベル B-NR　　　　　　　　　　　　　　　　（非無作為化）
- 1 件以上の綿密にデザインされ，適切に実施された非無作為化試験，観察研究，または症例登録試験から得られた質が中等度のエビデンス‡
- そのような試験のメタアナリシス

レベル C-LD　　　　　　　　　　　　　　　　（限定的なデータ）
- デザインまたは実施に限界がある無作為化または非無作為化観察研究または症例登録試験
- そのような試験のメタアナリシス
- ヒトを対象にした生理学的試験または反応機構研究

レベル C-EO　　　　　　　　　　　　　　　　（専門家の見解）
- 臨床経験に基づく専門家の見解のコンセンサス

COR および LOE は個別に決定する（COR と LOE のあらゆる組み合わせが可能）。

LOE C の推奨事項は，その推奨事項が弱いことを意味するわけではない。ガイドラインが扱っている重要な医療上の問題の多くは，臨床試験の対象となっていない。RCT が行われていなくても，特定の検査あるいは治療法の有用性／有効性について，臨床上非常に明確なコンセンサスが得られている場合がある。

* 介入の成果または結果を記述すべきである（臨床転帰の改善，または診断精度の向上，または予後情報の増加）。

† 比較に基づく有効性の推奨事項（COR 1 および 2a，LOE A および B のみ）に関してその推奨事項の裏付けとなる試験は，評価する治療または治療戦略を直接比較しているものでなければならない。

‡ 標準化され，広く用いられていて，望ましくは検証されている複数のエビデンス評価ツールを活用し，システマティックレビューについてはエビデンスレビュー委員会を設けるなど，質を評価する方法は進化している。

COR：推奨事項のクラス（Class of Recommendation），EO：専門家の見解（expert opinion），LD：限定的なデータ（limited data），LOE：エビデンスレベル（Level of Evidence），NR：非無作為化（nonrandomized），R：無作為化（randomized），RCT：無作為化比較試験（randomized controlled trial）。

高めるために，チームデブリーフィングと体系的なフィードバックに関する推奨事項も取り上げた。

「新型コロナウイルス感染症（COVID-19）ガイダンス」

AHA は他の専門学会と協力して，COVID-19 感染確定例または感染疑いのある成人，小児，新生児の一次救命処置と二次救命処置の暫定的ガイダンスを提供している。COVID-19 の状況に伴いエビデンスおよびガイダンスは変化し続けているため，この暫定的ガイダンスは ECC ガイドラインとは別に管理する。最新のガイダンスについては AHA の CPR および ECC の Web サイト（cpr.heart.orghttp://cpr.heart.org）を参照。1)

治療システム執筆グループの組織

治療システム執筆グループは，臨床医学，教育，研究，公衆衛生などさまざまな背景の専門家で構成されている。治療システムのガイドラインは主要執筆グループの資材を利用しているため，各執筆グループの委員長がその分野に関する専門家，AHA のスタッフ，AHA 上級科学編集者と協力して治療システムガイドラインを作成した。各勧告は，元の情報を担当した執筆グループが作成し，正式に承認した。

AHA は厳格な利益相反の方針と手順を有しており，ガイドライン策定中のバイアスや不適切な影響のリスクを最小限にしている。指名に先立ち，執筆グループのメンバーは商業的な関係

とその他の利益相反（知的財産含む）の可能性をすべて開示した。この手順は「第2章：エビデンス評価とガイドライン作成」[2]に詳細に記載されている。執筆グループメンバーの開示情報を付録1に列挙した。

方法論とエビデンスのレビュー

この治療システムガイドラインは，国際蘇生連絡委員会（International Liaison Committee on Resuscitation, ILCOR）および提携するILCOR加盟団体が協力して行った網羅的なエビデンス評価に基づいている。2020年のプロセスでは3種類のエビデンスレビュー（システマティックレビュー，スコーピングレビュー，エビデンスアップデート）を使用した。それぞれの結果はガイドラインの策定に使用した文献の記述として示した。これらの手法の詳細は「第2章：エビデンス評価とガイドライン作成」[2]に記載されている。

推奨事項のクラスおよびエビデンスレベル

他のAHAガイドラインと同様に，2020年版の各推奨事項はエビデンスの強さと一貫性，代替の治療選択肢，患者と社会に及ぼす影響によって推奨事項のクラス（COR）が割り当てられている。エビデンスレベル（LOE）は，有効なエビデンスの質と量，関連性，一貫性に基づいている（表1）。

「第7章：治療システム」の各推奨事項は，元の情報を担当した執筆グループが特定の推奨事項の文言とCORおよびLOEの割り当てを検討して承認した。CORを決定するときに，執筆グループはLOEに加えて，済的要素，公正性・受け入れ可能性・実施可能性などの倫理的要素も検討した。CORとLOEを決定する具体的な基準など，エビデンスレビューの方法は，「第2章：エビデンス評価とガイドライン作成」[2]に詳細に記載されている。治療システム執筆グループのメンバーは，これらの推奨事項の最終的な決定権を有し，正式に承認した。

ガイドラインの構成

ガイドライン2020は，特定のトピックや管理上の問題に関する情報を個々のモジュールにグループ化した「知識チャンク」で構成される[3]。各モジュールの知識チャンクには，AHAの標準的なCORとLOEの表記法に従って推奨事項表を示す。簡潔な導入もしくはと短い「概要」を示すことで，重要な背景情報や包括的な管理概念や，治療概念のある中での推奨事項を提示する。推奨事項に特化した内容で，推奨事項を裏付ける根拠と重要な研究データを明らかにする。必要に応じてフローチャートまたは補助的な表を掲載した。迅速なアクセスと確認のためにハイパーリンク付きの参考資料を提供する。

文書のレビューと承認

『AHA 心肺蘇生と救急心血管治療のためのガイドライン 2020』の各文書は，を盲検下での査読のため，AHAが指名した対象分野の専門家5人に提出された。指名に先立ち，査読者に対して，企業との関係およびその他の利益相反の可能性を開示するよう要求し，開示された情報をすべてAHAスタッフが確認した。査読者のフィードバックは，ガイドラインの草案と，さらに最終版に提出された。ガイドラインはすべてAHA Science Advisory and Coordinating CommitteeおよびAHA Executive Committeeの査読を受け，公開に関する承認を受けた。査読者の開示情報を，付録2に収載する。

略語

略語	意味／語句
ALS	二次救命処置（advanced life support）
AED	自動体外式除細動器（automated external defibrillator）
AHA	アメリカ心臓協会（American Heart Association）
BLS	一次救命処置（basic life support）
CAC	心停止治療センター（cardiac arrest center）
COR	推奨事項のクラス（Class of Recommendation）
CPR	心肺蘇生（cardiopulmonary resuscitation）
EMS	救急医療サービス（emergency medical services）
IHCA	院内心停止（in-hospital cardiac arrest）
ILCOR	国際蘇生連絡委員会（International Liaison Committee on Resuscitation）
LOE	エビデンスレベル（Level of Evidence）
MET	救急医療チーム（medical emergency team）
OHCA	院外心停止（out-of-hospital cardiac arrest）
OR	オッズ比（odds ratio）
PAD	市民による除細動（電気ショック）（public access defibrillation）
RCT	無作為化比較試験（randomized controlled trial）
ROSC	自己心拍再開（return of spontaneous circulation）
RR，aRR	相対リスク，調整後の相対リスク（relative risk, adjusted relative risk）
RRT	迅速対応チーム（rapid response team）
T-CPR	テレコミュニケーターによるCPRの指示（telecommunicator CPR instructions）

参考文献

1. American Heart Association. CPR & ECC. https://cpr.heart.org/. Accessed June 19, 2020.
2. Magid DJ, Aziz K, Cheng A, Hazinski MF, Hoover AV, Mahgoub M, Panchal AR, Sasson C, Topjian AA, Rodriguez AJ, et al. Part 2: evidence evaluation and guidelines development: 2020 American Heart Association Guidelines for Cardiopulmonary Resuscitation and Emergency Cardiovascular Care. Circulation. 2020;142(suppl 2):S358-S365. doi: 10.1161/CIR.0000000000000898

3. Levine GN, O'Gara PT, Beckman JA, Al-Khatib SM, Birtcher KK, Cigarroa JE, de Las Fuentes L, Deswal A, Fleisher LA, Gentile F, Goldberger ZD, Hlatky MA, Joglar JA, Piano MR, Wijeysundera DN. Recent innovations, modifications, and evolution of ACC/AHA clinical practice guidelines: an update for our constituencies: a report of the American College of Cardiology/American Heart Association Task Force on Clinical Practice Guidelines. Circulation. 2019;139:e879-e886. doi: 10.1161/CIR.0000000000000651

主要な概念
ウツタイン様式の救命

蘇生治療システムの開発と実装は，ウツタイン様式の救命[1]に基づいている。ウツタイン様式では，蘇生の救命は，医学の進歩（実現可能な最良のエビデンスに基づく蘇生ガイドライン）と普及：蘇生実施者や市民救助者の効果的な訓練などを含めた教育の有効性；蘇生のあらゆる段階と心拍再開後のケアに関与する治療者間のシームレスな協力を含んだ地域での実践（図1）。ガイドライン2020の第3章～第5章は，利用可能な最良の蘇生科学に基づくAHAの代表的なガイドラインである。「第6章：蘇生教育科学」でAHAは，心停止した傷病者を救護する医療専門家と一般市民の訓練技術を批判的に評価している。「第7章：治療システム」では，乳児，小児，成人の蘇生に共通するさまざまな蘇生のトピックを取り上げる。

AHAの救命の連鎖

1991年以来，AHAは蘇生科学とトレーニングを導入する際の調和のとれた取り組みである救命の連鎖の概念を強調してきた[2]。BLS，ALS，PALSの治療環境による若干の違いはあるものの，AHAの救命の連鎖は，心停止の早期認識，救急対応システムへの出動要請，早期の除細動，質の高いCPR，高度な蘇生技術，心停止後の治療を重視した。

救命の連鎖の概念はガイドラインの中で何度も改善を重ねてきた。心停止の原因と治療は成人と乳児／小児，IHCAとOHCAの間で異なるため，具体的な救命の連鎖は年齢層や状況に応じて策定している（図2）。また，各鎖は回復の鎖を追加することによって延長されている。新生児の「救命の連鎖」の概念（図には示されていない）はこれとはやや異なる。新生児の場合は，出生前に地域や施設で準備する機会が多くあり，新生児の蘇生チームが前もって警告したり，親を巻き込んだりできるためである。しかし，救命の連鎖の原則と救命の様式は共通して適用できる。この章では，一人の患者だけでなく傷病者全体の転帰を改善できるような，救命の連鎖全体にわたる幅広い介入の推奨事項に焦点を当てる。

集団や状況に応じて意図的に内容や順序を変えることはあるが，どの救命の連鎖にも以下の要素がある。

- **予防と準備**：救助者の訓練，心停止の早期認識，迅速な対応を含む
- **救急対応システムへの出動要請**：院内または院外
- **質の高いCPR**：心室細動と無脈性心室頻拍の早期の除細動を含む
- **高度な蘇生処置**：：投薬，高度な気道確保，体外循環補助を用いたCPRを含む
- **心拍再開後の治療**：集中治療，目標体温管理を含む
- **リカバリー**：身体的，認知的，感情的，家族のニーズに対する効果的なサポートを含む

予防：院外で心停止を予防する手段として，市民や個人の健康増進に加えて，急性冠症候群および心停止の症状と徴候を周知する啓発活動が挙げられる。院内での**準備**には，蘇生が必要となる患者の早期認識と早期対応（高リスク分娩への準備など），迅速対応チーム（「IHCAの予防」参照），個人や蘇生チームの訓練などがある。個人や蘇生チームの訓練の詳細は「第6章：蘇生教育科学」[3]でも取り上げている。一般市民が質の高いCPRを開始して早期の除細動を実施できるようにするための救急対応システムの開発，心停止の認識に対する市民救助者と通信指令員の訓練，地域社会のCPR訓練，広範なAEDの普及，テレコミュニケーターの指示はすべて院外での予防手順の重要な要素である。最近の技術革新として，CPRの訓練を受けた市民を招集する携帯電話技術の利用がある（「CPRを要する事態の発生をバイスタンダーに通知する携帯電話技術」参照）。「第5章：新生児の蘇生」[4]で述べたように，新生児の蘇生を成功させるには分娩前の準備が重要な要素である。

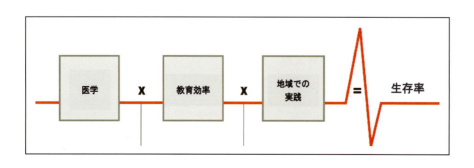

図1. ウツタイン様式の救命[1]

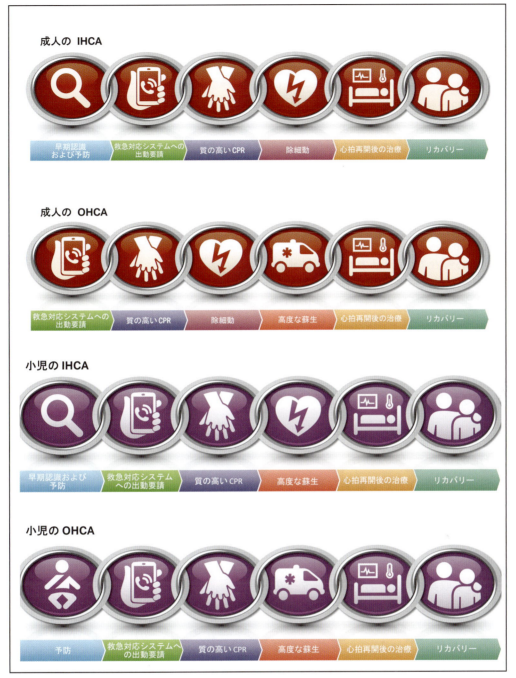

図 2. AHA の救命の連鎖の更新版
AHA：アメリカ心臓協会（American Heart Association），CPR：心肺蘇生，IHCA：院内心停止，OHCA：院外心停止

救急対応システムへの出動要請：救急対応システムへの出動要請は，大声で近くの人に助けを求めることから始まることが多い。院外では，ただちに次に行うべき手順は一般的な救急通報番号（119 番通報）に電話することや，最寄りの AED を取りに行くことである。IHCA の場合は，並行して院内の蘇生チームを呼び出す。

質の高い CPR：最小限の中断と連続的な質のモニタリングで実施する質の高い CPR と，心室細動や無脈性心室頻拍への**早期の除細動**は，現代の蘇生の基盤であり，いずれも良好な蘇生転帰に密接に関連する介入である。重要なのは，このような一刻を争う介入を，医療従事者に加えて市民救助者も提供できることである。同様に，オピオイドによる呼吸停止は，バイスタンダーまたは訓練された救助者によるナロキソンの早期投与によって救命できる。

高度な蘇生処置：薬物療法や高度な気道確保（気管挿管や声門上気道確保器具の挿入），体外循環補助を用いた CPR などの高度な蘇生処置も，特定の蘇生状況での転帰を改善する可能性がある。

心拍再開後の治療：心拍再開後の治療には，ルーチンの集中治療（機械的換気，血管収縮薬の静脈内投与など）に加えて，蘇生成功後に ROSC を得た患者の転帰を改善する目標体温管理などの

具体的なエビデンスに基づいた介入も含まれる。目標体温管理についての個別の推奨事項は，第3章，第4章，第5章に記載されており，それぞれ2020年版のAHAの成人[5]，小児[6]，新生児のガイドライン[4]である。神経学的転帰不良が避けられない患者を早期に特定する確実な方法がないため，現在の成人のガイドラインでは，蘇生後少なくとも72時間，および低体温療法からの復温後まで，場合によってはさらに長時間，救命処置を中止することを推奨していない[5,8,9]。神経保護の追加の戦略やROSC後の予後の良否を予測するバイオマーカーを開発する多くの研究が現在精力的に進められている。

リカバリー 心停止からのリカバリーは退院後も長期にわたって続く。リカバリーの重要な要素には，達成された転帰次第で，心停止の根本原因への対処方法，二次予防の心臓リハビリテーション，神経学的側面に注目したリハビリテーションケア，患者と家族への心理学的支援などがある。心停止からの生存者のための介入を検討する重要な研究がますます行われている[10]。

継続的改善のためのデータの利用

救命の連鎖は個々の患者のケアで重要な要素を中心に据えているが，将来のパフォーマンス改善に必要な手順は十分に取り上げられていない。例えば，蘇生活動後の体系的なチームデブリーフィングの実施，AHAの「Get With The Guidelines」の取り組みを通じて収集されたIHCAデータへの反応，ウツタインの枠組みを使用して収集したOHCAデータのレビューなどである（表2）。継続的改善を行うために，リーン，シックスシグマ，高信頼性組織の枠組み，Demingの改善モデルなど，公式のプロセス改善の枠組みが複数存在する。AHAおよびその他の組織は，蘇生の具体的なパフォーマンス改善に取り組む体系構築を推奨している。目標は，データを活用して準備と蘇生転帰を継続的に改善する「学習を続けるヘルスケアシステム」[11]にすることである。この概念を蘇生治療システムに適用することは以前から支持されており，多くの蘇生組織で実施中である[12,13]。

OHCAの場合，蘇生成功の主要因は早期の効果的なCPRと早期の除細動である。CPRの遅れを短縮し，CPRの有効性を向上し，ショック適応リズムの患者に確実に早期の除細動を実施するための対策は，このガイドラインの重要な要素である。

表2. システム改善のためのデータ活用例

活況を呈するオフィスビルの管理者は，職場でのAEDの役割に関する資料を読んだ後，AEDを設置して，スタッフ全員にハンズオンリーCPRの訓練を実施した。
公共図書館の本館でオピオイド過量投与が多いことを示すデータへの対応として，EMS機関は図書館スタッフにナロキソンキットを配布して訓練を実施した。
蘇生中に，気管チューブからバッグマスク換気をしている救助者が患者を過換気状態にしていることにチームリーダーが気づいた。チームリーダーは，バッグの圧迫を胸郭の上がりに十分な程度にするよう救助者を指導した。
一部の地区でのバイスタンダーによるCPR実施率の低さを示すデータに対応して，その地区のコミュニティセンターで無料のCPR講座を開催した。
困難であったが成功した小児の蘇生後のチームデブリーフィングで，エピネフリン用量のミスが発見された。根本的な原因は，プレッシャーのかかる状態で薬物量の計算が必要となることにあった。小児の体重別に蘇生薬物の標準量（mL）を列挙する参考資料を作成した。
女性が心停止をきたした場合に男性の場合よりもバイスタンダーによるCPRを受ける可能性が低いことを示す研究に対応して，この抵抗感の根本的な原因を特定するためにフォーカスグループ調査を実施し，この障壁に照準を合わせた訓練を調整した。
多くの新生児が蘇生に低体温になったことを示すデータに対応して，この合併症を防ぐための手順を確実に実施するために，分娩前のチェックリストを導入した。

AED：自動体外式除細動器，CPR：心肺蘇生，EMS：救急医療サービス

IHCAの場合も蘇生成功の主要因は同様であるが，医療専門家の存在が心停止を防ぐ可能性を高める。成人患者で入院からIHCAまでの期間の中央値は2日である[13]。非代償状態の患者の早期認識によって，心停止予防のための安定化を図ることができる。この介入にはリスクのある患者の特定と容態悪化を防ぐための早期介入の2つの手順があり，患者の現在の治療者または専用チームメンバーのいずれかが実施する。これらの疑問に対する成人と小児のエビデンスの基盤は異なるため，成人一次救命処置と二次救命処置の執筆グループと小児一次救命処置と二次救命処置の執筆グループが並行して，早期警告スコアシステムと迅速対応チーム（RRT）および救急医療チーム（MET）に関するエビデンスの評価を実施した。

参考文献

1. Søreide E, Morrison L, Hillman K, Monsieurs K, Sunde K, Zideman D, Eisenberg M, Sterz F, Nadkarni VM, Soar J, Nolan JP; Utstein Formula for Survival Collaborators. The formula for survival in resuscitation. Resuscitation. 2013;84:1487-1493. doi: 10.1016/j.resuscitation.2013.07.020
2. Cummins RO, Ornato JP, Thies WH, Pepe PE. Improving survival from sudden cardiac arrest: the "chain of survival" concept. A statement for health professionals from the Advanced Cardiac Life Support Subcommittee and the Emergency Cardiac Care Committee, American Heart Association. Circulation.1991;83:1832-1847. doi: 10.1161/01.cir.83.5.1832

3. Cheng A, Magid DJ, Auerbach M, Bhanji F, Bigham BL, Blewer AL, Dainty KN, Diederich E, Lin Y, Leary M, et al. Part 6: resuscitation education science: 2020 American Heart Association Guidelines for Cardiopulmonary Resuscitation and Emergency Cardiovascular Care.Circulation.2020;142 (suppl 2):S551-S579. doi: 10.1161/CIR.0000000000000903

4. Aziz K, Lee HC, Escobedo MB, Hoover AV, Kamath-Rayne BD, Kapadia VS, Magid DJ, Niermeyer S, Schmölzer GM, Szyld E, et al. Part 5: neonatal resuscitation: 2020 American Heart Association Guidelines for Cardiopulmonary Resuscitation and Emergency Cardiovascular Care.Circulation.2020;142 (suppl 2):S524-S550. doi: 10.1161/CIR.0000000000000902

5. Panchal AR, Bartos JA, Cabañas JG, Donnino MW, Drennan IR, Hirsch KG, Kudenchuk PJ, Kurz MC, Lavonas EJ, Morley PT, et al; on behalf of the Adult Basic and Advanced Life Support Writing Group. Part 3: adult basic and advanced life support: 2020 American Heart Association Guidelines for Cardiopulmonary Resuscitation and Emergency Cardiovascular Care.Circulation.2020;142 (suppl 2):S366-S468. doi: 10.1161/CIR.0000000000000916

6. Topjian AA, Raymond TT, Atkins D, Chan M, Duff JP, Joyner BL Jr, Lasa JJ, Lavonas EJ, Levy A, Mahgoub M, et al; on behalf of the Pediatric Basic and Advanced Life Support Collaborators. Part 4: pediatric basic and advanced life support: 2020 American Heart Association Guidelines for Cardiopulmonary Resuscitation and Emergency Cardiovascular Care.Circulation.2020;142 (suppl 2):S469-S523. doi: 10.1161/CIR.0000000000000901

7. Deleted in proof.

8. Callaway CW, Donnino MW, Fink EL, Geocadin RG, Golan E, Kern KB, Leary M, Meurer WJ, Peberdy MA, Thompson TM, et al. Part 8: post-cardiac arrest care: 2015 American Heart Association Guidelines Update for Cardiopulmonary Resuscitation and Emergency Cardiovascular Care.Circulation.2015;132 (suppl 2):S465-482. doi: 10.1161/cir.0000000000000262

9. Geocadin RG, Callaway CW, Fink EL, Golan E, Greer DM, Ko NU, Lang E, Licht DJ, Marino BS, McNair ND, Peberdy MA, Perman SM, Sims DB, Soar J, Sandroni C; American Heart Association Emergency Cardiovascular Care Committee. Standards for Studies of Neurological Prognostication in Comatose Survivors of Cardiac Arrest: a scientific statement from the American Heart Association.Circulation. 2019;140:e517-e542. doi: 10.1161/CIR.0000000000000702

10. Sawyer KN, Camp-Rogers TR, Kotini-Shah P, Del Rios M, Gossip MR, Moitra VK, Haywood KL, Dougherty CM, Lubitz SA, Rabinstein AA, Rittenberger JC, Callaway CW, Abella BS, Geocadin RG, Kurz MC; American Heart Association Emergency Cardiovascular Care Committee; Council on Cardiovascular and Stroke Nursing; Council on Genomic and Precision Medicine; Council on Quality of Care and Outcomes Research; and Stroke Council. Sudden Cardiac Arrest Survivorship: a scientific statement from the American Heart Association.Circulation. 2020;141:e654-e685. doi: 10.1161/CIR.0000000000000747

11. Institute of Medicine (US) Roundtable on Evidence-Based Medicine. Olsen LA, Aisner D, McGinnis JM, eds. Washington DC: National Academies Press; 2007.

12. Committee on the Treatment of Cardiac Arrest: Current Status and Future Directions; Board on Health Sciences Policy; Institute of Medicine. Strategies to Improve Cardiac Arrest Survival: A Time to Act. Graham R, McCoy MA, Schultz AM, eds. Washington DC; 2015. https://www.ncbi.nlm.nih.gov/pubmed/26225413. Accessed 2020/02/14.

13. Neumar RW, Eigel B, Callaway CW, Estes NA 3rd, Jollis JG, Kleinman ME, Morrison LJ, Peberdy MA, Rabinstein A, Rea TD, et al; on behalf of the American Heart Association. American Heart Association response to the 2015 Institute of Medicine report on strategies to improve cardiac arrest survival. Circulation.2015;132:1049-1070. doi: 10.1161/CIR.0000000000000233

14. Deleted in proof.

15. Nolan JP, Soar J, Smith GB, Gwinnutt C, Parrott F, Power S, Harrison DA, Nixon E, Rowan K; National Cardiac Arrest Audit. Incidence and outcome of in-hospital cardiac arrest in the United Kingdom National Cardiac Arrest Audit. Resuscitation.2014;85:987-992. doi: 10.1016/j.resuscitation.2014.04.002

病院前治療システム
CPR実施を推進する地域の取り組み

CPR実施を推進する地域の取り組みに対する推奨事項		
COR	LOE	推奨事項
2b	C-LD	1. 地域社会で認識向上とバイスタンダーによるCPRの実施率向上のための戦略を導入することは妥当である[1-12]。

「概要」

CPRおよびAEDの使用は救命のための介入であるが，バイスタンダーによる実施率は低い[13]。地域におけるバイスタンダーによるCPR実施率を改善するために，マスメディアのキャンペーン（広告，教育用資材の大量配布など），インストラクターによる訓練（インストラクター主導による少人数または大人数でのCPR訓練），様々な介入の併用などが検討されてきた[1-12]。複数の介入の併用には，救命の連鎖内のいくつかの鎖を改善する多面的なアプローチがあり，対象を定めた教育（郵便番号やリスク評価に基づく）や対象を定めない教育（大衆向け）教育がある。これらはインストラクター主導，同僚との訓練，デジタルメディア（ビデオなど）の利用，自己学習などを含む。状況に応じて，「地域」が指す範囲は近隣の住民のこともあれば，1つまたは複数の都市，町，地域，国全体のこともある[14]。

「推奨事項の裏付けとなる解説」

1. 2020年のILCORのシステマティックレビュー[14]によると，1件の無作為化比較試験（RCT）[15]と16件の観察研究[1-12,16-19]でバイスタンダーによるCPR実施率または生存転帰が報告されていた。バイスタンダーによるCPR実施率はこれらの研究のうち12件で改善していた[1-12]。

インストラクター主導の訓練：6件の観察研究がインストラクター主導の訓練の影響を評価していた[1-4,17-19]。4件中2件の研究で，インストラクター主導の訓練導入後に良好な神経学的転帰を伴う生存率の改善が認められた[1,2,17,18]。3件中2件の研究で生存退院率の改善が報告され[1,3,18]，1件でインストラクター主導の訓練導入後にROSCの改善が示された[3]。インストラクター主導の訓練は，4件の研究でバイスタンダーによるCPR実施率を10%～19%改善していた[1-4]。

マスメディアのキャンペーン：1件の観察研究で，バイスタンダーによるCPRを推進するテレビ広告のキャンペーン後にバイスタンダーによるCPR実施率が12%の絶対的増加を示したことが報告された[6]。しかし，10分間のCPR学習ビデオの8659世帯への大量配布（郵送による）では，ビデオを送付しなかった世帯と比較してバイスタンダーによるCPR実施率の有意な改善は

みられなかった（介入世帯で 47%，対照世帯で 53%）[15]。

複数の介入の併用：9 件の観察研究で，複数の介入の併用がバイスタンダーによる CPR 実施率と生存転帰に及ぼす影響を評価した[5,7,12,16,19]。バイスタンダーによる CPR 実施率は 7 件の研究で改善していた[4,5,7,12,16]。

上記の推奨事項は，AHA の蘇生教育科学執筆グループが作成し，2020 年の ILCOR システマティックレビューで支持された[14]。

参考文献

1. Fordyce CB, Hansen CM, Kragholm K, Dupre ME, Jollis JG, Roettig ML, Becker LB, Hansen SM, Hinohara TT, Corbett CC, Monk L, Nelson RD, Pearson DA, Tyson C, van Diepen S, Anderson ML, McNally B, Granger CB. Association of public health initiatives with outcomes for out-of-hospital cardiac arrest at home and in public locations. JAMA Cardiol. 2017;2:1226-1235. doi: 10.1001/jamacardio.2017.3471
2. Malta Hansen C, Kragholm K, Pearson DA, Tyson C, Monk L, Myers B, Nelson D, Dupre ME, Fosbol EL, Jollis JG, et al. Association of bystander and first-responder intervention with survival after out-of-hospital cardiac arrest in North Carolina, 2010-2013. JAMA.2015;314:255-264. doi: 10.1001/jama.2015.7938
3. Tay PJM, Pek PP, Fan Q, Ng YY, Leong BS, Gan HN, Mao DR, Chia MYC, Cheah SO, Doctor N, Tham LP, Ong MEH. Effectiveness of a community based out-of-hospital cardiac arrest (OHCA) interventional bundle: Results of a pilot study. Resuscitation.2020;146:220-228. doi: 10.1016/j.resuscitation.2019.10.015
4. Boland LL, Formanek MB, Harkins KK, Frazee CL, Kamrud JW, Stevens AC, Lick CJ, Yannopoulos D. Minnesota Heart Safe Communities: Are community-based initiatives increasing pre-ambulance CPR and AED use? Resuscitation.2017;119:33-36. doi: 10.1016/j.resuscitation.2017.07.031
5. Bergamo C, Bui QM, Gonzales L, Hinchey P, Sasson C, Cabanas JG. TAKE10: A community approach to teaching compression-only CPR to high-risk zip codes. Resuscitation.2016;102:75-79. doi: 10.1016/j.resuscitation.2016.02.019
6. Becker L, Vath J, Eisenberg M, Meischke H. The impact of television public service announcements on the rate of bystander CPR. Prehosp Emerg Care.1999;3:353-356. doi: 10.1080/10903129908958968
7. Hwang WS, Park JS, Kim SJ, Hong YS, Moon SW, Lee SW. A system-wide approach from the community to the hospital for improving neurologic outcomes in out-of-hospital cardiac arrest patients. Eur J Emerg Med.2017;24:87-95. doi: 10.1097/MEJ.0000000000000313
8. Ro YS, Shin SD, Song KJ, Hong SO, Kim YT, Lee DW, Cho SI. Public awareness and self-efficacy of cardiopulmonary resuscitation in communities and outcomes of out-of-hospital cardiac arrest: A multi-level analysis. Resuscitation.2016;102:17-24. doi: 10.1016/j.resuscitation.2016.02.004
9. Nielsen AM, Isbye DL, Lippert FK, Rasmussen LS. Persisting effect of community approaches to resuscitation. Resuscitation.2014;85:1450-1454. doi: 10.1016/j.resuscitation.2014.08.019
10. Møller Nielsen A, Lou Isbye D, Knudsen Lippert F, Rasmussen LS. Engaging a whole community in resuscitation. Resuscitation.2012;83:1067-1071. doi: 10.1016/j.resuscitation.2012.04.012
11. Wissenberg M, Lippert FK, Folke F, Weeke P, Hansen CM, Christensen EF, Jans H, Hansen PA, Lang-Jensen T, Olesen JB, Lindhardsen J, Fosbol EL, Nielsen SL, Gislason GH, Kober L, Torp-Pedersen C. Association of national initiatives to improve cardiac arrest management with rates of bystander intervention and patient survival after out-of-hospital cardiac arrest. JAMA.2013;310:1377-1384. doi: 10.1001/jama.2013.278483
12. Ro YS, Song KJ, Shin SD, Hong KJ, Park JH, Kong SY, Cho SI. Association between county-level cardiopulmonary resuscitation training and changes in Survival Outcomes after out-of-hospital cardiac arrest over 5 years: A multilevel analysis. Resuscitation.2019;139:291-298. doi: 10.1016/j.resuscitation.2019.01.012
13. Girotra S, van Diepen S, Nallamothu BK, Carrel M, Vellano K, Anderson ML, McNally B, Abella BS, Sasson C, Chan PS; CARES Surveillance Group and the HeartRescue Project. Regional Variation in Out-of-Hospital Cardiac Arrest Survival in the United States. Circulation.2016;133:2159-2168. doi: 10.1161/CIRCULATIONAHA.115.018175
14. Olasveengen TM, Mancini ME, Perkins GD, Avis S, Brooks S, Castrén M, Chung SP, Considine J, Couper K, Escalante R, et al; on behalf of the Adult Basic Life Support Collaborators. Adult basic life support: 2020 International Consensus on Cardiopulmonary Resuscitation and Emergency Cardiovascular Care Science With Treatment Recommendations. Circulation.2020;142 (suppl 1):S41-S91. doi: 10.1161/CIR.0000000000000892
15. Eisenberg M, Damon S, Mandel L, Tewodros A, Meischke H, Beaupied E, Bennett J, Guildner C, Ewell C, Gordon M. CPR instruction by videotape: results of a community project. Ann Emerg Med.1995;25:198-202. doi: 10.1016/s0196-0644(95)70324-1
16. Del Rios M, Han J, Cano A, Ramirez V, Morales G, Campbell TL, Vanden Hoek T. Pay it forward: high school video-based instruction can disseminate CPR knowledge in priority neighborhoods. West J Emerg Med. 2018;19:423-429. doi: 10.5811/westjem.2017.10.35108
17. Nishiyama C, Kitamura T, Sakai T, Murakami Y, Shimamoto T, Kawamura T, Yonezawa T, Nakai S, Marukawa S, Sakamoto T, Iwami T. Community-wide dissemination of bystander cardiopulmonary resuscitation and automated external defibrillator use using a 45-minute chest compression-only cardiopulmonary resuscitation training. J Am Heart Assoc. 2019;8:e009436. doi: 10.1161/JAHA.118.009436
18. Uber A, Sadler RC, Chassee T, Reynolds JC. Does non-targeted community CPR training increase bystander CPR frequency? Prehosp Emerg Care.2018;22:753-761. doi: 10.1080/10903127.2018.1459978
19. Isbye DL, Rasmussen LS, Ringsted C, Lippert FK. Disseminating cardiopulmonary resuscitation training by distributing 35,000 personal manikins among school children. Circulation.2007;116:1380-1385. doi: 10.1161/CIRCULATIONAHA.107.710616

市民による電気ショック

市民による除細動（電気ショック）に対する推奨事項		
COR	LOE	推奨事項
1	B-NR	1. 心停止リスクの高い地域社会で OHCA 患者に対する市民による電気ショックプログラムの導入は推奨される[1-33]。

「概要」

早期の除細動は OHCA からの生存率を有意に上昇させる[34-37]。市民による電気ショック（PAD）プログラムは，AED を公共の場所に設置し，市民が使用できるよう訓練することにより，除細動までの時間を短縮できるようデザインされている。PAD プログラムと併用しない従来の EMS システムと比較して，EMS システムと PAD プログラムが併用された状況で OHCA を経験した人は，ROSC 率が高く，生存退院率と OHCA から 30 日後の生存率が高く，退院時，OHCA から 30 日後，OHCA から 1 年後の良好な神経学的転帰での生存率が高かった[9,10,33]。このエビデンスに基づいて，心停止リスクのある人のいる地域で PAD を実施することを推奨する（オフィスビル，カジノ，マンション，人の集まる場所など）。PAD プログラムの有効性は既存のエビデンスで裏付けられているが，市民救助者による除細動器の使用率は依然として低い[38,39]。市民救助者による除細動器使用率を改善する戦略に関してはさらに研究が必要である。例えば，最寄りの AED を特定してその場所を通報者に通知する救急サービスの通信指令員の役割，AED の最適な配置，救助者が適時の除細動を実施する能力を高めるテクノロジーの利用などである[33,40]。

「推奨事項の裏付けとなる解説」

1. PAD プログラムの影響を評価した 31 件の研究のうち，27 件（RCT 1 件[20]，観察研究 26 件[1-3,5,7,8,11-19,21-23,25-28,30-32,41]）で転帰の改善が認められ，4 件の観察研究[4,6,24,29]では転帰に差はなかった。

2020年のILCORのシステマティックレビュー[33]によると，エビデンスの質は低いものの，PADプログラムを併用したシステムでは，PADプログラムを併用しない場合と比較して生存率の改善と良好な神経学的転帰が得られた。その結果は，1件の観察研究では1年後[4]（登録患者62例）（43% vs 0%，P=0.02），7件の観察研究では30日後[3,22,25,26,29,30,41]（登録患者43〜116例）（オッズ比[OR] 6.60，95%CI 3.54-12.28），8件の観察研究で退院時[1,2,4,7,11-13,24]（登録患者11〜837例）（OR 2.89，95%CI 1.79-4.66）に示された。

同レビューで，PADプログラムをの併したシステムでは，PADプログラムを併用しない場合と比較して生存率の改善が得られたという低〜中程度の質のエビデンスが得られた。その結果は，8件の観察研究では30日後[3,5,15,17,22,28-30]（登録患者85〜589例）（OR 3.66，95%CI 2.63-5.11），1件のRCT[20]（登録患者235例）（RR 2.0，95%CI 1.07-3.77）および16件の観察研究では退院時[1,2,6-8,11,13,14,16,18,19,21,24,27,31,32]（登録患者40〜243例）（OR 3.24，95%CI 2.13-4.92）に示された。

エビデンスの質は低いが，13件の観察研究[3-7,11,17,19,22,28-31]（登録患者95〜354例）から，EMSシステムとPADプログラムの併用で，PADプログラムを併用しない場合と比較してROSCが改善したという知見が示された（OR 2.45，95%CI 1.88-3.18）。

上記の推奨事項は，AHAの成人一次救命処置と二次救命処置の執筆グループが作成し，2020年のILCORシステマティックレビューで支持された[33]。

参考文献

1. Berdowski J, Blom MT, Bardai A, Tan HL, Tijssen JG, Koster RW. Impact of onsite or dispatched automated external defibrillator use on survival after out-of-hospital cardiac arrest. Circulation.2011;124:2225-2232. doi: 10.1161/CIRCULATIONAHA.110.015545
2. Fordyce CB, Hansen CM, Kragholm K, Dupre ME, Jollis JG, Roettig ML, Becker LB, Hansen SM, Hinohara TT, Corbett CC, Monk L, Nelson RD, Pearson DA, Tyson C, van Diepen S, Anderson ML, McNally B, Granger CB. Association of public health initiatives with outcomes for out-of-hospital cardiac arrest at home and in public locations. JAMA Cardiol.2017;2:1226-1235. doi: 10.1001/jamacardio.2017.3471
3. Fukuda T, Ohashi-Fukuda N, Kobayashi H, Gunshin M, Sera T, Kondo Y, Yahagi N. Public access defibrillation and outcomes after pediatric out-of-hospital cardiac arrest. Resuscitation.2017;111:1-7. doi: 10.1016/j.resuscitation.2016.11.010
4. Gianotto-Oliveira R, Gonzalez MM, Vianna CB, Monteiro Alves M, Timerman S, Kalil Filho R, Kern KB. Survival after ventricular fibrillation cardiac arrest in the Sao Paulo Metropolitan subway system: first successful targeted automated external defibrillator (AED) program in Latin America. J Am Heart Assoc. 2015;4:e002185. doi: 10.1161/JAHA.115.002185
5. Hansen SM, Hansen CM, Folke F, Rajan S, Kragholm K, Ejlskov L, Gislason G, Køber L, Gerds TA, Hjortshøj S, Lippert F, Torp-Pedersen C, Wissenberg M. Bystander defibrillation for out-of-hospital cardiac arrest in public vs residential locations. JAMA Cardiol.2017;2:507-514. doi: 10.1001/jamacardio.2017.0008
6. Nas J, Thannhauser J, Herrmann JJ, van der Wulp K, van Grunsven PM, van Royen N, de Boer MJ, Bonnes JL, Brouwer MA. Changes in automated external defibrillator use and survival after out-of-hospital cardiac arrest in the Nijmegen area. Neth Heart J. 2018;26:600-605. doi: 10.1007/s12471-018-1162-9
7. Pollack RA, Brown SP, Rea T, Aufderheide T, Barbic D, Buick JE, Christenson J, Idris AH, Jasti J, Kampp M, Kudenchuk P, May S, Muhr M, Nichol G, Ornato JP, Sopko G, Vaillancourt C, Morrison L, Weisfeldt M; ROC Investigators. Impact of bystander automated external defibrillator use on survival and functional outcomes in shockable observed public cardiac arrests. Circulation.2018;137:2104-2113. doi: 10.1161/CIRCULATIONAHA.117.030700
8. Weisfeldt ML, Sitlani CM, Ornato JP, Rea T, Aufderheide TP, Davis D, Dreyer J, Hess EP, Jui J, Maloney J, Sopko G, Powell J, Nichol G, Morrison LJ; ROC Investigators. Survival after application of automatic external defibrillators before arrival of the emergency medical system: evaluation in the resuscitation outcomes consortium population of 21 million. J Am Coll Cardiol.2010;55:1713-1720. doi: 10.1016/j.jacc.2009.11.077
9. Bækgaard JS, Viereck S, Møller TP, Ersbøll AK, Lippert F, Folke F. The effects of public access defibrillation on survival after out-of-hospital cardiac arrest: a systematic review of observational studies. Circulation.2017;136:954-965. doi: 10.1161/CIRCULATIONAHA.117.029067
10. Holmberg MJ, Vognsen M, Andersen MS, Donnino MW, Andersen LW. Bystander automated external defibrillator use and clinical outcomes after out-of-hospital cardiac arrest: A systematic review and meta-analysis. Resuscitation.2017;120:77-87. doi: 10.1016/j.resuscitation.2017.09.003
11. Andersen LW, Holmberg MJ, Granfeldt A, Løfgren B, Vellano K, McNally BF, Siegerink B, Kurth T, Donnino MW; CARES Surveillance Group. Neighborhood characteristics, bystander automated external defibrillator use, and patient outcomes in public out-of-hospital cardiac arrest. Resuscitation.2018;126:72-79. doi: 10.1016/j.resuscitation.2018.02.021
12. Aschieri D, Penela D, Pelizzoni V, Guerra F, Vermi AC, Rossi L, Torretta L, Losi G, Villani GQ, Capucci A. Outcomes after sudden cardiac arrest in sports centres with and without on-site external defibrillators. Heart. 2018;104:1344-1349. doi: 10.1136/heartjnl-2017-312441
13. Capucci A, Aschieri D, Piepoli MF, Bardy GH, Iconomu E, Arvedi M. Tripling survival from sudden cardiac arrest via early defibrillation without traditional education in cardiopulmonary resuscitation. Circulation.2002;106:1065-1070. doi: 10.1161/01.cir.0000028148.62305.69
14. Capucci A, Aschieri D, Guerra F, Pelizzoni V, Nani S, Villani GQ, Bardy GH. Community-based automated external defibrillator only resuscitation for out-of-hospital cardiac arrest patients. Am Heart J. 2016;172:192-200. doi: 10.1016/j.ahj.2015.10.018
15. Claesson A, Herlitz J, Svensson L, Ottosson L, Bergfeldt L, Engdahl J, Ericson C, Sandén P, Axelsson C, Bremer A. Defibrillation before EMS arrival in western Sweden. Am J Emerg Med.2017;35:1043-1048. doi: 10.1016/j.ajem.2017.02.030
16. Culley LL, Rea TD, Murray JA, Welles B, Fahrenbruch CE, Olsufka M, Eisenberg MS, Copass MK. Public access defibrillation in out-of-hospital cardiac arrest: a community-based study. Circulation.2004;109:1859-1863. doi: 10.1161/01.CIR.0000124721.83385.B2
17. Dicker B, Davey P, Smith T, Beck B. Incidence and outcomes of out-of-hospital cardiac arrest: A New Zealand perspective. Emerg Med Australas.2018;30:662-671. doi: 10.1111/1742-6723.12966
18. Edwards MJ, Fothergill RT. Exercise-related sudden cardiac arrest in London: incidence, survival and bystander response. Open Heart. 2015;2:e000281. doi: 10.1136/openhrt-2015-000281
19. Garcia EL, Caffrey-Villari S, Ramirez D, Caron JL, Mannhart P, Reuter PG, Lapostolle F, Adnet F. [Impact of onsite or dispatched automated external defibrillator use on early survival after sudden cardiac arrest occurring in international airports]. Presse Med.2017;46:e63-e68. doi: 10.1016/j.lpm.2016.09.027
20. Hallstrom AP, Ornato JP, Weisfeldt M, Travers A, Christenson J, McBurnie MA, Zalenski R, Becker LB, Schron EB, Proschan M; Public Access Defibrillation Trial Investigators. Public-access defibrillation and survival after out-of-hospital cardiac arrest. N Engl J Med.2004;351:637-646. doi: 10.1056/NEJMoa040566
21. Karam N, Marijon E, Dumas F, Offredo L, Beganton F, Bougouin W, Jost D, Lamhaut L, Empana JP, Cariou A, Spaulding C, Jouven X; Paris Sudden Death Expertise Center. Characteristics and outcomes of out-of-hospital sudden cardiac arrest according to the time of occurrence. Resuscitation.2017;116:16-21. doi: 10.1016/j.resuscitation.2017.04.024
22. Kiguchi T, Kiyohara K, Kitamura T, Nishiyama C, Kobayashi D, Okabayashi S, Shimamoto T, Matsuyama T, Kawamura T, Iwami T. Public-access defibrillation and survival of out-of-hospital cardiac arrest in public vs. residential locations in Japan. Circ J. 2019;83:1682-1688. doi: 10.1253/circj.CJ-19-0065.
23. Kim JH, Uhm TH. Survival to admission after out-of-hospital cardiac arrest in Seoul, South Korea. Open Access Emerg Med. 2014;6:63-68. doi: 10.2147/OAEM.S68758
24. Kuisma M, Castrén M, Nurminen K. Public access defibrillation in Helsinki-costs and potential benefits from a community-based pilot study. Resuscitation.2003;56:149-152. doi: 10.1016/s0300-9572(02)00344-1
25. Matsui S, Kitamura T, Sado J, Kiyohara K, Kobayashi D, Kiguchi T, Nishiyama C, Okabayashi S, Shimamoto T, Matsuyama T, Kawamura T, Iwami T, Tanaka R, Kurosawa H, Nitta M, Sobue T. Location of arrest and survival from out-of-hospital cardiac arrest among children in the public-access defibrillation era in Japan. Resuscitation.2019;140:150-158. doi: 10.1016/j.resuscitation.2019.04.045

26. Nakahara S, Tomio J, Ichikawa M, Nakamura F, Nishida M, Takahashi H, Morimura N, Sakamoto T. Association of bystander interventions with neurologically intact survival among patients with bystander-witnessed out-of-hospital cardiac arrest in Japan. JAMA.2015;314:247-254. doi: 10.1001/jama.2015.8068
27. Nehme Z, Andrew E, Bernard S, Haskins B, Smith K. Trends in survival from out-of-hospital cardiac arrests defibrillated by paramedics, first responders and bystanders. Resuscitation.2019;143:85-91. doi: 10.1016/j.resuscitation.2019.08.018
28. Ringh M, Jonsson M, Nordberg P, Fredman D, Hasselqvist-Ax I, Håkansson F, Claesson A, Riva G, Hollenberg J. Survival after public access defibrillation in Stockholm, Sweden-a striking success. Resuscitation.2015;91:1-7. doi: 10.1016/j.resuscitation.2015.02.032
29. Tay PJM, Pek PP, Fan Q, Ng YY, Leong BS, Gan HN, Mao DR, Chia MYC, Cheah SO, Doctor N, Tham LP, Ong MEH.Effectiveness of a community based out-of-hospital cardiac arrest (OHCA) interventional bundle: Results of a pilot study.Resuscitation.2020;146:220-228. doi: 10.1016/j.resuscitation.2019.10.015
30. Kitamura T, Kiyohara K, Sakai T, Matsuyama T, Hatakeyama T, Shimamoto T, Izawa J, Fujii T, Nishiyama C, Kawamura T, Iwami T. Public-access defibrillation and out-of-hospital cardiac arrest in Japan. N Engl J Med.2016;375:1649-1659. doi: 10.1056/NEJMsa1600011
31. Colquhoun MC, Chamberlain DA, Newcombe RG, Harris R, Harris S, Peel K, Davies CS, Boyle R. A national scheme for public access defibrillation in England and Wales: early results. Resuscitation.2008;78:275-280. doi: 10.1016/j.resuscitation.2008.03.226
32. Fleischhackl R, Roessler B, Domanovits H, Singer F, Fleischhackl S, Foitik G, Czech G, Mittlboeck M, Malzer R, Eisenburger P, Hoerauf K. Results from Austria's nationwide public access defibrillation (ANPAD) programme collected over 2 years. Resuscitation.2008;77:195-200. doi: 10.1016/j.resuscitation.2007.11.019
33. Olasveengen TM, Mancini ME, Perkins GD, Avis S, Brooks S, Castrén M, Chung SP, Considine J, Couper K, Escalante R, et al; on behalf of the Adult Basic Life Support Collaborators.Adult basic life support: 2020 International Consensus on Cardiopulmonary Resuscitation and Emergency Cardiovascular Care Science With Treatment Recommendations.Circulation.2020;142(suppl 1):S41-S91. doi: 10.1161/CIR.0000000000000892
34. Sasson C, Rogers MA, Dahl J, Kellermann AL. Predictors of survival from out-of-hospital cardiac arrest: a systematic review and meta-analysis.Circ Cardiovasc Qual Outcomes.2010;3:63-81. doi: 10.1161/CIRCOUTCOMES.109.889576
35. Wissenberg M, Lippert FK, Folke F, Weeke P, Hansen CM, Christensen EF, Jans H, Hansen PA, Lang-Jensen T, Olesen JB, Lindhardsen J, Fosbol EL, Nielsen SL, Gislason GH, Kober L, Torp-Pedersen C. Association of national initiatives to improve cardiac arrest management with rates of bystander intervention and patient survival after out-of-hospital cardiac arrest. JAMA.2013;310:1377-1384. doi: 10.1001/jama.2013.278483
36. Larsen MP, Eisenberg MS, Cummins RO, Hallstrom AP. Predicting survival from out-of-hospital cardiac arrest: a graphic model.Ann Emerg Med.1993;22:1652-1658. doi: 10.1016/s0196-0644(05)81302-2
37. Perkins GD, Handley AJ, Koster RW, Castren M, Smyth MA, Olasveengen T, Monsieurs KG, Raffay V, Grasner JT, Wenzel V, et al; on behalf of the adult basic life support and automated external defibrillation section collaborators. European Resuscitation Council guidelines for resuscitation 2015: Section 2: adult basic life support and automated external defibrillation. Resuscitation. 2015;95:81-99. doi: 10.1016/j.resuscitation.2015.07.015
38. Ringh M, Hollenberg J, Palsgaard-Moeller T, Svensson L, Rosenqvist M, Lippert FK, Wissenberg M, Malta Hansen C, Claesson A, Viereck S, Zijlstra JA, Koster RW, Herlitz J, Blom MT, Kramer-Johansen J, Tan HL, Beesems SG, Hulleman M, Olasveengen TM, Folke F; COSTA study group (research collaboration between Copenhagen, Oslo, STockholm, and Amsterdam). The challenges and possibilities of public access defibrillation. J Intern Med.2018;283:238-256. doi: 10.1111/joim.12730
39. Myat A, Baumbach A. Public-access defibrillation: a call to shock. Lancet.2020;394:2204-2206. doi: 10.1016/S0140-6736(19)32560-7
40. Mao RD, Ong ME. Public access defibrillation: improving accessibility and outcomes. Br Med J.2016;118:25-32. doi: 10.1093/bmb/ldw011
41. Takeuchi I, Nagasawa H, Jitsuiki K, Kondo A, Ohsaka H, Yanagawa Y. Impact of automated external defibrillator as a recent innovation for the resuscitation of cardiac arrest patients in an urban city of Japan. J Emerg Trauma Shock. 2018;11:217-220. doi: 10.4103/JETS.JETS_79_17

CPRを要する事態の発生をバイスタンダーに通知する携帯電話のテクノロジー

CPRを要する事態の発生をバイスタンダーに通知する携帯電話技術に対する推奨事項

COR	LOE	推奨事項
2a	B-NR	1. 救急通報システムで携帯電話技術を使用して，意欲のあるバイスタンダーに，CPRまたはAEDの使用を要する近隣の事象を通知することは妥当である[1-7]。

「概要」

OHCA転帰の改善における第1市民救助者の役割は認識されているものの，大部分の地域でバイスタンダーによるCPR実施率[8]およびAEDの使用率[1]は低い。テキストメッセージやスマートフォンアプリなどの携帯電話のテクノロジーは，OHCAの発生時にバイスタンダーの協力を要請するためにますます多く利用されている。例えば，スマートフォンアプリを使用すると，緊急医療のテレコミュニケーターは心停止が発生した現場近くにいるCPR訓練を受けた地域社会のメンバーに警告を送信し，マッピング技術によって最寄りのAEDの場所や心停止を起こした傷病者の場所を案内できる[2]。

ILCORのシステマティックレビュー[10]によると，スマートフォンアプリやテキストメッセージの警告を利用した市民救助者への通知は，バイスタンダーによる応答時間の短縮[2]，バイスタンダーによるCPR実施率の向上[5,6]，除細動までの時間の短縮[1]，OHCA患者の生存退院率の向上[3-5,7]に関連していた。現在は，携帯電話のテクノロジーを利用して，CPRや除細動が必要となる近隣の事象に意欲のあるバイスタンダーを招集する救急通報システムのためのテクノロジーが存在する。この種のテクノロジーがさらに普及するにつれて，救命の連鎖で果たす役割が拡大する可能性がある。無作為化比較試験や費用対効果の検討，この介入をさまざまな患者，地域，および地理的背景に応用する探索的な研究が必要となる。ケアの提供に市民を巻き込むことのバイスタンダーに対する心理学的影響は不明である。

「推奨事項の裏付けとなる解説」

1. 1件のシステマティックレビュー[9]によると，1件のRCT[6]と6件の観察研究[1-5,7]で，バイスタンダーの招集に携帯電話技術を利用することを支持する総じて肯定的なデータを報告している。4件の観察研究（登録されたOHCA事象2905件）を対象としたメタアナリシスで，携帯電話のテクノロジーによって市民救助者にOHCAを通知した場合に，通知しない場合と比較して生存退院率が向上することが示された（調整後の相対リスク［aRR］ 1.70, 95%CI 1.16-2.48）[3-5,7]。このエビデンスは，観察研究に

固有のバイアスのために確実性は低い。1件のRCT[6]（登録されたOHCA患者667例）では，携帯電話のテクノロジーによって市民救助者にOHCAを通知した場合に，バイスタンダーによるCPR実施率が14%向上したが（aRR 1.27, CI 1.10-1.46），ROSCと生存率は向上しなかった。1件の観察研究（登録されたOHCA事象1696件）では，テキストメッセージによって市民救助者に通知した場合に，バイスタンダーによるCPR実施率が16%向上したと報告された（aRR 1.29, CI 1.20-1.37）[5]。4件の観察研究（登録されたOHCA事象1833件）では，携帯電話のテクノロジーによって通知された市民救助者は救急車よりも3〜4分到着が早かったことが示された[1-3,7]。除細動を行うまでの時間は，市民救助者にテキストメッセージでAEDを持ってくるよう伝えた場合に，救急車の応答と比較して2分39秒短かった。[1] 市民への通知に関連する有害事象の発生を報告した研究はなかった。現在までのところ，重要な文化的および地理的な違いによってこの種のテクノロジーの効果が国や地域ごとに異なるという研究は北米では行われていない。有効性を確立するためにさらに多くの研究が必要である。

上記の推奨事項は，AHAの蘇生教育科学執筆グループが作成し，2020年のILCORシステマティックレビューで支持された[10]。

参考文献

1. Zijlstra JA, Stieglis R, Riedijk F, Smeekes M, van der Worp WE, Koster RW. Local lay rescuers with AEDs, alerted by text messages, contribute to early defibrillation in a Dutch out-of-hospital cardiac arrest dispatch system. Resuscitation.2014;85:1444-1449. doi: 10.1016/j.resuscitation.2014.07.020
2. Berglund E, Claesson A, Nordberg P, Djärv T, Lundgren P, Folke F, Forsberg S, Riva G, Ringh M. A smartphone application for dispatch of lay responders to out-of-hospital cardiac arrests. Resuscitation.2018;126:160-165. doi: 10.1016/j.resuscitation.2018.01.039
3. Caputo ML, Muschietti S, Burkart R, Benvenuti C, Conte G, Regoli F, Mauri R, Klersy C, Moccetti T, Auricchio A. Lay persons alerted by mobile application system initiate earlier cardio-pulmonary resuscitation: A comparison with SMS-based system notification. Resuscitation.2017;114:73-78. doi: 10.1016/j.resuscitation.2017.03.003
4. Pijls RW, Nelemans PJ, Rahel BM, Gorgels AP. A text message alert system for trained volunteers improves out-of-hospital cardiac arrest survival. Resuscitation.2016;105:182-187. doi: 10.1016/j.resuscitation.2016.06.006
5. Lee SY, Shin SD, Lee YJ, Song KJ, Hong KJ, Ro YS, Lee EJ, Kong SY. Text message alert system and resuscitation outcomes after out-of-hospital cardiac arrest: A before-and-after population-based study. Resuscitation.2019;138:198-207. doi: 10.1016/j.resuscitation.2019.01.045
6. Ringh M, Rosenqvist M, Hollenberg J, Jonsson M, Fredman D, Nordberg P, Järnbert-Pettersson H, Hasselqvist-Ax I, Riva G, Svensson L. Mobile-phone dispatch of laypersons for CPR in out-of-hospital cardiac arrest. N Engl J Med.2015;372:2316-2325. doi: 10.1056/NEJMoa1406038
7. Stroop R, Kerner T, Strickmann B, Hensel M. Mobile phone-based alerting of CPR-trained volunteers simultaneously with the ambulance can reduce the resuscitation-free interval and improve outcome after out-of-hospital cardiac arrest: A German, population-based cohort study. Resuscitation.2020;147:57-64. doi: 10.1016/j.resuscitation.2019.12.012
8. Girotra S, van Diepen S, Nallamothu BK, Carrel M, Vellano K, Anderson ML, McNally B, Abella BS, Sasson C, Chan PS; CARES Surveillance Group and the HeartRescue Project.Regional Variation in Out-of-Hospital Cardiac Arrest Survival in the United States.Circulation.2016;133:2159-2168. doi: 10.1161/CIRCULATIONAHA.115.018175
9. Semeraro F, Zace D, Bigham BL, Scapigliati A, Ristagno G, Bhanji F, Bray JE, Breckwoldt J, Cheng A, Duff JP, et al. First responder engaged by technology (EIT #878): systematic review: consensus on science with treatment recommendations. https://costr.ilcor.org/document/first-responder-engaged-by-technology-systematic-review. Accessed February 17, 2020.
10. Greif R, Bhanji F, Bigham BL, Bray J, Breckwoldt J, Cheng A, Duff JP, Gilfoyle E, Hsieh M-J, Iwami T, et al; on behalf of the Education, Implementation, and Teams Collaborators. Education, implementation, and teams: 2020 International Consensus on Cardiopulmonary Resuscitation and Emergency Cardiovascular Care Science With Treatment Recommendations.Circulation.2020;142(suppl 1):S222-S283. doi: 10.1161/CIR.0000000000000896

OHCAの管理におけるテレコミュニケーターの役割

「概要」

バイスタンダーによる早期の効果的なCPRはOHCAの救命の連鎖で重要な要素である。残念ながら，バイスタンダーによるCPR実施率は成人と小児のいずれも依然として低い。救急医療における一般市民と公共安全の最初の窓口として，テレコミュニケーターはOHCAの救命の連鎖の重要な鎖の1つである。OHCAをきたした成人および小児において，通報対応オペレーター（通称：通報対応オペレーターまたは通信指令員）がCPRの指示を出すことによって，バイスタンダーのCPR実施率の向上と患者転帰の改善がみられた。EMSシステムでテレコミュニケーターがCPRの指示を出す場合（T-CPR，あるいは通信指令員の指示によるCPR，DA-CPRともいう），成人と小児のOHCAのいずれもバイスタンダーによるCPR実施率が向上することが実証されている[1-3]。しかし，T-CPRが提供されている場合でも，小児のOHCAに対するバイスタンダーによるCPR実施率は依然として低い。バイスタンダーのCPRを受けるOHCA傷病者数を最大にするためにT-CPRプロセスを記述し，質向上の仕組みを定型化する必要がある。

この疑問に対するエビデンスの基盤は成人集団と小児集団で異なるため，AHAの成人一次救命処置と二次救命処置の執筆グループとAHAの小児一次救命処置と二次救命処置の執筆グループが別々にレビューした。

参考文献

1. Duff JP, Topjian AA, Berg MD, Chan M, Haskell SE, Joyner BL Jr, Lasa JJ, Ley SJ, Raymond TT, Sutton RM, et al. 2019 American Heart Association focused update on pediatric basic life support: an update to the American Heart Association guidelines for cardiopulmonary resuscitation and emergency cardiovascular care. Circulation.2019;140:e915-e921. doi: 10.1161/CIR.0000000000000736
2. Panchal AR, Berg KM, Cabañas JG, Kurz MC, Link MS, Del Rios M, Hirsch KG, Chan PS, Hazinski MF, Morley PT, Donnino MW, Kudenchuk PJ. 2019 American Heart Association focused update on systems of care: dispatcher-assisted cardiopulmonary resuscitation and cardiac arrest centers: an update to the American Heart Association Guidelines for Cardiopulmonary Resuscitation and Emergency Cardiovascular Care. Circulation.2019;140:e895-e903. doi: 10.1161/CIR.0000000000000733
3. Kurz MC BB, Buckingham J, Cabanas JG, Eisenberg M, Fromm P, Panczyk MJ, Rea T, Seaman K, Vaillancourt C. Telephone cardiopulmonary resuscitation: an advocacy statement from the American Heart Association. Circulation.2020;141:e686-e700. doi: 10.1161/CIR.0000000000000744

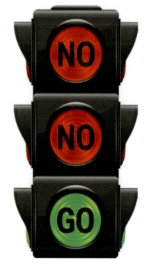

図 3. バイスタンダーによる CPR を開始する No-No-Go の暗記法
出典：From The Road to Recognition and Resuscitation: The Role of Telecommunicators and Telephone CPR Quality Improvement in Cardiac Arrest Survival. With permission from The Resuscitation Academy, Seattle, WA. CPR：心肺蘇生, T-CPR：電話による心肺蘇生

成人の OHCA におけるテレコミュニケーターの役割

テレコミュニケーターによる成人の心停止の認識に対する推奨事項

COR	LOE	推奨事項
1	C-LD	1. テレコミュニケーターは、OHCA を識別するための質問の前に、EMS 対応を同時に要請できるように、現場の場所の特定に必要な情報を得る必要がある[1,2]。
2a	C-LD	2. 異常な呼吸や、死戦期呼吸、または呼吸がなく反応がない場合は、救急の通信指令員がその患者を心停止状態にあるとみなすことは妥当である[3,4]。

「推奨事項の裏付けとなる解説」

1. 心停止が疑われる成人患者の緊急通報（119 番通報）を受けたテレコミュニケーターは、OHCA の認識と同時に適切な救急医療対応を手配できるように、まず緊急事態の現場の場所を聞く。[1] No-No-Go プロセスにある 2 つの質問をして（図 3）、傷病者に反応がなく、異常な呼吸があると判定した場合は、OHCA を起こしている人の最大 92％を識別できる可能性がある[2]。

2. 通報者からの情報により、成人の傷病者に反応がなく、無呼吸か異常な呼吸である場合、テレコミュニケーターは傷病者が OHCA を起こしつつあり、ただちに T-CPR の指示をする必要があると判断する[3,5]。OHCA の多様な症状に対処するため、テレコミュニケーターには、死戦期呼吸や短いミオクローヌスなどさまざまな状況で OHCA を識別する訓練が必要である[4]。上記の推奨事項は、AHA の成人一次救命処置と二次救命処置の執筆グループが作成し、「2019 AHA Focused Update on Systems of Care: Dispatcher-Assisted CPR and Cardiac Arrest Centers: An Update to the AHA Guidelines for CPR and ECC」、2018 年の ILCOR システマティックレビュー、2020 年の AHA の提言で支持された[3,5,6]。

心停止が疑われる成人の T-CPR 指示に対する推奨事項

COR	LOE	推奨事項
1	C-LD	1. 緊急派遣センターが CPR の指示を提供し、通信指令員が心停止中の成人患者のためにそのような指示を提供できるようにすることを推奨する[7]。
1	C-LD	2. テレコミュニケーターは、OHCA が疑われる成人患者に CPR を開始するよう通報者に指示する必要がある[7]。
1	C-LD	3. 通信指令員は通報者に対し、OHCA が疑われる成人に胸骨圧迫のみの CPR を実施するよう指示することを推奨する[7]。

「推奨事項の裏付けとなる解説」

1. 緊急出動センターを介した EMS への迅速な通報（119 番通報）と早期の CPR は、成人 OHCA の救命の連鎖のうち、最初の 2 つの鎖である。3 件の調整後の観察研究によると、T-CPR の使用は非使用と比較して、バイスタンダーによる CPR の実施率が 5 倍以上になり[8-10]、CPR が 7 分早く開始された[9]。

2. 救急対応の専門家が到着する前のバイスタンダーによる CPR の実施は，6 件の観察研究で生存と良好な神経学的転帰に関連していた[8,9,11-14]。2 件の研究では，複数の変数で調整した後でも，T-CPR の提供が退院から 1 カ月の生存率の向上と良好な神経学的転帰に関連していた。[9,12] したがって，緊急連絡センターは OHCA の傷病者が特定される全通報に適時の T-CPR 指示を与える必要がある[3]。

3. 通信指令員が指示する胸骨圧迫のみの CPR と従来の CPR を比較する 2 件の大規模無作為化試験のメタアナリシス（計 2496 例）によると，通信指令員が指示する胸骨圧迫のみの CPR は，胸骨圧迫および補助呼吸の指示と比較して，長期生存の有益性と関連していた[6,15]。

T-CPR の質向上に対する推奨事項		
COR	LOE	推奨事項
1	B-NR	1. T-CPR の指示の伝達は EMS システムの質向上プロセスの一環としてレビューし，評価する必要がある[16,17]。

「推奨事項の裏付けとなる解説」

1. T-CPR プログラムを成功させるには，T-CPR をできるだけ広範，迅速かつ適切に提供するために，OHCA 通報の音声記録のレビューなど，確実な質向上プロセスを備える必要がある[16,17]。

上記の推奨事項は，AHA の成人一次救命処置と二次救命処置の執筆グループが作成し，「2019 AHA Focused Update on Systems of Care: Dispatcher-Assisted CPR and Cardiac Arrest Centers: An Update to the AHA Guidelines for CPR and ECC」，2018 年の ILCOR システマティックレビュー，2020 年の AHA の提言で支持された[3,5,6]。

参考文献

1. Lerner EB, Rea TD, Bobrow BJ, Acker JE III, Berg RA, Brooks SC, Cone DC, Gay M, Gent LM, Mears G, Nadkarni VM, O'Connor RE, Potts J, Sayre MR, Swor RA, Travers AH; American Heart Association Emergency Cardiovascular Care Committee; Council on Cardiopulmonary, Critical Care, Perioperative and Resuscitation. Emergency medical service dispatch cardiopulmonary resuscitation prearrival instructions to improve survival from out-of-hospital cardiac arrest: a scientific statement from the American Heart Association. Circulation.2012;125:648-655. doi: 10.1161/CIR.0b013e31823ee5fc
2. Lewis M, Stubbs BA, Eisenberg MS. Dispatcher-assisted cardiopulmonary resuscitation: time to identify cardiac arrest and deliver chest compression instructions. Circulation.2013;128:1522-1530. doi: 10.1161/CIRCULATIONAHA.113.002627
3. Kurz MC BB, Buckingham J, Cabanas JG, Eisenberg M, Fromm P, Panczyk MJ, Rea T, Seaman K, Vaillancourt C. Telephone cardiopulmonary resuscitation: an advocacy statement from the American Heart Association. Circulation.2020;141:e686-e700. doi: 10.1161/CIR.0000000000000744
4. Bång A, Herlitz J, Martinell S. Interaction between emergency medical dispatcher and caller in suspected out-of-hospital cardiac arrest calls with focus on agonal breathing. A review of 100 tape recordings of true cardiac arrest cases.Resuscitation.2003;56:25-34. doi: 10.1016/s0300-9572 (02)00278-2
5. Panchal AR, Berg KM, Cabañas JG, Kurz MC, Link MS, Del Rios M, Hirsch KG, Chan PS, Hazinski MF, Morley PT, Donnino MW, Kudenchuk PJ.2019 American Heart Association focused update on systems of care: dispatcher-assisted cardiopulmonary resuscitation and cardiac arrest centers: an update to the American Heart Association Guidelines for Cardiopulmonary Resuscitation and Emergency Cardiovascular Care.Circulation.2019;140:e895-e903. doi: 10.1161/CIR.0000000000000733
6. Olasveengen TM, Mancini ME, Perkins GD, Avis S, Brooks S, Castrén M, Chung SP, Considine J, Couper K, Escalante R, et al; on behalf of the Adult Basic Life Support Collaborators.Adult basic life support: 2020 International Consensus on Cardiopulmonary Resuscitation and Emergency Cardiovascular Care Science With Treatment Recommendations.Circulation.2020;142 (suppl 1):S41-S91. doi: 10.1161/CIR.0000000000000892
7. Nikolaou N, Dainty KN, Couper K, Morley P, Tijssen J, Vaillancourt C; International Liaison Committee on Resuscitation's (ILCOR) Basic Life Support and Pediatric Task Forces. A systematic review and meta-analysis of the effect of dispatcher-assisted CPR on outcomes from sudden cardiac arrest in adults and children.Resuscitation.2019;138:82-105. doi: 10.1016/j.resuscitation.2019.02.035
8. Song KJ, Shin SD, Park CB, Kim JY, Kim DK, Kim CH, Ha SY, Eng Hock Ong M, Bobrow BJ, McNally B. Dispatcher-assisted bystander cardiopulmonary resuscitation in a metropolitan city: a before-after population-based study. Resuscitation.2014;85:34-41. doi: 10.1016/j.resuscitation.2013.06.004
9. Goto Y, Maeda T, Goto Y. Impact of dispatcher-assisted bystander cardiopulmonary resuscitation on neurological outcomes in children with out-of-hospital cardiac arrests: a prospective, nationwide, population-based cohort study. J Am Heart Assoc. 2014;3:e000499. doi: 10.1161/JAHA.113.000499
10. Fukushima H, Panczyk M, Hu C, Dameff C, Chikani V, Vadeboncoeur T, Spaite DW, Bobrow BJ. Description of abnormal breathing is associated with improved outcomes and delayed telephone cardiopulmonary resuscitation instructions. J Am Heart Assoc. 2017;6:e005058. doi: 10.1161/JAHA.116.005058
11. Besnier E, Damm C, Jardel B, Veber B, Compere V, Dureuil B. Dispatcher-assisted cardiopulmonary resuscitation protocol improves diagnosis and resuscitation recommendations for out-of-hospital cardiac arrest. Emerg Med Australas.2015;27:590-596. doi: 10.1111/1742-6723.12493
12. Harjanto S, Na MX, Hao Y, Ng YY, Doctor N, Goh ES, Leong BS, Gan HN, Chia MY, Tham LP, Cheah SO, Shahidah N, Ong ME; PAROS study group. A before-after interventional trial of dispatcher-assisted cardio-pulmonary resuscitation for out-of-hospital cardiac arrests in Singapore. Resuscitation.2016;102:85-93. doi: 10.1016/j.resuscitation.2016.02.014
13. Hiltunen PV, Silfvast TO, Jäntti TH, Kuisma MJ, Kurola JO; FINNRESUSCI Prehospital Study Group. Emergency dispatch process and patient outcome in bystander-witnessed out-of-hospital cardiac arrest with a shockable rhythm. Eur J Emerg Med.2015;22:266-272. doi: 10.1097/MEJ.0000000000000151
14. Takahashi H, Sagisaka R, Natsume Y, Tanaka S, Takyu H, Tanaka H. Does dispatcher-assisted CPR generate the same outcomes as spontaneously delivered bystander CPR in Japan? Am J Emerg Med.2018;36:384-391. doi: 10.1016/j.ajem.2017.08.034
15. Hüpfl M, Selig HF, Nagele P. Chest-compression-only versus standard cardiopulmonary resuscitation: a meta-analysis. Lancet.2010;376:1552-1557. doi: 10.1016/S0140-6736 (10)61454-7
16. Tanaka Y, Taniguchi J, Wato Y, Yoshida Y, Inaba H. The continuous quality improvement project for telephone-assisted instruction of cardiopulmonary resuscitation increased the incidence of bystander CPR and improved the outcomes of out-of-hospital cardiac arrests. Resuscitation.2012;83:1235-1241. doi: 10.1016/j.resuscitation.2012.02.013
17. Bobrow BJ, Spaite DW, Vadeboncoeur TF, Hu C, Mullins T, Tormala W, Dameff C, Gallagher J, Smith G, Panczyk M. Implementation of a regional telephone cardiopulmonary resuscitation program and outcomes after out-of-hospital cardiac arrest. JAMA Cardiol.2016;1:294-302. doi: 10.1001/jamacardio.2016.0251

乳児と小児のOHCAにおけるテレコミュニケーターの役割

T-CPRに対する推奨事項—：乳児および小児		
COR	LOE	推奨事項
1	C-LD	1. 緊急医療派遣センターでは，小児心停止が想定される場合にT-CPRの指示を与えることを推奨する[1-5]。
1	C-LD	2. バイスタンダーによるCPRが実施されていない場合，救急の通信指令員が小児の心停止に対するT-CPRの指示を与えることを推奨する[1-5]。

「推奨事項の裏付けとなる解説」

1. 最近のILCORのシステマティックレビューでは，T-CPRの使用はT-CPR不使用と比較して，小児および成人の患者転帰が改善するというエビデンスが示されている[6]。ある観察研究で，T-CPRと，OHCAをきたした小児の1カ月後の生存率向上の関連が報告された[1]。心停止をきたした患者5009例を登録した観察研究では，通信指令員が支援するCPRの提供は，1カ月後の生存率向上と関連していたが，1カ月後の良好な神経学的転帰とは関連していなかった。バイスタンダーによるCPRの実施は，通信指令員の指示の有無にかかわらず，バイスタンダーによるCPR非実施と比較して，生存オッズの改善および良好な神経学的転帰での生存と関連していた[2]。

2. 横断的な症例登録研究で，T-CPRと，支援を受けないバイスタンダーによるCPRはいずれも，バイスタンダーによるCPR非実施と比較して，退院時の良好な神経学的転帰の可能性が向上することが示された[3]。同じデータベースを使用したOHCAの小児の新しい横断研究では，通信指令員の支援の有無にかかわらず，バイスタンダーによるCPRによって退院時に神経学的機能が良好な生存が2倍以上になることが分かった[4]。

上記の推奨事項は，AHAの小児一次救命処置と二次救命処置の執筆グループが作成し，「2019 AHA Focused Update on Pediatric Basic Life Support: An Update to the AHA Guidelines for CPR and ECC」および2019年のILCORシステマティックレビューで支持された[6]。

参考文献

1. Akahane M, Ogawa T, Tanabe S, Koike S, Horiguchi H, Yasunaga H, Imamura T. Impact of telephone dispatcher assistance on the outcomes of pediatric out-of-hospital cardiac arrest. Crit Care Med.2012;40:1410-1416. doi: 10.1097/CCM.0b013e31823e99ae
2. Goto Y, Maeda T, Goto Y. Impact of dispatcher-assisted bystander cardiopulmonary resuscitation on neurological outcomes in children with out-of-hospital cardiac arrests: a prospective, nationwide, population-based cohort study.J Am Heart Assoc. 2014;3:e000499. doi: 10.1161/JAHA.113.000499
3. Ro YS, Shin SD, Song KJ, Hong KJ, Ahn KO, Kim DK, Kwak YH. Effects of Dispatcher-assisted Cardiopulmonary Resuscitation on Survival Outcomes in Infants, Children, and Adolescents with Out-of-hospital Cardiac Arrests. Resuscitation.2016;108:20-26. doi: 10.1016/j.resuscitation.2016.08.026
4. Chang I, Ro YS, Shin SD, Song KJ, Park JH, Kong SY. Association of dispatcher-assisted bystander cardiopulmonary resuscitation with survival outcomes after pediatric out-of-hospital cardiac arrest by community property value. Resuscitation.2018;132:120-126. doi: 10.1016/j.resuscitation.2018.09.008
5. Nikolaou N, Dainty KN, Couper K, Morley P, Tijssen J, Vaillancourt C; International Liaison Committee on Resuscitation's (ILCOR) Basic Life Support and Pediatric Task Forces.A systematic review and meta-analysis of the effect of dispatcher-assisted CPR on outcomes from sudden cardiac arrest in adults and children.Resuscitation.2019;138:82-105. doi: 10.1016/j.resuscitation.2019.02.035
6. Olasveengen TM, Mancini ME, Perkins GD, Avis S, Brooks S, Castrén M, Chung SP, Considine J, Couper K, Escalante R, et al; on behalf of the Adult Basic Life Support Collaborators. Adult basic life support: 2020 International Consensus on Cardiopulmonary Resuscitation and Emergency Cardiovascular Care Science With Treatment Recommendations.Circulation.2020;142(suppl 1):S41-S91. doi: 10.1161/CIR.0000000000000892

IHCAの予防

概要

IHCAからの生存率には依然としてばらつきがあり，特に成人で顕著である[1]。ほとんどの一般病棟でよくあることだが，モニタリングされていない，あるいは目撃者のいない状況で心停止した患者の転帰は最悪となる。小児のIHCA後の転帰は改善しており，生存率は38%という報告があり[2]，小児のIHCAの大多数はICUで起こっている[3]。院内の心停止または呼吸停止は，悪化している患者を認識してリソースを割り当てるシステムによって予防できる可能性がある。臨床ケアチームまたは家族によるMETまたはRRTの出動要請は，患者の容態の変化に反応して行われるのが理想的である。METやRRTのようなチームは，院内心肺停止や死亡を防ぐ取り組みとして，急激に生理機能が破綻する患者に対応する。迅速対応システムは広く採用されているが，転帰に関して一貫した研究結果は示されていない。迅速対応チームの構成やチームの出動要請と対応の一貫性，早期警告スコアシステムの構成要素は，医療施設によって大幅に異なるため，この種の介入の有効性に関して一般化した科学的な結論を下すのは困難である。

この疑問に対するエビデンスの基盤は成人集団と小児集団で異なるため，AHAの成人一次救命処置と二次救命処置の執筆グループとAHAの小児一次救命処置と二次救命処置の執筆グループが別々にレビューした。

参考文献

1. Virani SS, Alonso A, Benjamin EJ, Bittencourt MS, Callaway CW, Carson AP, Chamberlain AM, Chang AR, Cheng S, Delling FN, et al; on behalf of the American Heart Association Council on Epidemiology and Prevention Statistics Committee and Stroke Statistics Subcommittee. Heart disease and stroke statistics—2020 update: a report from the American Heart Association. Circulation. 2020;141:e139-e596. doi: 10.1161/CIR.0000000000000757
2. Holmberg MJ, Wiberg S, Ross CE, Kleinman M, Hoeyer-Nielsen AK, Donnino MW, Andersen LW. Trends in survival after pediatric in-hospital cardiac arrest in the United States. Circulation. 2019;140:1398-1408. doi: 10.1161/CIRCULATIONAHA.119.041667
3. Berg RA, Sutton RM, Holubkov R, Nicholson CE, Dean JM, Harrison R, Heidemann S, Meert K, Newth C, Moler F, Pollack M, Dalton H, Doctor A, Wessel D, Berger J, Shanley T, Carcillo J, Nadkarni VM; Eunice Kennedy Shriver National Institute of Child Health and Human Development Collaborative Pediatric Critical Care Research Network and for the American Heart Association's Get With the Guidelines–Resuscitation (formerly the National

成人のIHCAを予防する臨床早期警告システムと迅速対応チーム

COR	LOE	推奨事項
2a	C-LD	1. 入院中の成人では，迅速対応チームまたは救急医療チームなどの対応システムが，特に一般病棟における心停止の発生抑制に有効な可能性がある[1]。
2b	C-LD	2. 入院中の成人に対し，早期警告スコアシステムの利用を考慮してもよい[1]。

「推奨事項の裏付けとなる解説」

1. 最新のILCORのシステマティックレビューでは，RRT/METシステム導入の観察研究の結果に不一致がみられ，17件の研究では心停止発生率の有意な改善が示されたが，7件の研究ではそのような改善はみられなかった[1]。1件の大規模なRCTでは，心停止の発生率と死亡率にベネフィットが示されなかった[2]。このエビデンスによると，RRT/METシステムの導入は，ICU以外の心停止の減少に加えて死亡率の低下にも有効な可能性があるが，さらに詳細な評価が必要である。システムの強化（例えば，RRT/METの出動要請率の向上，RRT/METへの上級の医療スタッフ割り当てなど）は，さらに効果を高めると考えられる。研究デザインや状況，患者集団，対応チームの構成，チームの出動要請基準，研究対象の転帰の不均一性のため，研究間での意味のあるデータ解析は困難である。

2. システマティックレビューは主にRRT/METシステムの効果に着目しているが，早期警告システムの使用も対象とされている。成人のIHCA減少を具体的な目標とした早期警告スコアシステム使用に関するRCTは特定されなかった。レビュー対象となった1件の観察研究は，修正早期警告スコアのIHCA予測能力に一貫性がないことを指摘していた[1,3]。最近では，容態悪化の早期発見を支援する機械学習やその他のアプローチへの関心がますます高まっており，研究を進める十分な理由となる[4]。

上記の推奨事項は，AHAの成人一次救命処置と二次救命処置の執筆グループが作成し，RRT/MET導入に着目した2020年のILCORシステマティックレビューを拠り所としている[1]。

参考文献

1. Greif R, Bhanji F, Bigham BL, Bray J, Breckwoldt J, Cheng A, Duff JP, Gilfoyle E, Hsieh M-J, Iwami T, et al; on behalf of the Education, Implementation, and Teams Collaborators. Education, implementation, and teams: 2020 International Consensus on Cardiopulmonary Resuscitation and Emergency Cardiovascular Care Science With Treatment Recommendations. Circulation. 2020;142(suppl 1):S222-S283. doi: 10.1161/CIR.0000000000000896
2. Hillman K, Chen J, Cretikos M, Bellomo R, Brown D, Doig G, Finfer S, Flabouris A; MERIT study investigators. Introduction of the medical emergency team (MET) system: a cluster-randomised controlled trial. Lancet. 2005;365:2091-2097. doi: 10.1016/S0140-6736(05)66733-5
3. Subbe CP, Davies RG, Williams E, Rutherford P, Gemmell L. Effect of introducing the Modified Early Warning score on clinical outcomes, cardiopulmonary arrests and intensive care utilisation in acute medical admissions. Anaesthesia. 2003;58:797-802. doi: 10.1046/j.1365-2044.2003.03258.x
4. Kwon JM, Lee Y, Lee Y, Lee S, Park J. An algorithm based on deep learning for predicting in-hospital cardiac arrest. J Am Heart Assoc. 2018;7:e008678. doi: 10.1161/jaha.118.008678

乳児，小児，青年のIHCAを予防する臨床早期警告システムと迅速対応チーム

COR	LOE	推奨事項
2a	C-LD	1. 小児の迅速対応チーム／救急医療チームのシステムは，リスクの高い疾患を抱える小児が一般病棟にいる病院では効果的な可能性がある[1-4]。
2b	B-R	2. リスクの高い乳児や小児を発見して早期に上位レベルのケアに移行できるように，小児の迅速対応チーム／救急医療チームに加えて，小児の早期警告／トリガースコアを検討してもよい[1,5-9]。

「推奨事項の裏付けとなる解説」

1. RRT/METシステムは成人集団と小児集団の両方で院内の死亡率と心肺停止率の低下に関連している[1-3]。小児病院38施設の症例を登録した1件の観察研究では，RRT/METの導入に関連して，リスク調整後の死亡率に差は認められなかった[4]。小児の心停止を予防するRRT/METシステムの役割を評価するエビデンスは質と量ともに低い。主な限界は，小児の心停止発生率と死亡率が低いこと（特に，ICU外），患者集団が不均一なことである。

2. 国際共同，多施設共同，クラスター無作為化試験で，ベッドサイドの小児早期警告システムの導入は，市中病院の非三次医療病棟での臨床的に重要な容態悪化の減少と関連していたが，全死因による死亡率とは関連していなかった[5]。最近の4件のシステマティックレビューと1件のスコーピングレビューによると，小児早期警告システムの使用は容態悪化の減少につながるという限定的なエビデンスが示された[1,6-9]。1件のスコーピングレビューでは，限定的であるが，低または中所得国において小児早期警告システムの有用性を示唆するエビデンスが示された[8]。

上記の推奨事項は，AHA の小児一次救命処置と二次救命処置の執筆グループが作成し，2019 年の ILCOR のスコーピングレビューと 2020 年のエビデンスレビューを拠り所としている[10]。

参考文献

1. Maharaj R, Raffaele I, Wendon J. Rapid response systems: a systematic review and meta-analysis. Crit Care. 2015;19:254. doi: 10.1186/s13054-015-0973-y
2. Bonafide CP, Localio AR, Roberts KE, Nadkarni VM, Weirich CM, Keren R. Impact of rapid response system implementation on critical deterioration events in children. JAMA Pediatr. 2014;168:25-33. doi: 10.1001/jamapediatrics.2013.3266
3. Kolovos NS, Gill J, Michelson PH, Doctor A, Hartman ME. Reduction in mortality following pediatric rapid response team implementation. Pediatr Crit Care Med.2018;19:477-482. doi: 10.1097/PCC.0000000000001519
4. Kutty S, Jones PG, Karels Q, Joseph N, Spertus JA, Chan PS. Association of Pediatric Medical Emergency Teams With Hospital Mortality. Circulation.2018;137:38-46. doi: 10.1161/CIRCULATIONAHA.117.029535
5. Parshuram CS, Dryden-Palmer K, Farrell C, Gottesman R, Gray M, Hutchison JS, Helfaer M, Hunt EA, Joffe AR, Lacroix J, Moga MA, Nadkarni V, Ninis N, Parkin PC, Wensley D, Willan AR, Tomlinson GA; Canadian Critical Care Trials Group and the EPOCH Investigators. Effect of a pediatric early warning system on all-cause mortality in hospitalized pediatric patients: the EPOCH randomized clinical trial. JAMA.2018;319:1002-1012. doi: 10.1001/jama.2018.0948
6. Trubey R, Huang C, Lugg-Widger FV, Hood K, Allen D, Edwards D, Lacy D, Lloyd A, Mann M, Mason B, Oliver A, Roland D, Sefton G, Skone R, Thomas-Jones E, Tume LN, Powell C. Validity and effectiveness of paediatric early warning systems and track and trigger tools for identifying and reducing clinical deterioration in hospitalised children: a systematic review. BMJ Open. 2019;9:e022105. doi: 10.1136/bmjopen-2018-022105
7. Chapman SM, Wray J, Oulton K, Peters MJ. Systematic review of paediatric track and trigger systems for hospitalised children. Resuscitation.2016;109:87-109. doi: 10.1016/j.resuscitation.2016.07.230
8. Brown SR, Martinez Garcia D, Agulnik A. Scoping review of pediatric early warning systems (PEWS) in resource-limited and humanitarian settings. Front Pediatr. 2018;6:410. doi: 10.3389/fped.2018.00410
9. Lambert V, Matthews A, MacDonell R, Fitzsimons J. Paediatric early warning systems for detecting and responding to clinical deterioration in children: a systematic review. BMJ Open. 2017;7:e014497. doi: 10.1136/bmjopen-2016-014497
10. Maconochie IK, Aickin R, Hazinski MF, Atkins DL, Bingham R, Couto TB, Guerguerian A-M, Nadkarni VM, Ng K-C, Nuthall GA, et al; on behalf of the Pediatric Life Support Collaborators. Pediatric life support: 2020 International Consensus on Cardiopulmonary Resuscitation and Emergency Cardiovascular Care Science With Treatment Recommendations.Circulation.2020;142 (suppl 1):S140-S184. doi: 10.1161/CIR.0000000000000894

蘇生のパフォーマンス
蘇生の認知支援

COR	LOE	推奨事項
2b	C-LD	1. 心停止に対応する市民救助者への認知支援ツールの有効性は不明であり，広く普及させる前にさらに研究が必要がある[1-5]。
2b	C-LD	2. 心肺蘇生中に，医療従事者のチームパフォーマンスを改善するために認知支援ツールを利用することは妥当である[6-9]。

「概要」

認知支援によって緊急以外の状況での患者ケアは改善する[10,11]が，重大な状況での影響についてはほとんどわかってない。認知支援ツールが有用になるとしたらそれはいつ，どのような場合かを理解すると，市民救助者や医療従事者の蘇生の取り組みの改善に役立ち，引いては多くの人命の救助につなげることができる。認知支援については，望ましい行為，判断，転帰の可能性を高める情報を想起しやすくすることを目的とした支援の提供と考えられる[12]。例えば，チェックリスト，警報，携帯電話用アプリ，暗記法などが該当する。

ILCOR のシステマティックレビューでは，心停止シミュレーションにおいて市民救助者による認知支援の利用が CPR の開始を遅らせたことを示唆しており，実際の患者では非常に有害な影響が生じる可能性がある[14]。心停止時の市民救助者に対する認知支援を広く普及させる前に，さらに研究が必要である。心停止時の医療チーム間での認知支援ツールの利用を評価する研究は特定されなかった。外傷蘇生のエビデンスは，認知支援ツールの使用によって蘇生ガイドラインへの遵守が向上し，ミスが減り，重症患者の生存率が向上することを示唆している。心停止時に医療従事者に対して認知支援ツールを使用することは合理的と考えられる。関連性の高い分野から推定することは妥当であるが，さらに検討を要する。実際の心停止時に認知支援がツールバイスタンダーおよび医療従事者の行動を支援するかどうかは今後の研究で検討する必要がある。

「推奨事項の裏付けとなる解説」

1. 1 件のシステマティックレビュー[14]で特定された 4 件の無作為化試験[1-4]では，市民救助者に認知支援ツールを提供したときに CPR の開始に統計学的に有意かつ臨床的に意味のある遅延が示された（各試験の群間に 30 秒～70 秒の差）。CPR の開始後は，認知支援ツールを利用する救助者では何もしていない時間が短縮し[1,2,4,5,]行動する能力への自信が高まるようであり[4]，それは最終的に心停止に対応する市民救助者を支えるために重要となる可能性がある。
2. システマティックレビューでは，心停止時に認知支援ツールを利用した場合の生存退院率を解析している研究は特定されなかったが，外傷蘇生に関連する 3 つの研究が特定された（1 件の RCT[6] と 2 件の観察研究[7,9]。これらの観察研究によると，認知支援ツールを利用している場合に重症度が高い傷病者（重症度スコア 25 以上）の生存退院率が高かった[7,9]。この RCT には重症度の低い傷病者が登録されており，生存率に差はみられなかった[6]。蘇生のパフォーマンスの尺度（ミスの少なさ，一次および二次サーベイの完遂，タスク実施の速さなど)は，試験ごとに指標が一貫していなかったが，外傷蘇生で

認知支援ツールを利用したほうが概ね良好であった[6-9]。

上記の推奨事項は，AHA の蘇生教育科学執筆グループが作成し，2020 年の ILCOR システマティックレビューで支持された[14]。

参考文献

1. Hunt EA, Heine M, Shilkofski NS, Bradshaw JH, Nelson-McMillan K, Duval-Arnould J, Elfenbein R. Exploration of the impact of a voice activated decision support system (VADSS) with video on resuscitation performance by lay rescuers during simulated cardiopulmonary arrest. Emerg Med J. 2015;32:189-194. doi: 10.1136/emermed-2013-202867
2. Merchant RM, Abella BS, Abotsi EJ, Smith TM, Long JA, Trudeau ME, Leary M, Groeneveld PW, Becker LB, Asch DA. Cell telephone cardiopulmonary resuscitation: audio instructions when needed by lay rescuers: a randomized, controlled trial. Ann Emerg Med. 2010;55:538-543.e1. doi: 10.1016/j.annemergmed.2010.01.020
3. Paal P, Pircher I, Baur T, Gruber E, Strasak AM, Herff H, Brugger H, Wenzel V, Mitterlechner T. Mobile phone-assisted basic life support augmented with a metronome. J Emerg Med.2012;43:472-477. doi: 10.1016/j.jemermed.2011.09.011
4. Rössler B, Ziegler M, Hüpfl M, Fleischhackl R, Krychtiuk KA, Schebesta K. Can a flowchart improve the quality of bystander cardiopulmonary resuscitation? Resuscitation.2013;84:982-986. doi: 10.1016/j.resuscitation.2013.01.001
5. Hawkes GA, Murphy G, Dempsey EM, Ryan AC. Randomised controlled trial of a mobile phone infant resuscitation guide. J Paediatr Child Health.2015;51:1084-1088. doi: 10.1111/jpc.12968
6. Fitzgerald M, Cameron P, Mackenzie C, Farrow N, Scicluna P, Gocentas R, Bystrzycki A, Lee G, O'Reilly G, Andrianopoulos N, Dziukas L, Cooper DJ, Silvers A, Mori A, Murray A, Smith S, Xiao Y, Stub D, McDermott FT, Rosenfeld JV. Trauma resuscitation errors and computer-assisted decision support. Arch Surg. 2011;146:218-225. doi: 10.1001/archsurg.2010.333
7. Bernhard M, Becker TK, Nowe T, Mohorovicic M, Sikinger M, Brenner T, Richter GM, Radeleff B, Meeder PJ, Büchler MW, Böttiger BW, Martin E, Gries A. Introduction of a treatment algorithm can improve the early management of emergency patients in the resuscitation room. Resuscitation.2007;73:362-373. doi: 10.1016/j.resuscitation.2006.09.014
8. Kelleher DC, Carter EA, Waterhouse LJ, Parsons SE, Fritzeen JL, Burd RS. Effect of a checklist on advanced trauma life support task performance during pediatric trauma resuscitation. Acad Emerg Med.2014;21:1129-1134. doi: 10.1111/acem.12487
9. Lashoher A, Schneider EB, Juillard C, Stevens K, Colantuoni E, Berry WR, Bloem C, Chadbunchachai W, Dharap S, Dy SM, Dziekan G, Gruen RL, Henry JA, Huwer C, Joshipura M, Kelley E, Krug E, Kumar V, Kyamanywa P, Mefire AC, Musafir M, Nathens AB, Ngendahayo E, Nguyen TS, Roy N, Pronovost PJ, Khan IQ, Razzak JA, Rubiano AM, Turner JA, Varghese M, Zakirova R, Mock C. Implementation of the World Health Organization Trauma Care Checklist program in 11 centers across multiple economic strata: effect on care process measures. World J Surg. 2017;41:954-962. doi: 10.1007/s00268-016-3759-8
10. de Vries EN, Prins HA, Crolla RM, den Outer AJ, van Andel G, van Helden SH, Schlack WS, van Putten MA, Gouma DJ, Dijkgraaf MG, Smorenburg SM, Boermeester MA; SURPASS Collaborative Group. Effect of a comprehensive surgical safety system on patient outcomes. N Engl J Med.2010;363:1928-1937. doi: 10.1056/NEJMsa0911535
11. Haynes AB, Weiser TG, Berry WR, Lipsitz SR, Breizat AH, Dellinger EP, Herbosa T, Joseph S, Kibatala PL, Lapitan MC, Merry AF, Moorthy K, Reznick RK, Taylor B, Gawande AA; Safe Surgery Saves Lives Study Group. A surgical safety checklist to reduce morbidity and mortality in a global population. N Engl J Med.2009;360:491-499. doi: 10.1056/NEJMsa0810119
12. Fletcher KA, Bedwell WL. Cognitive aids: design suggestions for the medical field. Proc Int Symp Human Factors Ergonomics Health Care. 2014;3:148-152. doi: 10.1177/2327857914031024
13. Deleted in proof.
14. Greif R, Bhanji F, Bigham BL, Bray J, Breckwoldt J, Cheng A, Duff JP, Gilfoyle E, Hsieh M-J, Iwami T, et al; on behalf of the Education, Implementation, and Teams Collaborators. Education, implementation, and teams: 2020 International Consensus on Cardiopulmonary Resuscitation and Emergency Cardiovascular Care Science With Treatment Recommendations.Circulation.2020;142 (suppl 1):S222-S283. doi: 10.1161/CIR.0000000000000896

心拍再開後の治療
心停止治療センター

心停止治療センターに対する推奨事項		
COR	LOE	推奨事項
2a	C-LD	1. 急性期の蘇生患者を専門の心停止治療センターへ直接搬送することを含む，心拍再開後の治療に対する地域化アプローチは，地域の施設で心拍再開後の包括的治療ができない場合に妥当である[1-10]。

「概要」

心停止治療センター（CAC）は，他の専門センターのような正式な施設基準はまだないが，エビデンスに基づいた包括的な心拍再開後の治療を提供する専門施設であり，緊急の心臓カテーテル検査，目標体温管理，血行動態サポート，神経学的評価などを実施する。CAC は，ガイドラインを遵守したケアを確実に実施するためにプロトコルや質向上プログラムを備えている。体外膜型人工肺やその他の方式の循環補助を実施する能力も備えた CAC がますます増えている。患者は蘇生中または ROSC 後に EMS により直接 CAC に搬送されることもあれば，ROSC 後に別の病院から CAC に搬送されることもある。この意思決定プロセスでの重要な考慮事項として，搬送時間，患者の安定，搬送サービスが必要なケアを提供する能力などが挙げられる。

心拍再開後の包括的治療の裏付けとなるエビデンスはほとんどが観察研究のものであり（特に，専門センターでケアバンドル（包括的治療）としてまとめて実施された場合），研究の結果も一貫していないが，それにもかかわらず CAC は蘇生の成功と最終的な生存の間に理にかなった臨床的な関わりを有している。外傷，脳卒中，ST 上昇型急性心筋梗塞など他の緊急事態に対する地域の取り組みでの経験と併せて，心拍再開後のサービスを補完する適切な医療が地域で利用できない場合に，そのようなサポートを提供する地域のセンターに蘇生後の患者を直接搬送することは有益であり，実現可能であれば合理的なアプローチである。

「推奨事項の裏付けとなる解説」

1. エビデンスに基づく包括的な心拍再開後の治療は，蘇生後の患者にとってきわめて重要である。2 件の観察研究の調整後の解析によると，AC での治療は 30 日後の良好な神経学的転帰での生存率上昇に関連していなかったが[2,3]，他の 2 件の研究では，CAC への入院は良好な神経学的転帰での生存退院率の改善に関連していた[4,7]。CAC での治療は CAC 以外での治療と比較して，30 日後の生存率向上[5,6]および生存退院率[4,7-10] と関連していた。CAC への迅速な搬送を評価する無作為

化試験の実現可能性中間報告（患者 40 例）では臨床転帰に差は示されなかったが，この報告は予備的なものであり，この転帰の検出力も不足していた[11]。

上記の推奨事項は，AHA の成人一次救命処置と二次救命処置の執筆グループが作成し，2019 年の ILCOR システマティックレビューで支持された[12]。

参考文献

1. Panchal AR, Berg KM, Cabañas JG, Kurz MC, Link MS, Del Rios M, Hirsch KG, Chan PS, Hazinski MF, Morley PT, Donnino MW, Kudenchuk PJ. 2019 American Heart Association focused update on systems of care: dispatcher-assisted cardiopulmonary resuscitation and cardiac arrest centers: an update to the American Heart Association Guidelines for Cardiopulmonary Resuscitation and Emergency Cardiovascular Care. Circulation. 2019;140:e895–e903. doi: 10.1161/CIR.0000000000000733
2. Matsuyama T, Kiyohara K, Kitamura T, Nishiyama C, Nishiuchi T, Hayashi Y, Kawamura T, Ohta B, Iwami T. Hospital characteristics and favourable neurological outcome among patients with out-of-hospital cardiac arrest in Osaka, Japan. Resuscitation. 2017;110:146–153. doi: 10.1016/j.resuscitation.2016.11.009
3. Tagami T, Hirata K, Takeshige T, Matsui J, Takinami M, Satake M, Satake S, Yui T, Itabashi K, Sakata T, Tosa R, Kushimoto S, Yokota H, Hirama H. Implementation of the fifth link of the chain of survival concept for out-of-hospital cardiac arrest. Circulation. 2012;126:589–597. doi: 10.1161/CIRCULATIONAHA.111.086173
4. Kragholm K, Malta Hansen C, Dupre ME, Xian Y, Strauss B, Tyson C, Monk L, Corbett C, Fordyce CB, Pearson DA, et al. Direct transport to a percutaneous cardiac intervention center and outcomes in patients with out-of-hospital cardiac arrest. Circ Cardiovasc Qual Outcomes. 2017;10:e003414. doi: 10.1161/CIRCOUTCOMES.116.003414
5. Harnod D, Ma MHM, Chang WH, Chang RE, Chang CH. Mortality factors in out-of-hospital cardiac arrest patients: a nationwide population-based study in Taiwan. Int J Gerontology. 2013;7:216-220.
6. Søholm H, Wachtell K, Nielsen SL, Bro-Jeppesen J, Pedersen F, Wanscher M, Boesgaard S, Møller JE, Hassager C, Kjaergaard J. Tertiary centres have improved survival compared to other hospitals in the Copenhagen area after out-of-hospital cardiac arrest. Resuscitation. 2013;84:162–167. doi: 10.1016/j.resuscitation.2012.06.029
7. Spaite DW, Bobrow BJ, Stolz U, Berg RA, Sanders AB, Kern KB, Chikani V, Humble W, Mullins T, Stapczynski JS, Ewy GA; Arizona Cardiac Receiving Center Consortium. Statewide regionalization of postarrest care for out-of-hospital cardiac arrest: association with survival and neurologic outcome. Ann Emerg Med. 2014;64:496-506.e1. doi: 10.1016/j.annemergmed.2014.05.028
8. Cournoyer A, Notebaert É, de Montigny L, Ross D, Cossette S, Londei-Leduc L, Iseppon M, Lamarche Y, Sokoloff C, Potter BJ, Vadeboncoeur A, Larose D, Morris J, Daoust R, Chauny JM, Piette É, Paquet J, Cavayas YA, de Champlain F, Segal E, Albert M, Guertin MC, Denault A. Impact of the direct transfer to percutaneous coronary intervention-capable hospitals on survival to hospital discharge for patients with out-of-hospital cardiac arrest. Resuscitation. 2018;125:28–33. doi: 10.1016/j.resuscitation.2018.01.048
9. Lick CJ, Aufderheide TP, Niskanen RA, Steinkamp JE, Davis SP, Nygaard SD, Bemenderfer KK, Gonzales L, Kalla JA, Wald SK, Gillquist DL, Sayre MR, Osaki Holm SY, Oski Holm SY, Oakes DA, Provo TA, Racht EM, Olsen JD, Yannopoulos D, Lurie KG. Take Heart America: A comprehensive, community-wide, systems-based approach to the treatment of cardiac arrest. Crit Care Med. 2011;39:26–33. doi: 10.1097/CCM.0b013e3181fa7ce4
10. Stub D, Smith K, Bray JE, Bernard S, Duffy SJ, Kaye DM. Hospital characteristics are associated with patient outcomes following out-of-hospital cardiac arrest. Heart. 2011;97:1489–1494. doi: 10.1136/hrt.2011.226431
11. Patterson T, Perkins GD, Joseph J, Wilson K, Van Dyck L, Robertson S, Nguyen H, McConkey H, Whitbread M, Fothergill R, Nevett J, Dalby M, Rakhit R, MacCarthy P, Perera D, Nolan JP, Redwood SR. A randomised trial of expedited transfer to a cardiac arrest centre for non-ST elevation ventricular fibrillation out-of-hospital cardiac arrest: The ARREST pilot randomised trial. Resuscitation. 2017;115:185–191. doi: 10.1016/j.resuscitation.2017.01.020
12. Yeung J, Matsuyama T, Bray J, Reynolds J, Skrifvars MB. Does care at a cardiac arrest centre improve outcome after out-of-hospital cardiac arrest? A systematic review. Resuscitation. 2019;137:102–115. doi: 10.1016/j.resuscitation.2019.02.006

臓器提供

臓器提供に対する推奨事項

COR	LOE	推奨事項
1	B-NR	1. 心停止から蘇生した後に死亡に至ったすべての患者に，臓器提供に対する評価を行うことを推奨する[1]。
2b	B-NR	2. 臓器提供プログラムがある現場では，蘇生努力後に ROSC に至らず，本来ならば蘇生が中止される患者を，臓器提供の可能性があるとみなしてもよい[1]。

「概要」

臓器提供は神経学的基準による死亡後または循環的基準による死亡後に行われる。循環的死亡後の臓器提供はコントロール下と非コントロール下で実施される。管理下の循環的死亡後の臓器提供は，一般に病院で救命処置の中止後に発生する。非管理下の心停止後臓器提供は，徹底的な蘇生努力で ROSC に至らなかったのち，通常，救急部で発生する。いかなる状況の臓器提供でも重要な倫理的問題が生じる。蘇生処置終了や生命維持手段の中止の決定は臓器提供のプロセスから独立していなければならない。

2015 年に，ILCOR の二次救命処置タスクフォースは，CPR を受けたドナーが臓器機能に及ぼす影響のエビデンスをレビューした。一般的な 2 つの比較は，1) 管理下の臓器提供で，CPR を受けて ROSC を得られたドナーと CPR を受けていないドナーの臓器を使用する際の比較と，2) 非管理下の臓器提供で，CPR を継続中だが蘇生に効果がないと考えられるドナーとそれ以外のタイプのドナーの臓器を使用する際の比較であり[1]，管理下の提供と非管理下の提供の状況で取得された臓器が生存や合併症に影響を及ぼすかどうかという疑問がある。

「推奨事項の裏付けとなる解説」

1 および 2. 提供前に CPR の成功したドナーの臓器と提供前に CPR を受けていないドナーの臓器とで移植後の臓器機能を比較した研究は，移植された臓器の機能に差がないことを明らかにした[2-6]。研究結果には，移植直後，移植 1 年後，移植 5 年後の臓器機能を含む。また，CPR で ROSC に至らなかった成人ドナーから摘出された腎臓および肝臓において（非管理下の臓器提供），それ以外のタイプのドナーから摘出された臓器と比べ，移植後の予後不良を示す所見を明

らかにした研究はなかった[7-9]。蘇生処置中止の決定と臓器提供遂行の決定は独立した当事者が行う必要があるというコンセンサスが広く得られている[10-13]。

上記の推奨事項は，AHAの成人一次救命処置と二次救命処置の執筆グループが作成し，2015年の系統的エビデンスレビューで支持された[1,14]。包括的なILCORのレビューは2020年に実施される予定である。

参考文献

1. Soar J, Callaway CW, Aibiki M, Böttiger BW, Brooks SC, Deakin CD, Donnino MW, Drajer S, Kloeck W, Morley PT, et al; on behalf of the Advanced Life Support Chapter Collaborators. Part 4: advanced life support: 2015 International Consensus on Cardiopulmonary Resuscitation and Emergency Cardiovascular Care Science With Treatment Recommendations. Resuscitation.2015;95:e71-e120. doi: 10.1016/j.resuscitation.2015.07.042
2. Orioles A, Morrison WE, Rossano JW, Shore PM, Hasz RD, Martiner AC, Berg RA, Nadkarni VM. An under-recognized benefit of cardiopulmonary resuscitation: organ transplantation. Crit Care Med.2013;41:2794-2799. doi: 10.1097/CCM.0b013e31829a7202
3. Adrie C, Haouache H, Saleh M, Memain N, Laurent I, Thuong M, Darques L, Guerrini P, Monchi M. An underrecognized source of organ donors: patients with brain death after successfully resuscitated cardiac arrest. Intensive Care Med.2008;34:132-137. doi: 10.1007/s00134-007-0885-7
4. Quader MA, Wolfe LG, Kasirajan V. Heart transplantation outcomes from cardiac arrest-resuscitated donors. J Heart Lung Transplant. 2013;32:1090-1095. doi: 10.1016/j.healun.2013.08.002
5. Pilarczyk K, Osswald BR, Pizanis N, Tsagakis K, Massoudy P, Heckmann J, Jakob HG, Kamler M. Use of donors who have suffered cardiopulmonary arrest and resuscitation in lung transplantation. Eur J Cardiothorac Surg.2011;39:342-347. doi: 10.1016/j.ejcts.2010.06.038
6. Southerland KW, Castleberry AW, Williams JB, Daneshmand MA, Ali AA, Milano CA. Impact of donor cardiac arrest on heart transplantation. Surgery.2013;154:312-319. doi: 10.1016/j.surg.2013.04.028
7. Fondevila C, Hessheimer AJ, Flores E, Ruiz A, Mestres N, Calatayud D, Paredes D, Rodríguez C, Fuster J, Navasa M, Rimola A, Taurá P, García-Valdecasas JC. Applicability and results of Maastricht type 2 donation after cardiac death liver transplantation. Am J Transplant. 2012;12:162-170. doi: 10.1111/j.1600-6143.2011.03834.x
8. Alonso A, Fernández-Rivera C, Villaverde P, Oliver J, Cillero S, Lorenzo D, Valdés F. Renal transplantation from non-heart-beating donors: a single-center 10-year experience. Transplant Proc.2005;37:3658-3660. doi: 10.1016/j.transproceed.2005.09.104
9. Morozumi J, Matsuno N, Sakurai E, Nakamura Y, Arai T, Ohta S. Application of an automated cardiopulmonary resuscitation device for kidney transplantation from uncontrolled donation after cardiac death donors in the emergency department. Clin Transplant. 2010;24:620-625. doi: 10.1111/j.1399-0012.2009.01140.x
10. Dalle Ave AL, Shaw DM, Gardiner D. Extracorporeal membrane oxygenation (ECMO) assisted cardiopulmonary resuscitation or uncontrolled donation after the circulatory determination of death following out-of-hospital refractory cardiac arrest-An ethical analysis of an unresolved clinical dilemma. Resuscitation.2016;108:87-94. doi: 10.1016/j.resuscitation.2016.07.003
11. Steinbrook R. Organ donation after cardiac death. N Engl J Med.2007;357:209-213. doi: 10.1056/NEJMp078066
12. Gallagher TK, Skaro AI, Abecassis MM. Emerging ethical considerations of donation after circulatory death: getting to the heart of the matter. Ann Surg.2016;263:217-218. doi: 10.1097/SLA.0000000000001585
13. Truog RD, Miller FG, Halpern SD. The dead-donor rule and the future of organ donation. N Engl J Med.2013;369:1287-1289. doi: 10.1056/NEJMp1307220
14. Mancini ME, Diekema DS, Hoadley TA, Kadlec KD, Leveille MH, McGowan JE, Munkwitz MM, Panchal AR, Sayre MR, Sinz EH. Part 3: ethical issues: 2015 American Heart Association Guidelines Update for Cardiopulmonary Resuscitation and Emergency Cardiovascular Care.Circulation.2015;132(suppl 2):S383-S396. doi: 10.1161/CIR.0000000000000254

蘇生パフォーマンスの向上
デブリーフィング

臨床デブリーフィングに対する推奨事項

COR	LOE	推奨事項
2a	B-NR	1. 心停止後のパフォーマンスを中心とした救助者のデブリーフィングは，院外の治療システムに有効である[1]。
2a	B-NR	2. 心停止後のパフォーマンスを中心とした救助者のデブリーフィングは，院内の治療システムに有効である[1-3]。
2a	B-NR	3. 蘇生活動後のデブリーフィングで客観的かつ定量的な蘇生データをレビューすることは有効である[1-5]。
2a	C-EO	4. 確立したデブリーフィングプロセスに精通した医療専門家がデブリーフィングのファシリテーターをつとめることは妥当である[1-5]。

「概要」

イベント発生後のデブリーフィングを「2名以上が参加し，パフォーマンスの各局面を分析してディスカッションするもの」と定義し[6]，将来の臨床診療の改善をその目標とする[7]。デブリーフィングでは，蘇生チームメンバーは治療のプロセスと質（アルゴリズムの遵守など）について議論し，事象発生中に収集した定量的データ（CPR指標など）をレビューし，チームワークやリーダーシップの問題に反映し，事象に対する感情的な反応に対処する[8-13]。ファシリテーターは通常は医療専門家がつとめ，パフォーマンス改善のための機会と戦略の特定に的を絞った議論を主導する[8,9,11,13,14]。デブリーフィングは，蘇生活動の直後（ホットデブリーフィング）に実施しても，後日（コールドデブリーフィング）実施してもよい[7,9,15]。デブリーフィングは個別に振り返りの面談を行ったり[1,4]，大規模な多職種による蘇生チーム内でグループディスカッションを行ったりすることもある[2,3]。我々は，プロセスの指標（CPRの質など）や患者転帰（生存など）で，蘇生活動後の臨床デブリーフィングの効果を評価した。トラウマ後ストレス症候群の予防や抑制を意図したプロセスである，緊急事態ストレスデブリーフィング（心理学的デブリーフィング）に関連する研究はレビューからは除外したが，別の場所で十分にレビューした[16]。心停止後にデータを提示して行うプロバイダーのデブリーフィングは，院内と院

外の治療システムのいずれでも有益である。医療専門家がファシリテーターをつとめるのが理想的である[1-4]。

「推奨事項の裏付けとなる解説」

1. 病院前救護者の OHCA 後のデブリーフィングに関する 1 件の前向き観察研究で，蘇生の質の向上（すなわち，胸骨圧迫の割合の増加，中断時間の短縮）が示されたが，生存退院率は向上しなかった[1]。パフォーマンスの良し悪しが議論で取り上げられた。
2. 集学的蘇生チームメンバーの IHCA 後のデブリーフィングを対象とした 3 件の前向き観察研究では，結果が一貫していなかった[2-4]。これらの研究のメタアナリシスでは，デブリーフィング実施後の期間に ROSC および平均の胸骨圧迫の深さの改善が示された。2 件の研究で蘇生の質（胸骨圧迫の深さ，胸骨圧迫の割合，中断時間，優れた CPR）と生存転帰（ROSC，良好な神経学的転帰良好での生存率）の改善が示されたが[2,3]，1 件の研究で患者またはプロセスに焦点を当てた転帰の改善が示されなかった[4]。
3. プロバイダーのイベントの記憶やパフォーマンスの自己評価はしばしば正確さに欠けるため[9,17,18]，デブリーフィングで CPR の質のパフォーマンスデータ（胸骨圧迫の速さ，深さ，割合，テレメトリおよび除細動器の記録，呼気終末 CO_2 の記録，蘇生の記録[1-4]）などの客観的で定量的なデータの説明によって補足する必要がある。
4. 査読された全ての研究において，推奨されるデブリーフィングのプロセスまたは構造に精通した医療専門家がデブリーフィングのファシリテーターをつとめ，一部では認知支援ツールやチェックリストが補助的に使用された[1-4]。議論は参加者のタイプとグループの大きさに応じて調整し，イベント発生時のパフォーマンスの性質に合わせて個別化した。

上記の推奨事項は，AHA の蘇生教育科学執筆グループが作成し，2019 年の ILCOR システマティックレビューで支持された[19]。

参考文献

1. Bleijenberg E, Koster RW, de Vries H, Beesems SG. The impact of post-resuscitation feedback for paramedics on the quality of cardiopulmonary resuscitation. Resuscitation.2017;110:1-5. doi: 10.1016/j.resuscitation.2016.08.034
2. Wolfe H, Zebuhr C, Topjian AA, Nishisaki A, Niles DE, Meaney PA, Boyle L, Giordano RT, Davis D, Priestley M, Apkon M, Berg RA, Nadkarni VM, Sutton RM. Interdisciplinary ICU cardiac arrest debriefing improves survival outcomes. Crit Care Med. 2014;42:1688-1695. doi: 10.1097/CCM.0000000000000327
3. Edelson DP, Litzinger B, Arora V, Walsh D, Kim S, Lauderdale DS, Vanden Hoek TL, Becker LB, Abella BS. Improving in-hospital cardiac arrest process and outcomes with performance debriefing.Arch Intern Med.2008;168:1063-1069. doi: 10.1001/archinte.168.10.1063
4. Couper K, Kimani PK, Davies RP, Baker A, Davies M, Husselbee N, Melody T, Griffiths F, Perkins GD. An evaluation of three methods of in-hospital cardiac arrest educational debriefing: The cardiopulmonary resuscitation debriefing study. Resuscitation.2016;105:130-137. doi: 10.1016/j.resuscitation.2016.05.005
5. Cheng A, Nadkarni VM, Mancini MB, Hunt EA, Sinz EH, Merchant RM, Donoghue A, Duff JP, Eppich W, Auerbach M, Bigham BL, Blewer AL, Chan PS, Bhanji F; American Heart Association Education Science Investigators; and on behalf of the American Heart Association Education Science and Programs Committee, Council on Cardiopulmonary, Critical Care, Perioperative and Resuscitation; Council on Cardiovascular and Stroke Nursing; and Council on Quality of Care and Outcomes Research. Resuscitation education science: educational strategies to improve outcomes from cardiac arrest: a scientific statement from the American Heart Association. Circulation.2018;138:e82-e122. doi: 10.1161/CIR.0000000000000583
6. Cheng A, Eppich W, Grant V, Sherbino J, Zendejas B, Cook DA. Debriefing for technology-enhanced simulation: a systematic review and meta-analysis. Med Educ.2014;48:657-666. doi: 10.1111/medu.12432
7. Kronick SL, Kurz MC, Lin S, Edelson DP, Berg RA, Billi JE, Cabanas JG, Cone DC, Diercks DB, Foster JJ, et al. Part 4: systems of care and continuous quality improvement: 2015 American Heart Association Guidelines Update for Cardiopulmonary Resuscitation and Emergency Cardiovascular Care.Circulation.2015;132(suppl 2):S397-S413. doi: 10.1161/CIR.0000000000000258
8. Kessler DO, Cheng A, Mullan PC. Debriefing in the emergency department after clinical events: a practical guide. Ann Emerg Med.2015;65:690-698. doi: 10.1016/j.annemergmed.2014.10.019
9. Mullan PC, Cochrane NH, Chamberlain JM, Burd RS, Brown FD, Zinns LE, Crandall KM, O'Connell KJ. Accuracy of postresuscitation team debriefings in a pediatric emergency department. Ann Emerg Med.2017;70:311-319. doi: 10.1016/j.annemergmed.2017.01.034
10. Mullan PC, Kessler DO, Cheng A. Educational opportunities with postevent debriefing. JAMA.2014;312:2333-2334. doi: 10.1001/jama.2014.15741
11. Zinns LE, O'Connell KJ, Mullan PC, Ryan LM, Wratney AT. National survey of pediatric emergency medicine fellows on debriefing after medical resuscitations. Pediatr Emerg Care.2015;31:551-554. doi: 10.1097/PEC.0000000000000196
12. Eppich W, Cheng A. Promoting Excellence and Reflective Learning in Simulation (PEARLS): development and rationale for a blended approach to health care simulation debriefing. Simul Healthc.2015;10:106-115. doi: 10.1097/SIH.0000000000000072
13. Couper K, Salman B, Soar J, Finn J, Perkins GD. Debriefing to improve outcomes from critical illness: a systematic review and meta-analysis. Intensive Care Med.2013;39:1513-1523. doi: 10.1007/s00134-013-2951-7
14. Rose S, Cheng A. Charge nurse facilitated clinical debriefing in the emergency department. CJEM.2018;20:781-785. doi: 10.1017/cem.2018.369
15. Sweberg T, Sen AI, Mullan PC, Cheng A, Knight L, Del Castillo J, Ikeyama T, Seshadri R, Hazinski MF, Raymond T, Niles DE, Nadkarni V, Wolfe H; pediatric resuscitation quality (pediRES-Q) collaborative investigators. Description of hot debriefings after in-hospital cardiac arrests in an international pediatric quality improvement collaborative. Resuscitation.2018;128:181-187. doi: 10.1016/j.resuscitation.2018.05.015
16. Rose SC, Bisson J, Churchill R, Wessely S. Psychological debriefing for preventing post traumatic stress disorder (PTSD). Cochrane Database Syst Rev. 2002; doi: 10.1002/14651858.CD000560
17. Cheng A, Overly F, Kessler D, Nadkarni VM, Lin Y, Doan Q, Duff JP, Tofil NM, Bhanji F, Adler M, Charnovich A, Hunt EA, Brown LL; International Network for Simulation-based Pediatric Innovation, Research, Education (INSPIRE) CPR Investigators. Perception of CPR quality: Influence of CPR feedback, Just-in-Time CPR training and provider role. Resuscitation.2015;87:44-50. doi: 10.1016/j.resuscitation.2014.11.015
18. Cheng A, Kessler D, Lin Y, Tofil NM, Hunt EA, Davidson J, Chatfield J, Duff JP; International Network for Simulation-based Pediatric Innovation, Research and Education (INSPIRE) CPR Investigators. Influence of cardiopulmonary resuscitation coaching and provider role on perception of cardiopulmonary resuscitation quality during simulated pediatric cardiac arrest. Pediatr Crit Care Med.2019;20:e191-e198. doi: 10.1097/PCC.0000000000001871
19. Greif R, Bhanji F, Bigham BL, Bray J, Breckwoldt J, Cheng A, Duff JP, Gilfoyle E, Hsieh M-J, Iwami T, et al; on behalf of the Education, Implementation, and Teams Collaborators.Education, implementation, and teams: 2020 International Consensus on Cardiopulmonary Resuscitation and Emergency Cardiovascular Care Science With Treatment Recommendations.Circulation.2020;142(suppl 1):S222-S283. doi: 10.1161/CIR.0000000000000896

システムパフォーマンス向上のためのデータレジストリ

COR	LOE	推奨事項
2a	C-LD	1. 心停止患者の治療を行う組織が、治療プロセスデータおよび転帰を収集することは妥当である[1-6]。

「概要」

医療を含む多くの業種で、品質を評価し改善の機会を特定するために、パフォーマンスデータを収集して評価する。心停止に関連する治療プロセス（CPR パフォーマンスデータ、除細動の回数、ガイドラインの遵守）および治療転帰（ROSC、生存）の情報を収集するデータレジストリへの参加を通じて、各施設、地域、または国レベルでデータを収集することができる。AHA の「Get With The Guidelines-Resuscitation」レジストリは、IHCA のプロセスと転帰を捕捉し、分析し、報告する取り組みの 1 つである。

最近の ILCOR のシステマティックレビュー[7]によると、データレジストリの効果を評価する研究の大部分は、指公的な報告の有無を問わず、そのようなシステム導入後に心停止からの生存転帰が改善したことを示している[1-6,8-21]。病院は他の状況で記録された指標に基づいて行動するが、この種の分析に対応して正確にどのような変化が起こるかは不明である。パフォーマンスおよび生存データの収集と報告や、パフォーマンス改善計画の実施は、公的な報告の有無を問わず、システムのパフォーマンス改善につながり、最終的に患者に利益をもたらす可能性がある。特定のニーズをもった地域への介入を目標としたレジストリの使用が関心の対象であり、将来のそのようなシステムの最適な実施戦略を知るためにさらに研究が必要である。

「推奨事項の裏付けとなる解説」

1. 最近の ILCOR のシステマティックレビュー[7]によると、6 件の観察研究で、心停止レジストリの実施によって時間経過とともに生存率および重要なパフォーマンス指標の遵守（CPR プロセスの指標、除細動器使用までの時間、ガイドラインの遵守）が向上することが示された[1-6]。

IHCA 患者 104,732 例を登録したレジストリの観察研究では、病院のレジストリ参加年数が増えるごとに経時的に心停止からの生存が延長した（OR 参加年数ごとに 1.02、CI 1.00-1.04、P＝0.046）[1]。米国の複数の州で OHCA 64,988 例を登録したレジストリの観察研究では、レジストリ開始後に全てのリズム における生存率が 2 倍になった（レジストリ開始前 8.0%、レジストリ開始後 16.1%、P＜0.001）[6]。患者 15,145 名を登録したある州の OHCA レジストリでは、10 年間で生存退院率が向上した（8.6%-16%）[5]。OHCA 128,888 例を登録し、転帰の公的な報告が義務付けられている別の研究では、生存率が 10 年間で 1.2%から 4.1%に上昇した[4]。

上記の推奨事項は、AHA の蘇生教育科学執筆グループが作成し、2020 年の ILCOR システマティックレビューで支持された[7]。

参考文献

1. Bradley SM, Huszti E, Warren SA, Merchant RM, Sayre MR, Nichol G. Duration of hospital participation in Get With the Guidelines-Resuscitation and survival of in-hospital cardiac arrest. Resuscitation.2012;83:1349–1357. doi: 10.1016/j.resuscitation.2012.03.014
2. Nehme Z, Bernard S, Cameron P, Bray JE, Meredith IT, Lijovic M, Smith K. Using a cardiac arrest registry to measure the quality of emergency medical service care: decade of findings from the Victorian Ambulance Cardiac Arrest Registry. Circ Cardiovasc Qual Outcomes. 2015;8:56–66. doi: 10.1161/CIRCOUTCOMES.114.001185
3. Stub D, Schmicker RH, Anderson ML, Callaway CW, Daya MR, Sayre MR, Elmer J, Grunau BE, Aufderheide TP, Lin S, Buick JE, Zive D, Peterson ED, Nichol G; ROC Investigators. Association between hospital post-resuscitative performance and clinical outcomes after out-of-hospital cardiac arrest. Resuscitation.2015;92:45–52. doi: 10.1016/j.resuscitation.2015.04.015
4. Kim YT, Shin SD, Hong SO, Ahn KO, Ro YS, Song KJ, Hong KJ. Effect of national implementation of utstein recommendation from the global resuscitation alliance on ten steps to improve outcomes from Out-of-Hospital cardiac arrest: a ten-year observational study in Korea. BMJ Open. 2017;7:e016925. doi: 10.1136/bmjopen-2017-016925
5. Grunau B, Kawano T, Dick W, Straight R, Connolly H, Schlamp R, Scheuermeyer FX, Fordyce CB, Barbic D, Tallon J, et al. Trends in care processes and survival following prehospital resuscitation improvement initiatives for out-of-hospital cardiac arrest in British Columbia, 2006–2016. Resuscitation.2018;125:118–125. doi: 10.1016/j.resuscitation.2018.01.049
6. van Diepen S, Girotra S, Abella BS, Becker LB, Bobrow BJ, Chan PS, Fahrenbruch C, Granger CB, Jollis JG, McNally B, et al. Multistate 5-year initiative to improve care for out-of-hospital cardiac arrest: primary results from the heartrescue project. J Am Heart Assoc. 2017;6:e005716. doi: 10.1161/JAHA.117.005716
7. Greif R, Bhanji F, Bigham BL, Bray J, Breckwoldt J, Cheng A, Duff JP, Gilfoyle E, Hsieh M-J, Iwami T, et al; on behalf of the Education, Implementation, and Teams Collaborators. Education, implementation, and teams: 2020 International Consensus on Cardiopulmonary Resuscitation and Emergency Cardiovascular Care Science With Treatment Recommendations.Circulation.2020;142(suppl 1):S222–S283. doi: 10.1161/CIR.0000000000000896
8. Hostler D, Everson-Stewart S, Rea TD, Stiell IG, Callaway CW, Kudenchuk PJ, Sears GK, Emerson SS, Nichol G; Resuscitation Outcomes Consortium Investigators. Effect of real-time feedback during cardiopulmonary resuscitation outside hospital: prospective, cluster-randomised trial. BMJ. 2011;342:d512. doi: 10.1136/bmj.d512
9. Wolfe H, Zebuhr C, Topjian AA, Nishisaki A, Niles DE, Meaney PA, Boyle L, Giordano RT, Davis D, Priestley M, Apkon M, Berg RA, Nadkarni VM, Sutton RM. Interdisciplinary ICU cardiac arrest debriefing improves survival outcomes*. Crit Care Med. 2014;42:1688–1695. doi: 10.1097/CCM.0000000000000327
10. Couper K, Kimani PK, Abella BS, Chilwan M, Cooke MW, Davies RP, Field RA, Gao F, Quinton S, Stallard N, Woolley S, Perkins GD; Cardiopulmonary Resuscitation Quality Improvement Initiative Collaborators. The system-wide effect of real-time audiovisual feedback and postevent debriefing for in-hospital cardiac arrest: the cardiopulmonary resuscitation quality improvement initiative. Crit Care Med.2015;43:2321–2331. doi: 10.1097/CCM.0000000000001202
11. Knight LJ, Gabhart JM, Earnest KS, Leong KM, Anglemyer A, Franzon D. Improving code team performance and survival outcomes: implementation of pediatric resuscitation team training. Crit Care Med.2014;42:243–251. doi: 10.1097/CCM.0b013e3182a6439d

12. Davis DP, Graham PG, Husa RD, Lawrence B, Minokadeh A, Altieri K, Sell RE. A performance improvement–based resuscitation programme reduces arrest incidence and increases survival from in-hospital cardiac arrest. Resuscitation.2015;92:63-69. doi: 10.1016/j.resuscitation.2015.04.008
13. Hwang WS, Park JS, Kim SJ, Hong YS, Moon SW, Lee SW.A system-wide approach from the community to the hospital for improving neurologic outcomes in out-of-hospital cardiac arrest patients.Eur J Emerg Med.2017;24:87-95. doi: 10.1097/MEJ.0000000000000313
14. Pearson DA, Darrell Nelson R, Monk L, Tyson C, Jollis JG, Granger CB, Corbett C, Garvey L, Runyon MS. Comparison of team-focused CPR vs standard CPR in resuscitation from out-of-hospital cardiac arrest: Results from a statewide quality improvement initiative. Resuscitation.2016;105:165-172. doi: 10.1016/j.resuscitation.2016.04.008
15. Sporer K, Jacobs M, Derevin L, Duval S, Pointer J. Continuous quality improvement efforts increase survival with favorable neurologic outcome after out-of-hospital cardiac arrest. Prehosp Emerg Care.2017;21:1-6. doi: 10.1080/10903127.2016.1218980
16. Park JH, Shin SD, Ro YS, Song KJ, Hong KJ, Kim TH, Lee EJ, Kong SY. Implementation of a bundle of Utstein cardiopulmonary resuscitation programs to improve survival outcomes after out-of-hospital cardiac arrest in a metropolis: A before and after study. Resuscitation.2018;130:124-132. doi: 10.1016/j.resuscitation.2018.07.019
17. Hubner P, Lobmeyr E, Wallmüller C, Poppe M, Datler P, Keferböck M, Zeiner S, Nürnberger A, Zajicek A, Laggner A, Sterz F, Sulzgruber P. Improvements in the quality of advanced life support and patient outcome after implementation of a standardized real-life post-resuscitation feedback system. Resuscitation.2017;120:38-44. doi: 10.1016/j.resuscitation.2017.08.235
18. Anderson ML, Nichol G, Dai D, Chan PS, Thomas L, Al-Khatib SM, Berg RA, Bradley SM, Peterson ED; American Heart Association's Get With the Guidelines-Resuscitation Investigators. Association between hospital process composite performance and patient outcomes after in-hospital cardiac arrest care. JAMA Cardiol.2016;1:37-45. doi: 10.1001/jamacardio.2015.0275
19. Del Rios M, Weber J, Pugach O, Nguyen H, Campbell T, Islam S, Stein Spencer L, Markul E, Bunney EB, Vanden Hoek T. Large urban center improves out-of-hospital cardiac arrest survival. Resuscitation.2019;139:234-240. doi: 10.1016/j.resuscitation.2019.04.019
20. Ewy GA, Sanders AB. Cardiocerebral resuscitation improves survival of patients with out-of-hospital cardiac arrest.J Am Coll Cardiol.2013;61:113-118. doi: 10.1016/j.jacc.2012.06.064
21. Hopkins CL, Burk C, Moser S, Meersman J, Baldwin L, Youngquist ST. Implementation of pit crew approach and cardiopulmonary resuscitation metrics for out-of-hospital cardiac arrest improves patient survival and neurological outcome. J Am Heart Assoc. 2016;5 doi: 10.1161/JAHA.115.002892

今後の課題と研究の優先順位

蘇生科学は，統合された治療システムについての理解と併せて発展を続けている。優先順位の高い多くの未解決の問題のうち一部を以下に挙げる。

- 地域社会の CPR および AED プログラムの臨床的な効果は十分に確立されているが，この種の介入の費用対効果が高い集団と状況については，さらに検討が必要である。
- ドローンによる AED 運搬の予備的な研究は期待が持てる結果である[1,2]。一刻を争う除細動にもたらす利益を考慮すると，ジャストインタイムの AED 運搬のためにこの構想やその他の手段をさらに検討すべきである。
- RRT/MET の概念は有望と考えられるが，現在のデータは確固とした結論の裏付けとするには不均一である。体系的なデータ収集によって，RRT/MET によって利益が得られる介入のタイプや患者特性，および成功するチームの構成と活動への理解が進むと予想される。
- 同様に，承認されている臨床的基準は，おそらく機械学習技術によって開発されており，IHCA リスクのある患者を特定して介入を指示するのに役立つであろう。
- 概念は理にかなっているが，CPR を実施するバイスタンダーを支援する（T-CPR 以外の）認知支援ツールはまだ効果が証明されていない。スマートフォンの普及とスマートフォンアプリのプラットフォームの革新性を考えると，さらに研究を進める十分な理由となる。
- バイスタンダーによる CPR 実施率は，女性や小児，マイノリティー集団に所属する人に対して依然として低いままである。これらの集団に対するバイスタンダーの反応を改善する取り組みを実施して，有効性を評価すべきである。
- 行動する文化を作り上げることは，バイスタンダーのにとって重要な部分である。バイスタンダーを動かして CPR の実施や AED の使用を促すために重要な要素を理解するためには，さらに研究を要する。
- 蘇生チームのパフォーマンスを向上させるために，OHCA および IHCA を遂行する医療従事者とチームを補助する認知支援ツールに関して，さらに研究が必要である。
- 即時のフィードバック（チームのデブリーフィングなど）とデータに基づくシステムのフィードバックの価値は十分に確立されているが，明確で効果の高いフィードバックの要素はまだ特定されていない。
- 院内と院外の両方で心停止患者に関するデータと質の向上を促進させるテクノロジーの利用方法を解明するためにはさらに研究を要する。

参考文献

1. Boutilier JJ, Brooks SC, Janmohamed A, Byers A, Buick JE, Zhan C, Schoellig AP, Cheskes S, Morrison LJ, Chan TCY; Rescu Epistry Investigators. Optimizing a drone network to deliver automated external defibrillators. Circulation.2017;135:2454-2465. doi: 10.1161/CIRCULATIONAHA.116.026318
2. Cheskes S, Snobelen P, McLeod S, Brooks S, Vaillancourt C, Chan T, Dainty KN, Nolan M. AED on the fly: a drone delivery feasibility study for rural and remote out-of-hospital cardiac arrest [abstract 147]. Circulation. 2019;140:A147. doi:10.1161/circ.140.suppl_2.147

文献情報

アメリカ心臓協会（American Heart Association）は，本書が以下のとおりに引用されることを要請する。Berg KM, Cheng A, Panchal AR, Topjian AA, Aziz K, Bhanji F, Bigham BL, Hirsch KG, Hoover AV, Kurz MC, Levy A, Lin Y, Magid DJ, Mahgoub M, Peberdy MA, Rodriguez AJ, Sasson C, Lavonas EJ; on behalf of the Adult Basic and Advanced Life Support, Pediatric Basic and Advanced Life Support, Neonatal Life Support, and Resuscitation Education Science Writing Groups. Part 7: systems of care: 2020 American Heart Association Guidelines for Cardiopulmonary Resuscitation and Emergency Cardiovascular Care. Circulation. 2020;142 (suppl 2):S580-S604. doi: 10.1161/CIR.0000000000000899

謝辞

著者らは，Monica Kleinman 博士 の献身に心より感謝し，その意をここに表す。

情報開示

付録 1. 執筆グループの情報開示

執筆グループメンバー	所属	研究助成金	その他の研究支援	講演／謝礼金	鑑定人	株式所有	コンサルタント／顧問	その他
Katherine M. Berg	Beth Israel Deaconess Medical Center	NHLBI Grant K23 HL128814†	なし	なし	なし	なし	なし	なし
Khalid Aziz	University of Alberta (Canada)	なし	なし	なし	なし	なし	なし	University of Alberta (Professor of Pediatrics)†
Farhan Bhanji	McGill University (Canada)	なし	なし	なし	なし	なし	なし	なし
Blair L. Bigham	McMaster University (Canada)	なし	なし	なし	なし	なし	なし	なし
Adam Cheng	Alberta Children's Hospital (Canada)	なし	なし	なし	なし	なし	なし	なし
Karen G. Hirsch	Stanford University	American Heart Association (cardiac arrest research)*	なし	なし	Stroke and TBI cases (not cardiac arrest)*	なし	なし	なし
Amber V. Hoover	American Heart Association	なし	なし	なし	なし	なし	なし	なし
Michael C. Kurz	University of Alabama at Birmingham	DOD (DSMB for Pre-Hospital Airway Control Trial [PACT])*; NIH (Co-PI for R21 examining mast-cell degranulation in OHCA)*	なし	Zoll Medical Corp*	なし	なし	Zoll Circulation, Inc†	Zoll Circulation, Inc†
Eric J. Lavonas	Denver Health Emergency Medicine	BTG Pharmaceuticals（Denver Health（Lavonas 博士の雇用者）には，BTG Pharmaceuticals との研究，コールセンター，コンサルティング，および教育の各契約がある。BTG はジゴキシンの解毒剤（DigiFab）を製造している。Lavonas 博士はボーナスやインセンティブ報酬を受け取らず，これらの契約は無関係な製品を対象とする。これらのガイドラインの作成時に，Lavonas 博士はジゴキシン中毒に関わる考察に関与しなかった）†	なし	なし	なし	なし	なし	アメリカ心臓協会（上級科学編集者）†
Arielle Levy	University of Montreal (Canada)	なし	なし	なし	なし	なし	なし	なし
Yiqun Lin	Alberta Children's Hospital (Canada)	なし	なし	なし	なし	なし	なし	なし
David J. Magid	University of Colorado	NIH†; NHLBI†; CMS†; AHA†	なし	なし	なし	なし	なし	アメリカ心臓協会（上級科学編集者）†
Melissa Mahgoub	American Heart Association	なし	なし	なし	なし	なし	なし	なし
Ashish R. Panchal	The Ohio State University	なし	なし	なし	なし	なし	なし	なし
Mary Ann Peberdy	Virginia Commonwealth University	なし	なし	なし	なし	なし	なし	なし

（続き）

付録 1. 続き

執筆グループメンバー	所属	研究助成金	その他の研究支援	講演／謝礼金	鑑定人	株式所有	コンサルタント／顧問	その他
Amber J. Rodriguez	American Heart Association	なし	なし	なし	なし	なし	なし	なし
Comilla Sasson	American Heart Association	なし	なし	なし	なし	なし	なし	なし
Alexis A. Topjian	The Children's Hospital of Philadelphia	NIH (POCCA trial site PI)*	なし	なし	なし	なし	なし	なし

　この表は，執筆グループの全メンバーに回答および提出が求められる情報開示アンケート（Disclosure Questionnaire）の結果に基づき実在の利益相反または合理的に認定できる利益相反とみなされる可能性のある，執筆グループメンバーの関係を示している。メンバーと該当団体との関係が「顕著」であると考えられるのは，次のいずれかの状況が存在する場合である。（a）当該メンバーが団体から受領した金額が過去いずれの 12 か月間に $10,000 以上であるか，メンバーの総収入の 5％以上である，（b）団体の議決権株式の 5％以上，またはその団体の公正市場価値の $10,000 以上を保有している。この定義において「重大」に相当するレベルに満たない場合，その関係は「軽度」とみなされる。

　*軽度
　†重大

付録 2. レビューアーの情報開示

レビューアー	所属	研究助成金	その他の研究支援	講演／謝礼金	鑑定人	株式所有	コンサルタント／顧問	その他
Alix Carter	Dalhousie University (Canada)	Maritime Heart*	なし	なし	なし	なし	なし	なし
Henry Halperin	Johns Hopkins University	Zoll Medical†; NIH†	なし	なし	なし	なし	なし	なし
Jonathan Jui	Oregon Health and Science University	NIH*	なし	なし	なし	なし	なし	なし
Fred Severyn	Denver Health and Hospital Authority and University of Colorado Anschutz Medical Campus; University of Arkansas	なし	なし	なし	なし	なし	なし	なし
Robert A. Swor	William Beaumont Hospital	なし	なし	なし	なし	なし	なし	なし
Andrew H. Travers	Emergency Health Services (Canada)	なし	なし	なし	なし	なし	なし	なし

　この表は，執筆グループの全メンバーに回答および提出が求められる情報開示アンケート（Disclosure Questionnaire）の結果に基づき実在の利益相反または合理的に認定できる利益相反とみなされる可能性のある，執筆グループメンバーの関係を示している。メンバーと該当団体との関係が「顕著」であると考えられるのは，次のいずれかの状況が存在する場合である。（a）当該メンバーが団体から受領する金額が過去いずれの 12 か月間に $10,000 以上であるか，メンバーの総収入の 5％以上である，（b）団体の議決権株式の 5％以上，またはその団体の公正市場価値の $10,000 以上を保有している。この定義において「重大」に相当するレベルに満たない場合，その関係は「軽度」とみなされる。

　*軽度
　†重大